MEDICINES

MEDICINES

THE COMPREHENSIVE GUIDE

Third Edition

BLOOMSBURY

This completely revised edition first published 1995

Text and database copyright © 1995
Dr I K M Morton, Dr J M Hall
and book Creation Services Limited, London

Bloomsbury Publishing Limited,
2 Soho Square, London W1V 6HB

British Library Cataloguing in Publication Data

A CIP catalogue for this book is available
from The British Library

ISBN 0 7475 2095 X

10 9 8 7 6 5 4 3 2

Edited by Sam Merrell

Designed and typeset by
Book Creation Services Limited
21 Carnaby Street
London W1V 1PH

Printed and bound by
Cox & Wyman Ltd
Reading

CONTENTS

PREFACE

This is the third edition of Medicines: The Comprehensive Guide – a dictionary-style reference source-book for the range of medicines that are available in the UK today. The text is so extensively revised – to take account of the many new drugs, both generic and proprietary, that have been developed and marketed since publication of the second edition in 1991, along with those that remain on the market – that from all practical points of view this is an almost entirely new publication.

The purpose of the book is to give straightforward information on the constituent drug components of medicines, describing their actions clearly and explaining how they work and what side-effects they may have.

It has been our aim to provide as full a list as possible and practical in such a changeable industry, of the generic drugs and most of the proprietary medical preparations of drugs currently available.

There are some categories of preparations we have not felt it was either possible or appropriate to include, however. The following three are the main ones. Preparations of vitamins and minerals that are part of a normal balanced diet are not included, although there are entries on medicines where vitamins or minerals are used medically to correct clinical deficiencies (for example, iron preparations for anaemia, folic acid vitamin supplements in pregnancy, and so on). Homoeopathic or herbal remedies do not fall within the scope of the book, but nevertheless there are many entries on the valuable drugs of plant and natural origin, and standardized plant extracts, that are part of everyday medicine. The 'social' and non-medical use of drugs is also not covered, although some medicines used to treat drug-overdose and drug-dependence (addiction) are included.

Finally, it is important to note that the dictionary is not intended to be a guide to the prescription or administration of drugs, and it gives neither doses nor recommendations regarding which drugs to use in particular circumstances. A qualified practitioner should be consulted before any medicine is taken.

IKMM
JMH
King's College London

HOW TO USE THIS BOOK

Hopefully the layout of the book is sufficiently clear for it to be used without further instructions, but in any event some words of explanation may be useful.

The main section of this book contains entries on the medicinal drugs available in the UK, listed A-Z. Drugs are listed under their generic and proprietary names. There are also articles covering the major drug families that explain in more detail how they work and what they are used for. These are indicated by an *asterisk in front of the name.

The A-Z is cross-referenced within the text of one entry to further related entries. These cross-references are indicated when the drug name is printed in the text in CAPITALS. The side-effects or warnings to be borne in mind when taking a drug are indicated by symbols (✚ for side-effects and ▲ for warnings) in articles about generic drugs. At the end of entries on generic drugs there is a list of related entries (indicated by the symbol ✪), which leads to proprietary preparations that contain that drug.

Following common practice, drugs are usually named in two ways:

The generic name, without an initial capital letter, is the official (simplified) chemical name of a drug, which unambiguously describes an active constituent of a medicine. The generic name is now routinely used in everyday medicine and doctors are encouraged to refer to and prescribe drugs by their generic names, because this is less likely to be misunderstood, and generic forms of drugs are often cheaper.

The proprietary name, normally with an initial capital letter, is a brand name, which is a preparation of a drug, or a mixture of drugs, that represents a particular formulation from a particular manufacturer.

For instance, the generic name paracetamol refers to an established and familiar standard drug. In the case of a particular generic formulation such as paracetamol tablets, even details such as purity, time for the tablets to dissolve, and accuracy of dose are all subject to strict control as laid out in the British Pharmacopoeia or other official standards.

The doctor may prescribe paracetamol described simply as 'paracetamol'; but in practice, common non-prescription medicines such as paracetamol are available not just under the generic name, but also as proprietary preparations under a variety of trade names.

Drugs are also often prescribed or sold in a variety of forms (tablets, capsules, effervescent tablets, powders for solution, suppositories, etc) and sometimes in different strengths (the stronger versions usually have a distinguishing name such as Extra, Plus, or Ultra).

To add to these complexities, an analgesic (painkiller) such as paracetamol is also available for non-prescription (over-the-counter, or OTC) sale, alone or in combination with other drugs.

For instance, there are compound analgesic preparations that contain two or more analgesics (eg paracetamol with codeine), and compound preparations (eg paracetamol with caffeine; or 'cold-cures' such as paracetamol with a decongestant or a cough-suppressant drug).

This potentially confusing system of describing and marketing medicines can be understood through the system of entry types and cross-references used in this book.

Step by step

The following examples highlight the most common points where confusion can arise and illustrate how this dictionary can help. For example, begin by supposing you have bought a proprietary medicine (eg Nurofen), and want to learn more about its constituents, their uses, side-effects, and the circumstances when it should not be used. Then take the following steps:

[1] *Discover the generic name(s) of the constituents*
This information can be obtained by reading the labels on the medicine or by looking up the entry in this dictionary. An entry gives a list of the generic constituents together with their pharmacological class (eg analgesic), the form it is available in (eg modified-release tablet), and a word or two about uses.

It also gives the manufacturer's name, which is a useful cross-check of the identity of the preparation. Although readers should be warned that the major pharmaceutical companies may label particular medicines either under their own familiar name, or that of a subsidiary company. The latter is especially common with over-the-counter 'healthcare' products.

[2] *Turn to the generic name or names*
Generic entries contain substantially more detail (eg '...is a (NSAID) non-narcotic analgesic and antirheumatic drug which is used to treat serious rheumatic and arthritic complaints, musculoskeletal pain and postoperative pain').

The generic drug entry has further important information about the drug: the main side-effects (✚) and warnings (▲) relating to its use. The list of possible side-effects is extensive, starting with the common and most-often experienced symptoms, running on to relatively infrequent side-effects, and sometimes finishing with rarely reported effects.

To complement the information on side-effects there are specific warnings about the circumstances when the drugs may be unsafe to use.

The warnings commonly refer to use in pregnancy or when breast-feeding. Other warnings relate to special circumstances, such as kidney or liver disorders, which may prevent the drug being metabolized and excreted normally, or to inherited disorders such as porphyria, which may precipitate adverse interactions.

Warnings do not necessarily apply to all users, however, and skilful prescribing can minimize discomfort and risk. But they do serve to emphasize the importance of seeking professional medical advice. For more information about side-effects, see later in this introduction.

[3] *For more information read the cross-references*
Capitalization of keywords in the text of each entry indicates that more information can be found in another article. For example, the cross-reference ANTIRHEUMATIC leads to an article discussing some other classes of

drugs that are used in treating rheumatoid arthritis and osteoarthritis. The reference to non-narcotic analgesic leads to an entry explaining that the drugs called analgesics are used to treat pain, and they can be conveniently split (on the basis of the way they work and whether or not they cause drug-dependence) into the (opioid) narcotic analgesic and the (NSAID) non-narcotic analgesic classes.

Finally, the **NSAID** (non-steroidal anti-inflammatory drug) heading, is the most important, since it is here the reader will find details of side-effects (✚) and warnings (▲) for this class of analgesic as a whole.

[4] *Going from generic drug names to proprietary preparations*
If you wish to travel in the opposite direction, from generic name to proprietary preparations that contain the drug in question, then the journey is also straightforward. Under the **Related entry** subheading, every generic drug entry has, a list of proprietary preparations that contain this generic drug. This way of using the A-Z is particularly useful when it is clear what you want a particular drug for.

Taking paracetamol as an example, once again, if you are suffering from a cold with headache and fever, you might want a simple paracetamol preparation, and a number of these are described in the book. On the other hand, if you have a congested nose as well, you could find out about a proprietary compound preparation that contains a nasal decongestant, possibly a sympathomimetic vasoconstrictor such as ephedrine and/or an antihistamine such as promethazine.

If you are concerned whether the generic constituents included in these 'cold-cures' have adverse effects in your particular situation, a glance at the entries would remind you, for instance, that a sympathomimetic vasoconstrictor should under no circumstances be taken on top of a prescription for monoamine-oxidase inhibitor (MAOI) antidepressants (as your doctor would have warned you), and that antihistamines cause drowsiness to the extent that they should not be taken if you intend to drive or operate potentially dangerous machinery, but could be taken before sleep at night.

These examples illustrate that gaining an understanding of how prescribed drugs work is not necessarily difficult, and such understanding can only assist the partnership in health care that a patient establishes with his or her doctor. In addition, outside that partnership, making an appropriate choice of non-prescription medication that is both suitable and safe requires a reliable and flexible source of information, which the authors hope this book provides.

INTRODUCTION

The sweeping changes that have occurred – and are still occurring – in the ways the pharmaceutical industry develops and promotes its products in the UK have meant that this new edition, of what has become one of the most successful books on this subject ever published, had to be updated so extensively that not one entry remains unchanged from the second edition. What are these changes and why have they occurred? And most significantly, what do they mean for those of us who buy and use these medicines?

The pharmaceutical industry and new drug development

The drug industry is one of the most rapidly expanding areas of commerce of the twentieth century. Although pharmaceutical companies are increasingly international in their organisation, many (whether British- or foreign-owned) have a strong base in the UK.

In research and development (R&D), scientists in the UK have an enviable record of innovation. Also, in the later stages of drug development involving clinical trials, and ultimately the approval and continuing licensing of drugs for use in patients, our Committee on Safety of Medicines and other parts of the Medicines Control Agency set world standards for authoritative assessment of safety and efficacy of drugs.

Currently, we have one of the most restrictive legislations in relation to limiting the majority of drugs to prescription-only use – although this is now beginning to move towards European practice and standards as discussed below.

One outcome of the last couple of decades, the most buoyant period ever in the history of the pharmaceutical industry, has been the emergence of many new generic drugs. These have not simply been further examples of existing drugs or drug types, often derogatorily called 'me-too' drugs, but entirely new classes of drugs. Some of these have now become famous, such as the beta-blocker 'heart-drugs' and the ulcer-healing H_2-antagonist drugs, which are both British inventions.

The second edition of this book saw the introduction of new types of drugs that are treat cardiovascular-related diseases, including the calcium-channel blockers and the ACE inhibitors. In this third edition, development work within the pharmaceutical industry has now yielded considerable numbers of different generic drugs, each with its individual virtues, within these and other groups.

For instance, there are described in this book some 19 different generic beta-blocker drugs, which are marketed in 89 different proprietary preparations.

This edition also sees the introduction of several promising new types of drug, including so-called angiotensin-receptor blockers and potassium-channel activators, which are used to treat cardiovascular disorders.

Future developments

Will this rapid progress continue? Many people within the industry are not optimistic because of escalating costs of drug development – to produce just one new drug can take years and cost millions. However, new research strategies, many involving the emerging science of molecular biology, may prove cheaper and more effective.

There are also several major targets for drug therapy towards which progress has been slow. For instance, in the early days of pharmacology researchers in the area of chemotherapeutics once dreamed of the 'magic bullet' whereby the cause of disease was 'hit' leaving the patient unharmed. Antibiotics have realized this dream in the treatment of infections caused by bacteria and other micro-organisms. However, in use against malignant cells or viruses the battle is not yet won.

This book lists some 45 anticancer drugs and 11 antiviral drugs, but it should be realized that unfortunately most of these leave a lot to be desired in terms of efficacy and freedom from side-effects. Overall, however, there is more cause for hope than pessimism, and perhaps the next edition of this book will be able to report some new breakthroughs in the treatment of such diseases.

Partnerships between patients, doctors and pharmacists

Successful medical therapy has always depended on a partnership between the patient and medical professionals. Every patient is different and requires individual treatment – a truth that is often easy to forget in a world where mass production and standardization of products and practice is regarded as the norm.

Medicines are prepared and tested according to the most rigorous criteria of standardization, for the sake of safety as well as for economic efficiency. But because the people who use the medicines are all likely to be different to some degree, either in their basic physiological make-up or in the circumstances surrounding the condition they are seeking to treat, an individual's response to a certain drug must therefore be taken into account.

Where prescribed medicines are concerned, the doctor can help interpret specific needs and situations, and prescribe accordingly. But an increasingly wide range of medicines are now becoming available without prescription and can be purchased directly from a pharmacy.

Associated with this is a growing trend to give an increasing share of the advisory role to the pharmacist, who has years of training to qualify him or her to provide this important service.

Although the doctor will know important details of a patient's history and present condition, the pharmacist cannot be aware of such privileged information.

Consequently, this trend towards making more medicines available without prescription places a substantial responsibility for choosing the correct medication on the patient, or on carers in the case of children, the elderly, and those who are too ill to co-operate.

The move to non-prescription drugs

The number of drugs switched each year from prescription-only to an over-the-counter (non-prescription) status is accelerating at a remarkable rate. Whereas there were only 11 such changes in individual generic drugs or their indicated uses during the period from 1983 to 1992, there were 15 between 1993 and 1994, and have already been 10 in the first half of 1995.

This switch has perhaps its greatest overall effect in the area of marketing. For example, the analgesic ibuprofen was one of the 11 prescription drugs that changed status between 1983 and 1992; now there are 32 proprietary preparations of it listed in this book.

Types of drugs are also affected; between the second and third editions of this book members of several major drug groups have changed their status from prescription-only to over-the-counter. For example, the ulcer-healing drugs of the H_2-antagonist group (although only for the treatment of dyspepsia), a number of corticosteroids for topical use, and antifungal antibiotic treatments for thrush infections.

As more medicines become readily available without prescription, authorities in the UK expect patients to become more skilled at knowing when they should seek expert advice. For much the same reasons, the list of drugs that may be prescribed by nurses and dentists has also been extended, and it is likely that various healthcare workers will be empowered in future either to prescribe or to recommend medication for the patient to buy.

Not all healthcare professionals welcome this rapidly moving trend towards deregulation, and are worried that aspects of it will be detrimental both to the health of an individual and the community as a whole.

For instance, in other parts of the world the excessive and often inappropriate use of antibiotics obtained without prescription (OTC) is a major reason for the now widespread emergence of antibiotic-resistant strains of bacteria that cause major diseases such as tuberculosis and gonorrhoea.

It is to be hoped that in this country, with co-operation and appropriate health education, some of these dangers can be avoided.

Cost considerations
In part, these changes are motivated by financial considerations. On the one hand the cost of drugs is the biggest single item of the National Health Service annual bill, so the government is looking to shed some of this load. On the other hand, nearly half of all prescriptions actually cost less than the standard prescription charge.

The move to European practices
These changes are part of a gradual evolution towards a common standard in Europe. Currently the UK has one of the most restrictive pharmaceutical legislations in the world, and those who travel widely may already be aware that a very high proportion of the drugs listed in this dictionary as prescription-only are available over-the-counter in Europe, and to an even greater extent in the Americas and in the East.

Drugs and the traveller
The traveller should note that generic names of drugs differ

little between countries. This dictionary lists the new European standard names, and major American names, both as separate cross-indexes and in brackets after the UK generic name.

Because it is cheaper in some cases to buy proprietary drugs in Europe and dispense them here – so called 'parallel imports' – it is not uncommon to have a prescription for a generic drug supplied by the pharmacist in packaging showing an unfamiliar foreign spelling of the usual British proprietary name.

Proprietary names used by a manufacturer for the same generic drug are today less likely to be totally different according to the country in which it is marketed, although there may be minor variations in spelling to accommodate local requirements.

The protective shield: what should the patient know?

It is clear from consideration of these changing circumstances that, in the future, patients and their carers will be playing an increasingly large part in the decision-making processes relating to drug therapy. This is also the case in other branches of medicine and is seen by most people as a welcome democratization of medical practice.

In the case of drugs, however, the lowering of the protective shield afforded by the older scheme – where virtually all the drugs that were potentially harmful were available only on prescription – has obvious dangers. In order to avoid these dangers, members of the public will need to understand more and more about the medicines they are prescribed or purchase.

However, it is reassuring to remember that the drugs of today are far safer than their forebears. The strictest safety criteria must now be satisfied before a new drug can be introduced into medical use, and many of the more dangerous drugs that were in everyday use not so very long ago, have now been withdrawn or are reserved for special circumstances.

While this dictionary is emphatically not a guide to self-medication, it is definitely intended to help in this process by providing a comprehensive source of easily understandable information about the medicines themselves.

Other publications

Healthcare professionals use a number of similar guides. The British National Formulary (BNF), which is issued twice a year by the British Medical Association and the Pharmaceutical Society of Great Britain, serves as the standard, impartial and authoritative guide. Along with MIMS (Monthly Index of Medical Specialities, a commercial compendium), the BNF is circulated to prescribing medical practitioners. Over-the-counter drugs are covered by the OTC Directory, published by PAGB, the Proprietary Association of Great Britain, and issued to healthcare professionals.

Detailed information on proprietary drugs is also available to professionals from manufacturers, and is published annually in the ABPI Handbook (Association of British Pharmaceutical Industry). Independent comment on drug-related matters is available to all, including members of the public, in the Drug and Therapeutics Bulletin published by the Consumers Association.

There are a number of useful guides to self-medication. Both the Guide to Drugs and Medicines published by the British Medical Association, and Which Medicine?, from the Consumers Association, deal with drugs under disease-related headings. Medicines: The Comprehensive Guide can act as a complementary reference source to these.

What are side-effects and why do they occur?

One of the biggest problems associated with taking medicines relates to the side-effects they may have. Drugs act by having specific effects on the body, usually to attack the cause or relieve the symptoms of an illness.

However, while dealing with the conditions they were designed to
treat, many drugs may also affect the body in other, undesirable ways that are incidental to their primary purpose.

These actions, or side-effects, may be so mild as to be barely noticeable or so severe as to be life-threatening, depending on the drug and the person taking it.
Side-effects are of two basic kinds. 'Type 1' side-effects are inherent in the way the drug acts pharmacologically, and may be largely inevitable and very difficult to circumvent. The side-effect of drowsiness and sedation, for instance, is so common with the antihistamines used in the treatment of hay fever that it is accepted by most sufferers as inevitable. Similarly, 'sleeping pills' taken at night tend to reduce alertness in the morning.

Because pharmacologists who study the action of drugs, and design new ones, and the pharmaceutical industry in general are aware of the inconvenience of side-effects, attempts are continually being made to minimize their action. For example, more recently developed examples of antihistamine drugs are altered chemically to restrict the drug's access to the brain. Similarly, sleeping pills have been developed using shorter-acting benzodiazepine drugs in order to minimize the 'morning-after' effect. It is important to be aware that such developments are occurring so that, where undesirable side-effects are experienced, discussion with a physician may result in finding a more individually acceptable treatment.

'Type 2' side-effects are less predictable, and are often referred to as 'idiosyncratic'. One example of an idiosyncratic or Type 2 side-effect is a true allergic reaction to a drug by the body's immune system. A sensitivity reaction of this kind can present a serious threat to the patient, and the dangers can only be minimized if the patient is aware of the danger because of an earlier reaction to a drug of that class. Physicians routinely ask whether the patient is allergic to antibiotics or local anaesthetics before prescribing them – and each individual must know his or her own idiosyncratic responses.

However, some antibiotics, local anaesthetics, and other drugs that cause allergic reactions, are now available over-the-counter for non-prescription use, so it is vitally important to read the Patient Information Leaflet (PIL) that comes with a medicine.

Reporting side-effects

Both doctors and the pharmaceutical industry are constantly aware of the challenge to safe and acceptable medication posed by the incidence of side-effects of drugs. When information is available about the incidence of a particular drug's side-effect – perhaps in relation to dose and duration of treatment, interactions with other drugs or foodstuffs, or the medical history and individual characteristics of patients exhibiting adverse reactions – then it becomes easier to treat individual patients more safely.

Armed with such information, a doctor will be in a position to decide whether to use that drug for a given individual, to adjust the dose so side-effects are tolerable, to watch out for potentially serious adverse reactions, or to switch to a similar drug that may be better tolerated.

In practice, much information about adverse reactions to drugs is gained during the pre-marketing, clinical-trial phase of testing, and at this stage it is often possible to identify factors that predispose towards individual side-effects.

Once a drug is in use, there are various forms of reporting that continue to track patients on a particular medication. In addition, the UK has a 'yellow card' reporting system, whereby all medical practitioners are issued with supplies of cards which they use to report to the Committee on Safety of Medicines any adverse effects in any drug as they are noticed. Such later procedures help identify rarer adverse reactions and lead to specific warnings being issued about the type of patient for whom the drug should not be prescribed.

How safe are drugs?

Questions about drug safety only make sense on a risks-to-benefit basis. In other words, does the severity of the condition warrant risking certain known side-effects?

At one end of the scale, is a certain individual's headache sufficiently severe that it is worth risking the known side-effects of the humble aspirin tablet? If the individual is in good health with no history of intolerance to NSAID drugs, and no form of stomach upset, then the answer may well be Yes. On the other hand if the individual is a child, or has a predisposition towards gastric ulcers, or asthma, then the answer will be No. For further information on this topic, see the NSAID entry in this book. In the case of headaches, an alternative drug can readily be found (in this example, it will probably be paracetamol).

At the other end of the scale of risks-to-benefit scale, however, if the patient has a life-threatening infection, or cancer, then the physician may discuss with the patient whether to treat the condition with drugs that would be too toxic to use for less serious conditions.

How serious is serious?

Looking at the list of side-effects and warnings for some generic drugs entries, the reader may gain the impression that patients would be ill-advised to take any of them.

At one extreme, certainly, on the basis of the risk-to-benefit ratio, it is true that any unnecessary taking of drugs should always be avoided.

Nevertheless, most people accept that in some circumstances the use of drugs is unavoidable. The risks or undesirability of an unplanned pregnancy may outweigh the known risks of taking the 'pill'. The seasonal hay fever sufferer may be willing to put up with the short-term side-effects of antihistamines to gain relief from the misery of sneezing and rhinitis. And when it comes to serious illness, benefits can outweigh risks by a considerable margin.

A short course of antibiotics may achieve a complete and permanent cure of infections that without them could prove fatal (eg meningitis), and the side-effects of such a course may be no worse than occasional diarrhoea.

Even more effective is vaccination, which at its most successful can, by treating the most vulnerable sectors of the population, completely eliminate some infectious diseases. Smallpox infection no longer exists in the world population, and poliomyelitis may soon follow it, both as a result of worldwide vaccination programmes.

In the UK, MMR vaccination of children has been introduced with the intention of eliminating mumps, measles, and rubella (also called German measles). Although there may be very rare incidences of serious adverse reactions, most people accept that these risks are far outweighed by the considerable threat to children of contracting the infections themselves. And in any vaccination programme, it is important that all, rather than just a selection of children are vaccinated, or the diseases may regenerate in the unvaccinated group and so become re-established in the population.

When interpreting the listed side-effects of individual drugs, it is important to understand that the longer the period a drug has been in use, the longer the list of possible side-effects is likely to be.

Conversely, new drugs may appear to be free of side-effects because relatively little is known about them as they are still going through the yellow card and other reporting processes. In the listings in this book, the most frequent side-effects appear first, while those at the end of the list are likely to be rare.

Similarly the warnings are based on doctors' accumulated experience in using that drug. As already mentioned, many drugs need to be used with special care if the drug is not metabolized or excreted as rapidly as normal, and so causing the drug to build up to toxic levels. This is most likely to happen in patients with certain kidney or liver disorders, and in the elderly: when the physician is aware of the circumstances, using a lower dosage often avoids any potential problems.

It can also be seen that the majority of the drugs in this book should be avoided by women who are pregnant or breast-feeding, because, although it is not known for certain that they are dangerous, the lessons of the thalidomide disaster have not been forgotten, and it is better to be careful than sorry.

Individuals at risk of adverse reaction
People suffering from the following conditions are particularly susceptible to certain drugs or forms of drug therapy. Although the conditions are generally rare, it is very important to be aware of them, and reminders to this effect appear throughout the book under the lists of Warnings.

Inherited conditions
Porphyria appears as a 'should not use' warning in many entries. This fairly rare inherited condition, which causes abnormal metabolism of blood pigments, is serious in its own right, but is potentially lethal in combination with a wide range of drugs – some of which are commonly available and otherwise harmless. Normally individuals who have

porphyria know it, but the condition is sufficiently serious that relatives of patients should also be screened for a tendency to porphyria.

G6PD deficiency (glucose 6-phosphate dehydrogenase enzyme deficiency) is relatively common in African, Indian, and some Mediterranean races. It is a genetically inherited condition with a widely different frequency in different biological groups. Serious adverse reactions occur with quite a few drugs – for instance the antimalarial drug primaquine causes blood red cell haemolysis in 5–10% of black males, leading to severe anaemia.

Slow acetylators are mentioned only a few times. Similar to G6PD, this describes an inherited condition where an enzyme that breaks down drugs within the body has low activity, so it is important that lower doses of such drugs are taken.

Non-inherited conditions

Age needs to be taken into account as a factor in drug doses. The elderly metabolize drugs slowly, so lower doses usually need to be used; the elderly are also more likely to become confused with many drugs that act on the brain.

Kidney disorders slow down the excretion of drugs and so active constituents may remain in the body for longer than is intended, so doses should be adjusted to take account of this.

Liver disorders slows down the body's metabolism of drugs, so lower doses may be needed.

Alcoholism is likely to have caused damage to the liver, so the same considerations apply as to liver disease.

Heart disease requires special care when drugs are prescribed, and more usually patients need special advice in the safe use of medicines.

Pregnancy requires special care and, as mentioned already, it is best to avoid taking any drugs during pregnancy if this is practicable. Even before becoming pregnant it is best to discontinue use of some drugs as well as alcohol to avoid the residual effects of these. Not all drugs are damaging in pregnancy, however, and the Department of Health now agree that supplements of the vitamin folic acid help prevent neural tube defects when taken before and during pregnancy. *In breast-feeding*, specific information is now available on which drugs are of concern because they pass to the baby in the mother's milk or effect milk production. Here too, however, as a general rule it is best to avoid all drugs if possible, and if not a doctor should be consulted in every case.

Drug interactions: good or bad?

One of the greatest inherent dangers in the use of either prescription or non-prescription drugs lies in the unpredictability of the interactions between two or more different drugs, or even in the interaction between drugs and foodstuffs or environmental factors.

The risk of serious interactions between monoamine-oxidase inhibitor (MAOI) antidepressants and certain foodstuffs and decongestant drugs is well known. Most people will be aware of the additive or potentiating action that ingestion of alcohol has on the sedative or sleep-enhancing effects of many drugs ranging from benzodiazepine anxiolytics to antihistamines and components of 'cold-cures'.

An interaction called synergy, which is the additive effect that occurs when two drugs with the same sort of action are taken together, may be a considerable problem. But opposing interactions may be just as significant and potentially just as or even more dangerous.

There is a widely held belief that antibiotics and alcohol 'do not mix'. In fact certain antibiotics (eg azole antimicrobials such as metronidazole) interfere with the metabolism of alcohol so that it produces a toxic metabolite, called acetaldehyde, in the body, and this may make the subject feel very ill indeed (see the entry on disulfiram).

Details of some of the more worrying drug interactions are given under individual generic entries. However, by no means all interactions between two drugs are detrimental, and two drugs may be specifically prescribed to be taken together for a variety of reasons. For example, one of a pair of drugs may inhibit the break down or excretion of the other drug, so prolonging its beneficial effects (eg probenicid prolongs the duration of action of some penicillin antibiotics). Another reason for taking two drugs simultaneously is where one drug counteracts the adverse effects of the other; this can occur in the treatment of Parkinson's disease and other diseases of the central nervous system.

In general, however, drug interactions are complex and sometimes difficult to predict. The doctor or pharmacist will have detailed charts of known interactions, and in all cases should be consulted if the patient is worried, and expert opinion should always be taken if more than one drug is to be used at a time.

Drugs in sport

It should be noted that drugs that are available and/or legal for everyday use are not necessarily legal in competitive sports. Athletes should be aware that banned drugs include constituents of over-the-counter medicines including 'cold-cures' (eg ephedrine, phenylpropanolamine, pseudoephedrine) and prescribed drugs common in asthma treatment (eg fenoterol, isoprenaline).

In summary

It is often argued that a little knowledge is a dangerous thing. However, the combination of current changes in prescribing habits in the UK with the increasing availability of powerful medicines over-the-counter suggests that ignorance too, is dangerous.

Sweeping deregulation is lowering the protective shield afforded by the older prescription-only approach to drug therapy, and as a result greater responsibility is being thrown on the individual.

To prepare for this, each of us must become conversant with some basic facts about our own individual reactions to the basic types of drugs. We must know when to seek advice from the healthcare professionals and what to ask them.

Good medical therapy depends on a partnership between the patient and medical professionals, and it is the authors' hope that this book will provide some of the basic facts about drugs, their characteristics and their uses, which will help with such a partnership.

IKMM
JMH
King's College London
September 1995

MEDICINES

A-Z

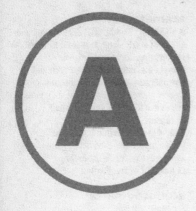

AC Vax
(SmithKline Beecham) is a proprietary, prescription-only VACCINE preparation. It can be used to give protection against the organism meningococcus (*Neisseria meningitidis* groups A and C), which can cause serious infection such as meningitis. It is available in a form for injection.
✚▲ side-effects/warning: see MENINGOCOCCAL POLYSACCHARIDE VACCINE

acarbose
is an ENZYME INHIBITOR that interferes with the conversion in the intestine of starch and sucrose (sugar) to glucose and is used in DIABETIC TREATMENT. It has recently been introduced for the treatment of Type II diabetes (non-insulin-dependent diabetes mellitus; NIDDM; maturity-onset diabetes). It may be of value in patients where other drugs, or diet control, have not been successful. It is available as tablets to be taken immediately before food.
✚ side-effects: gastrointestinal disturbances, including diarrhoea, flatulence and distension.
▲ warning: because of side-effects it should not be used if there are certain types of intestinal disease. Do not use in pregnancy and when breast-feeding, or when there are certain kidney or liver disorders. Monitor blood glucose and enzymes.
✪Related entry: Glucobay

Accupro
(Parke-Davis) is a proprietary, prescription-only preparation of the ACE INHIBITOR quinapril. It can be used as an ANTIHYPERTENSIVE and in HEART FAILURE TREATMENT. It is available as tablets.
✚▲ side-effects/warning: see QUINAPRIL

Accuretic
(Parke-Davis) is a proprietary, prescription-only COMPOUND PREPARATION of the ACE INHIBITOR quinapril and the (THIAZIDE) DIURETIC drug

A

hydrochlorothiazide. It can be used as an ANTIHYPERTENSIVE treatment and is available as tablets.

✚▲ side-effects/warning: see HYDROCHLOROTHIAZIDE; QUINAPRIL

*ACE inhibitors

(angiotensin-converting enzyme inhibitors) are drugs used in ANTIHYPERTENSIVE treatment and in HEART FAILURE TREATMENT. They work by inhibiting the conversion of the natural circulating HORMONE angiotensin I to angiotensin II; and because the latter is a potent VASOCONSTRICTOR, the overall effect is vasodilation (see VASODILATOR) with a HYPOTENSIVE action. This action is of value when the blood pressure is raised (as in hypertension) and also in the treatment of heart failure. There has been a considerable increase recently in the use of ACE inhibitors in moderate hypertension and in severe hypertension when other treatments are not suitable or successful. They are usually used in conjunction with other antihypertension treatments, especially DIURETICS.
See: CAPTOPRIL; CILAZAPRIL; ENALAPRIL MALEATE; FOSINOPRIL; LISINOPRIL; PERINDOPRIL; QUINAPRIL; RAMIPRIL; TRANDOLAPRIL

acebutolol

is a BETA-BLOCKER drug. It can be used as an ANTIHYPERTENSIVE treatment for raised blood pressure, as an ANTI-ANGINA treatment to relieve symptoms and to improve exercise tolerance and as an ANTI-ARRHYTHMIC to regularize heartbeat and to treat myocardial infarction (damage to heart muscle, usually due to a heart attack). Administration is oral in the form of tablets or sustained-release capsules. It is also available, as an antihypertensive treatment, in the form of COMPOUND PREPARATIONS with DIURETICS.

✚▲ side-effects/warning: see PROPRANOLOL HYDROCHLORIDE

❂ Related entries: Secadrex; Sectral

32

acemetacin

is a (NSAID) NON-NARCOTIC ANALGESIC and ANTIRHEUMATIC drug. It is used to treat serious rheumatic and arthritic complaints, musculoskeletal pain and postoperative pain. Chemically, it is closely related to indomethacin (it is its glycolic acid ester) and is available as capsules.

✚▲ side-effect/warning: see under indomethacin. It should not be administered to patients who are breast-feeding.

❂ Related entry: Emflex

acenocoumarol

See NICOUMALONE

acetaminophen

is the standard name used in the USA for PARACETAMOL.

acetazolamide

is a CARBONIC ANHYDRASE INHIBITOR that has quite wide-ranging actions in the body. It can be used as a GLAUCOMA TREATMENT because it reduces the formation of aqueous humour in the eye. It acts as a DIURETIC and so can be used to treat oedema, especially when associated with congestive heart failure. It has also been used as an ANTI-EPILEPTIC to assist in the prevention of certain types of epileptic seizures, especially in children.

Additionally, it can be used to treat the symptoms of premenstrual syndrome and to prevent motion sickness. It is available as tablets, a powder for reconstitution as a medium for injection or infusion and as capsules.

✚ side-effects: there may be numbness and tingling of the hands and feet. Rarely, there may be blood disorders or lowered blood potassium.

▲ warning: it should be administered with caution to patients who are pregnant; and avoid its use in patients with certain severe kidney disorders.

❂ Related entry: Diamox

Acetoxyl 2.5 Acne Gel

(Stiefel) is a proprietary, non-prescription preparation of the KERATOLYTIC and ANTIMICROBIAL drug benzoyl peroxide (2.5%). It can be used to treat acne and is available as a gel.

+▲ side-effects/warning: see BENZOYL PEROXIDE

Acetoxyl 5 Acne Gel

(Stiefel) is a proprietary, non-prescription preparation of the KERATOLYTIC and ANTIMICROBIAL drug benzoyl peroxide (5%). It can be used to treat acne and is available as a gel.

+▲ side-effects/warning: see BENZOYL PEROXIDE

acetylcholine

is a NEUROTRANSMITTER in the body. It has a number of important roles in both the central and peripheral nervous systems, relaying messages between nerves or from nerve to innervated organs. In medicine, it is rarely used as a drug because it is rapidly broken down in the body by cholinesterase enzymes.

However, in the form of ACETYLCHOLINE CHLORIDE it can be administered in solution to the eyes for cataract surgery and other ophthalmic procedures requiring rapid constriction of the pupil. Although acetylcholine itself is not used therapeutically, a considerable number of drugs work by mimicking, exaggerating, or blocking its actions.

PARASYMPATHOMIMETICS are a class of drugs with effects similar to those of the parasympathetic nervous system and work by mimicking the actions of acetylcholine. Important parasympathomimetic actions include slowing of the heart, vasodilation, constriction of the pupil and altered focusing of the eye. *Direct-acting* parasympathomimetics act at *muscarinic* RECEPTORS for acetylcholine (eg CARBACHOL and PILOCARPINE). *Indirect-acting* parasympathomimetics prolong the duration of action of naturally released acetylcholine by inhibiting cholinesterase enzymes (eg NEOSTIGMINE).

Certain SKELETAL MUSCLE RELAXANT drugs act to interfere with neurotransmission by acetylcholine at so-called *nicotinic* receptors, which lie at the junction between nerves and voluntary (skeletal) muscles and are called *neuromuscular blocking drugs*. They are used in surgical operations to paralyse skeletal muscles that are normally under voluntary nerve control and so allow lighter levels of anaesthesia to be administered. These drugs are of one or two sorts: *non-depolarizing* skeletal muscle relaxants (eg GALLAMINE TRIETHIODIDE and TUBOCURARINE CHLORIDE); or *depolarizing* skeletal muscle relaxants (eg SUXAMETHONIUM CHLORIDE). The action of the non-depolarizing blocking drugs can be reversed at the end of an operation by administering an anticholinesterase drug.

GANGLION-BLOCKER drugs block the transmission of acetylcholine in the peripheral autonomic nervous system at the junctions called ganglia. The ganglion-blockers are now rarely used in medicine because they have very widespread actions. However, TRIMETAPHAN CAMSYLATE is used as a HYPOTENSIVE drug for controlling blood pressure during bloodless surgery.

Drugs that mimic acetylcholine through the stimulation of nicotinic receptors also have only a limited use in medicine, because their actions have unacceptable side-effects and are too widespread. Indeed, NICOTINE, as adsorbed into the body by the use of tobacco products, causes such widespread and undesirable effects, for example an increase in blood pressure, heart rate and blood sugar levels and also a release of adrenaline (which contributes to many of these effects).

In the brain, nicotine acts at nicotinic receptors and causes further stimulation and euphoria, which are all factors in

A

making it such a powerfully habituating (addictive) drug.

Although some ANTICHOLINERGIC drugs act at nicotinic receptors, there is an important group that work by blocking the actions of acetylcholine at muscarinic receptors. The ANTIMUSCARINIC drugs have extensive uses in medicine and it is because they are used so extensively that the term *antimuscarinic* is often used synonymously for *anticholinergic* (even though this is incorrect). Antimuscarinic drugs tend to relax smooth muscle, reduce the secretion of saliva, digestive juices and sweat and to dilate the pupils of the eyes. They can also be used as ANTISPASMODICS and ANTIPARKSONISM drugs (in the treatment of some of the symptoms of Parkinson's disease), or as ANTINAUSEANTS, or ANTI-EMETICS, in the treatment of motion sickness, peptic ulcers, in ophthalmic examinations and in antagonizing adverse effects of ANTICHOLINESTRASES (in medicine, agricultural accidental poisoning, or in warfare). Examples of antimuscarinic drugs include ATROPINE SULPHATE, BENZHEXOL HYDROCHLORIDE and HYOSCINE HYDROBROMIDE.

acetylcholine chloride

is a PARASYMPATHOMIMETIC drug, which is rarely used therapeutically because it is rapidly broken down in the body. However, it can be applied in solution to the eye for cataract surgery, iridectomy and other types of surgery requiring rapid miosis (constriction of the pupil). Administration is by topical application as a solution. (ACETYLCHOLINE is the natural NEUROTRANSMITTER released from cholinergic nerves in the body.)
✚▲ side-effects/warning: see under PILOCARPINE
◑ Related entry: Miochol

acetylcysteine

is a MUCOLYTIC drug, which reduces the viscosity of sputum and so can be used as

an EXPECTORANT in patients with disorders of the upper respiratory airways, such as chronic asthma and bronchitis. It is also used to treat abdominal complications associated with cystic fibrosis and in the eye to increase lacrimation (the production of tears) and mucus secretion.

It is also used as an ANTIDOTE to treat overdose poisoning by the NON-NARCOTIC ANALGESIC drug paracetamol. The initial symptoms of poisoning usually settle within 24 hours, but give way to a serious toxic effect on the liver which takes some days to develop.

It is to prevent these latter effects that treatment is directed and is required immediately after overdose, normally in hospital. Administration as an antidote is by intravenous infusion and for other purposes it is either topical as eye-drops or oral as a solution.
✚ side-effects: the type and severity of any side-effects depends on the route of administration, but there may be headache, tinnitus (ringing in the ears) and gastrointestinal irritation.
▲ warning: administer with caution to patients who are asthmatics.
◑ Related entries: Fabrol; Ilube; Parvolex

Acezide

(Squibb) is a proprietary, prescription-only COMPOUND PREPARATION of the ACE INHIBITOR quinapril and the (THIAZIDE) DIURETIC drug hydrochlorothiazide. It can be used as an ANTIHYPERTENSIVE treatment and is available as tablets.
✚▲ side-effects/warning: see QUINAPRIL; HYDROCHLOROTHIAZIDE

Achromycin

(Lederle) is a proprietary, prescription-only preparation of the broad-spectrum ANTIBACTERIAL and (TETRACYCLINE) ANTIBIOTIC drug tetracycline (as hydrochloride). It can be used to treat many types of infection and is available as tablets, capsules, as an ointment (for skin,

eye, or ear) and in a form for infusion.
✚▲ side-effects/warning: see TETRACYCLINE

aciclovir
See ACYCLOVIR

Aci-Jel
(Cilag) is a proprietary, non-prescription
ANTIMICROBIAL preparation of acetic acid.
It can be used to treat non-specific vaginal
infections and to restore acidity to the
vagina. It is available as a jelly, which is
supplied with a special applicator.

acipimox
is used as a LIPID-LOWERING DRUG in
hyperlipidaemia to reduce the levels, or
change the proportions, of various lipids
in the bloodstream. It is thought to act in
a similar way to NICOTINIC ACID, by
inhibiting synthesis of lipids in the liver.
Generally, it is administered only to
patients in whom a strict and regular
dietary regime, alone, is not having the
desired effect. Administration is oral
in the form of capsules.
✚ side-effects: there may be flushing, itching,
rashes and reddening of the skin; nausea and
abdominal pain; diarrhoea; malaise;
headache.
▲ warning: it should not be administered to
patients who are pregnant, or have peptic
ulcers; and should be administered with
caution to those with impaired kidney
function.
○ Related entry: Olbetam

acitretin
is chemically a retinoid (it is a metabolite
of etretinate, which is a derivative of
RETINOL or vitamin A) and has a marked
effect on the cells that make up the skin
epithelium. It can be taken over a period
of weeks to relieve severe psoriasis that is
resistant to other treatments and for other
skin conditions (including severe Darier's
disease). Treatment is under strict medical
supervision and administration is oral in
the form of capsules.

✚ side-effects: these include dryness of skin,
cracked lips and mucous membrane, muscle
and joint ache, hair loss, reversible visual
disturbances, nausea, headache, sweating,
changes in liver function, blood upsets, mood
changes and drowsiness.
▲ warning: do not use in patients who are
pregnant (and exclude pregnancy before
starting and after treatment) or breast-
feeding, or who have certain liver or kidney
disorders. Avoid excessive exposure to
sunlight.
○ Related entry: Neotigason

Aclacin
(Lundbeck) is a proprietary, prescription-
only preparation of the (CYTOTOXIC)
ANTICANCER drug aclarubicin. It is used to
treat certain leukaemias and is available in
a form for injection.
✚▲ side-effects/warning: see ACLARUBICIN

aclarubicin
is a recently introduced CYTOTOXIC DRUG
(an ANTIBIOTIC in origin) with properties
similar to doxorubicin. It is used as an
ANTICANCER drug, particularly to treat
acute non-lymphocytic leukaemia in
patients who have not responded to, or
who have relapsed from, other forms of
chemotherapy. Administration is by
injection.
✚▲ side-effects/warning: see CYTOTOXIC
DRUGS. Administer with caution to patients
with kidney or liver impairment; it is irritant
to tissues.
○ Related entry: Aclacin

Acnecide
(Novex) is a proprietary, non-prescription
preparation of the KERATOLYTIC and
ANTIMICROBIAL drug benzoyl peroxide. It
can be used to treat acne and is available
as a gel.
✚▲ side-effects/warning: see
BENZOYL PEROXIDE

Acnegel
(Stiefel) is a proprietary, non-prescription

A

preparation of the KERATOLYTIC and ANTIMICROBIAL drug benzoyl peroxide (5%). It can be used to treat acne and is available as a gel. It is not normally used for children under 12 years, except on medical advice.

+▲ side-effects/warning: see BENZOYL PEROXIDE

Acnegel Forte

(Stiefel) is a proprietary, non-prescription preparation of the KERATOLYTIC and ANTIMICROBIAL drug benzoyl peroxide (10%). It can be used to treat acne and is available as a gel. It is not normally used for children under 12 years, except on medical advice.

+▲ side-effects/warning: see BENZOYL PEROXIDE

Acnidazil

(Cilag) is a proprietary, non-prescription COMPOUND PREPARATION of the ANTIFUNGAL drug miconazole (as nitrate) and the KERATOLYTIC and ANTIMICROBIAL drug benzoyl peroxide. It can be used to treat acne and is available as a cream.

+▲ side-effects/warning: see BENZOYL PEROXIDE; MICONAZOLE

Acnisal

(Euroderma) is a proprietary, non-prescription preparation of the KERATOLYTIC agent salicylic acid. It can be used to treat acne and is available as a solution for topical application.

+▲ side-effects/warning: see SALICYLIC ACID

acrivastine

is an ANTIHISTAMINE drug, which has only recently been developed and has less sedative side-effects than some of the older antihistamines. It can be used for the symptomatic relief of allergic conditions such as hay fever and urticaria (itchy skin rash). Administration is oral in the form of capsules.

+▲ side-effects/warning: see under ANTIHISTAMINE; but the incidence of sedative and anticholinergic effects is low. Avoid its use in patients with kidney impairment.

✪ Related entry: Semprex

acrosoxacin

(rosoxacin) is an ANTIBACTERIAL and (QUINOLONE) ANTIBIOTIC drug. It is used to treat the sexually transmitted disease gonorrhoea in patients who are allergic to penicillin, or whose gonorrhoea is resistant to penicillin-type antibacterials. Administration is oral in the form of a capsule.

+ side-effects: nausea, vomiting, abdominal pain, diarrhoea, headache, dizziness, sleep disorders, rash, pruritus, fever, photosensitivity, increase in blood creatinine and urea, transient disturbances in liver enzymes and bilirubin, joint and muscle pains, blood disorders. Less frequently, there may be anaphylaxis, anorexia, confusion, hallucinations and sensory disturbances.

▲ warning: administer with caution to children or adolescents; to patients with epilepsy, kidney or liver impairment; or who are pregnant or breast-feeding. There is a risk of convulsions being precipitated in those showing no previous tendencies (eg by NSAIDs).

✪ Related entry: Eradacin

Actal Tablets

(Sterling Health) is a proprietary, non-prescription preparation of the ANTACID alexitol sodium. It can be used for the relief of hyperacidity, dyspepsia and indigestion. It is available as tablets and is not normally given to children under 12 years, except on medical advice.

+▲ side-effects/warning: see ALEXITOL SODIUM

Act-HIB

(Merieux) is a proprietary, prescription-only VACCINE preparation for *Haemophilus influenzae* infection and is available in a form for injection.

+▲ side-effects/warning: see HAEMOPHILUS INFLUENZAE TYPE B VACCINE

Actifed Compound Linctus

(Wellcome) is a proprietary, non-prescription preparation of the ANTIHISTAMINE triprolidine hydrochloride, the SYMPATHOMIMETIC and DECONGESTANT drug pseudoephedrine hydrochloride and the (OPIOID) NARCOTIC ANALGESIC and ANTITUSSIVE drug dextromethorphan hydrobromide.

It can be used for the symptomatic relief of unproductive cough and congestion of the upper respiratory tract, including allergic conditions. It is available as a liquid and is not normally given to children under two years, except on medical advice.

+▲ side-effects/warning: see DEXTROMETHORPHAN HYDROBROMIDE; PSEUDOEPHEDRINE HYDROCHLORIDE; TRIPROLIDINE HYDROCHLORIDE

Actifed Expectorant

(Wellcome) is a proprietary, non-prescription COMPOUND PREPARATION of the ANTIHISTAMINE drug triprolidine hydrochloride, the SYMPATHOMIMETIC and DECONGESTANT drug pseudoephedrine hydrochloride and the EXPECTORANT guaiphenesin.

It can be used for the symptomatic relief of upper respiratory tract disorders accompanied by productive cough. It is available as a liquid and is not normally given to children under two years, except on medical advice.

+▲ side-effects/warning: see GUAIPHENESIN; PSEUDOEPHEDRINE HYDROCHLORIDE; TRIPROLIDINE HYDROCHLORIDE

Actifed Junior Cough Relief

(Wellcome) is a proprietary, non-prescription COMPOUND PREPARATION of the ANTIHISTAMINE drug triprolidine hydrochloride and the ANTITUSSIVE drug dextromethorphan hydrobromide. It can be used for the symptomatic relief of upper respiratory tract disorders accompanied by unproductive cough and other cold symptoms in children.

It is available as a liquid and is not normally given to children under one year, except on medical advice.

+▲ side-effects/warning: see DEXTROMETHORPHAN HYDROBROMIDE; TRIPROLIDINE HYDROCHLORIDE

Actifed Syrup

(Wellcome) is a proprietary, non-prescription COMPOUND PREPARATION of the ANTIHISTAMINE drug triprolidine hydrochloride and the SYMPATHOMIMETIC and DECONGESTANT drug pseudoephedrine hydrochloride.

It can be used for congestion of the upper airways and sinuses and for the symptomatic treatment of colds, hay fever and rhinitis. It is available as a liquid and is not normally given to children under two years, except on medical advice.

+▲ side-effects/warning: see PSEUDOEPHEDRINE HYDROCHLORIDE; TRIPROLIDINE HYDROCHLORIDE

Actifed Tablets

(Wellcome) is a proprietary, non-prescription COMPOUND PREPARATION of the ANTIHISTAMINE drug triprolidine hydrochloride and the SYMPATHOMIMETIC and DECONGESTANT drug pseudoephedrine hydrochloride.

It can be used for congestion of the upper airways and sinuses and for the symptomatic treatment of colds, hay fever and rhinitis. It is available as a liquid and is not normally given to children under 12 years, except on medical advice.

+▲ side-effects/warning: see PSEUDOEPHEDRINE HYDROCHLORIDE; TRIPROLIDINE HYDROCHLORIDE

Actilyse

(Boehringer Ingelheim) is a proprietary, prescription-only preparation of the FIBRINOLYTIC drug alteplase. It can be used to treat myocardial infarction and is available in a form for injection.

+▲ side-effects/warning: see ALTEPLASE

A

Actinac

(Roussel) is a proprietary, prescription-only COMPOUND PREPARATION of the broad-spectrum ANTIBACTERIAL and ANTIBIOTIC drug chloramphenicol and the ANTI-INFLAMMATORY and CORTICOSTEROID drug hydrocortisone (as acetate). It can be used by topical application to treat acne and is available as a lotion.

+▲ side-effects/warning: see CHLORAMPHENICOL; HYDROCORTISONE

actinomycin D

See DACTINOMYCIN

activated charcoal

is an adsorbent material. Its primary use is for soaking up poisons in the stomach or small intestine, especially drug overdoses in cases where only a small quantity of the drug may be extremely toxic (eg some ANTIDEPRESSANTS). It can help prevent the effects of drug overdose by increasing the elimination of certain drugs even after they have been absorbed (eg ASPIRIN and BARBITURATES). It is available as a powder to be taken in solution as often as necessary. It can also be used as a constituent in ANTIDIARRHOEAL preparations – it is effective in binding together faecal matter – and can relieve flatulence.

۞ Related entries: Carbomix; Medicoal

Actron

(Bayer) is a proprietary, non-prescription COMPOUND PREPARATION of the (NSAID) NON-NARCOTIC ANALGESIC drug para-cetamol, the (NSAID) non-narcotic and ANTIRHEUMATIC drug aspirin, the ANTACID sodium bicarbonate, citric acid and the STIMULANT caffeine. It can be used for general aches and pains and for headache with upset stomach. It is available as effervescent tablets and is not normally given to children under 12 years, except on medical advice.

+▲ side-effects/warning: see ASPIRIN; CAFFEINE; PARACETAMOL; SODIUM BICARBONATE

Acupan

(3M Health Care) is a proprietary, prescription-only preparation of the NON-NARCOTIC ANALGESIC drug nefopam hydrochloride. It can be used to treat moderate pain and is available as tablets and in a form for injection.

+▲ side-effects/warning: see NEFOPAM HYDROCHLORIDE

acyclovir

(aciclovir) is an ANTIVIRAL drug. It is used specifically to treat infection by the herpes viruses (eg shingles, chickenpox, cold sores, genital herpes and herpes infections of the eye and mouth). It works by inhibiting the action of two enzymes in human cells that are used by the virus to replicate itself. To be effective, however, treatment must begin early. It can be valuable in immunocompromised patients. The drug can also be used prophylactically to prevent individuals at risk from contracting a herpes disease. Administration can be oral as tablets or a suspension, or as a variety of topical preparations (ointments and creams), or by intravenous infusion.

+ side-effects: when applied topically, there may be a temporary burning or stinging sensation; some patients experience a localized drying of the skin. When taken orally, it may give rise to gastrointestinal disturbance and various blood-cell deficiencies. There may also be fatigue, rash, headache, tremor and effects on mood.

▲ warning: administer with caution to patients who are pregnant or breast-feeding; or who have impaired kidney function. Adequate fluid intake must be maintained.

۞ Related entry: Zovirax

Adalat

(Bayer) is a proprietary, prescription-only preparation of the CALCIUM-CHANNEL BLOCKER nifedipine. It can be used as an ANTI-ANGINA treatment in the prevention of attacks, as an ANTIHYPERTENSIVE treatment and as a VASODILATOR in peripheral

A

vascular disease (Raynaud's phenomenon). It is available as capsules.
+▲ side-effects/warning: see NIFEDIPINE

Adalat LA

(Bayer) is a proprietary, prescription-only preparation of the CALCIUM-CHANNEL BLOCKER nifedipine. It can be used as an ANTIHYPERTENSIVE treatment and is available as modified-release tablets in two doses: *Adalat LA 30* and *Adalat LA 60*.
+▲ side-effects/warning: see NIFEDIPINE

Adalat Retard

(Bayer) is a proprietary, prescription-only preparation of the CALCIUM-CHANNEL BLOCKER nifedipine. It can be used as an ANTIHYPERTENSIVE and an ANTI-ANGINA treatment in the prevention of attacks. It is available as modified-release tablets in two doses: *Adalat Retard 10* and *Adalat Retard 20*.
+▲ side-effects/warning: see NIFEDIPINE

Adcortyl

(Squibb) is a proprietary, prescription-only preparation of the CORTICOSTEROID and ANTI-INFLAMMATORY drug triamcinolone acetonide. It can be used to treat skin conditions such as eczema and psoriasis that are unresponsive to other corticosteroids. It is available as a cream and an ointment.
+▲ side-effects/warning: see TRIAMCINOLONE ACETONIDE

Adcortyl in Orabase

(Squibb) is a proprietary, prescription-only preparation of the CORTICOSTEROID and ANTI-INFLAMMATORY drug triamcinolone acetonide. It can be used to treat mouth ulcers and inflammation and is available as an oral paste.
+▲ side-effects/warning: see TRIAMCINOLONE ACETONIDE

Adcortyl Intra-articular/Intradermal

(Squibb) is a proprietary, prescription-only preparation of the CORTICOSTEROID and ANTI-INFLAMMATORY drug triamcinolone acetonide. It can be administered by intradermal injection to relieve some skin lesions, or by injection directly into soft tissue or a joint to relieve pain, swelling and stiffness (eg tennis elbow).
+▲ side-effects/warning: see TRIAMCINOLONE ACETONIDE

Adcortyl with Graneodin

(Squibb) is a proprietary, prescription-only COMPOUND PREPARATION of the ANTI-INFLAMMATORY and CORTICOSTEROID drug triamcinolone acetonide and the ANTIBACTERIAL and ANTIBIOTIC drugs neomycin sulphate and gramicidin. It can be used to treat inflammatory skin conditions with infection, such as psoriasis and eczema. It is available as a cream.
+▲ side-effects/warning: see GRAMICIDIN; NEOMYCIN SULPHATE; TRIAMCINOLONE ACETONIDE

Adenocor

(Sanofi Winthrop) is a proprietary, prescription-only preparation of the ANTI-ARRHYTHMIC drug adenosine. It can be used to correct heart irregularities and is available as tablets and in a form for injection.
+▲ side-effects/warning: see ADENOSINE

adenosine

can be used as an ANTI-ARRHYTHMIC drug. It corrects certain abnormal rhythms (eg Wolff-Parkinson-White syndrome) and helps in the diagnosis of certain arrhythmias (complex supraventricular tachycardias). Administration is by injection.
+ side-effects: flushes of the face; shortness of breath, choking and bronchospasm; nausea and light-headedness; extreme slowing of the heart and chest pain.
▲ warning: it should be administered with caution in certain heart conditions and is not

A

to be given to patients with asthma.
○ Related entry: Adenocor

ADH (antidiuretic hormone)
See VASOPRESSIN

Adifax
(Servier) is a proprietary, prescription-only preparation of the APPETITE SUPPRESSANT dexfenfluramine hydrochloride. It can be used to treat obesity and is available as capsules.
✚▲ side-effects/warning: see
DEXFENFLURAMINE HYDROCHLORIDE

Adizem-60
(Napp) is a proprietary, prescription-only preparation of the CALCIUM-CHANNEL BLOCKER diltiazem hydrochloride. It can be used as an ANTIHYPERTENSIVE treatment and as an ANTI-ANGINA drug in the prevention of attacks. It is available as modified-release tablets.
✚▲ side-effects/warning: see
DILTIAZEM HYDROCHLORIDE

Adizem-SR
(Napp) is a proprietary, prescription-only preparation of the CALCIUM-CHANNEL BLOCKER diltiazem hydrochloride. It can be used as an ANTIHYPERTENSIVE treatment and as an ANTI-ANGINA drug in the prevention of attacks. It is available as long-acting, modified-release tablets and capsules.
✚▲ side-effects/warning: see
DILTIAZEM HYDROCHLORIDE

Adizem-XL
(Napp) is a proprietary, prescription-only preparation of the CALCIUM-CHANNEL BLOCKER diltiazem hydrochloride. It can be used as an ANTIHYPERTENSIVE treatment and as an ANTI-ANGINA drug in the prevention of attacks. It is available as long-acting, modified-release capsules.
✚▲ side-effects/warning: see DILTIAZEM
HYDROCHLORIDE

adrenaline
is chemically called a catecholamine (in the USA it is known as *epinephrine* or *Adrenalin*). It is secreted into the bloodstream (along with the closely related substance NORADRENALINE) as an endocrine HORMONE by the adrenal glands, from the region called the medulla (the central core; hence adrenomedullary hormone).

The adrenal glands constitute an important part of the sympathetic nervous system. Together with noradrenaline (which also acts as a NEUROTRANSMITTER, being released from nerve-endings by electrical signals travelling from the central nervous system via nerves in the body), adrenaline activates or inhibits a wide variety of muscles, exocrine glands and metabolic processes in the body.

The responses of the body to stimulation of the sympathetic nervous system are primarily concerned with reactions to stress. In the face of stress, or the need for exertion, the body uses adrenaline and noradrenaline to cause constriction of some blood vessels while dilating others, with the net effect that the two catecholamines increase blood flow to the skeletal muscles and heart. The heart rate is raised and there is relaxation of the smooth muscles of the intestine and bronchioles.

There is also a rise in concentration of energy supplying glucose and free fatty-acids in the bloodstream. The actions of noradrenaline and adrenaline are similar. Adrenaline itself is not greatly used therapeutically because its actions are so widespread.

In emergencies, however, it may be injected (in the form of adrenaline acid tartrate) in cardiac arrest, to treat the circulatory collapse and bronchoconstriction of anaphylactic shock and in angio-oedema. More commonly, adrenaline is included in several LOCAL ANAESTHETIC preparations, because its pronounced VASOCONSTRICTOR actions considerably prolong anaesthesia by preventing the local anaesthetic from being removed in the bloodstream. Also, it is administered in solution in eye-drops to treat glaucoma. Administration of adrenaline is by subcutaneous, intramuscular or intravenous injection (as well as various specialized methods with local anaesthetics), by inhalation, or by eye-drops.

✚ side-effects: depending on the method of administration, there may be an increase in heart rate and irregular rhythms; dry mouth, anxiety or fear and coldness in the fingertips and toes. High dosage may lead to tremor, the accumulation of fluid in the lungs and cerebral haemorrhage. Adrenaline in eye-drops may cause redness and smarting of the eye.

▲ warning: it should be administered with caution to patients who suffer from ischaemic heart disease or hypertension, from diabetes, or from over-activity of the thyroid gland (hyperthyroidism). There may be severe drug interactions in those already taking a number of other drugs, especially antidepressants and beta-blockers.

○ Related entries: Epipen; Eppy; Ganda; Marcain with Adrenaline; Medihaler-epi; Min-I-Jet Adrenaline; Min-I-Jet Lignocaine Hydrochloride with Adrenaline; Simplene

*adrenergic-neurone blocker

drugs act to prevent the release of NORADRENALINE from the nerves of the sympathetic nervous system, which is involved in controlling involunary functions such as blood pressure, heart rate and the activity of muscles of internal organs (eg blood vessels, intestines and secretions).

Noradrenaline is the main NEUROTRANSMITTER of the sympathetic nervous system and therefore adrenergic-neurone blocker drugs cause an overall ANTISYMPATHETIC action with a fall in blood pressure.

Consequently, the main use of such drugs is in ANTIHYPERTENSIVE therapy. However, because of quite marked side-effects, they are not drugs-of-choice in the treatment of moderate to severe high blood pressure. See: BETHANIDINE SULPHATE; BRETYLIUM TOSYLATE; DEBRISOQUINE; GUANETHIDINE MONOSULPHATE

adrenocorticotrophlc hormone (ACTH)

See CORTICOTROPHIN

Adsorbed Diphtheria and Tetanus Vaccine

(District Health Authorities) (DT/Vac/Ads) is a non-proprietary, prescription-only VACCINE preparation that combines (toxoid) vaccines for diphtheria and TETANUS VACCINE adsorbed onto a mineral carrier. It is available in a form for injection.

✚▲ side-effects/warning: see DIPHTHERIA VACCINES; TETANUS VACCINE

Adsorbed Diphtheria and Tetanus Vaccine for Adults and Adolescents

(District Health Authorities) (DT/Vac/Ads for Adults) is a non-proprietary, prescription-only VACCINE preparation that combines (toxoid) vaccines for diphtheria and TETANUS VACCINE adsorbed onto a mineral carrier. It is available in a form for injection.

✚▲ side-effects/warning: see DIPHTHERIA VACCINES; TETANUS VACCINE

Adsorbed Diphtheria Vaccine

(District Health Authorities) (Dip/Vac/Ads) is a non-proprietary, prescription-only VACCINE preparation of (toxoid) vaccines for diphtheria adsorbed onto a mineral carrier. It is available in a form for injection.

✚▲ side-effects/warning: see DIPHTHERIA VACCINES

A Adsorbed Diphtheria Vaccine for Adults

(Dip/Vac/Ads for Adults) is a non-proprietary, prescription-only VACCINE preparation of (toxoid) vaccines for diphtheria adsorbed onto a mineral carrier. It is available in a form for injection.

+▲ side-effects/warning: see DIPHTHERIA VACCINES

Adsorbed Diphtheria, Tetanus and Pertussis Vaccine

(District Health Authorities) (DTPer/Vac/Ads) is a non-proprietary, prescription-only VACCINE preparation, commonly referred to as *triple vaccine*, that combines (toxoid) vaccines for diphtheria and pertussis (whooping cough) with TETANUS VACCINE adsorbed onto a mineral carrier. It is available in a form for injection.

+▲ side-effects/warning: see DIPHTHERIA VACCINES; PERTUSSIS VACCINE; TETANUS VACCINE

Adsorbed Tetanus Vaccine

(Evans) (Tet/Vac/Ads) is a non-proprietary, prescription-only VACCINE preparation of adsorbed tetanus vaccine. It can be used for active IMMUNIZATION against tetanus and is available in a form for injection.

+▲ side-effects/warning: see ADSORBED TETANUS VACCINE

adsorbed diphtheria and tetanus vaccine

(DT/Vac/Ads) is a VACCINE used for IMMUNIZATION against diphtheria and tetanus and is adsorbed onto a mineral carrier. This combination of DIPHTHERIA VACCINE and TETANUS VACCINE is used for the primary immunization of children and as an alternative to ADSORBED DIPHTHERIA, TETANUS and PERTUSSIS VACCINE (DTPer/Vac/Ads) for children who can not be given the pertussis vaccine. It is also used as a reinforcing vaccination at school entry. It is administered by intramuscular or subcutaneous injection.

+▲ side-effects/warning: see under DIPHTHERIA VACCINE; TETANUS VACCINE

✪ Related entries: Adsorbed Diphtheria and Tetanus Vaccine; Adsorbed Diphtheria and Tetanus Vaccine for Adults and Adolescents; Diftavax

adsorbed diphtheria vaccine

(Dip/Vac/Ads) is a VACCINE used for IMMUNIZATION against diphtheria and is adsorbed onto a mineral carrier. This form of DIPHTHERIA VACCINE is administered to those who come into contact with a diphtheria case or a carrier. It is available in a form for intramuscular or subcutaneous injection.

+▲ side-effects/warning: see DIPHTHERIA VACCINE

✪ Related entries: Adsorbed Diphtheria Vaccine; Adsorbed Diphtheria Vaccine for Adults

adsorbed diphtheria, tetanus and pertussis vaccine

(DTPer/Vac/Ads) is a VACCINE used for IMMUNIZATION against diphtheria, tetanus and pertussis (whooping cough). It consists of DIPHTHERIA VACCINE, TETANUS VACCINE and PERTUSSIS VACCINE adsorbed onto a mineral carrier. This *triple vaccine* is used for the primary immunization of children and is administered by intramuscular or subcutaneous injection.

+▲ side-effects/warning: see DIPHTHERIA VACCINE; PERTUSSIS VACCINE; TETANUS VACCINE

✪ Related entries: Adsorbed Diphtheria, Tetanus and Pertussis Vaccine; Trivac-AD

adsorbed tetanus vaccine

(Tet/Vac/Ads) is a VACCINE used for IMMUNIZATION against tetanus and is adsorbed onto a mineral carrier. This

A

form of TETANUS VACCINE is used where a combined vaccine such as *triple vaccine* has not been given, or as a booster in later life. Administration is by intramuscular or subcutaneous injection.

○ **Related entries: Adsorbed Tetanus Vaccine**

AcroBec

(3M Health Care) is a proprietary, prescription-only preparation of the CORTICOSTEROID and ANTI-ASTHMATIC drug beclomethasone dipropionate. It can be used to prevent asthmatic attacks and is available in aerosols for inhalation as *AeroBec 50 Autohaler* and *AeroBec 100 Autohaler*.

✚▲ side-effects/warning: see BECLOMETHASONE DIPROPIONATE

AeroBec Forte

(3M Health Care) is a proprietary, prescription-only preparation of the CORTICOSTEROID and ANTI-ASTHMATIC drug beclomethasone dipropionate. It can be used to prevent asthmatic attacks and is available in an aerosol for inhalation.

✚▲ side-effects/warning: see BECLOMETHASONE DIPROPIONATE

Aerocrom

(Fisons) is a proprietary, prescription-only COMPOUND PREPARATION of the ANTI-ALLERGIC drug sodium cromoglycate and the BETA-RECEPTOR STIMULANT salbutamol (as salbutamol sulphate), which is used as an ANTI-ASTHMATIC. It is important that it is used for the prevention (prophylaxis) of asthma symptoms rather than the acute treatment of asthma attacks. It is available as an aerosol.

✚▲ side-effects/warning: see SALBUTAMOL; SODIUM CROMOGLYCATE

Aerolin Autohaler

(3M Health Care) is a proprietary, prescription-only preparation of the BETA-RECEPTOR STIMULANT salbutamol (as salbutamol sulphate). It can be used as a

BRONCHODILATOR in reversible obstructive airways disease, as an ANTI-ASTHMATIC treatment in severe acute asthma, or for the alleviation of symptoms of chronic bronchitis and emphysema. It is available as a breath-actuated metered aerosol inhalant.

✚▲ side-effects/warning: see SALBUTAMOL

Afrazine

(Schering-Plough) is a proprietary, non-prescription preparation of the NASAL DECONGESTANT drug oxymetazoline hydrochloride. It can be used for the relief of nasal congestion associated with a wide variety of upper respiratory tract disorders. It is available as a nasal spray and is not normally given to children under five years, except on medical advice.

✚▲ side-effects/warning: see OXYMETAZOLINE HYDROCHLORIDE

Agarol

(Warner Wellcome) is a proprietary, non-prescription COMPOUND PREPARATION of the (*stimulant*) LAXATIVE phenolphthalein and the (*faecal softener*) laxative liquid paraffin. It can be used to relieve temporary constipation and is available as an emulsion. It is not normally given to children under five years, except on medical advice.

✚▲ side-effects/warning: see LIQUID PARAFFIN; PHENOLPHTHALEIN

Akineton

(Knoll) is a proprietary, prescription-only preparation of the ANTICHOLINERGIC drug biperiden. It can be used in the treatment of parkinsonism and is available as tablets and in a form for injection.

✚▲ side-effects/warning: see BIPERIDEN

Aknemin

(Merck) is a proprietary, prescription-only preparation of the ANTIBACTERIAL and (TETRACYCLINE) ANTIBIOTIC drug minocycline. It can be used to treat a wide range of infections and is available as capsules.

✚▲ side-effects/warning: see MINOCYCLINE

albendazole

is an ANTHELMINTIC drug. It is used to provide cover during surgery for the removal of cysts caused by the tapeworm *Echinococcus* and as treatment when surgery is not possible. Administration is oral in the form of tablets.

✚ side-effects: there may be headache, dizziness, gastrointestinal disturbances, hair loss, rash and fever. Blood disorders have been reported.

▲ warning: it is not to be given to pregnant women and administer with care to those who are breast-feeding. Blood and liver function tests are advisable.

○ Related entry: Eskazole

alclometasone dipropionate

is a CORTICOSTEROID with ANTI-INFLAMMATORY properties. It is used in the treatment of inflammatory skin disorders, particularly eczema. Administration is by topical application as a cream or an ointment.

✚▲ side-effects/warning: see under HYDROCORTISONE

○ Related entry: Modrasone

Alcobon

(Roche) is a proprietary, prescription-only preparation of the ANTIFUNGAL drug flucytosine. It can be used to treat systemic infections by yeasts (eg candidiasis) and it is available in a form for infusion.

✚▲ side-effects/warning: see FLUCYTOSINE

Alcoderm

(Novex) is a proprietary, non-prescription preparation of liquid paraffin and a number of other EMOLLIENT agents. It can be used for dry or itchy skin and is available as a lotion.

✚▲ side-effects/warning: see LIQUID PARAFFIN

alcohol

is the name of a class of compounds that are derived from hydrocarbons. The best-known alcohol is ethyl alcohol, or ethanol. Although not normally used as a medicine, the actions of ethanol are similar to a number of drugs that depress the central nervous system and it is therefore similar to SEDATIVES or HYPNOTICS. The apparent stimulation experienced by many users is usually due to the loss of social inhibitions. Although it *can* be used as a hypnotic drug, it can also cause rebound wakefulness during the night.

Ethanol has quite a strong DIURETIC action, which can also lead to a disrupted night's sleep. There is also a marked dilation of blood vessels (particularly of the face) which can lead to a profound and potentially dangerous loss of body heat in cold weather. An equally dangerous and sometimes lethal side-effect, is that vomiting is stimulated at higher doses and a protective reflex is inhibited which can lead to the inhalation of vomit. For medical purposes, a strong solution of ethanol can be used as an ANTISEPTIC (particularly to prepare skin before injection) or as a preservative.

Aldactide 25

(Searle) is a proprietary, prescription-only COMPOUND PREPARATION of the (*aldosterone-antagonist* and *potassium-sparing*) DIURETIC drug spironolactone and the (THIAZIDE-type) diuretic drug hydroflumethiazide (a combination called co-flumactone 25/25). It can be used for congestive HEART FAILURE TREATMENT and is available as tablets.

✚▲ side-effects/warning: see HYDROFLUMETHIAZIDE; SPIRONOLACTONE

Aldactide 50

(Searle) is a proprietary, prescription-only COMPOUND PREPARATION the (*aldosterone-antagonist* and *potassium-sparing*) DIURETIC drug spironolactone and the (THIAZIDE-type) diuretic drug hydroflumethiazide (a combination called co-flumactone 50/50). It can be used for congestive HEART FAILURE TREATMENT and is available as tablets.

+▲ side-effects/warning: see HYDROFLUMETHIAZIDE; SPIRONOLACTONE

Aldactone

(Searle) is a proprietary, prescription-only preparation of the (*aldosterone antagonist* and *potassium-sparing*) DIURETIC drug spironolactone, which can be used in conjunction with other types of diuretic, such as the THIAZIDES, that cause loss of potassium. It can be used to treat oedema associated with aldosteronism, for congestive HEART FAILURE TREATMENT, kidney disease and fluid retention and ascites caused by cirrhosis of the liver. It is available as tablets.

+▲ side-effects/warning: see SPIRONOLACTONE

aldesleukin

interleukin-2, is an ANTICANCER drug, which is mainly used for treating metastatic renal cell carcinoma. Administration is by injection.

+▲ side-effects/warning: it has widespread toxicity, including oedema (accumulation of fluid in the tissues) and hypotension and adverse actions on the bone marrow, kidneys, liver, thyroid gland and central nervous system.

✿ Related entry: Proleukin

Aldomet

(Merck, Sharp & Dohme) is a proprietary, prescription-only preparation of the ANTISYMPATHETIC drug methyldopa. It can be used in ANTIHYPERTENSIVE treatment and is available as tablets, an oral suspension and in a form for injection (as methyldopate hydrochloride).

+▲ side-effects/warning: see METHYLDOPA

Alexan

(Pfizer) is is a proprietary, prescription-only preparation of the (CYTOTOXIC)

ANTICANCER drug cytarabine. It can be used in the treatment of acute leukaemia and is available in a form for injection.

+▲ side-effects/warning: see CYTARABINE

Alexan 100

(Pfizer) is a proprietary, prescription-only preparation of the (CYTOTOXIC) ANTICANCER drug cytarabine. It can be used in the treatment of acute leukaemia and is available in a form for injection.

+▲ side-effects/warning: see CYTARABINE

alexitol sodium

is an aluminium-containing salt that is used as an ANTACID for the relief of hyperacidity, dyspepsia and indigestion. It is available as tablets.

✿ Related entries: Actal Tablets; Magnatol

alfacalcidol

(1α-hydroxycholecalciferol) is a synthesized form of CALCIFEROL (VITAMIN D). It is used to make up vitamin D deficiency, particularly in the treatment of types of hypoparathyroidism and rickets. Administration is oral in the form of capsules or solution.

✿ Related entry: One-Alpha

alfentanil

is an (OPIOID) NARCOTIC ANALGESIC drug, which is used for short surgical operations, outpatient surgery, in combination to enhance the effect of GENERAL ANAESTHETICS and to suppress breathing in patients receiving artificial ventilation. Administration is by intravenous infusion. Its proprietary form is on the Controlled Drugs List.

+▲ side-effect/warning: see under OPIOID

✿ Related entry: RAPIFEN

alfuzosin

is an ALPHA-ADRENOCEPTOR BLOCKER that is used to treat urinary retention because of its SMOOTH MUSCLE RELAXANT properties (for example, in benign prostatic

A

hyperplasia). Administration is oral in the form of tablets.

✚ side-effects: postural hypotension (fall in blood pressure on standing); dizziness; sedation and lack of energy, headache, nausea, urinary frequency, sweating; dry mouth and nasal congestion; failure to ejaculate; tachycardia and palpitations. There may be depression and drowsiness.

▲ warning: initially, it may cause marked postural hypotension, so the patient should lie down, or doses should be given on retiring to bed. Administer with caution to patients with certain kidney or liver disorders, or in the elderly. It may cause drowsiness, so the ability to drive or operate machinery may be impaired.

○ Related entry: Xatral

Algesal

(Duphar) is a proprietary, non-prescription preparation of diethylamine salicylate, which has a COUNTER-IRRITANT, or RUBEFACIENT, action. It can be applied to the skin for the symptomatic relief of musculoskeletal rheumatic conditions and is available as a cream.

✚▲ side-effects/warning: see DIETHYLAMINE SALICYLATE

Algicon

(Rhône-Poulenc Rorer) is a proprietary, non-prescription COMPOUND PREPARATION of the ANTACID aluminium hydroxide combined with magnesium carbonate, potassium bicarbonate, magnesium alginate (a protectant in reflux oesophagitis) and sucrose (as a sweetener). It can be used for the symptomatic relief of heartburn associated with gastric reflux, reflux oesophagitis, hiatus hernia and hyperacidity (it can be used to relieve these symptoms in pregnancy). It is available as tablets and a suspension.

✚▲ side-effects/warning: see ALUMINIUM HYDROXIDE; MAGNESIUM CARBONATE

alginic acid

usually in the form of alginate (magnesium alginate or sodium alginate), is extracted from seaweed. It has a viscous, sticky consistency and is used as a DEMULCENT in certain ANTACID preparations to protect against reflux oesophagitis (regurgitation of acid and enzymes into the oesophagus). It is also incorporated in some mouthwashes or gargles to protect and soothe mucous membranes within the mouth.

○ Related entries: Algitec; Bisodol Heartburn; Gastrocote; Gastron; Gaviscon 250; Gaviscon Liquid; Infant Gaviscon Liquid; Topal

Algipan Rub

(Whitehall) is a proprietary, non-prescription COMPOUND PREPARATION of capsicum oleoresin, methyl nicotinate and glycol salicylate, which all have COUNTER-IRRITANT, or RUBEFACIENT, actions. It can be applied to the skin for the symptomatic relief of muscle pain and stiffness in backache, lumbago, sciatica and fibrosis rheumatic pain. It is available as a cream.

✚▲ side-effects/warning: see CAPSICUM OLEORESIN; GLYCOL SALICYLATE; METHYL NICOTINATE

Algipan Spray

(Whitehall) is a proprietary, non-prescription COMPOUND PREPARATION of ethyl nicotinate and glycol salicylate, which have COUNTER-IRRITANT, or RUBEFACIENT, actions. It can be applied to the skin for the symptomatic relief of muscle pain and stiffness in backache, lumbago, sciatica and fibrosis rheumatic pain. It is available as a spray and is not normally used for children under six years, except on medical advice.

✚▲ side-effects/warning: see GLYCOL SALICYLATE; METHYL NICOTINATE

Algitec

(SmithKline Beecham) is a proprietary COMPOUND PREPARATION of the H_2-

ANTAGONIST drug cimetidine and the DEMULCENT alginic acid. It is usually only available on prescription, but it can be obtained without a prescription in a limited amount and for short-term use only. It is used as an ULCER-HEALING DRUG for benign peptic ulcers (in the stomach or duodenum), gastro-oesophageal reflux, dyspepsia and associated conditions. It is available as chewable tablets (*Chewtab*) and a suspension.

✚▲ side-effects/warning: see ALGINIC ACID; CIMETIDINE

alimemazine tartrate
See TRIMEPRAZINE TARTRATE

Alimix
(Cilag) is a proprietary, prescription-only preparation of the MOTILITY STIMULANT drug cisapride. It can be used to stimulate the stomach and intestine in a number of conditions and is available as tablets.

✚▲ side-effects/warning: see CISAPRIDE

*alkaloid
is a chemical term applied to a group of compounds that are used as drugs. The majority of alkaloids were originally extracted from plants and are chemically heterocyclic, often complex, organic compounds with basic (alkali) properties and in medicine they are usually administered in the form of their salts. Examples still in medical use include the BELLADONNA ALKALOIDS from *Atropa belladonna* plant and related species (eg ATROPINE SULPHATE and HYOSCINE HYDROBROMIDE); the alkaloids of opium from the poppy *Papaver somniferum* (eg CODEINE PHOSPHATE, MORPHINE SULPHATE and PAPAVERINE); ERGOT ALKALOIDS (eg ERGOMETRINE MALEATE and ERGOTAMINE TARTRATE); the CINCHONA ALKALOIDS QUINIDINE and QUININE from the bark of the cinchona tree; the VINCA ALKALOIDS (eg VINBLASTINE SULPHATE, VINCRISTINE SULPHATE and VINDESINE SULPHATE); EPHEDRINE HYDROCHLORIDE from ancient Chinese plants of the *Ephedra* species; NICOTINE from *Nicotiana tabacum*; TUBOCURARINE CHLORIDE, originally a South American arrow-poison from *Chondrodendron tomentosum* and other species; PILOCARPINE from a South American *Pilocarpus* shrub; and IPECACUANHA, which contains emetine and cephaeline from ipecac ('Brazil root').

Alka-Seltzer Original
(Bayer) is a proprietary, non-prescription COMPOUND PREPARATION of the (NSAID) NON-NARCOTIC ANALGESIC and ANTIRHEUMATIC drug aspirin, citric acid and the ANTACID sodium bicarbonate. It can be used for general aches and pains and for headache with upset stomach. It is available as effervescent tablets and also as *Alka-Seltzer Lemon Flavour*. It is not normally given to children under 12 years, except on medical advice.

✚▲ side-effects/warning: see ASPIRIN; SODIUM BICARBONATE

Alkeran
(Wellcome) is a proprietary, prescription-only preparation of the (CYTOTOXIC) ANTICANCER drug melphalan. It can be used in the treatment of myelomatosis and is available as tablets and in a form for injection.

✚▲ side-effects/warning: see MELPHALAN

Allegron
(Dista) is a proprietary, prescription-only preparation of the (TRICYCLIC) ANTIDEPRESSANT drug nortriptyline hydochloride. It can be used to treat depressive illness and also to stop children bed-wetting at night. It is available as tablets.

✚▲ side-effects/warning: see NORTRIPTYLINE HYDROCHLORIDE

Aller-eze
(Intercare Products) is a proprietary, non-prescription preparation of the ANTIHISTAMINE drug clemastine (as

A

hydrogen fumarate). It can be used to treat the symptoms of allergic disorders such as hay fever and urticaria. It is available as tablets and is not normally given to children under three years, except on medical advice.

✚▲ side-effects/warning: see CLEMASTINE

Aller-eze Plus

(Intercare Products) is a proprietary, non-prescription COMPOUND PREPARATION of the ANTIHISTAMINE drug clemastine (as hydrogen fumarate) and the SYMPATHOMIMETIC and DECONGESTANT drug phenylpropanolamine. It can be used to treat the symptoms of allergic disorders such as hay fever, urticaria and nasal congestion. It is available as tablets and is not normaly given to children, except on medical advice.

✚▲ side-effects/warning: see CLEMASTINE; PHENYLPROPANOLAMINE HYDROCHLORIDE

allopurinol

is an ENZYME INHIBITOR. It is a XANTHINE OXIDASE INHIBITOR that inhibits the action of the enzyme xanthine oxidase, which produces uric acid and so can be used to treat excess uric acid in the blood (hyperuricaemia). It is used to prevent attacks of gout and to treat uric acid and calcium oxalate stones in the urinary tract (renal stones). Administration is oral in the form of tablets.

✚ side-effects: a rash (which may mean that treatment should be stopped), gastrointestinal disorders, fever, skin reactions; rarely, malaise, headache, vertigo, drowsiness, hypertension, taste disturbance, xanthine deposits in muscle, hair loss, liver toxicity and peripheral nerve disorders.

▲ warning: it is not be used in patients with acute gout; concurrent treatment is required with other drugs (eg colchicine and a NSAID, but not aspirin) and an adequate fluid intake must be maintained.

⊕ Related entries: Caplenal; Cosuric; Hamarin; Rimapurinol; Xanthomax; Zyloric

Almevax

(Evans) is a proprietary, prescription-only VACCINE preparation for the prevention of rubella (German measles). It is available in a form for injection.

✚▲ side-effects/warning: see RUBELLA VACCINE

Almodan

(Berk) is a proprietary, prescription-only preparation of the broad-spectrum ANTIBACTERIAL and (PENICILLIN) ANTIBIOTIC drug amoxycillin. It can be used to treat systemic bacterial infections, infections of the upper respiratory tract, of the ear, nose and throat and of the urinogenital tracts. It is available as capsules and as an oral suspension.

✚▲ side-effects/warning: see AMOXYCILLIN

aloin

is a *stimulant* LAXATIVE that is incorporated into some proprietary preparations for the relief of constipation.

✚▲ side-effects/warning: see under SENNA

⊕ Related entries: Alophen Pills; Beecham Pills

Alophen Pills

(Warner Wellcome) is a proprietary, non-prescription COMPOUND PREPARATION of the (*stimulant*) LAXATIVES aloin and phenolphthalein. It can be used to relieve constipation and is available as tablets. It is not normally given to children, except on medical advice.

✚▲ side-effects/warning: see ALOIN; PHENOLPHTHALEIN

aloxiprin

is a (NSAID) NON-NARCOTIC ANALGESIC and ANTIRHEUMATIC drug that is incorporated into some proprietary COMPOUND ANALGESIC preparations.

⊕ Related entries: Askit Capsules; Askit Powders

Alpha VIII

(Alpha) is a proprietary, prescription-only

preparation of dried human factor VIII fraction, which acts as a HAEMOSTATIC drug to reduce or stop bleeding. It can be used in the treatment of disorders in which bleeding is prolonged and potentially dangerous (mainly haemophilia A). It is available in a form for infusion or injection.
✚▲ side-effects/warning: see
FACTOR VIII FRACTION, DRIED

Alpha Keri Bath

(Bristol-Myers) is a proprietary, non-prescription COMPOUND PREPARATION of liquid paraffin and lanolin oils, which have EMOLLIENT properties. It can be used for dry or itchy skin and is available as a bath oil.
✚▲ side-effects/warning: see
LIQUID PARAFFIN; LANOLIN

alpha tocopheryl acetate

is a form of vitamin E (TOCOPHEROL). It is used to treat deficiency due to malabsorption, such as in abetalipoproteinaemia in young children with congenital cholestasis or cystic fibrosis and as a vitamin supplement. Administration is oral in the form of an oral suspension.
✚ side-effects: diarrhoea, abdominal pain.
▲ warning: use with care if there is a predisposition to thrombosis (clot formation).
✪ Related entry: Vitamin E Suspension

alpha-adrenoceptor antagonists

See ALPHA-ADRENOCEPTOR BLOCKERS

*alpha-adrenoceptor blockers

(alpha-blockers; alpha-adrenoceptor antagonists) are drugs that inhibit some actions of the alpha receptor-stimulant drugs, such as the HORMONE ADRENALINE (released from the adrenal gland) and the NEUROTRANSMITTER NORADRENALINE (which is released from sympathetic nerves). They also inhibit some actions of

the SYMPATHOMIMETIC drugs that are used therapeutically (many are chemically catecholamines). The alpha-adrenoceptor blocking drugs work by blocking the receptor sites called alpha-adrenoceptors, thereby preventing the action of adrenaline-like agents. A major use of alpha-blockers is in ANTIHYPERTENSIVE treatment, where they lower blood pressure by preventing VASOCONSTRICTOR actions of noradrenaline and adrenaline (including in the treatment of phaeochromocytoma). They are also used to treat urinary retention in benign prostatic hyperplasia (through an action on the blood circulation within the prostate). See: INDORAMIN; PHENTOLAMINE MESYLATE; PHENOXYBENZAMINE; PRAZOSIN HYDROCHLORIDE; TERAZOSIN

alpha-blockers

See ALPHA-ADRENOCEPTOR BLOCKERS

Alphaderm

(Procter & Gamble) is a proprietary, prescription-only COMPOUND PREPARATION of the CORTICOSTEROID and ANTI-INFLAMMATORY drug hydrocortisone and the HYDRATING AGENT urea. It can be used to treat mild inflammation of the skin such as eczema and is available as a cream for topical application.
✚▲ side-effects/warning: see
HYDROCORTISONE; UREA

Alphanine

(Alpha) is a proprietary, prescription-only preparation of factor IX fraction, dried, which is prepared from human blood plasma. It can be used in treating patients with a deficiency in factor IX (haemophilia B) and is available in a form for infusion.
✚▲ side-effects/warning: see
FACTOR IX FRACTION, DRIED

Alphavase

(Ashbourne) is a proprietary, prescription-only preparation of the ALPHA-ADRENOCEPTOR BLOCKER prazosin hydrochloride. It can be used in ANTIHYPERTENSIVE treatment and is available as tablets.

✚▲ side-effects/warning: see PRAZOSIN HYDROCHLORIDE

Alphosyl

(Stafford-Miller) is a proprietary, non-prescription preparation of coal tar (with allantoin). It can be used to treat eczema and psoriasis and is available as a cream and a lotion.

✚▲ side-effects/warning: see COAL TAR

Alphosyl 2 in 1 Shampoo

(Stafford-Miller) is a proprietary, non-prescription preparation of coal tar. It can be used for the treatment of psoriasis, seborrhoeic dermatitis, scaling, dandruff and itching.

✚▲ side-effects/warning: see COAL TAR

Alphosyl HC

(Stafford-Miller) is a proprietary, prescription-only COMPOUND PREPARATION of the CORTICOSTEROID and ANTI-INFLAMMATORY drug hydrocortisone and coal tar (with allantoin). It can be used to treat eczema and psoriasis and is available as a cream.

✚▲ side-effects/warning: see COAL TAR; HYDROCORTISONE

alprazolam

is a BENZODIAZEPINE drug, which is used as an ANXIOLYTIC drug in the short-term treatment of anxiety. Administration is oral in the form of tablets.

✚▲ side-effects/warning: see under BENZODIAZEPINE

✪ Related entry: Xanax

alprostadil

is a PROSTAGLANDIN (PGE_1), which is used to maintain babies born with congenital heart defects (to maintain patency of ductus arteriosus), while emergency preparations are being made for corrective surgery and intensive care;

administration is by infusion. In men, it is used to treat erectile dysfunction when it is given by intracavernosal injection into the penis.

✚ side-effects: in babies, breathing difficulties (particularly if small); fever, flushing, diarrhoea, blood-clotting problems, convulsions. In men, testicular pain during erection (especially where there is deformation), haematoma at injection site and a variety of local actions. Other effects have been reported on the cardiovascular system, as well as dizziness and headache.

▲ warning: in babies, monitoring of arterial pressure is essential; a close watch must also be kept for haemorrhage, hypotension and slow or fast heart rate, high temperature and flushing. Prolonged use may cause bone deformity and damage to the pulmonary artery. It should not be administered to babies whose lungs are imperfectly expanded (hyaline membrane disease). In men, it should not be given when there is a predisposition to prolonged erection (myeloma, sickle-cell anaemia, leukaemia); it should not be given to men who have deformed penises.

✪ Related entries: Caverject; Prostin VR

Alrheumat

(Bayer) is a proprietary, prescription-only preparation of the (NSAID) NON-NARCOTIC ANALGESIC and ANTIRHEUMATIC drug ketoprofen. It can be used to relieve arthritic and rheumatic pain and to treat other musculoskeletal disorders. It is available as capsules.

✚▲ side-effects/warning: see KETOPROFEN

Altacite Plus

(Roussel) is a proprietary, non-prescription COMPOUND PREPARATION of the ANTACID hydrotalcite and the ANTIFOAMING AGENT dimethicone. It can be used for the relief of hyperacidity, flatulence, gastritis and dyspepsia and is available as an oral suspension.

✚▲ side-effects/warning: see DIMETHICONE; HYDROTALCITE

Altacite Suspension

(Roussel) is a proprietary, non-prescription preparation of the ANTACID hydrotalcite. It can be used for the relief of hyperacidity, gastritis and dyspepsia and is available as an oral suspension.

✚▲ side-effects/warning: see HYDROTALCITE

Altacite Tablets

(Roussel) is a proprietary, non-prescription preparation of the ANTACID hydrotalcite. It can be used for the relief of hyperacidity, gastritis and dyspepsia and is available as chewable tablets.

✚▲ side-effects/warning: see HYDROTALCITE

alteplase

(tissue-type plasminogen activator; rt-PA) is used therapeutically as a FIBRINOLYTIC drug, because it has the property of breaking up blood clots. It is used in serious conditions such as myocardial infarction (damage to heart muscle, usually after a heart attack).
Administration is by injection or infusion.
✚ side-effects: nausea, vomiting and bleeding. There may be allergic reaction, such as a rash and a high temperature.
▲ warning: it should not be administered to patients with disorders of coagulation, or after recent surgery; who are liable to bleed (vaginal bleeding, peptic ulceration, recent trauma, or surgery); with acute pancreatitis, or oesophageal varices. Administer with caution to patients who are pregnant.
✪ Related entry: Actilyse

Alu-Cap

(3M Health Care) is a proprietary, non-prescription preparation of the ANTACID aluminium hydroxide, for the relief of hyperacidity and dyspepsia It is available as capsules. It is not normally given to children, except on medical advice.
✚▲ side-effects/warning: see ALUMINIUM HYDROXIDE

Aludrox Liquid

(Charwell Healthcare) is a proprietary, non-prescription preparation of the ANTACID aluminium hydroxide. It can be used for the relief of hyperacidity and dyspepsia and is available as a liquid gel. It is not normally given to children under six years, except on medical advice.
✚▲ side-effects/warning: see ALUMINIUM HYDROXIDE

Aludrox Tablets

(Charwell Healthcare) is a proprietary, non-prescription COMPOUND PREPARATION of the ANTACIDS aluminium hydroxide and magnesium hydroxide. It can be used for the relief of hyperacidity and dyspepsia and is available as tablets. It is not normally given to children under six years, except on medical advice.
✚▲ side-effects/warning: see ALUMINIUM HYDROXIDE; MAGNESIUM CARBONATE

aluminium acetate

is an ASTRINGENT that is used primarily to clean sites of infection and inflammation, particularly weeping or suppurating wounds or sores, eczema and infections of the outer ear. Administration is in the form of a lotion or as ear-drops.

aluminium chloride

is a powerful ANTIPERSPIRANT with ASTRINGENT properties. It can be used to treat hyperhidrosis (excessive sweating). Administration is topical in the form of a solution, a roll-on applicator, or a spray.
✚ side-effects: skin irritation
▲ warning: keep away from the eyes; do not shave the armpits or use hair-removing creams for 12 hours after application.
✪ Related entries: Anhydrol Forte; Driclor

aluminium hydroxide

is an ANTACID, which, because it is relatively insoluble in water, has a long duration of action when retained in the stomach. It can be used to for the symptomatic relief of dyspepsia, hyperacidity, gastritis, peptic ulcers and

A oesophageal reflux (regurgitation of acid and enzymes into the oesophagus). It can also be used to treat elevated levels of phosphates in the blood (hyperphosphataemia). Administration is oral in the form of tablets for chewing or sucking, as a gel, or in a liquid.

▲ warning: it should not be administered to patients with hypophosphataemia (low blood phosphates); and use with caution in those with porphyria.

❍ Related entries: Algicon; Alu-Caps; Aludrox Liquid; Aludrox Tablets; Asilone Liquid; Asilone Suspension; Asilone Tablets; Caved-S; Dijex; Dijex Tablets; Diovol; Gastrocote; Gastron; Gaviscon 250; Kolanticon Gel; Maalox Plus Suspension; Maalox Plus Tablets; Maalox Suspension; Maalox TC Suspension; Maclean Indigestion Tablets; Morland Tablets; Mucaine; Mucogel Suspension; Topal

Alupent

(Boehringer Ingelheim) is a proprietary, prescription-only preparation of the BETA-RECEPTOR STIMULANT drug orciprenaline sulphate. It can be used as a BRONCHODILATOR in reversible obstructive airways disease, as an ANTI-ASTHMATIC treatment in severe acute asthma, or for the alleviation of symptoms of chronic bronchitis and emphysema. It is available as tablets, as an aerosol spray (*Alupent Aerosol*), or as a sugar-free syrup (*Alupent Syrup*).

✚▲ side-effects/warning: see ORCIPRENALINE SULPHATE

Alvercol

(Norgine) is a proprietary, non-prescription COMPOUND PREPARATION of the ANTISPASMODIC drug alverine citrate and the (*bulking agent*) LAXATIVE sterculia. It can be used to treat irritable bowel syndrome and is available as oral granules.

✚▲ side-effects/warning: see ALVERINE CITRATE; STERCULIA

alverine citrate

is an ANTISPASMODIC drug. It is used to treat spasm in the gastrointestinal tract and in dysmenorrhoea (menstrual discomfort). It is available as capsules and soluble granules.

✚ warning: it should not be administered to patients who suffer from paralytic ileus; and administer with care to pregnant women.

❍ Related entries: Alvercol; Spasmonal

amantadine hydrochloride

is a prescription-only ANTIPARKINSONISM drug, but is not used to treat the parkinsonian symptoms induced by drugs. It also has some ANTIVIRAL activity and has been used orally to prevent infection with the influenza A_2 virus (but not other influenza viruses) and in the treatment of herpes zoster (shingles). Administration is oral as capsules or a dilute syrup.

✚ side-effects: restlessness and inability to concentrate; there may also be dizziness and insomnia, gastrointestinal disturbances, oedema, blood disorders, skin discolouration, anorexia, hallucinations and blurred vision.

▲ warning: it should not be administered to patients who suffer from gastric ulcers or from epilepsy. Administer with caution to patients who suffer from certain heart, liver, or kidney disorders, psychosis, or long-term eczema; who are pregnant or breast-feeding; who are in a state of confusion; or who are elderly. Withdrawal of treatment in Parkinson's disease must be gradual. It may effect performance of skilled tasks such as driving.

❍ Related entry: Symmetrel

Ambaxin

(Upjohn) is a proprietary, prescription-only preparation of the broad-spectrum ANTIBACTERIAL and (PENICILLIN) ANTIBIOTIC drug bacampicillin hydrochloride.

It can be used to treat systemic bacterial infections, infections of the upper respiratory tract, of the ear, nose and throat and of the urinogenital tracts. It is available as tablets.

A

+▲ side-effects/warning: see
BACAMPICILLIN HYDROCHLORIDE

AmBisome

(Vestar) is a proprietary, prescription-only
preparation of the ANTIFUNGAL and
ANTIBIOTIC drug amphotericin, which is in
an unusual lipid formulation
(encapsulated in liposomes) that is
intended to minimize toxicity (particularly
to the kidney), so that it can be used for
severe systemic or deep-seated fungal
infections. It is available in a form for
infusion.
+▲ side-effects/warning: see AMPHOTERICIN

amethocaine hydrochloride

is a LOCAL ANAESTHETIC drug. It is used to
treat localized pain and irritation and in
ophthalmic treaments. Administration is
by topical application as a throat spray or
eye-drops.
+▲ side-effects/warning: see under
LIGNOCAINE HYDROCHLORIDE. Hypersensitivity
reactions have been reported. It is absorbed
rapidly through mucous membranes and so
should not be applied to inflamed,
traumatized, or highly vascular surfaces.
○ Related entries: Eludril Spray;
Minims Amethocaine Hydrochloride

Amfipen

(Yamanouchi) is a proprietary,
prescription-only preparation of the
broad-spectrum ANTIBACTERIAL and
(PENICILLIN) ANTIBIOTIC drug ampicillin. It
can be used to treat systemic bacterial
infections, infections of the upper
respiratory tract, of the ear, nose and
throat and of the urinogenital tracts. It is
available as capsules and an oral
suspension.
+▲ side-effects/warning: see AMPICILLIN

amikacin

is a broad-spectrum ANTIBACTERIAL and
(AMINOGLYCOSIDE) ANTIBIOTIC drug.
Although it does have activity against
Gram-positive bacteria, it is used primarily

against serious infections caused by Gram-
negative bacteria that prove to be resistant
to the more widely used aminoglycoside
GENTAMICIN. Administration is by injection
or infusion.
+▲ side-effects/warning: see under
GENTAMICIN
○ Related entry: Amikin

Amikin

(Bristol-Myers) is a proprietary,
prescription-only preparation of the
ANTIBACTERIAL and (AMINOGLYCOSIDE)
ANTIBIOTIC drug amikacin (as sulphate). It
can be used to treat several serious
bacterial infections, particularly those that
prove to be resistant to the more widely
used aminoglycoside GENTAMICIN. It is
available in forms for injection and
infusion.
+▲ side-effects/warning: see AMIKACIN

Amil-Co

(Baker Norton) is a proprietary,
prescription-only COMPOUND PREPARATION
of the (*potassium-sparing*) DIURETIC
drug amiloride hydrochloride and the
(THIAZIDE) diuretic drug
hydrochlorothiazide (a combination
called co-amilozide 5/50). It can be used
to treat oedema and as an
ANTIHYPERTENSIVE treatment. It is available
as tablets.
+▲ side-effects/warning: see AMILORIDE
HYDROCHLORIDE; HYDROCHLOROTHIAZIDE

amiloride hydrochloride

is a weak, *potassium-sparing* DIURETIC
drug that retains potassium in the body
and is therefore used as an alternative to,
or commonly in combination with, other
diuretics such as the THIAZIDES and *loop
diuretics* (which normally cause a loss of
potassium from the body). It can be used
to treat oedema (accumulation of fluid in
the tissues), ascites in liver cirrhosis (fluid
in the abdomen), as an ANTIHYPERTENSIVE
treatment (in combination with other
drugs such as the BETA-BLOCKERS) and in

53

A

congestive HEART FAILURE TREATMENT. Administration is oral as tablets or a solution.

✚ side-effects: gastrointestinal upsets, skin rashes, dry mouth, confusion (particularly in the elderly), postural hypotension (fall in blood pressure on standing); raised blood potassium and lowered blood sodium.

▲ warning: it should not be administered to patients who have high blood potassium levels, who are taking potassium supplements, or who have kidney failure. Administer with care to patients who are pregnant, have diabetes, or are elderly.

○ Related entries: Amil-Co; Amilospare; Berkamil; Delvas Fru-Co; Frumil; Frumil Forte; Frumil LS; Kalten; Lasoride; Midamor; Moduret-25; Moducren; Moduretic; Navispare

Amilospare

(Ashbourne) is a proprietary, prescription-only preparation of the (*potassium-sparing*) DIURETIC drug amiloride hydrochloride. It can be used to treat oedema, ascites in cirrhosis of the liver, congestive heart failure (in conjunction with other diuretics) and as an ANTIHYPERTENSIVE. It is available as tablets.

✚▲ side-effects/warning: see AMILORIDE HYDROCHLORIDE

aminacrine hydrochloride

is an ANTISEPTIC agent incorporated into preparations that are used to treat mouth ulcers.

○ Related entries: Bonjela Antiseptic Pain-Relieving Pastilles

aminobenzoic acid

is an unusual drug, sometimes classed as one of the B complex vitamins. It is also used as a SUNSCREEN because it helps to protect the skin from ultraviolet radiation. For this reason, aminobenzoic acid is present in many suntan lotions and also in some barrier preparations to ward off the harmful effects of repeated radiotherapy.

Administration is topical in the form of creams and lotions.

▲ warning: protection is temporary, so creams and lotions must be reapplied every so often. It has been suggested that some preparations containing aminobenzoates may cause photosensitivity reactions.

○ Related entries: Spectraban Lotion; Spectraban Ultra; Sun E45

aminoglutethimide

is a drug used to treat breast cancer. It is thought to work as an indirect HORMONE ANTAGONIST, by inhibiting the conversion of the sex hormone ANDROGEN to the sex hormone OESTROGEN. It may also be used to treat Cushing's syndrome caused by cancer of the adrenal gland, which results in the excessive release of CORTICOSTEROID hormones in the body, by inhibiting the formation of corticosteroids. Administration is oral in the form of tablets.

✚ side-effects: there may be drowsiness, lethargy, unsteadiness, rashes and allergic manifestations, nausea and diarrhoea, thyroid gland disturbances and blood disorders.

▲ warning: It should not be given to pregnant or breast-feeding women; administer with caution to patients with porphyria.

○ Related entry: Orimeten

*aminoglycoside

drugs are a class of ANTIBIOTICS with ANTIBACTERIAL activity and are all *bactericidal* (that is, they kill bacteria rather than merely inhibiting their growth). Although they can be used against some Gram-positive bacteria, they are used primarily to treat serious infections caused by Gram-negative bacteria.

Aminoglycosides are not absorbed from the gut (unless there is damage), so they must be administered by injection, or by topical application in the case of the toxic members (eg NEOMYCIN SULPHATE). However, they all share a number of common toxic properties (i.e. side-effects) and, because they are excreted via the kidneys, a potentially dangerous accumulation can occur in patients with impaired kidney function. Toxic effects are related to the dose and one of the the most serious is ototoxicity (impaired hearing and balance). See: AMIKACIN; GENTAMICIN; KANAMYCIN; NETILMICIN; STREPTOMYCIN; TOBRAMYCIN

aminophylline
is a BRONCHODILATOR drug that is used as an acute ANTI-ASTHMATIC or a bronchitis treatment for severe acute attacks. It is chemically classed as a xanthine and is a chemical combination of theophylline (with ethylenediamine to make it more water-soluble). Administration can be oral in the form of tablets or by injection.
✚▲ side-effects/warning: see under THEOPHYLLINE; but the ethylenediamine can cause allergic reactions in the skin.
⊙ Related entries: Amnivent; Min-I-Jet Aminophylline; Pecram; Phyllocontin Continus

aminosalicylate
drugs contain a 5-aminosalicylic acid component. They are used primarily to treat active Crohn's disease and to induce and maintain remission of the symptoms of ulcerative colitis and also sometimes to treat rheumatoid arthritis.

The drugs in this group include MESALAZINE, which is 5-aminosalicylic acid itself, OLSALAZINE SODIUM, which is two molecules of 5-aminosalicylic acid joined together and SULPHASALAZINE, which combines within the one chemical both 5-aminosalicylic acid and the (SULPHONAMIDE) ANTIBACTERIAL drug sulphapyridine.

The aminosalicylate component causes characteristic side-effects such as diarrhoea, salicylate hypersensitivity and kidney effects (interstitial nephritis); whereas sulphasalazine also has sulphonamide-related side-effects,

including rashes, blood disorders, azoospermia (lack of sperm) and lupoid syndrome. The sensitivity of individual patients to one or other chemical component partly determines the most suitable treatment.

amiodarone hydrochloride
is a potentially toxic drug, which is used as an ANTI-ARRHYTHMIC to treat certain severe irregularities of the heartbeat, especially in cases where, for one reason or another, alternative drugs cannot be used. Administration can be oral in the form of tablets or by injection.
✚ side-effects: these are many and include: photosensitivity, deposits on the cornea; neurological effects; nausea, vomiting; blood disturbances, rashes and impaired vision.
▲ warning: it should not be administered to patients with certain heart irregularities; thyroid disorders; certain liver and kidney disorders; or to those who are pregnant or breast-feeding. There should be regular testing of thyroid, liver and lung function.
⊙ Related entry: Cordarone X

amitriptyline hydrochloride
is an ANTIDEPRESSANT drug of the TRICYCLIC group. It has quite marked SEDATIVE properties, which may be of benefit to agitated or violent patients. Along with other members of this class, it has pronounced ANTICHOLINERGIC side-effects. An alternative use is to prevent bed-wetting by children. Administration is oral as tablets, capsules, or a dilute mixture, or alternatively by injection.
✚ side-effects: common effects include loss of intricacy in movement or thought (affecting driving ability), dry mouth, blurred vision and constipation; there may also be difficulty in urinating, sweating, irregular heartbeat, behavioural disturbances, a rash, a state of confusion and changes in appetite and libido. Rarely, there are also blood disorders.
▲ warning: it should not be administered to patients who suffer from certain heart

A

disorders, severe liver disorders, psychosis or mania. It should be administered with caution to patients who suffer from diabetes, epilepsy, liver or thyroid disease, closed-angle glaucoma, or urinary retention; or who are pregnant or breast-feeding. Withdrawal of treatment must be gradual.
○ Related entries: Domical; Elavil; Lentizol; Tryptizol

Amix

(Ashbourne) is a proprietary, prescription-only preparation of the broad-spectrum ANTIBACTERIAL and (PENICILLIN) ANTIBIOTIC drug amoxycillin. It can be used to treat systemic bacterial infections, infections of the upper respiratory tract, of the ear, nose and throat and of the urinogenital tracts. It is available as capsules and an oral suspension.
✚▲ side-effects/warning: see AMOXYCILLIN

amlodipine besylate

is a CALCIUM-CHANNEL BLOCKER drug. It can be used as an ANTIHYPERTENSIVE treatment and as an ANTI-ANGINA drug in the prevention of attacks. Administration is oral as tablets.
✚ side-effects: flushing, dizziness, headache, oedema (accumulation of fluid in tissues) and fatigue. There may be an excessive growth of the gums and blood upsets.
▲ warning: administer with caution to patients with certain liver disorders, or who are pregnant or breast-feeding.
○ Related entry: Istin

ammonia and ipecacuanha mixture, BP

is a non-proprietary COMPOUND PREPARATION of the EXPECTORANT drugs ammonium bicarbonate and ipecacuanha tincture (together with liquorice liquid extract). It can be used to promote the expulsion of excess bronchial secretions and is administered orally as a liquid preparation.
✚▲ side-effects/warning: see IPECACUANHA

ammonium chloride

is used as an EXPECTORANT and is sometimes incorporated into cough treatments, though evidence of its efficacy is lacking. It can cause metabolic acidosis and so can be used to correct metabolic alkalosis. It has been used as a DIURETIC and has some use in the therapeutic acidification of urine, which increases the rate of the excretion of some drugs and poisons and is therefore effectively an ANTIDOTE.
○ Related entries: BN Liniment; Penetrol Catarrh Lozenges

ammonium salicylate

is a soluble (NSAID) NON-NARCOTIC ANALGESIC and ANTIRHEUMATIC drug. It is used to treat rheumatic and other musculoskeletal disorders. Administration is oral in the form of a non-proprietary liquid mixture.
See also: SALICYLATES; SALICYLIC ACID
✚▲ side-effects/warning: see under NSAID
○ Related entries: Aspellin; Radian B Heat Spray; Radian B Muscle Lotion

Amnivent

(Ashbourne) is a proprietary, non-prescription preparation of the BRONCHODILATOR drug aminophylline. It can be used as an ANTI-ASTHMATIC and bronchitis treatment and is available as modified-release tablets.
✚▲ warning/side-effects: see AMINOPHYLLINE

*amoebicidal

drugs are ANTIMICROBIAL drugs that are used to treat infection by the microscopic protozoan organisms known as amoebae, which cause such disorders as amoebic dysentery and hepatic amoebiasis. The best-known and most-used amoebicidal drug is the (AZOLE) METRONIDAZOLE. See also: DILOXANIDE FUROATE; TINIDAZOLE.

Amoram

(Eastern) is a proprietary, prescription-

only preparation of the broad-spectrum ANTIBACTERIAL and (PENICILLIN) ANTIBIOTIC drug amoxycillin. It can be used to treat systemic bacterial infections, infections of the upper respiratory tract, of the ear, nose and throat and of the urinogenital tracts. It is available as capsules and an oral suspension.
✚▲ side-effects/warning: see AMOXYCILLIN

amorolfine

is a recently introduced ANTIFUNGAL drug that differs chemically from other antifungals. It can be used topically to treat fungal skin infections such as foot mycosis. It is available as a cream and a nail lacquer.
✪ Related entry: LOCERYL

amoxapine

is an ANTIDEPRESSANT drug of the TRICYCLIC group. It can be used to treat depressive illness. Administration is oral as tablets.
✚▲ side-effects/warning: see under amitriptyline hydrochloride; but has less sedative actions. There may also be menstrual irregularities, breast enlargement in men, change in libido and, rarely, tardive dyskinesia.
✪ Related entry: Asendis

amoxicillin

See AMOXYCILLIN

Amoxil

(Bencard) is a proprietary, prescription-only preparation of the broad-spectrum ANTIBACTERIAL and (PENICILLIN) ANTIBIOTIC drug amoxycillin. It can be used to treat systemic bacterial infections, infections of the upper respiratory tract, of the ear, nose and throat and of the urinogenital tracts.

It is available as capsules, sugar-free soluble tablets, chewable tablets, a syrup for dilution, an oral suspension for children, a powder in sachets, a sugar-free powder in sachets. It is also available in a form for injection.
✚▲ side-effects/warning: see AMOXYCILLIN

amoxycillin

(amoxicillin) is a broad-spectrum, penicillin-like ANTIBACTERIAL and ANTIBIOTIC drug, which is closely related to AMPICILLIN. It is readily absorbed orally (better than ampicillin) and is used to treat many infections (due to both Gram-positive and Gram-negative bacteria), especially infections of the urinogenital tracts, the upper respiratory tract and the middle ear.

It is also sometimes used to prevent infection following dental surgery, to prevent endocarditis, to treat Lyme disease in children and (in combination with other drugs) to treat long-standing *Helicobacter pylori* infection associated with peptic ulcers.

However, it is not *penicillinase-resistant*, as it is inactivated by penicillinase enzymes produced by Gram-positive bacteria such as *Stapylococcus aureus* and common Gram-negative bacteria such as *Escherichia Coli*.

For this reason, it is sometimes combined with CLAVULANIC ACID, which is an inhibiter of penicillinase enzymes. Administration can be oral in the form of tablets, capsules, sachets, suspensions (including paediatric versions) or syrups, or by injection.
✚▲ side-effects/warning: see under AMPICILLIN
✪ Related entries: Almodan; Amix; Amoram; Amoxil; Amoxymed; Amrit; Augmentin; Flemoxin Solutab; Galenamox; Rimoxallin

Amoxymed

(Medipharma) is a proprietary, prescription-only preparation of the broad-spectrum ANTIBACTERIAL and (PENICILLIN) ANTIBIOTIC drug amoxycillin. It can be used to treat systemic bacterial infections, infections of the upper respiratory tract, of the ear, nose and

A

A

throat and of the urinogenital tracts. It is available as capsules and an oral suspension.

+▲ side-effects/warning: see AMOXYCILLIN

Amphocil

(Zeneca) is a proprietary, prescription-only preparation of the ANTIFUNGAL and ANTIBIOTIC drug amphotericin, which has an unusual formulation as a lipid colloidal dispersion (with sodium cholesteryl sulphate) that is intended to minimize toxicity (particularly to the kidney), so that it can be used for severe systemic or deep-seated fungal infections. It is available in a form for infusion.

+▲ side-effects/warning: see AMPHOTERICIN

amphotericin

(amphotericin B) is a broad-spectrum ANTIFUNGAL drug, which is one of the polyene ANTIBIOTICS. It can be used particularly to treat infection by most fungi and yeasts and is an extremely important drug in the treatment of systemic fungal infections. However, it is a toxic drug and side-effects are common. There have been recent attempts to minimize toxicity (particularly to the kidney) by making a lipid formulation (encapsulated in liposomes; *AmBisome*) and a colloidal dispersion (with sodium cholesteryl sulphate; *Amphocil*) so that amphotericin can be used for severe systemic or deep-seated fungal infections. Administration can be oral in the form of tablets, lozenges or an oral liquid suspension, or by infusion.

+ side-effects: treatment by infusion may cause nausea, vomiting, anorexia, abdominal pain, headache, muscle and joint pain, kidney, heart, hearing, liver and blood disorders; and rash.

▲ warning: during treatment by infusion, tests on kidney and blood function are essential. Administer with care to patients who are pregnant or breast-feeding.

✪ Related entries: AmBisome; Amphocil; Fungilin; Fungizone

amphotericin B

See AMPHOTERICIN

ampicillin

is a broad-spectrum, penicillin-type ANTIBACTERIAL and ANTIBIOTIC drug. It is taken orally (though absorption is reduced by the presence of food in the stomach or intestines) and is used to treat many infections (due to both Gram-positive and Gram-negative bacteria), especially infections of the urinogenital tracts, the upper respiratory tract, the middle ear and also gonorrhoea and invasive salmonellosis. It is sometimes given as a COMPOUND PREPARATION with CLOXACILLIN, which is a combination called CO-FLUAMPICIL. Administration can be oral as capsules, an oral suspension (including paediatric versions) or syrup, or by injection.

+ side-effects: diarrhoea is common; nausea; rarely, sensitivity reactions such as rashes (particularly in patients suffering from glandular fever, leukaemia, or have HIV infection), high temperature and joint pain. Allergic patients may suffer anaphylactic shock.

▲ warning: it should not be administered to patients who are known to be allergic to penicillin-type antibiotics in case anaphylactic shock ensues. It should be administered with caution to those with impaired kidney function.

✪ Related entries: Amfipen; Ampiclox; Ampiclox Neonatal; Flu-Amp; Magnapen; Penbritin; Rimacillin; Vidopen

Ampiclox

(Beecham) is a proprietary, prescription-only COMPOUND PREPARATION of the broad-spectrum ANTIBACTERIAL and (PENICILLIN) ANTIBIOTIC drug ampicillin and the *penicillinase-resistant*, antibacterial and (penicillin) antibiotic cloxacillin. It can be used to treat systemic bacterial infections, infections of the upper respiratory tract, of the ear, nose and throat and of the urinogenital tracts. It is available as capsules, a syrup and in a form for injection.

+▲ side-effects/warning: see AMPICILLIN; CLOXACILLIN

Ampiclox Neonatal

(Beecham) is a proprietary, prescription-only COMPOUND PREPARATION of the broad-spectrum ANTIBACTERIAL and (PENICILLIN) ANTIBIOTIC drug ampicillin and the *penicillinase-resistant*, antibacterial and (penicillin) antibiotic cloxacillin. It can be used to treat systemic bacterial infections, infections of the upper respiratory tract, of the ear, nose and throat and of the urinogenital tracts. It is available as capsules, an oral suspension and in a form for injection.

+▲ side-effects/warning: see AMPICILLIN; CLOXACILLIN

Amrit

(BHR) is a proprietary, prescription-only preparation of the broad-spectrum ANTIBACTERIAL and (PENICILLIN) ANTIBIOTIC drug amoxycillin. It can be used to treat systemic bacterial infections, infections of the upper respiratory tract, of the ear, nose and throat and of the urinogenital tracts. It is available as capsules and an oral suspension.

+▲ side-effects/warning: see AMOXYCILLIN

amsacrine

is a (CYTOTOXIC) ANTICANCER drug, which is used specifically in the treatment of acute myeloid leukaemia. Administration is by intravenous infusion.

+▲ side-effects/warning: see under CYTOTOXIC DRUGS; there may also be heartbeat irregularities.

✪ Related entry: Amsidine

Amsidine

(Parke-Davis) is a proprietary, prescription-only preparation of the (CYTOTOXIC) ANTICANCER drug amsacrine. It can be used to treat acute myeloid

leukaemia and is available in a form for intravenous infusion.

+▲ side-effects/warning: see AMSACRINE

amylobarbitone

is a BARBITURATE drug. It is used as a HYPNOTIC, but only when absolutely necessary, to treat severe and intractable insomnia in patients who are already taking barbiturates. Administration is oral as tablets or capsules, or by injection. Preparations containing amylobarbitone are on the Controlled Drugs List.

+▲ side-effects/warning: see under BARBITURATE

✪ Related entries: Amytal; Sodium Amytal; Tuinal

Amytal

(Lilly) is a proprietary, prescription-only preparation of the BARBITURATE drug amylobarbitone and is on the Controlled Drugs List. It can be used as a HYPNOTIC to treat persistent and intractable insomnia and is available as tablets.

+▲ side-effects/warning: see AMYLOBARBITONE

Anacal Rectal Ointment

(Panpharma) is a proprietary, non-prescription preparation of heparinoids (with lauromacrogol). It can be used for the symptomatic relief of haemorrhoids, perianal eczema, itching and anal fissure. It is available as an ointment and is not normally used for children under five years, except on medical advice.

+▲ side-effects/warning: see HEPARINOID

Anacal Suppositories

(Panpharma) is a proprietary, non-prescription preparation of heparinoids (with lauromacrogol). It can be used for the symptomatic relief of haemorrhoids, perianal eczema, itching and anal fissure. It is available as suppositories and is not normally used for children under five years, except on medical advice.

+▲ side-effects/warning: see HEPARINOID

A

Anadin Analgesic Caplets

(Whitehall Laboratories) is a proprietary, non-prescription COMPOUND PREPARATION of the (NSAID) NON-NARCOTIC ANALGESIC and ANTIRHEUMATIC drug aspirin and the STIMULANT caffeine. It can be used for the treatment of mild to moderate pain and for symptomatic relief of feverish colds and flu. It is available as capsule-shaped tablets (*Caplets*) and is not normally given to children under 12 years, except on medical advice.
✚▲ side-effects/warning: see ASPIRIN; CAFFEINE

Anadin Analgesic Capsules, Maximum Strength

(Whitehall Laboratories) is a proprietary, non-prescription COMPOUND PREPARATION of the (NSAID) NON-NARCOTIC ANALGESIC and ANTIRHEUMATIC drug aspirin and the STIMULANT caffeine. It can be used for the treatment of mild to moderate pain and for symptomatic relief of colds and flu. It is available as capsules and is not normally given to children under 12 years, except on medical advice.
✚▲ side-effects/warning: see ASPIRIN; CAFFEINE

Anadin Extra

(Whitehall Laboratories) is a proprietary, non-prescription COMPOUND PREPARATION of the (NSAID) NON-NARCOTIC ANALGESIC and ANTIRHEUMATIC drug aspirin, the non-narcotic analgesic drug paracetamol and the STIMULANT caffeine. It can be used for the treatment of pain, especially headaches, period, dental and rheumatic pain and also to relieve cold and flu symptoms. It is available as capsules and is not normally given to children, except under medical supervision.
✚▲ side-effects/warning: see ASPIRIN; CAFFEINE; PARACETAMOL

Anadin Extra Soluble Tablets

(Whitehall Laboratories) is a proprietary,

non-prescription COMPOUND PREPARATION of the (NSAID) NON-NARCOTIC ANALGESIC and ANTIRHEUMATIC drug aspirin, the non-narcotic analgesic drug paracetamol and the STIMULANT caffeine. It can be used to treat mild to moderate pain, relieve swelling, stiffness and cold and flu symptoms. It is available as soluble tablets and is not normally given to children under 12 years, except on medical advice.
✚▲ side-effects/warning: see ASPIRIN; CAFFEINE; PARACETAMOL

Anadin Paracetamol Tablets

(Whitehall Laboratories) is a proprietary, non-prescription preparation of the NON-NARCOTIC ANALGESIC drug paracetamol. It can be used for the treatment of headache, migraine, period pain and dental pain and to relieve the symptoms of colds and flu. It is available as tablets.
✚▲ side-effects/warning: see PARACETAMOL

*anaemia treatment

involves the use of drugs to correct a deficiency of the oxygen-carrying blood pigment haemoglobin (anaemia). The type of treatment depends on the cause of the anaemia.

For example, the drugs administered to treat iron-deficient anaemia are mainly salts of IRON and are used where there is deficiency of iron in the form of haemoglobin in blood and a similar oxygen-carrier in muscles.

Dietary deficiency of iron in the diet and disease states that prevent its proper absorption can both lead to forms of anaemia. Iron supplements may be administered orally in one of several forms, as FERROUS FUMARATE, FERROUS GLUCONATE, FERROUS GLYCINE SULPHATE, or FERROUS SULPHATE (and other salts), or by injection or intravenous infusion in the form of iron dextran and other preparations. Iron supplements are also used where there is deficiency of iron during pregnancy.

*anaesthetic

drugs are used to reduce sensations, especially pain. LOCAL ANAESTHETIC drugs (eg LIGNOCAINE HYDROCHLORIDE) affect a specific area and do not cause a loss of consciousness. GENERAL ANAESTHETIC drugs (eg HALOTHANE) do cause a loss of consciousness and the loss of sensation is a result of this. Local anaesthetics are a logical choice for minor and local surgical procedures, such as in dental surgery, because their duration of action can be short and they is less discomfort and medical risk.

However, local anaesthetics can also achieve a more extensive loss of sensation with nerve block (eg injected near to the nerve supplying a limb), or with spinal anaesthesia (eg epidural injection in childbirth) where loss of sensation in whole areas of the body allows major surgery. Local anaesthetics are particularly valuable in situations where general anaesthesia carries a high risk, or the conscious co-operation of the patient is required. General anaesthetic drugs are normally used for more extensive surgical procedures. In modern anaesthetic practice, ANALGESIC, SEDATIVE, or SKELETAL MUSCLE RELAXANT drugs are used in premedication or during the operation so that quite low doses of general anaesthetic are needed. See also NARCOTIC ANALGESIC.

Anaflex

(Geistlich) is a proprietary, non-prescription preparation of the ANTIFUNGAL and ANTIBACTERIAL drug polynoxylin. It can be used topically to treat minor skin infections and is available as a cream.

+▲ side-effects/warning: see POLYNOXYLIN

Anafranil

(Geigy) is a proprietary, prescription-only preparation of the (TRICYCLIC) ANTIDEPRESSANT drug clomipramine hydrochloride. It can be used to relieve the symptoms of depressive illness and as an additional treatment in phobic and obsessional states. It is available as capsules, modified-release tablets (*Anafranil SR*), a syrup and in a form for injection.

+▲ side-effects/warning: see CLOMIPRAMINE HYDROCHLORIDE

*analgesic

is a drug that relieves pain. There are many ways that drugs can be used to relieve pain. In this book the term analgesic is restricted to two main classes of drug.

The first class is the NARCOTIC ANALGESICS (eg MORPHINE SULPHATE), which have powerful actions on the central nervous system and alter the perception of pain. Because of the numerous possible side-effects, the most important of which is drug dependence (habituation or addiction), this class is usually used under strict medical supervision and preparations are normally available only on prescription. Other notable side-effects include depression of respiration, nausea and vomiting, sometimes hypotension, constipation, inhibition of coughing (ANTITUSSIVE action) and constriction of the pupils (miosis).

Other members of this class, also known as OPIOIDS (or OPIATES), include DIAMORPHINE HYDROCHLORIDE (heroin), PENTAZOCINE, METHADONE HYDROCHLORIDE, PETHIDINE HYDROCHLORIDE and CODEINE PHOSPHATE. Narcotic analgesics are used for different types and severities of pain. It is now recognized that the characteristic pharmacology of the narcotic analgesics follows from their action as mimics of the natural opioid NEUROTRANSMITTERS (enkephalins, endorphins, dynorphins) in nerves in the brain.

The second class is the NON-NARCOTIC ANALGESICS, which are drugs that have no tendency to produce dependence, for example ASPIRIN, but are by no means free

A

of side-effects. This class is referred to by many names, including *weak analgesics* (something of a misnomer in view of their powerful actions in treating inflammatory pain); and, in medical circles, a very large number are referred to as *non-steroidal, anti-inflammatory drugs*, abbreviated to NSAID. The latter term refers to the valuable anti-inflammatory action of some members of this class. These drugs are used for a variety of purposes, ranging from mild aches and pains (at lower dosages), to the treatment of rheumatoid arthritis (at higher dosages).

PARACETAMOL does not have strong anti-inflammatory actions, but is non-narcotic and, along with other drugs in this class, has ANTIPYRETIC action (the ability to lower raised body temperature). The non-narcotic analgesics work by altering the synthesis of prostaglandins (natural LOCAL HORMONES within the body) that tend to enhance pain.

Although this class of drugs has important actions and uses, all its members have side-effects of concern, which for aspirin-like drugs include gastrointestinal upsets ranging from dyspepsia to serious haemorrhage. Other examples of non-narcotic analgesics include IBUPROFEN and INDOMETHACIN. Often drugs in this class are used in combination with other analgesics (eg paracetamol with codeine), or with drugs of other classes (eg caffeine).

Apart from these two main classes, there are other drugs that are sometimes referred to as analgesic because of their ability to relieve pain. For example, LOCAL ANAESTHETICS are referred to as *local analgesics* in the USA; also, RUBEFACIENTS, or COUNTER IRRITANTS, are sometimes called analgesics.

Anapolon 50

(Syntex) is a proprietary, prescription-only preparation of the (*anabolic*) STEROID oxymetholone. It can be used to treat aplastic anaemia in particular

and is available as tablets.
+▲ side-effects/warning: see OXYMETHOLONE

Anbesol Liquid

(Whitehall) is a proprietary, non-prescription COMPOUND PREPARATION of the LOCAL ANAESTHETIC drug lignocaine hydrochloride and the ANTISEPTIC agent cetylpyridinium chloride (with chlorocresol). It can be used for the temporary relief of pain caused by teething, mouth ulcers and denture irritation. It is available as a liquid for topical application.
+▲ side-effects/warning: see CETYLPYRIDINIUM CHLORIDE; LIGNOCAINE HYDROCHLORIDE

Anbesol Teething Gel

(Whitehall) is a proprietary, non-prescription COMPOUND PREPARATION of the LOCAL ANAESTHETIC drug lignocaine hydrochloride and the ANTISEPTIC agent cetylpyridinium chloride (with chlorocresol). It can be used for the temporary relief of pain caused by teething, mouth ulcers and denture irritation. It is available as a gel for topical application.
+▲ side-effects/warning: see CETYLPYRIDINIUM CHLORIDE; LIGNOCAINE HYDROCHLORIDE

ancrod

is an effective ANTICOAGULANT derived from an enzyme that is a constituent of the venom of the Malaysian pit viper. It works by depleting the protein fibrinogen, which is necessary for the formation of blood clots.

It is used in the treatment of deep-vein thrombosis (blood clots), especially the sort that occur following surgery, or to prevent thrombosis. It is no longer commonly used and is available only on a 'named-patient' basis. Administration is by injection.
✪ Related entry: Arvin

Andrews Answer

(Sterling Health) is a proprietary, non-prescription COMPOUND PREPARATION of the NON-NARCOTIC ANALGESIC drug paracetamol and the ANTACID sodium bicarbonate. It can be used for headache with upset stomach and other general pain. It is available as effervescent granules and is not normally given to children under 18 years, except on medical advice.

+▲ side-effects/warning: see PARACETAMOL; SODIUM BICARBONATE

Andrews Antacid

(Sterling Health) is a proprietary, non-prescription COMPOUND PREPARATION of the ANTACIDS calcium carbonate and magnesium carbonate. It can be used for the relief of upset stomach, heartburn, indigestion and trapped wind. It is available as chewable tablets and also in a flavoured version called *Andrews Antacid Fruit Flavour*. It is not normally given to children, except on medical advice.

+▲ side-effects/warning: see CALCIUM CARBONATE; MAGNESIUM CARBONATE

Androcur

(Schering Health) is a proprietary, prescription-only preparation of the ANTI-ANDROGEN cyproterone acetate, which is a SEX HORMONE ANTAGONIST. It can be used to treat severe hypersexuality and sexual deviation in men and is available as tablets.

+▲ side-effects/warning: see CYPROTERONE ACETATE

androgen

is the term used to describe the predominantly male (STEROID) SEX HORMONES, which stimulate the development of male sex organs and male secondary sexual characteristics. In men, they are produced primarily by the testes and the main form is called TESTOSTERONE. However androgens are produced in both men and women by the adrenal glands and in women small quantities are also secreted by the ovaries. An excessive amount in women causes masculinization. Forms of the natural hormones and a number of synthetic androgens are used therapeutically (eg forms of testosterone and MESTEROLONE) to correct hormonal deficiency, for example, delayed puberty and can also be used as ANTICANCER treatments for cancers linked to sex hormones (eg breast cancer in women). ANTI-ANDROGENS are drugs that inhibit the actions of androgens and are also used in medicine.

+ side-effects: oedema (fluid retention in the tissues) leading to weight gain. Increased levels of calcium in the body may cause bone growth (and in younger patients may fuse bones before fully grown), there may be enlargement of the prostate gland, priapism in men, reduced production of sperm in men and masculinization in women.

▲ warning: they should not be administered to male patients who suffer from nephrosis, cancer of the prostate gland, or cancer of the breast; or to female patients who are pregnant or breast-feeding. Administer with caution to those with impaired function of the heart, liver, or kidney, certain circulatory disorders and/or hypertension, epilepsy or diabetes, thyroid disorders, or migraine.

androgen antagonists

See ANTI-ANDROGENS

Anectine

(Wellcome) is a proprietary, prescription-only preparation of the (*depolarizing*) SKELETAL MUSCLE RELAXANT drug suxamethonium chloride. It can be used to induce muscle paralysis during surgery and is available in a form for injection.

+▲ side-effects/warning: see SUXAMETHONIUM CHLORIDE

Anestan Bronchial Tablets

(Seton Healthcare) is a proprietary, non-prescription COMPOUND PREPARATION of the SYMPATHOMIMETIC and DECONGESTANT

A

drug ephedrine hydrochloride and the BRONCHODILATOR drug theophylline (anhydrous). It can be used as an ANTI-ASTHMATIC for reversible bronchospasm. It is not normally given to children under 12 years, except on medical advice.

✚▲ side-effects/warning: see EPHEDRINE HYDROCHLORIDE; THEOPHYLLINE

Anexate

(Roche) is a proprietary, prescription-only preparation of the BENZODIAZEPINE antagonist drug flumazenil. It can be used to reverse the effects of benzodiazepines and is available in a form for intravenous injection or infusion.

✚▲ side-effects/warning: see FLUMAZENIL

Angettes 75

(Bristol-Myers) is a proprietary, non-prescription preparation of the ANTIPLATELET aggregation drug aspirin. It can be used to help prevent the formation of thrombi (blood clots) and is used particularly for problems relating to blocked blood vessels, such as following and to prevent, heart attacks. It is available as tablets.

✚▲ side-effects/warning: see ASPIRIN

Angilol

(DDSA Pharmaceuticals) is a proprietary, prescription-only preparation of the BETA-BLOCKER drug propranolol hydrochloride. It can be used as an ANTIHYPERTENSIVE treatment for raised blood pressure, as an ANTI-ANGINA treatment to relieve symptoms and to improve exercise tolerance and as an ANTI-ARRHYTHMIC to regularize heartbeat and to treat myocardial infarction. It may also be used as an ANTITHYROID drug for short-term treatment of thyrotoxicosis, as an ANTIMIGRAINE treatment to prevent attacks, as an ANXIOLYTIC treatment, particularly for symptomatic relief of tremor and palpitations and, with an ALPHA-ADRENOCEPTOR BLOCKER, in the acute treatment of phaeochromocytoma. It is

available as tablets.

✚▲ side-effects/warning: see PROPRANOLOL HYDROCHLORIDE

Angiopine

(Ashbourne) is a proprietary, prescription-only preparation of the CALCIUM-CHANNEL BLOCKER drug nifedipine. It can be used as an ANTI-ANGINA drug in the prevention of attacks, as an ANTIHYPERTENSIVE treatment and as a VASODILATOR in peripheral vascular disease (Raynaud's phenomenon). It is available as capsules.

✚▲ side-effects/warning: see NIFEDIPINE

angiotension-converting enzyme inhibitors

See ACE INHIBITORS

*angiotensin-receptor blocker

drugs work by blocking angiotensin receptors. Angiotensin II is a circulating HORMONE that is a powerful VASOCONSTRICTOR and blocking its effects leads to a fall in blood pressure. LOSARTAN POTASSIUM is a recently introduced drug of this type and can be used as an ANTIHYPERTENSIVE agent.

Angiozem

(Ashbourne) is a proprietary, prescription-only preparation of the CALCIUM-CHANNEL BLOCKER drug diltiazem hydrochloride. It can be used as an ANTIHYPERTENSIVE treatment and as an ANTI-ANGINA drug in the prevention of attacks. It is available as modified-release tablets.

✚▲ side-effects/warning: see DILTIAZEM HYDROCHLORIDE

Anhydrol Forte

(Dermal) is a proprietary, non-prescription preparation of aluminium chloride (as hexahydrate), which can be used as an ANTIPERSPIRANT to treat hyperhidrosis (excessive sweating). It is

available in a roll-on applicator.
+▲ side-effects/warning: see ALUMINIUM
CHLORIDE

anistreplase

is used therapeutically as a FIBRINOLYTIC
drug because it has the property of
breaking up blood clots. It is used rapidly
in serious conditions such as myocardial
infarction (damage to heart muscle,
usually after a heart attack).
Administration is by injection or infusion.
+▲ side-effects/warning: see under
ALTEPLASE
⊕ Related entry: Eminase

Anodesyn

(Seton Healthcare) is a proprietary, non-
prescription preparation of the LOCAL
ANAESTHETIC drug lignocaine
hydrochloride (with allantoin). It can be
used for the symptomatic relief of the pain
and itching of haemorrhoids and is
available as an ointment and as
suppositories. It is not normally given to
children, except on medical advice.
+▲ side-effects/warning: see LIGNOCAINE
HYDROCHLORIDE

Anquil

(Janssen) is a proprietary, prescription-
only preparation of the ANTIPSYCHOTIC
drug benperidol. It can be used to treat
and tranquillize psychotic patients,
especially those with antisocial and deviant
sexual behaviour. It is available as tablets.
+▲ side-effects/warning: see BENPERIDOL

Antabuse 200

(CP Pharmaceuticals) is a proprietary,
prescription-only preparation of the
ENZYME INHIBITOR disulfiram. It can be
used to assist in the treatment of
alcoholism, because, in combination with
the consumption of even small quantities
of alcohol, it causes unpleasant reactions:
flushing, headache, palpitations, nausea
and vomiting. It is available as tablets.
+▲ side-effects/warning: see DISULFIRAM

*antacid

drugs are used to neutralize the
hydrochloric acid that the stomach
produces as part of the normal digestion
of food. Over-production of acid
(hyperacidity) can cause the symptoms of
dyspepsia (indigestion), which can be
exacerbated by alcohol and NSAID drugs.
Antacids give symptomatic relief of the
dyspepsia and gastritis associated with
peptic ulcers (gastric or duodenal ulcer),
but allow little actual healing of ulcers. A
further painful condition is when there is
regurgitation of acid and enzymes into the
oesophagus (oesophageal reflux), which
in the short term causes heartburn and in
the long term can cause inflammation
(reflux oesophagitis: common in hiatus
hernia and pregnancy). Antacids taken
alone effectively reduce acidity, but are
commonly combined with other drugs (eg
ULCER-HEALING DRUGS, DEMULCENTS and
ANTIFOAMING AGENTS). Antacids themselves
have side-effects; bicarbonates and
carbonates tend to cause flatulence and
some aluminium-containing antacids
cause constipation, whereas magnesium-
containing antacids can cause diarrhoea
(so are often used in combination). See:
ALUMINIUM HYDROXIDE; CALCIUM
CARBONATE; MAGNESIUM CARBONATE;
MAGNESIUM HYDROXIDE; MAGNESIUM
TRISILICATE; SODIUM BICARBONATE

*antagonist

drugs have no pharmacological actions in
their own right, but have profound actions
because they actually block (physically
occupy) RECEPTORS that normally allow
natural mediators, or sometimes synthetic
drugs, to have an effect. Many of the most
widely used drugs in medicine are
antagonists. Their most important
property is that they can be used to
prevent the actions of mediators within the
body, including within the brain and can
therefore be used to 'switch-off' systems
within the body that are not functioning
correctly, for instance in a disease state

A

caused by excessive amounts of NEUROTRANSMITTERS, LOCAL HORMONES and HORMONES. This very valuable property can be used in a range of applications from changing mood and psychological states of mind, through to preventing allergic responses. Some examples will illustrate this point.

BETA-BLOCKERS (beta-adrenoceptor blocking drugs) are antagonists drugs that prevent the action of ADRENALINE and NORADRENALINE by blocking the receptors called beta-adrenoceptors. They may be used as ANTIHYPERTENSIVES, in ANTI-ARRHYTHMIC and ANTI-ANGINA treatment for the heart and in ANXIOLYTIC, ANTITHYROID and GLAUCOMA TREATMENT. The best-known and most-used beta-blockers include ACEBUTOLOL, OXPRENOLOL, PROPRANOLOL and SOTALOL and as a class they are probably the single most used drugs in medicine.

ANTIHISTAMINES (H_1-antagonists) are drugs that inhibit the effects in the body of the local hormone histamine by blocking receptors called H_1 receptors. Histamine is released, for instance, as an allergic reaction to a substance such as pollen, insect bites and stings, contact with some metal objects and certain foods. Antihistamines can be given by mouth, or applied topically, to block many of the unpleasant or dangerous actions of histamine.

There is a second group of drugs that also inhibit histamine effects, but block a quite different class of receptor called the (H_2) receptor, which is involved in (stomach) gastric acid secretion. This group is referred to as H_2-ANTAGONISTS and they are used as ULCER-HEALING DRUGS, for example, in the treatment of peptic ulcers. The H_2-antagonist drug RANITIDINE is probably the most prescribed individual drug in the world.

Other examples of antagonist drugs include ANTICHOLINERGIC drugs, ANTI-ANDROGENS, ANTI-OESTROGENS and OPIOID ANTAGONISTS.

antazoline

is an ANTIHISTAMINE drug, which can be used for the symptomatic relief of allergic symptoms such as allergic conjunctivitis in the eye. Administration is in the form of eye-drops.

✚▲ side-effects/warning: see under ANTIHISTAMINE. Avoid its use in patients with kidney impairment.

○ Related entry: Otrivine-Antistin

Antepsin

(Wyeth) is a proprietary, prescription-only preparation of the CYTOPROTECTANT drug sucralfate. It can be used to treat gastric and duodenal ulcers and is available as tablets.

✚▲ side-effects/warning: see SUCRALFATE

*anthelmintic drugs

are used to treat infections by parasitic organisms of the helminth (worm) family. The threadworm, roundworm and tapeworm are the most common helminths responsible for infection in the UK. In warmer countries illnesses caused by helminths are a major problem, eg hookworm disease (caused by hookworms), bilharziasis (caused by schistosomes) and elephantiasis (caused by filaria). Most worms infest the intestines and diagnosis is often made by finding the worms in the faeces.

Drugs can then be administered and the worms are killed or anaesthetized and then excreted. Complications arise if the worms migrate within the body, in which case the treatment becomes very unpleasant for the patient. In the case of threadworms, medication should be combined with hygienic measures (eg short fingernails) and the whole family should be treated. Among the most-useful and best-known anthelmintic drugs are PIPERAZINE, MEBENDAZOLE, NICLOSAMIDE and THIABENDAZOLE.

Anthranol

(Stiefel) is a proprietary, non-prescription

COMPOUND PREPARATION of dithranol and salicylic acid. It can be used for subacute and chronic psoriasis and is available as an ointment.
+▲ side-effects/warning: see DITHRANOL; SALICYLIC ACID

Anthrax Vaccine
(Public Health Laboratory Service) is a non-proprietary, prescription-only VACCINE preparation, which can be used to protect individuals exposed to anthrax-infected materials. It is available in a form for injection.

anthrax vaccine
for IMMUNIZATION is required only by individuals who are exposed to anthrax-infected hides and carcasses, or who handle imported bone meal, fish meal and other feedstuffs. The VACCINE is a precipitate of antigen from *Bacillus anthracis*, which causes anthrax and can be administered by a course of intramuscular injection.

*anti-allergic
drugs relieve the symptoms of an allergic reaction that follows exposure to specific substances to which a patient is allergic. These substances may be endogenous (in the patients body), or they may be exogenous (present in the environment). Because allergic reactions generally cause the release of the natural LOCAL HORMONE histamine within the body, ANTIHISTAMINES are often very effective for providing symptomatic relief.

For example, allergic skin reactions to foreign proteins, contact dermatitis and insect stings and bites, show characteristic symptoms – including pruritus (itching), urticaria (an itchy skin rash) and erythema (reddening of the skin) – and these often respond well to treatment with antihistamines (including local application in a cream). However, because allergic responses cause an inflammatory effect, many anti-allergic drugs also have ANTI-INFLAMMATORY properties. For example, in the treatment of atopic (allergic) bronchial asthma, chronic (long-term) inhalation of CORTICOSTEROIDS may prevent asthma attacks and the associated bronchoconstriction and congested airways. Similar anti-inflammatory protection from the symptoms of allergic asthma may be achieved by chronic inhalation of SODIUM CROMOGLYCATE, which prevents the release of histamine and other substances (though exactly how it works is not clear). In the acute treatment of anaphylactic shock (an extreme and generalized reaction, sometimes life-threatening; with release of histamine causing general swelling (oedema; accumulation of fluid in the tissues), bronchoconstriction (narrowing of the airways), heart failure and collapse of the blood circulation), immediate treatment with three types of drugs is often required: an injection of a SYMPATHOMIMETIC such as ADRENALINE to dilate the bronchioles and stimulate the cardiovascular circulation; and administration of corticosteroids and antihistamines to counter other serious allergic reactions. In general, corticosteroids will suppress or mask inflammatory responses at most sites (including the skin), but these drugs have quite marked and serious side-effects and are only given systemically in serious conditions and are normally used topically only for short-term alleviation of symptoms.

*anti-androgens
(androgen antagonists) are a class of drugs that are HORMONE ANTAGONISTS, which usually act directly to prevent the actions of the male sex HORMONE TESTOSTERONE at its target tissues. Other anti-androgens act indirectly to prevent the formation, or inhibit the release, of the hormones and are known as indirect hormone antagonists. Examples of drugs acting by the direct mechanism include

A CYPROTERONE ACETATE and FLUTAMIDE; and those that act through the indirect mechanism include BUSERELIN.

*anti-angina

drugs are used to relieve the pain of angina pectoris, which is an intense pain originating from the heart and due to ischaemia (insufficient blood supply to the heart muscle) and is especially pronounced in *exercise angina*. The disease state often results from atheroma, which is a degeneration of the lining of the arteries of the heart due to a build up of fatty deposits. The objective of drug treatment is to reduce the heart's workload and to prevent spasm or to dilate the arteries of the heart (the coronary arteries). Unloading can be achieved by stopping exercise, preventing the speeding of the heart and by dilating the coronary arteries.

BETA-BLOCKERS are drugs that, by blocking the effect of ADRENALINE and NORADRENALINE on the heart, prevent the normal increase in heart rate seen in exercise and are very effective in preventing anginal pain. Examples of beta-blocker drugs include: ACEBUTOLOL, ATENOLOL, METOPROLOL TARTRATE, NADOLOL, OXPRENOLOL HYDROCHLORIDE, PINDOLOL, PROPRANOLOL HYDROCHLORIDE, SOTALOL HYDROCHLORIDE and TIMOLOL MALEATE.

VASODILATORS are drugs (many of which are SMOOTH MUSCLE RELAXANTS) that dilate blood vessels and thereby increase blood flow. For the acute treatment of anginal pain (and to a lesser extent in preventing angina attacks) the NITRATES (eg GLYCERYL TRINITRATE, ISOSORBIDE DINITRATE, ISOSORBIDE MONONITRATE and PENTAERYTHRITOL TETRANITRATE) are widely used.

CALCIUM-CHANNEL BLOCKERS are a recently introduced anti-angina treatment. They dilate the coronary arteries and peripheral small arteries, which helps to reduce the workload on the heart. If drug treatment is not sufficient, then a coronary bypass operation may be needed. See also: AMLODIPINE BESYLATE; DILTIAZEM HYDROCHLORIDE; NICARDIPINE HYDROCHLORIDE; NIFEDIPINE; VERAPAMIL HYDROCHLORIDE

*anti-arrhythmic drugs

(antidysrrhythmic drugs) strengthen and regularize a heartbeat that has become unsteady and is not showing its usual patter of activity. But because there are many ways in which the heartbeat can falter – atrial tachycardia, ventricular tachycardia, atrial flutter or fibrillation and the severe heartbeat irregularity that may follow a heart attack (myocardial infarction) – there is a variety of drugs available, each for a fairly specific use. The best-known and most-used anti-arrhythmic drugs include DIGOXIN (a CARDIAC GLYCOSIDE), VERAPAMIL (a CALCIUM-CHANNEL BLOCKER) and LIGNOCAINE (a LOCAL ANAESTHETIC, especially used for ventricular arrhythmia); also extremely effective are the BETA-BLOCKERS (which are also used to treat high blood pressure and angina pectoris).

*anti-asthmatic

drugs relieve the symptoms of bronchial asthma or prevent recurrent attacks. The symptoms of asthma include bronchoconstriction (a narrowing of the bronchioles of the airways, with consequent difficulty in exhaling), often with over-secretion of fluid by glands within the bronchioles, with coughing and breathing difficulties. Two main types of drugs are used: one group treat acute attacks; and the second prevent attacks (as prophylaxis). BRONCHODILATOR drugs, which are SMOOTH MUSCLE RELAXANTS, work by dilating and relaxing the bronchioles. The most commonly used are the BETA-RECEPTOR STIMULANT drugs (which are SYMPATHOMIMETICS), notably SALBUTAMOL and TERBUTALINE SULPHATE.

antibiotics

A

The beta-receptor stimulant drugs, normally inhaled, are mostly used for treating acute attacks (or immediately before exertion in exercise asthma) and are largely of a type that does not normally adversely stimulate the heart. Other bronchodilator drugs that work directly on the bronchioles include smooth muscle relaxants such as THEOPHYLLINE.

The second group of anti-asthmatic drugs do not directly cause bronchodilation, but because of their ANTI-INFLAMMATORY action they prevent the release of local inflammatory mediators, which contribute to attacks; so preventing asthma attacks and providing symptomatic relief. Examples of this group of anti-inflammatory drugs include the CORTICOSTEROIDS and SODIUM CROMOGLYCATE. These drugs are almost always taken over a period of time, both to prevent attacks and to reverse pathological changes and preferably are inhaled so as to deliver the drug to where it is required and which helps limit side-effects. Indeed, a great deal of research has been done to design delivery devices that are able to more efficiently deliver the inhaled droplets, or particles, of bronchodilator or anti-inflammatory drugs into the airways, particularly in an attempt to reach the narrower bronchioles.

There are some other drugs, such as KETOTIFEN and IPRATROPIUM BROMIDE, that are occasionally used to treat asthma (for instance, when the other types of drug are ineffective for some reason). ANTIHISTAMINES, however, are now thought to be of no value, but are useful as ANTI-ALLERGIC treatments for hay fever or rashes.

*antibacterial

drugs are used to treat infections caused by bacteria, on which they have a selective toxic action. They can be used both topically (that is, on the skin or the eye) to treat infections of superficial tissues or systemically (carried by the blood after being swallowed or injected to the site of the infection).

A distinction can be made between *bacteriostatic* drugs, which act primarily by arresting bacterial growth (eg SULPHONAMIDES, TETRACYCLINES and CHLORAMPHENICOL) and the *bactericidal* agents, which act primarily by killing bacteria (eg PENICILLINS, CEPHALOSPORINS, AMINOGLYCOSIDES, ISONIAZID and RIFAMPICIN). As bacteria are the largest and most diverse group of pathogenic (disease-causing) micro-organisms, antibacterials form the major constituent group of ANTIMICROBIAL drugs.

*antibiotics

are, strictly speaking, natural products secreted by micro-organisms into their environment where they inhibit the growth of competing micro-organisms of different types. But in common usage the term is often applied to any drug, natural or synthetic, that has a selectively toxic action on bacteria or similar non-nucleated, single-celled micro-organisms (including chlamydia, rickettsia and mycoplasma) – but not viruses.

However, the more accurate term for these drugs is ANTIMICROBIALS. Most modern antibiotics are, in fact, either completely or partly synthetic and not produced by natural organisms, but nevertheless they are generally modelled on natural substances.

When administered by an appropriate route, such as topically (eg to the skin or eyes) orally, by injection, or by infusion, antibiotics kill micro-organisms such as bacteria – *bactericidal action* – or inhibit their growth – *bacteriostatic action*. The selectively toxic action on invading micro-organism exploits differences between bacteria and their human host cells. Major target sites are the bacterial cell wall located outside the cell membrane (human cells have only a cell membrane) and the bacterial ribosome (the protein-synthesizing

A organelle within its cell), which in micro-organisms is different to human cells. Antibiotics of the PENICILLIN and CEPHALOSPORIN families (collectively known as BETA-LACTAM antibiotics) attack the bacterial cell wall, whereas AMINOGLYCOSIDE and TETRACYCLINE antibiotics attack the ribosomes.

Viruses, which lack both cell walls and ribosomes, are therefore resistant to these and other similar antibiotics. Because there is such a diversity of pathogenic (disease-causing) micro-organisms, it is not surprising that specific infections are best treated using specific antibiotics developed to combat them.

Unfortunately, because of the widespread use of antibiotics certain strains of common bacteria have developed resistance to antibiotics that were once effective against them and this is has become a major problem. A mechanism by which bacteria become resistant is by the development of enzymes called PENICILLINASES, which break down penicillins and so limit an antibiotic's action. It has proved possible both to use drugs that inhibit these enzymes and, more directly, to develop *penicillinase-resistant* antibiotics. Another problem is the occurrence of *superinfections*, in which the use of a broad-spectrum antibiotic disturbs the normal, harmless bacterial population in the body, as well as the pathogenic ones.

In mild cases this may allow, for example, an existing but latent oral or vaginal thrush infection to become worse, or mild diarrhoea to develop. In rare cases the superinfection that develops is more serious than the disorder for which the antibiotic was administered.

*anticancer
drugs are used to treat cancer and most of them are CYTOTOXIC, that is, they work by interfering with cell replication or production, so preventing the growth of new cancerous tissue. Inevitably, this means that normal cell production is also affected, which causes serious side-effects. They are usually administered in combination in a series of treatments known collectively as *chemotherapy*.

In cases where the growth of a tumour is linked to the presence of a sex hormone (as with some cases of breast cancer or cancer of the prostate gland), treatment with sex hormones opposite to the patient's own sex can be extremely beneficial – though side-effects may be psychologically stressful. The CORTICOSTEROID drug PREDNISONE is also used as an anticancer drug in the treatment of the lymphatic cancer Hodgkin's disease and other forms of lymphoma and may also be helpful in halting the progress of hormone-linked breast cancer.

*anticholinergic
drugs inhibit the action, release, or production of the NEUROTRANSMITTER ACETYLCHOLINE, which plays an important part in the nervous system. The term is commonly used synonymously with ANTIMUSCARINIC (drugs that block the actions of acetylcholine at *muscarinic* RECEPTORS). Anticholinergic drugs (of the antimuscarinic type) tend to relax smooth (involuntary) muscle, reduce the secretion of saliva, digestive juices and sweat and dilate the pupil of the eye (mydriasis).

They can therefore be used as ANTISPASMODICS in the treatment of parkinsonian symptoms, peptic ulcer and to dilate the pupil for ophthalmic examinations.

Other uses include reversal of the adverse effects of overdose with anticholinesterases (in medicine, agricultural accidental poisoning, or warfare). However, the administration of such drugs is usually accompanied by side-effects, including dry mouth, dry skin, blurred vision, an increased heart rate, constipation and difficulty in urinating.

A number of other types of drug, for instance ANTIHISTAMINES, can also cause *anticholinergic side-effects*.

Examples of drugs used in medicine for their anticholinergic actions include: ATROPINE SULPHATE, BENZHEXOL HYDROCHLORIDE, BENZTROPINE MESYLATE, BIPERIDEN, CO-PHENOTROPE, CYCLOPENTOLATE HYDROCHLORIDE, FLAVOXATE HYDROCHLORIDE, GLYCOPYRRONIUM BROMIDE, HYOSCINE BUTYLBROMIDE, HYOSCINE HYDROBROMIDE, IPRATROPIUM BROMIDE, MEBEVERINE HYDROCHLORIDE, MEPENZOLATE BROMIDE, ORPHENADRINE CITRATE, ORPHENADRINE HYDROCHLORIDE, PIPENZOLATE BROMIDE, PIRENZEPINE, POLDINE METHYLSULPHATE, PROCYCLIDINE HYDROCHLORIDE, PROPANTHELINE BROMIDE and TROPICAMIDE.

The other main groups of anticholinergic drugs work at sites where acetylcholine interacts with *nicotinic* receptors (such as in the autonomic ganglia, skeletal neuromuscular junction and central nervous system) and have quite different actions. See: GANGLION-BLOCKERS and the SKELETAL MUSCLE RELAXANT

*anticholinesterase

is an ENZYME INHIBITOR drug. It inhibits certain enzymes (called cholinesterases) that are normally involved in the rapid breakdown of the natural NEUROTRANSMITTER acetylcholine.

Acetylcholine is released from *cholinergic* nerves and has many actions in the body. Consequently, since anticholinesterase drugs enhance the effects of acetylcholine on its release from these nerves, they may have a very wide range of actions and can be used for a variety of purposes.

In respect of their actions at the junction of nerves with skeletal (voluntary) muscles, anticholinesterases are used in the diagnosis and treatment of the muscle-weakness disease myesthenia

gravis. At the end of surgical operations in which SKELETAL MUSCLE RELAXANTS have been used, the anaesthetist is able to reverse the muscle paralysis by injecting an anticholinesterase.

In organs innervated by parasympathetic division of the autonomic nervous system, anticholinesterases cause an exaggeration of the nerves' actions – referred to as PARASYMPATHOMIMETIC actions – and they can be used for a number of purposes. These include stimulation of the bladder (in urinary retention), the intestine (in paralytic ileus) and the pupil of the eye (on local application in GLAUCOMA TREATMENT). However, anticholinesterases have a number of generally undesirable side-effects, such as slowing of the heart, constriction of the airways with excessive production of secretions and actions in the brain.

In anticholinesterase poisoning, their diverse actions can be life-threatening. Chemicals with anticholinesterase properties are used as insecticides (and in chemical warfare), so ANTIDOTES are required (eg PRALIDOXIME MESYLATE and ATROPINE SULPHATE). See: DISTIGMINE BROMIDE; NEOSTIGMINE; PYRIDOSTIGMINE; PHYSOSTIGMINE SULPHATE.

*anticoagulant

drugs prevent the clotting of blood and break up blood clots that have formed. The blood's own natural anticoagulant is HEPARIN, which is probably still the most effective anticoagulant known. Synthetic anticoagulants, such as WARFARIN SULPHATE, NICOUMALONE and PHENINDIONE, take longer to act.

Therapeutically, anticoagulants are used to prevent the formation of and to treat blood clots in, conditions such as thrombosis and embolism, especially following surgery. They are also used to prevent blood clots in patients fitted with a heart pacemaker or who have certain heart disorders.

*anticonvulsant

drugs are used to prevent the onset of epileptic seizures or to reduce their severity if they do occur. The best-known and most-used anticonvulsant is SODIUM VALPROATE, which is used to treat all forms of epilepsy. Other examples include CARBAMAZEPINE and PHENYTOIN, which are used to treat grand mal forms of epilepsy and ETHOSUXIMIDE, which is used to treat petit mal. In every case, dosage must be adjusted to the requirements of each individual patient. Anticonvulsant drugs may also be used to treat other types of convulsions, for instance, in drug or chemical poisoning. However, some of these drugs, such as CHLORPROMAZINE HYDROCHLORIDE and DIAZEPAM, are not effective or suitable for treating epilepsy. See ANTI-EPILEPTIC

*antidepressant

drugs are used to relieve the symptoms of depressive illness and are divided into three main groups.

The first and oldest, group are the TRICYCLIC antidepressants (named after the chemical structure of the original members), such as AMITRIPTYLINE HYDROCHLORIDE, IMIPRAMINE HYRDOCHLORIDE and DOXEPIN. They are effective in alleviating a number of depressive symptoms, but have ANTICHOLINERGIC side-effects. Most drugs of this class also have SEDATIVE properties, which in some is quite pronounced (especially amitriptyline hydrochloride, which may be beneficial in some anxious and agitated patients).

The second group consists of the MONOAMINE-OXIDASE INHIBITORS (MAOIs) eg ISOCARBOXAZID, TRANYLCYPROMINE and PHENELZINE, which are now used less frequently because they have severe side-effects, particularly through interaction with constituents of foodstuffs.

The third type of antidepressant and the most recently developed, is the SSRIs, for example FLUOXETINE, which are named after their mechanisms of action (*selective serotonin re-uptake inhibitors*).

Also used is the amino acid TRYPTOPHAN, which may sometimes be administered when other classes of antidepressant have not been effective and LITHIUM, which is used to treat manic-depression and related illnesses and for preventing certain types of recurrent depression.

The ANTIPSYCHOTIC drug FLUPENTHIXOL is occasionally used (at a much lower dose) as an antidepressant. Electroconvulsive therapy is sometimes very effective in severe depression. Treatment with antidepressant drugs often takes some weeks to show maximal beneficial effects. (See individual class entries for more detail.)

*antidiarrhoeal

drugs prevent the onset of diarrhoea, or assist in treating it if already present. The main medical treatment while diarrhoea lasts, however, is always the replacement of fluids and minerals.
Because there is a perceived need on the part of the general public, antidiarrhoeal preparations are generally available without prescription. Many are adsorbent mixtures that bind faecal material into solid masses.

These mixtures include preparations containing KAOLIN or METHYLCELLULOSE, which may also be useful in controlling faecal consistency for patients who have undergone colostomy or ileostomy. Other antidiarrhoeals, such as ANTIMOTILITY drugs, work by reducing peristalsis (the movement of the intestine), which slows down the movement of faecal material. OPIOIDS such as CODEINE PHOSPHATE and MORPHINE SULPHATE are efficient at this.

Diarrhoea caused by inflammatory disorders, such as irritable bowel syndrome, ulcerative colitis and Crohn's disease may be relieved by treatment with CORTICOSTEROIDS or AMINOSALICYLATES.

antidiuretic hormone
See VASOPRESSIN

*antidote
drugs are used to counteract poisons or overdose with other drugs. They are used in a wide variety of circumstances and can work in many ways. First, the most straightforward and commonly used method is where the poison works by stimulating, or over-stimulating, a distinct pharmacological RECEPTOR, since here the appropriate receptor ANTAGONIST can be used to reduce or completely block the effects of the poison. For example, NALOXONE HYDROCHLORIDE is an OPIOID ANTAGONIST and can be used as an antidote to an overdose of an (OPIOID) NARCOTIC ANALGESIC (including DIAMORPHINE; heroin) and being quick-acting it effectively reverses the respiratory depression, coma, or convulsions that result from such an overdose. It can also be used at the end of operations to reverse respiratory depression caused by narcotic analgesics and in newborn babies where mothers have been administered large amounts of opioid (such as pethidine) for pain relief during labour.

Second, poisoning by some agents is best counteracted by using an antidote that binds to the poison, rendering it relatively inert and facilitating its excretion from the body. For example, a CHELATING AGENT is used as an antidote to metal poisoning because it chemically binds to certain metallic ions and other substances, making them less toxic and allowing their excretion from the body. Chelating agents are used to treat too high levels of metals due to external origin (accidental or environmental), abnormal metabolism (eg high levels of copper in Wilson's disease), or a disease (eg penicillamine in rheumatoid arthritis). Examples of chelating agents are: DESFERRIOXAMINE MESYLATE, DICOBALT EDETATE, DIMERCAPROL, PENICILLAMINE and SODIUM CALCIUMEDETATE.

An ANTIVENOM is an antidote to the poison in a snakebite, a scorpion's sting, or a bite from any other poisonous creature (such as a spider). Normally, it is an ANTISERUM and is injected into the bloodstream for immediate relief (though it has its own adverse side-effects).

DIGIBIND is a proprietary drug that comprises antibody fragments that react with the glycosides and is used in the emergency treatment of an overdose of CARDIAC GLYCOSIDES, eg DIGOXIN and DIGITOXIN.

ACETYLCYSTEINE and METHIONINE are used as antidotes to treat overdose poisoning by the ANALGESIC paracetamol. The initial symptoms of paracetamol poisoning usually settle within 24 hours, but give way to serious toxic effect on the liver which takes some days to develop. It is to prevent these latter effects that treatment is directed and is required immediately after overdose. The antidotes work by chemically reacting with toxic products made by the liver from paracetamol when it is taken in excessive amounts.

A different principle is used with ANTICHOLINESTERASE poisoning. These ENZYME INHIBITOR drugs are used in medicine, as insecticides and in chemical warfare. PRALIDOXIME MESYLATE is an antidote that actually reactivates the cholinesterase enzyme after it has been poisoned and is highly effective (taken in conjunction with other drugs) in preventing the life-endangering chemical changes to the anticholinesterase enzymes.

In all cases of poisoning, prompt action in using an antidote is necessary.

anti-D (Rh₀) immunoglobulin
(anti-D immunoglobulin) for IMMUNIZATION is a SPECIFIC IMMUNOGLOBULIN that is used to prevent rhesus-negative mothers from making antibodies against foetal rhesus-positive cells that may pass into the mother's

A

circulation during childbirth or abortion, so protecting a future child from haemolytic disease of the newborn. Anti-D (Rh$_0$) immunoglobulin should be injected within a few days of birth.

○ Related entry: Partobulin

antidysrrhythmic drugs
See ANTI-ARRHYTHMIC DRUGS

*anti-emetic
drugs prevent actual vomiting, whereas ANTINAUSEANT drugs are used to reduce or prevent the *sensation* of nausea that very often precedes the physical process of vomiting. Anti-emetic drugs are used to help reduce the vomiting that accompanies radiotherapy and chemotherapy by actually preventing vomiting and helping the passage of food out of the stomach; that is, they act as gastric MOTILITY STIMULANTS (eg METOCLOPRAMIDE and CISAPRIDE).

*anti-epileptic
drugs are used to prevent the occurrence of epileptic seizures. In order to achieve this an effective concentration of the drug must be maintained in the plasma and so the dose varies according to each patient's requirements.

Generally, only one drug is required at any one time and the drug of choice depends on the type and severity of the epilepsy. CARBAMAZEPINE, PHENYTOIN and SODIUM VALPROATE are the drugs of choice for *tonic-clonic seizures* (grand mal) as part of a syndrome of primary generalized epilepsy; ETHOSUXIMIDE and sodium valproate are used for *absence seizures* (petit mal); and CLONAZEPAM, ethosuximide and sodium valproate for *myoclonic seizures*.

For other types of seizure such as atypical absence, atonic and tonic seizures (often in childhood), phenytoin, sodium valproate, clonazepam, phenobarbitone, or ethosuximide are often used. See also ANTICONVULSANT

*antifoaming agent
is a chemical incorporated into ANTACID preparations in order to lower surface tension so that small bubbles of froth coalesce into large bubbles, which allows the remedy to pass more easily through the intestine. The most effective are silicone polymers such as DIMETHICONE.

*antifungal
drugs are ANTIMICROBIAL drugs that are used to treat infections caused by fungal micro-organisms and are often ANTIBIOTICS that are produced naturally or synthetically. Fungal infections are usually not a major problem in healthy, well-nourished individuals.

However, superficial, localized infections such as thrush (caused by *Candida albicans*), athlete's foot and ringworm (caused by fungi of the dermatophyte group) are common. Severe infections occur most frequently in situations where the host's immunity is low, for example following immunosuppression for transplant surgery.

Under such conditions fungi that are not normally pathogenic (disease-causing) can exploit their host's altered state and cause infection.

Unfortunately, the most potent antifungal drugs also tend to be highly toxic and therefore severe systemic fungal infections remain an ever present danger. NYSTATIN and IMIDAZOLE drugs, such as CLOTRIMAZOLE, are often used for local treatment. AMPHOTERICIN and FLUCYTOSINE are reserved for systemic fungal infections. The commonest form of fungal infection in childhood is thrush, which usually occurs in the mouth and nappy area of infants and is usually treated with the topical application of MICONAZOLE.

*antihistamine
(H$_1$-antagonist) drugs inhibit the effects of histamine in the body. Histamine is

antihypertensive

A

released naturally as the result of a patient coming into contact with a substance to which he or she is allergically sensitive (i.e. allergic to) and causes various symptoms such as hay fever, urticaria (itchy skin rash), itching (pruritus), or even asthma-like bronchoconstriction.

Many agents can act as triggers for histamine release, including inhalation of pollen, insect bites and stings, contact with some metal objects, food constituents, food dye additives, a number of drug types (notably penicillin ANTIBIOTICS, LOCAL ANAESTHETICS, MORPHINE and, potentially, all drugs of a protein or peptide nature) and many environmental factors. Consequently, antihistamines may be used for many purposes, but particularly for the symptomatic relief of allergy such as hay fever and urticaria and in the acute treatment of anaphylactic shock (an extreme and generalized reaction, sometimes life-threatening, with the release of histamine causing general swelling (oedema), bronchoconstriction (narrowing of the airways), heart failure and collapse of the blood circulation).

Many antihistamines also have ANTI-EMETIC properties and are therefore used to prevent vomiting associated with travel sickness, vertigo, or the effects of chemotherapy. All but some recently developed antihistamines produce drowsiness and this SEDATIVE action may be used to help induce sleep.

Conventionally, only the older antihistamine drugs, which act on histamine H_1-receptors, are referred to by the general name *antihistamines* without qualification. However, somewhat confusingly, the newer and extensively prepscribed drugs that can be used as ULCER-HEALING DRUGS (eg CIMETIDINE and RANITIDINE) are also antihistamines, but they act on H_2-receptors that are involved in gastric secretion and so are referred to as H_2-ANTAGONISTS.

✚ side effects: following oral or systemic administration, there is commonly drowsiness, headache, impaired muscular co-ordination or dizziness, anticholinergic effects (dry mouth, blurred vision, urinary retention, gastrointestinal disturbances), occasional rashes and photosensitivity, palpitations and heart arrhythmias. Rarely, there may be paradoxical stimulation, especially in children, hypersensitivity reactions, blood disorders, liver disturbances, depression, sleep disturbances and hypotension.

▲ warning: administer with caution to patients with epilepsy, hypertrophy of the prostate gland, glaucoma, liver disease, or porphyria; or who are pregnant or breast-feeding. Those antihistamines with sedative actions may impair the performance of skilled tasks such as driving; and the sedative effect is enhanced by alcohol.

See: ACRIVASTINE; ANTAZOLINE; ASTEMIZOLE; AZATADINE MALEATE; AZELASTINE HYDROCHLORIDE; BROMPHENIRAMINE MALEATE; BUCLIZINE HYDROCHLORIDE; CETIRIZINE; CHLORPHENIRAMINE MALEATE; CINNARIZINE; CLEMASTINE; CYCLIZINE; CYPROHEPTADINE HYDROCHLORIDE; DIMENHYDRINATE; DIPHENHYDRAMINE HYDROCHLORIDE; DIPHENYLPYRALINE HYDROCHLORIDE; DIPIPANONE; DOXYLAMINE SUCCINATE; HYDROXYZINE HYDROCHLORIDE; KETOTIFEN; LORATADINE; MECLOZINE HYDROCHLORIDE; MEQUITAZINE; OXATOMIDE; PHENINDAMINE TARTRATE; PHENIRAMINE MALEATE; PIZOTIFEN; PROMETHAZINE HYDROCHLORIDE; PROMETHAZINE THEOCLATE; TERFENADINE; TRIMEPRAZINE TARTRATE; TRIPROLIDINE HYDROCHLORIDE.

*antihypertensive

drugs reduce hypertension (an elevation of arterial blood pressure above the normal range expected in a particular age group and sex and having several different causes) and so reduce a patient's risk of heart attacks, kidney failure, or stroke. Many are also used to treat angina pectoris (heart pain). There are several large groups of drugs used as antihypertensives, each with a specific

A

mode of action, but before any drugs are administered a check should be made on the patient's diet and lifestyle to see if therapy without drugs can be advised. DIURETIC drugs act as antihypertensives and often a mild diuretic may be all that is required.

If further treatment is necessary, any of the BETA-BLOCKERS may be used, with or without simultaneous administration of a diuretic. Other treatments include the use of a VASODILATOR, such as a CALCIUM-CHANNEL BLOCKER (eg NIFEDIPINE) or HYDRALAZINE HYDROCHLORIDE. Some antihypertensive drugs act on the brain centre responsible for controlling blood pressure (eg METHYLDOPA) and ADRENERGIC NEURONE BLOCKING DRUGS (eg DEBRISOQUINE) reduce the release of noradrenaline from sympathetic nerves, which are involved in controlling blood pressure. Individuals having antihypertensive treatment require regular medical checks and blood-pressure monitoring.

*anti-inflammatory

drugs are used to reduce inflammation – the body's response to injury. Although inflammation is essentially a normal defensive mechanism (eg a reaction to tissue injury, infection, or inhalation of foreign proteins), the manifestations may be so serious and inappropriate, or involve such discomfort, that treatment with anti-inflammatory drugs is required. Inflammatory conditions can be acute (eg insect strings) or chronic (eg chronic asthma, dermatitis and other skin conditions).

The NSAID (non-steroidal anti-inflammatory) drugs, such as ASPIRIN and IBUPROFEN, can give effective relief from inflammatory pain, tissue swelling, joint immobilization and can also lower raised body temperature, which means that they are often the first choice of treatment. They work by inhibiting the production and release in the body of

pro-inflammatory LOCAL HORMONE mediators (the PROSTAGLANDINS) and, used with care, they can be relatively free of side-effects. For more serious conditions, CORTICOSTEROID drugs may be required, but they can cause so many complications that they are normally only given by local application (eg as creams, or by inhalation into the lungs for asthma) with systemic injection reserved for emergencies such as *anaphylactic shock* (an extreme and generalized reaction, sometimes life-threatening; with the release of histamine causing general swelling (oedema; accumulation of fluid in the tissues), bronchoconstriction (narrowing of the airways), heart failure and collapse of blood circulation).

There are a number of other types of anti-inflammatory drugs, including SODIUM CROMOGLYCATE, the ANTIRHEUMATIC drugs (which are used to relieve the pain and inflammation of rheumatoid arthritis and osteoarthritis) and gold (in the form of PENICILLAMINE and SODIUM AUROTHIOMALATE).

The IMMUNOSUPPRESSANT drugs (eg CYCLOPHOSPHAMIDE, CYCLOSPORIN and METHOTREXATE) are reserved for the prevention of tissue rejection (eg in transplants) and are sometimes used to treat autoimmune diseases, such as rheumatoid arthritis and lupus, when they are unresponsive to less toxic drugs.

*antimalarial

drugs are used to treat or prevent malaria. Malaria is caused by infection of the red blood cells by a small organism called a protozoan (of the genus *Plasmodium*), which is carried by several species of mosquito of the genus *Anopheles*. Infection occurs as a result of a mosquito's bite. The class of drug most commonly used to treat or prevent infection are the quinidines, of which CHLOROQUINE is the standard. However, in some parts of the world certain forms of the protozoan that causes malaria are resistant to chloroquine. In such cases, QUININE, the traditional remedy for malaria, is used. It may also be used in patients who cannot tolerate chloroquine. Although the prevention of malaria by drugs cannot be guaranteed, administration of antimalarial drugs before, during and for a period after, travelling to a tropical place is recommended for protection. See: HALOFANTRINE HYDROCHLORIDE; MEFLOQUINE; PRIMAQUINE; PROGUANIL HYDROCHLORIDE; PYRIMETHAMINE

*antimania

drugs are used to treat manic-depressive illness, which is characterized by periods of mood normality punctuated by episodes of *mania* and bouts of *depression*. Because of these mood swings around the norm, the disorder is sometimes called *bipolar disorder*. The manic phase most often requires acute treatment and initially ANTIPSYCHOTIC drugs (eg PHENOTHIAZINE DERIVATIVES are usually administered. Thereafter, a very different psychoactive drug, LITHIUM, may gradually be substituted in most patients and this can prevent or reduce the frequency and severity of attacks.

*antimicrobials

are drugs used to treat infections caused by microbes (micro-organisms), which includes the major classes of pathogenic (disease-causing) micro-organisms covered in this book – viruses, mycoplasma, rickettsia, chlamydia, protozoa, bacteria and fungi (but not helminths; worms). The term therefore embraces ANTIBACTERIALS, ANTIBIOTICS, ANTIPROTOZOALS, ANTIVIRALS and ANTIFUNGALS

*antimigraine

drugs are used to treat migraine, which is a specific, clinically recognized form of headache and not simply a particularly severe headache. Migraine attacks vary in

form, but common characteristics include the following, a throbbing confined to one side of the head (*unilateral headache*), nausea and vomiting and a forewarning of an attack (an *aura*) consisting of visual disturbances and weakness or numbness of the limbs.

Drugs are used to help migraine sufferers (and also the related condition called 'cluster headache') in two quite distinct ways. One group of drugs is given chronically (i.e. long-term) in order to help prevent attacks (prophylactic use), for example, CALCIUM-CHANNEL BLOCKER drugs (eg NIFEDIPINE and VERAPAMIL HYDROCHLORIDE), BETA-BLOCKERS (eg METOPROLOL TARTRATE, NADOLOL, PROPANOLOL HYDROCHLORIDE and TIMOLOL MALEATE), CYPROHEPTADINE HYDROCHLORIDE and METHYSERGIDE.

All these drugs affect blood vessels in some way. In migraine attacks, blood vessels in the head and scalp are thought to narrow (constrict) before an attack and then widen (dilate) causing the pain during an attack. A second group of drugs may be used either at the *aura* stage or during the attack itself and for maximum effect speed of administration and subsequent absorption of the drug is an all-important factor. A number of ANALGESICS can be used to offset the pain of an attack (eg ASPIRIN, CODEINE PHOSPHATE and PARACETAMOL) and are often incorporated into COMPOUND PREPARATIONS together with a variety of drugs and drug types (eg CAFFEINE, BUCLIZINE HYDROCHLORIDE, DOXYLAMINE SUCCINATE, ISOMETHEPTENE MUCATE and PIZOTIFEN).

Sometimes drugs with ANTINAUSEANT or ANTI-EMETIC properties are included (eg CYCLIZINE and METOCLOPRAMIDE HYDROCHLORIDE). Drugs that affect blood vessels can also be used during the attack stage, including the widely used drug ERGOTAMINE TARTRATE and the recently introduced drug SUMATRIPTAN, which can be self-injected to achieve a rapid onset of

A action. In all cases, the appropriate combination of drugs will vary from individual to individual and also a certain amount of experimentation may be necessary to identify the factors that trigger a migraine attack (eg certain foods).

*antimuscarinic

drugs are one of the main classes that make up the ANTICHOLINERGIC group of drugs. All the anticholinergic drugs act by inhibiting the action, release, or production of the NEUROTRANSMITTER ACETYLCHOLINE, which plays an important part in the central and peripheral nervous systems. The term *anticholinergic* is commonly and incorrectly, used synonymously with antimuscarinic drugs because so many antimuscarinics are used in medicine.

Drugs that block the actions of acetylcholine at *muscarinic* RECEPTORS (i.e. antimuscarinic drugs) tend to relax smooth muscle, reduce the secretion of saliva, digestive juices and sweat and dilate the pupil of the eye. They may be used as ANTISPASMODICS, ANTIPARKINSONIAN drugs (in the treatment of some symptoms of parkinsonian disease), as ANTINAUSEANTS or ANTI-EMETICS in the treatment of motion sickness, to treat peptic ulcers, in ophthalmic examinations and in antagonizing adverse effects of ANTICHOLINESTERASES (in medicine, agricultural accidental poisoning, or warfare).

Examples of antimuscarinic anticholinergic drugs include: ATROPINE SULPHATE, ATROPINE METHONITRATE, BENZHEXOL HYDROCHLORIDE, BENZTROPINE MESYLATE, BIPERIDEN, CO-PHENOTROPE, CYCLOPENTOLATE HYDROCHLORIDE, FLAVOXATE HYDROCHLORIDE, GLYCOPYRRONIUM BROMIDE, HYOSCINE BUTYLBROMIDE, HYOSCINE HYDROBROMIDE, IPRATROPIUM BROMIDE, MEPENZOLATE BROMIDE, ORPHENADRINE CITRATE, ORPHENADRINE HYDROCHLORIDE, PIPENZOLATE BROMIDE, PIRENZEPINE, POLDINE METHYLSULPHATE, PROCYCLIDINE HYDROCHLORIDE, PROPANTHELINE BROMIDE and TROPICAMIDE.

The other main groups of anticholinergic drugs are the SKELETAL MUSCLE RELAXANTS (eg TUBOCURARINE CHLORIDE) and the GANGLION-BLOCKERS. These drugs interact with *nicotinic* cholinergic receptors (at which NICOTINE is a powerful stimulant) rather than with *muscarinic* cholinergic receptors (which are powerfully stimulated by the plant ALKALOID muscarine; derived from the poisonous mushroom *Amanita muscaria*).

*antinauseant

drugs are used to prevent or minimize the feeling of nausea and to reduce any subsequent vomiting. The type of drug used and the likelihood of its success, depends on the mechanism and origin of the nausea, which can be triggered in a number of ways. Motion sickness, or travel sickness, can often be prevented by taking antinauseants like HYOSCINE HYDROBROMIDE, MECLOZINE HYDROCHLORIDE and DIMENHYDRATE before travelling.

Similar drugs may be used to treat nausea and other symptoms of labyrinthine disease (where the vestibular balance mechanisms of the inner ear are disturbed, eg Ménière's disease), though other drugs may also be necessary, such as CINNARIZINE and PHENOTHIAZINE DERIVATIVES like CHLORPROMAZINE HYDROCHLORIDE and PROCHLORPERAZINE.

A number of chemicals and drugs induce nausea and vomiting by an action involving the so-called *chemoreceptor trigger zone* within the brain; for instance, this is the most common side-effect when using the (OPIOID) NARCOTIC ANALGESIC drug morphine and so it may be combined with cinnarizine. The nausea and vomiting that is caused by chemotherapy and radiotherapy can be difficult to treat.

A

However, some ANTI-EMETIC drugs, such as MOTILITY STIMULANTS (eg METOCLOPRAMIDE and CISAPRIDE), may be of some use by preventing vomiting and helping food out of the stomach.

Alternatively, there are some recently developed drugs that can also be effective, for instance certain inhibitors of the actions of the mediator SEROTONIN (5-HT$_3$ antagonists) such as GRANISETRON, ONDANSETRON and TROPISETRON. The cannabis derivative NABILONE may be administered in difficult cases.

*anti-oestrogen
(oestrogen antagonists) drugs are a class of HORMONE ANTAGONISTS that usually act directly to prevent the actions of female SEX HORMONES, the OESTROGENS (OESTRADIOL and OESTRIOL), at their target tissues; although they sometimes act indirectly to prevent the formation, or inhibit the release, of the hormones. An example of a drug that acts by the direct mechanism is TAMOXIFEN and of those that act indirectly are AMINOGLUTETHIMIDE and FORMESTANE.

*antiparkinsonism
drugs are used to treat parkinsonism, which is the name used to describe the symptoms of several disorders of the central nervous system, including muscle tremor and rigidity (extrapyramidal symptoms), especially in the limbs. It is caused by an imbalance in the actions of NEUROTRANSMITTERS such as ACETYLCHOLINE and DOPAMINE. In classic Parkinson's disease this is due to the degeneration of dopamine-containing nerves. However, what are known as parkinsonian extrapyramidal side-effects may be caused by treatment with several types of drugs, especially ANTIPSYCHOTICS (eg HALOPERIDOL).

Treatment of parkinsonism may be by ANTICHOLINERGIC drugs (eg BENZHEXOL HYDROCHLORIDE, BENZTROPINE MESYLATE, BIPERIDEN and PROCYCLIDINE

HYDROCHLORIDE), or by drugs that increase the effects of dopamine (eg LEVODOPA, BROMOCRIPTINE and PERGOLIDE). The former class is more useful for controlling fine tremor, including that induced by drugs and the latter class for overcoming difficulty in commencing movement and slowness brought about by degenerative disease. It is a difficult and often lengthy process to achieve the optimum dose in each patient and there are certain side-effects (such as confusion in the elderly) that occur with all the various treatments.

*antiperspirant
substances help to prevent sweating. Medically, they are required only in cases of severe hyperhidrosis (excessive sweating), when some disorder of the sweat glands causes constant and streaming perspiration. In such cases, ALUMINIUM CHLORIDE solution is an effective treatment and dusting powders may also be useful to dry the skin.

*antiplatelet
drugs (also known as antithrombotic drugs) prevent the formation of blood clots (thrombi), that is, they reduce platelet aggregation. These drugs can be used as a preventive treatment (prophylactic use) in patients who are at risk, for instance, after a heart attack or bypass operation. However, this same action may also increase bleeding time and so patients receiving ANTICOAGULANT drugs should not normally have antiplatelet drugs as well. The antiplatelet drug DIPYRIDAMOLE does not act as an anticoagulant, but instead seems to work by stopping platelets sticking together (or to surgically inserted tubes or artificial heart valves). EPOPROSTENOL (PROSTACYCLIN) is a naturally occurring prostaglandin present in the walls of blood vessels, which has antiplatelet activity when administered therapeutically by intravenous infusion.

A

Antipressan

(Berk) is a proprietary, prescription-only preparation of the BETA-BLOCKER drug atenolol. It can be used as an ANTIHYPERTENSIVE treatment for raised blood pressure, as an ANTI-ANGINA treatment to relieve symptoms and improve exercise tolerance and as an ANTI-ARRHYTHMIC to regularize heartbeat and to treat myocardial infarction. It is available as tablets.

+▲ side-effects/warning: see ATENOLOL

*antiprotozoal

drugs are used to treat or prevent infections caused by micro-organisms called protozoa. The most important protozoa, in terms of illness and death, are those of the genus *Plasmodium*, which cause malaria (see ANTIMALARIAL). Other major protozoal diseases found in tropical countries include trypanosomiasis, leishmaniasis and amoebic dysentery. Protozoal infections more familiar in this country include toxoplasmosis, trichomoniasis and giardiasis. A common form of pneumonia is caused in immunosuppressed patients (including those suffering from AIDS) by the protozoan *Pneumocystis carinii*. The drugs used to treat amoebic-protozoal infections are commonly referred to as AMOEBICIDAL drugs.

*antipsychotic

or neuroleptic, drugs calm and soothe patients without impairing consciousness. They are used mainly to treat psychologically disturbed patients, particularly those who manifest the complex behavioural patterns of schizophrenia. In the short-term, they can also be used to treat severe anxiety. They may also worsen, or help to alleviate, depression because they can affect mood. Antipsychotics work by acting in the brain, especially through an effect (inhibition) involving the NEUROTRANSMITTER DOPAMINE. They can cause many

side-effects, including abnormal face and body movements and restlessness, which often resemble the symptoms of the condition being treated. The use of other drugs may be required to control these side-effects. Notable examples of antipsychotic drugs include FLUPENTHIXOL, HALOPERIDOL and the PHENOTHIAZINE DERIVATIVES (especially CHLORPROMAZINE HYDROCHLORIDE and THIORIDAZINE). BENPERIDOL is used mostly to control antisocial sexual behaviour or hyperactivity. Those antipsychotics with markedly depressant side-effects are also, somewhat misleadingly, known as *major tranquillizers*.

*antipyretic

drugs reduce raised body temperature, for example in fever, but they do not lower normal body temperature. Best-known and most-used antipyretic drugs include certain NON-NARCOTIC ANALGESICS such as ASPIRIN, PARACETAMOL and IBUPROFEN. See also: NSAID

Antirabies Immunoglobulin Injection

See RABIES IMMUNOGLOBULIN

*antirheumatic

drugs are used to relieve the pain and inflammation of rheumatism and arthritis (particularly rheumatoid arthritis and osteoarthritis and so they are also known as *anti-arthritic drugs*) and sometimes of other musculoskeletal disorders. The primary form of treatment is with NON-STEROIDAL ANTI-INFLAMMATORY (NSAID) NON-NARCOTIC ANALGESICS such as ASPIRIN, SODIUM SALICYLATE, the aspirin-paracetamol ester BENORYLATE, INDOMETHACIN, FENOPROFEN, IBUPROFEN and PHENYLBUTAZONE. The CORTICOSTEROIDS can also be used because they are anti-inflammatory (eg PREDNISOLONE and TRIAMCINOLONE). Finally, there are some drugs that seem to halt the progression of musculoskeletal disorders, for example AURANOFIN and SODIUM AUROTHIOMALATE (which both contain gold) and PENICILLAMINE. However, some of these drugs have unpleasant side-effects and others can take up to six months to have any effect. In cases where there is an autoimmune element to the disease, IMMUNOSUPPRESSANT drugs (eg AZATHIOPRINE, CHLORAMBUCIL, CYCLOPHOSPHAMIDE, CYCLOSPORIN and METHOTREXATE) can also be used.

Antirubella Immunoglobulin Injection
See RUBELLA IMMUNOGLOBULIN

*antiseborrhoeic
drugs are used to treat seborrhoea, which is an excessive secretion of the oily substance sebum from the sebaceous glands of the skin and the glands are often enlarged, especially beside the nose. Over-secretion is common in adolescence and often results in acne or seborrhoeic eczema. Dandruff often appears during the development of seborrhoeic eczema.

*antiseptic
is an agent that destroys micro-organisms or inhibits their activity to such an extent that they are less, or no longer, harmful to health. Antiseptics can be applied to the skin, burns, or wounds to prevent infections and to limit the spread of pathogenic (disease-causing) micro-organisms. The term is often used synonymously with DISINFECTANT. However, the latter term can also apply to agents used on inanimate objects (such as surgical equipment, catheters, etc.), as well as to agents used on the skin and other living tissue.

*antiserum
is a general term that is used to describe certain preparations of blood serum rich in particular antibodies. Antiserum preparations (*antisera*) are used to provide what is called *passive immunity* to diseases, or some measure of treatment if the disease has already been contracted.

The common term used to describe that part of a disease-causing entity which is recognized by the immune system is *antigen*. If an antigen is injected into an animal, the animal produces *antibodies* in response. An antiserum is a preparation of animal blood serum containing these antibodies. Most antisera are prepared from the blood of antigen-treated horses, which are then purified and administered to humans to immunize them against disease. However, because they are *foreign* proteins, serious hypersensitivity reactions may result and, at the most extreme, cause anaphylactic shock. For this reason, such animal preparations are now rarely used and have to a large extent been replaced by preparations of human antibodies from human antiserum preparations, usually referred to simply as as *immunoglobulins*.

However, DIPHTHERIA ANTITOXIN prepared from horses is still used for passive immunization in circumstances where contraction of the disease is suspected.

⊙ Related entry: ZAGREB ANTIVENOM

*antispasmodic
or spasmolytic, drugs relieve spasm in smooth muscle (involuntary muscles, eg muscles in the respiratory tract and the intestinal walls) and form part of the group of drugs known collectively as SMOOTH MUSCLE RELAXANTS. Some are used as BRONCHODILATORS while others are used to relieve abdominal pain due to intestinal colic. They include the ANTICHOLINERGIC drugs such as ATROPINE SULPHATE and agents such as MEBEVERINE HYDROCHLORIDE which act directly on smooth muscle.

*antisympathetic
drugs act at some site or other within the sympathetic nervous system to reduce its

A

overall effect. Since activity within this division of the (autonomic) nervous system controls blood pressure and heart rate, then drugs that act to reduce its activity cause a fall in blood pressure and so the main use of such drugs is in ANTIHYPERTENSIVE treatment.

There are a number of sites and mechanisms by which such drugs act. For example, METHYLDOPA acts in the brain itself to reduce the activity of the sympathetic nervous system, while METIROSINE inhibits the enzymes that produce NORADRENALINE (the sympathetic NEUROTRANSMITTER) within the nerves. The ADRENERGIC NEURONE BLOCKER DRUGS (BETHANIDINE SULPHATE, BRETYLIUM TOSYLATE, DEBRISOQUINE and GUANETHIDINE MONOSULPHATE) interfere with the storage and release of noradrenaline and the drug CLONIDINE HYDROCHLORIDE decreases the amount that is released.

All these drugs have quite marked side-effects and some of them may be administered in comjunction with other classes of antihypertensive drugs, for instance the DIURETICS.

Antitetanus Immunoglobulin Injection
See TETANUS IMMUNOGLOBULIN

*antithrombotic
drugs prevent formation of blood clots (thrombi). See ANTIPLATELET

*antithyroid
drugs are used in the treatment of over-activity of the thyroid gland (hyperthyriodism; thyrotoxicosis). In thyrotoxicosis there is an excess secretion of THYROID HORMONES and this results in an exaggeration of the normal activity of the gland, which causes increased metabolic rate, raised body temperature, sweating, increased sensitivity to heat, nervousness, tremor, raised heart rate, tendency to fatigue and sometimes loss of

body weight with an increased appetite.

How the disease is treated depends on its origin, but if it is severe the surgical removal of part of the gland may be necessary, though more commonly the gland is treated with radioactive iodine to reduce the number of cells.

In any event, drugs are used to either control the symptoms in the long term, or in the short term to prepare the gland for more radical intervention. BETA-BLOCKERS (eg METOPROLOL TARTRATE, NADOLOL, PROPRANOLOL HYDROCHLORIDE and SOTALOL HYDROCHLORIDE) are widely used in the prevention of a number of the signs and symptoms of thyrotoxicosis and work by blocking the effects of over-stimulation of the release of ADRENALINE and NORADRENALINE by thyroid hormones, but do not treat the gland itself.

Some other drugs (chemically thionamides, eg CARBIMAZOLE and PROPYLTHIOURACIL) act directly on the thyroid gland to reduce the production of the thyroid hormones, so treating the excess of thyroid hormones in the blood. Iodine itself, which is chemically incorporated into the thyroid hormones THYROXINE and TRIIODOTHYRONINE, can be given (as AQUEOUS IODINE ORAL SOLUTION, or Lugol's solution) to suppress gland activity prior to thyroid surgery.

*antitubercular
(or antituberculous) drugs are used in combination to treat tuberculosis. The initial phase of treatment usually involves three drugs (commonly ISONIAZID, RIFAMPICIN and PYRAZINAMIDE) in order to tackle the disease as efficiently as possible, while reducing the risk of encountering bacterial resistance.

If, after about two months, the first phase is successful, treatment usually continues with only two of the initial three drugs (one of which is often isoniazid or rifampicin).

If the first line of treatment is not successful, for example because the patient suffered intolerable side-effects or because the disease was resistant to the drugs, then other drugs are used.

Treatment of tuberculosis with drugs is only necessary where the far more effective public health measure of vaccination has, for some reason, failed (see BCG VACCINE).

antituberculous
See ANTITUBERCULAR

*antitussive
drugs assist the treatment of coughs. The term is usually used to describe only those drugs that suppress coughing, rather than drugs used to treat the cause of coughing. Cough suppressants include OPIATES such as DEXTROMETHORPHAN HYDROBROMIDE, CODEINE PHOSPHATE and METHADONE HYDROCHLORIDE. They tend to cause constipation as a side-effect and so should not be used for prolonged periods.

Other antitussive preparations are EXPECTORANTS and DEMULCENTS. Expectorants are drugs used to decrease the viscosity of mucus or to increase the secretion of liquid mucus in dry, irritant, unproductive coughs. Expectorants include AMMONIUM CHLORIDE, GUAIPHENESIN and IPECACUANHA; and these are incorporated into many proprietary compound cough medicines. Demulcents also help to reduce the viscosity of mucus and relieve dry, unproductive coughs. All of these drugs are used to soothe coughs rather than to treat the underlying cause, such as an infection.

Antivaricella-Zoster Immunoglobulin
See VARICELLA-ZOSTER IMMUNOGLOBULIN (VZIG)

antivenin
See ANTIVENOM

*antivenom
(antivenin) is an antidote to the poison in a snakebite, a scorpion's sting, or a bite from any other poisonous creature (such as a spider).

Normally, it is an ANTISERUM and is injected into the bloodstream for immediate relief. Identification of the poisonous creature is important so that the right antidote can be selected.

In the UK the only indigenous poisonous snake is the adder (*Vipera berus*), the poison of which can usually be treated by medical supportive therapy, but on occasion require treatment with ZAGREB ANTIVENOM. Antivenoms have been prepared internationally for many foreign snakes, insects and spiders. Some of these are available in the UK for emergency use and are available from regional centres in London, Liverpool and Oxford).

+▲ side-effects/warning: because antivenoms are themselves foreign proteins, hypersensitivity reactions are not uncommon and may compound the symptoms and distress caused by the bite itself, therefore antivenoms should not be used except where symptoms are severe.

*antiviral
drugs are used to treat infections caused by viruses. There are relatively few antivirals and their effectiveness is often restricted to preventive or disease-limitation treatment. Some antiviral drugs can be life-savers, especially in immunocompromised patients. Infections due to the herpes viruses (eg cold sores, genital herpes, shingles and chickenpox) may be prevented or contained by early treatment with ACYCLOVIR. Serious cytomegaloviral infections may also be contained by treatment with GANCICLOVIR. ZIDOVUDINE (azidothymidine; AZT) is an antiviral drug that is used in the management of AIDS.

Anturan
(Geigy) is a proprietary, prescription-only preparation of the drug sulphinpyrazone. It can be used to treat and prevent gout

A

and hyperurea. It is available as tablets.
+▲ side-effects/warning: see
SULPHINPYRAZONE

Anugesic-HC

(Parke-Davis) is a proprietary,
prescription-only COMPOUND PREPARATION
of the CORTICOSTEROID and ANTI-
INFLAMMATORY drug hydrocortisone (as
acetate) and the ASTRINGENT agents zinc
oxide and bismuth oxide, benzyl benzoate
(with Peru balsam) and the LOCAL
ANAESTHETIC drug pramoxine
hydrochloride. It can be used to treat
haemorrhoids and inflammation in the
anal region. It is available as a cream and
suppositories.
+▲ side-effects/warning: see
BENZYL BENZOATE; BISMUTH OXIDE;
HYDROCORTISONE; ZINC OXIDE

Anusol

(Parke-Davis) is a proprietary, non-
prescription COMPOUND PREPARATION of
the ASTRINGENT agents bismuth oxide and
zinc oxide (with Peru balsam). It can be
used to treat haemorrhoids and
discomfort in the anal region. It is
available as a cream, an ointment and as
suppositories.
+▲ side-effects/warning: see
BISMUTH OXIDE; ZINC OXIDE

Anusol-HC

(Parke-Davis) is a proprietary,
prescription-only COMPOUND PREPARATION
of the CORTICOSTEROID and ANTI-
INFLAMMATORY drug hydrocortisone
(as acetate) and the ASTRINGENT and
ANTISEPTIC agents benzyl benzoate,
bismuth oxide, bismuth subgallate and
zinc oxide (with Peru Balsam). It can be
used to treat haemorrhoids and
inflammation in the anal region. It is
available as an ointment and
suppositories.
+▲ side-effects/warning: see
BENZYL BENZOATE; BISMUTH OXIDE; BISMUTH
SUBGALLATE; HYDROCORTISONE; ZINC OXIDE

*anxiolytic

drugs relieve medically diagnosed anxiety
states and are prescribed only for patients
whose anxiety is actually hindering its
resolution by other therapies, such as
pyschotherapy. They are also used to
relieve acute anxiety, for instance before
surgery. Treatment should be at the lowest
dose effective and must not be prolonged,
because psychological dependence and
physical dependence (addiction) readily
occurs and may make withdrawal difficult.

The best-known and most-used
anxiolytics are the BENZODIAZEPINES (eg
CHLORDIAZEPOXIDE, CLOBAZAM, DIAZEPAM
and LORAZEPAM) and other drugs such as
MEPROBAMATE and some of the
ANTIPSYCHOTIC drugs (at low doses).
Additionally, BETA-BLOCKERS are sometimes
used to treat anxiety by preventing the
physical symptoms such as palpitations of
the heart, sweating and tremor, which
helps the patient to stop the chain reaction
of worry to fear to panic.

The benzodiazepines are occasionally
administered for the relief of withdrawal
symptoms of addiction to other drugs
(such as alcohol). Some of these drugs
take time to work and careful adjusting of
the dose is required. Drugs of this class
are sometimes, somewhat misleadingly,
referred to as *minor tranquillizers*.

Apisate

(Wyeth) is a proprietary, prescription-only
preparation of the APPETITE SUPPRESSANT
diethylpropion hydrochloride (which is on
the Controlled Drugs List) and a vitamin
supplement of vitamins B_1, B_2, B_6 and the
B-vitamin NICOTINAMIDE. Treatment is
short term and under strict medical
supervision. It is available as modified-
release tablets.
+▲ side-effects/warning: see
DIETHYLPROPION HYDROCHLORIDE

apomorphine hydrochloride

is an ANTIPARKINSONISM drug that has

similar actions to BROMOCRIPTINE and is used in a patient's *off* periods, which are not controlled by the drug levodopa. It is chemically related to MORPHINE, though it is not an ANALGESIC and has been used as an EMETIC. Administration is by injection.

✚ side-effects: dyskinesias (movement disorders) during *on* periods, impaired speech and balance, nausea and vomiting, confusion, euphoria, light-headedness and hallucinations; postural hypotension, blood disorders, cognitive impairment. Pain at site of injection.

▲ warning: it should not be administered to patients with central nervous system or respiratory depression, hypersensitivity to opioids, psychiatric disorders and dementia; or who are pregnant or breast-feeding. Administer with caution to those with respiratory, cardiovascular and hormone disorders, kidney impairment and the elderly.

❍ Related entry: Britaject

*appetite suppressant

is a term used for two types of drug. The first type works by acting on the brain and a number of these drugs are related to amphetamine, consequently psychological dependence readily occurs.

Treatment with these drugs should be short term only and there is also a growing doubt among experts over the medical value of such a treatment. Examples of these drugs include DEXFENFLURAMINE HYDROCHLORIDE, DIETHYLPROPION HYDROCHLORIDE, FENFLURAMINE HYDROCHLORIDE and PHENTERMINE. The proprietary preparations of these drugs are on the Controlled Drugs List.

The second type works by bulking out the food eaten so that the body feels it has actually taken more than it has. Bulking agents include METHYLCELLULOSE and STERCULIA.

Both types of drug are intended to assist in the medical treatment of obesity, where the primary therapy is an appropriate diet.

apraclonidine

is a SYMPATHOMIMETIC drug, which is chemically a derivative of clonidine. It can be used to control or prevent postoperative elevation of intraocular pressure (pressure in the eyeball) after laser surgery. Administration is topical as eye-drops.

✚ side-effects: eyelid retraction, hyperaemia (excess blood in vessels in the eye), whitening of the conjunctiva; dilated pupil, systemic effects (for instance on the cardiovascular system) if a sufficient quantity of the drug is absorbed through the eye.

▲ warning: avoid its use in patients with severe cardiovascular disease (including hypertension); administer with care to those with a history of vagovagal attacks, or who are pregnant or breast-feeding.

❍ Related entry: Lopidine

Apresoline

(Ciba) is a proprietary, prescription-only preparation of the VASODILATOR drug hydralazine hydrochloride. It can be used in long-term ANTIHYPERTENSIVE treatment and in hypertensive crisis. It is available as tablets and in a form for injection.

✚▲ side-effects/warning: see HYDRALAZINE HYDROCHLORIDE

Aprinox

(Boots) is a proprietary prescription-only preparation of the (THIAZIDE) DIURETIC drug bendrofluazide. It can be used, either on its own or in conjunction with other diuretics or drugs, in the treatment of oedema, in congestive HEART FAILURE TREATMENT and as an ANTIHYPERTENSIVE. It is available as tablets.

✚▲ side-effects/warning: see BENDROFLUAZIDE

aprotinin

is an inhibitor of proteolytic enzymes and has antifibrinolytic activity, because it prevents thrombosis by an action on the blood clot formation system. It can be used to prevent life-threatening clot

A formation, for instance in open-heart surgery, removal of tumours and in surgical procedures in patients with certain blood disorders (eg hyperplasminaemias).

✚ side-effects: hypersensitivity reactions and occasionally inflammation of vein walls.

◔ **Related entry: Trasylol**

Apsifen

(APS) is a proprietary, prescription-only preparation of the (NSAID) NON-NARCOTIC ANALGESIC and ANTIRHEUMATIC drug ibuprofen, which also has valuable ANTIPYRETIC properties. It can be used to relieve pain, particularly of rheumatic disease and other musculoskeletal disorders. It is available as tablets.

✚▲ side-effects/warning: see IBUPROFEN

Apsin

(APS) is a proprietary, prescription-only preparation of the ANTIBACTERIAL and (PENICILLIN) ANTIBIOTIC drug phenoxymethylpenicillin. It is particularly effective in treating tonsillitis, infection of the middle ear, certain skin infections and in preventing recurrent streptococcal throat infection, which can lead to episodes of rheumatic fever. It is available as tablets and an oral solution (as the potassium salt).

✚▲ side-effects/warning: see PHENOXYMETHYLPENICILLIN

Apsolol

(APS) is a proprietary, prescription-only preparation of the BETA-BLOCKER drug propranolol hydrochloride. It can be used as an ANTIHYPERTENSIVE treatment for raised blood pressure, as an ANTI-ANGINA treatment to relieve symptoms and improve exercise tolerance and as an ANTI-ARRHYTHMIC to regularize heartbeat and to treat myocardial infarction. It can also be used as an ANTITHYROID drug for the short-term treatment of thyrotoxicosis, as an ANTIMIGRAINE treatment to prevent attacks, as an ANXIOLYTIC treatment,

particularly for symptomatic relief of tremor and palpitations and, with an ALPHA-ADRENOCEPTOR BLOCKER, in the acute treatment of phaeochromocytoma. It is available as tablets.

✚▲ side-effects/warning: see PROPRANOLOL HYDROCHLORIDE

Apsolox

(APS) is a proprietary, prescription-only preparation of the BETA-BLOCKER drug oxprenolol hydrochloride. It can be used as an ANTIHYPERTENSIVE treatment for raised blood pressure, as an ANTI-ANGINA treatment to relieve symptoms and improve exercise tolerance and as an ANTI-ARRHYTHMIC to regularize heartbeat and to treat myocardial infarction. It can also be used as an ANTITHYROID drug for the short-term treatment of thyrotoxicosis, as an ANTIMIGRAINE treatment to prevent attacks, as an ANXIOLYTIC treatment, particularly for symptomatic relief of tremor and palpitations and, with an ALPHA-ADRENOCEPTOR BLOCKER, in the acute treatment of phaeochromocytoma. It is available as tablets.

✚▲ side-effects/warning: see OXPRENOLOL HYDROCHLORIDE

Apstil

(APS) is a proprietary, prescription-only preparation of the SEX HORMONE stilboestrol, a synthetic OESTROGEN. It can be used as an ANTICANCER drug to treat prostate cancer and breast cancer. It is available in the form of tablets.

✚▲ side-effects/warning: see STILBOESTROL

Aquadrate

(Procter & Gamble) is a proprietary, non-prescription preparation of the HYDRATING AGENT urea. It can be used for dry, scaling, or itching skin and is available as a cream.

✚▲ side-effects/warning: see UREA

aqueous iodine oral solution

(or Lugol's solution) is a non-proprietary,

freshly made solution of iodine and potassium iodide in water. It is used by patients suffering from an excess of THYROID HORMONES in the bloodstream (thyrotoxicosis) prior to thyroid surgery. It is administered by mouth after being diluted with milk or water.
✚▲ side-effects/warning: see IODINE

arachis oil

is peanut oil and is used primarily as an EMOLLIENT in treating crusts on skin surfaces in conditions such as dandruff or cradle cap. It is also used as a LAXATIVE to lubricate and soften impacted faeces in order to promote bowel movement. It is available as a shampoo, an enema and a liquid.
✿ Related entries: Cerumol; Fletchers' Arachis Oil Retention Enema; Hydromol; Kamillosan; Massé Breast Cream; Oilatum

Aramine

(Merck, Sharp & Dohme) is a proprietary, prescription-only preparation of the SYMPATHOMIMETIC and VASOCONSTRICTOR drug metaraminol. It is most often used to raise blood pressure in a patient under general anaesthesia, or in conditions of severe hypotensive shock. It is available in a form for injection or infusion.
✚▲ side-effects/warning: see METARAMINOL

Arbralene

(Berk) is a proprietary, prescription-only preparation of the BETA-BLOCKER drug metoprolol tartrate. It can be used as an ANTIHYPERTENSIVE treatment for raised blood pressure, as an ANTI-ANGINA treatment to relieve symptoms and improve exercise tolreance and as an ANTI-ARRHYTHMIC to regularize the heartbeat and to treat mycocardial infection. It can also be used as an ANTITHYROID drug for short-term treatment of thyrotoxicosis, or as an ANTIMIGRAINE treatment to prevent attacks. It is available as tablets.

✚▲ side-effects/warning: see METOPROLOL TARTRATE

Aredia

(Ciba) is a recently introduced, proprietary, prescription-only preparation of the drug disodium pamidronate. It is used to treat high calcium levels associated with malignant tumours and is available in a form for intravenous infusion.
✚▲ side-effects/warning: see DISODIUM PAMIDRONATE

Arelix

(Hoechst) is a proprietary prescription-only preparation of the (*loop*) DIURETIC drug piretanide. It can be used, either on its own or in conjunction with other drugs, as an ANTIHYPERTENSIVE. It is available as capsules.
✚▲ side-effects/warning: see PIRETANIDE

Arfonad

(Cambridge) is a proprietary, prescription-only, preparation of the GANGLION BLOCKER drug trimetaphan camsylate. It can be used as a HYPOTENSIVE for controlled blood pressure during surgery and is available in a form for injection and infusion.
✚▲ side-effects/warning: see TRIMETAPHAN CAMSYLATE

Arilvax

(Evans) is a proprietary, prescription-only VACCINE preparation. It can be used to prevent infection by yellow fever and is available in a form for injection.
✚ warning: see YELLOW FEVER VACCINE

Arpicolin

(RP Drugs) is a proprietary, prescription-only preparation of the ANTICHOLINERGIC drug procyclidine hydrochloride. It can be used in the treatment of parkinsonism and is available as a syrup.
✚▲ side-effects/warning: see PROCYCLIDINE HYDROCHLORIDE

A

Arpimycin

(RP Drugs) is a proprietary, prescription-only preparation of the ANTIBACTERIAL and (MACROLIDE) ANTIBIOTIC drug erythromycin. It can be used to treat and prevent many forms of infection and is available as a liquid oral mixture.
✚▲ side-effects/warning: see ERYTHROMYCIN

Arret

(Janssen) is a proprietary, non-prescription preparation of the (OPIOID) ANTIDIARRHOEAL drug loperamide hydrochloride. It can be used for the relief of acute diarrhoea and its associated pain and discomfort. It is available as capsules.
✚▲ side-effects/warning: see LOPERAMIDE HYDROCHLORIDE

Artane

(Lederle) is a proprietary, prescription-only preparation of the ANTICHOLINERGIC drug benzhexol hydrochloride. It can be used in the treatment of parkinsonism and to control tremor and involuntary movement. It is available as tablets.
✚▲ side-effects/warning: see BENZHEXOL HYDROCHLORIDE

Arthrofen

(Ashbourne) is a proprietary, prescription-only preparation of the (NSAID) NON-NARCOTIC ANALGESIC and ANTIRHEUMATIC drug ibuprofen. It can be used to relieve pain, particularly that of rheumatic disease and other musculoskeletal disorders. It is available as tablets.
✚▲ side-effects/warning: see IBUPROFEN

Arthrosin

(Ashbourne) is a proprietary, prescription-only preparation of the (NSAID) NON-NARCOTIC ANALGESIC and ANTIRHEUMATIC drug naproxen. It can be used to relieve pain, particularly rheumatic and arthritic pain and to treat other musculoskeletal

disorders. It is available as tablets.
✚ side-effects/warning: see NAPROXEN

Arthrotec

(Searle) is a proprietary, prescription-only COMPOUND PREPARATION of the powerful (NSAID) NON-NARCOTIC ANALGESIC and ANTIRHEUMATIC drug diclofenac sodium and an ULCER-HEALING DRUG the PROSTAGLANDIN misoprostol. It can be used to treat pain and inflammation in rheumatic disease. This preparation has a novel approach to minimizing the gastrointestinal side-effects of the NSAID by adding prostaglandin, which is the LOCAL HORMONE whose production has been reduced by the NSAID. Prostaglandins are necessary for correct blood circulation in the gastrointestinal tract and if their level is reduced gastrointestinal side-effects (such as ulceration) may occur. It is available as tablets.
✚▲ side-effects/warning: see DICLOFENAC SODIUM; MISOPROSTOL

Arthroxen

(CP) is a proprietary, prescription-only preparation of the (NSAID) NON-NARCOTIC ANALGESIC and ANTIRHEUMATIC drug naproxen. It can be used to relieve pain and inflammation, particularly in rheumatism, arthritis and other musculoskeletal disorders. It is available as tablets.
✚ side-effects/warning: see NAPROXEN

*artificial saliva

is used to make up a deficiency of saliva in conditions that cause a dry mouth. Common preparations include viscous constituents such as CARMELLOSE SODIUM, SORBITOL, gastric mucin, gum acacia, MALIC ACID and electrolytes, including potassium chloride, sodium chloride and potassium phosphates.

Artracin

(DDSA Pharmaceuticals) is a proprietary, prescription-only preparation of the

(NSAID) NON-NARCOTIC ANALGESIC and ANTIRHEUMATIC drug indomethacin. It can be used to relieve pain and inflammation, particularly in rheumatism, arthritis and other musculoskeletal disorders. It is available as tablets.

✚▲ side-effects/warning: see INDOMETHACIN

Arvin

(Knoll) is a proprietary, prescription only preparation of the ANTICOAGULANT drug ancrod. It is not in common use and is available only on a 'named-patient' basis. Administration is by injection.

✚▲ side-effects/warning: see ANCROD

Arythmol

(Knoll) is a proprietary, prescription-only preparation of the ANTI-ARRHYTHMIC drug propafenone hydrochloride. It can be used to prevent and treat irregularities of the heartbeat and is available as tablets.

✚▲ side-effects/warning: see PROPAFENONE HYDROCHLORIDE

Asacol

(SmithKline Beecham) is a proprietary, prescription-only preparation of the AMINOSALICYLATE drug mesalazine. It can be used to treat patients who suffer from ulcerative colitis but who are unable to tolerate the more commonly used drug sulphasalazine. It is available as tablets, a foam enema and as suppositories.

✚▲ side-effects/warning: see MESALAZINE

Ascabiol Emulsion

(Rhône-Poulenc Rorer) is a proprietary, non-prescription preparation of benzyl benzoate in suspension, which is an insecticidal drug used as a PEDICULICIDAL for lice infestations, or as a SCABICIDAL for infestation by mites. It is available as an emulsion.

✚▲ side-effects/warning: see BENZYL BENZOATE

ascorbic acid

(Vitamin C) is a VITAMIN that is essential for the development and maintenance of cells and tissues. It cannot be synthesized within the body and must be found in the diet (good food sources are vegetables and citrus fruits). Deficiency eventually leads to scurvy, but before that there is a lowered resistance to infection and other disorders may develop, particularly in the elderly. However, vitamin C supplements are rarely necessary with a normal, well-balanced diet. There have been claims that pharmacological doses help prevent colds and because of this it is incorporated into a number of cold remedies. Administration is oral in the form of tablets and liquids.

✚ warning: it is destroyed by over-cooking or through the action of ultraviolet light (i.e. sunlight).

✪ Related entries: Beechams Hot Lemon; Beechams Hot Lemon and Honey; Children's Vitamin Drops; Coldrex Powders, Blackcurrant; Coldrex Tablets; Lemsip; Redoxon; Serfolic SV

Asendis

(Novex) is a proprietary, prescription-only preparation of the (TRICYCLIC) ANTIDEPRESSANT drug amoxapine. It can be used to treat depressive illness and is available as tablets.

✚▲ side-effects/warning: see AMOXAPINE

Aserbine

(Forley) is a proprietary, non-prescription COMPOUND PREPARATION of the ANTISEPTIC and KERATOLYTIC agents, MALIC ACID, BENZOIC ACID and SALICYLIC ACID. It can be used as a desloughing agent in the treatment of superficial ulcers, burns and bedsores so that natural healing can take place. It is available as an ointment and a solution.

▲ warning: avoid contact with the eyes.

Asilone Liquid

(Seton Healthcare) is a proprietary, non-prescription COMPOUND PREPARATION of the ANTACIDS aluminium hydroxide and

A

magnesium oxide and the ANTIFOAMING AGENT dimethicone (as simethicone). It can be used to treat dyspepsia, flatulence and associated abdominal distension, heartburn (including heartburn that occurs with hiatus hernia, pregnancy and reflux oesophagitis) and to soothe the symptoms of peptic ulcers. It is available as tablets and is not normally given to children, except on medical advice.
✚▲ side-effects/warning: see ALUMINIUM HYDROXIDE, DIMETHICONE

Asilone Suspension

(Seton Healthcare) is a proprietary, non-prescription COMPOUND PREPARATION of the ANTACIDS aluminium hydroxide and magnesium oxide and the ANTIFOAMING AGENT dimethicone (as simethicone). It can be used to treat dyspepsia, flatulence and associated abdominal distension, heartburn (including heartburn that occurs with hiatus hernia, pregnancy and reflux oesophagitis) and to soothe the symptoms of peptic ulcers. It is available as a suspension and is not normally given to children, except on medical advice.
✚▲ side-effects/warning: see ALUMINIUM HYDROXIDE; DIMETHICONE

Asilone Tablets

(Seton Healthcare) is a proprietary, non-prescription COMPOUND PREPARATION of the ANTACID aluminium hydroxide and the ANTIFOAMING AGENT dimethicone (as simethicone). It can be used to treat dyspepsia, flatulence and associated abdominal distension, heartburn (including heartburn that occurs with hiatus hernia, pregnancy and reflux oesophagitis) and to soothe the symptoms of peptic ulcers. It is available as tablets and is not normally given to children under 12 years, except on medical advice.
✚▲ side-effects/warning: see ALUMINIUM HYDROXIDE; DIMETHICONE

Askit Capsules

(Roche) is a proprietary, non-prescription COMPOUND PREPARATION of the (NSAID) NON-NARCOTIC ANALGESIC, ANTIRHEUMATIC and ANTIPYRETIC drugs aspirin and aloxiprin (a buffered form of aspirin) and the STIMULANT caffeine. It can be used to treat mild to moderate pain (including rheumatic pain), to relieve swelling, flu symptoms and other feverish conditions. It is available as capsules and is not normally given to children under 12 years, except on medical advice.
✚▲ side-effects/warning: see ALOXIPRIN; ASPIRIN; CAFFEINE

Askit Powders

(Roche) is a proprietary, non-prescription COMPOUND PREPARATION of the (NSAID) NON-NARCOTIC ANALGESIC, ANTIRHEUMATIC and ANTIPYRETIC drugs aspirin and aloxiprin (a buffered form of aspirin) and the STIMULANT caffeine. It can be used to treat mild to moderate pain (including rheumatic pain), to relieve swelling, flu symptoms and other feverish conditions. It is available as a powder and is not normally given to children under 12 years, except on medical advice.
✚▲ side-effects/warning: see ALOXIPRIN; ASPIRIN; CAFFEINE

Asmaven

(Berk) is a proprietary, prescription-only preparation of the BETA- RECEPTOR STIMULANT salbutamol (as salbutamol sulphate). It can be used as a BRONCHODILATOR in reversible obstructive airways disease, as an ANTI-ASTHMATIC treatment in severe acute asthma, or for the alleviation of symptoms of chronic bronchitis and emphysema. It may also be used to delay premature labour. It is available as tablets.
✚▲ side-effects/warning: see SALBUTAMOL

Aspav

(Roussel) is a proprietary, prescription-only preparation of the COMPOUND ANALGESIC containing the (NSAID) NON-NARCOTIC ANALGESIC drug aspirin and the

mixed (OPIOID) NARCOTIC ANALGESIC alkaloids (including morphine, codeine and papaverine). It can be used to relieve pain and is available as soluble tablets.
+▲ side-effects/warning: see ASPIRIN; CODEINE PHOSPHATE; OPIOID; PAPAVERINE

Aspellin

(Fisons) is a proprietary, non-prescription COMPOUND PREPARATION of menthol, camphor, methyl salicylate, ethyl salicylate and ammonium salicylate. It has a COUNTER-IRRITANT, or RUBEFACIENT, action and can be applied to the skin for symptomatic relief of underlying muscle or joint pain. It is available as a liniment.
+▲ side-effects/warning: see AMMONIUM SALICYLATE; CAMPHOR; ETHYL SALICYLATE; MENTHOL; METHYL SALICYLATE

aspirin

or acetylsalicylic acid, is a well-known and widely used non-steroidal anti-inflammatory (NSAID), NON-NARCOTIC ANALGESIC and ANTIRHEUMATIC drug. As an analgesic it relieves mild to moderate pain, particularly headache, toothache and period pain.

It is a useful ANTIPYRETIC for reducing raised body temperature in the treatment of the common cold, fevers, or influenza. Aspirin reduces platelet aggregation, which allows its prophylactic (preventive) use, at a lower dose, as an ANTIPLATELET treatment in those at risk (such as those who have already suffered a heart attack or following bypass surgery). However, this same action may also increase bleeding time, so those taking ANTICOAGULANT drugs must avoid aspirin. In tablet form, aspirin irritates the stomach lining and may cause bleeding and ulceration; consequently forms of soluble aspirin are preferred.

Many proprietary forms combine aspirin with such drugs as codeine, paracetamol and ibuprofen. Administration is normally oral. Medicines containing aspirin are now no longer normally given to children under 12 years (except for juvenile arthritis, Still's disease and on medical advice), because of a link with the rare, but serious, condition called Reye's Syndrome (which causes inflammation of the brain and liver). Aspirin can produce the same allergic-like symptoms (including bronchospasm) that occur in many patients after taking NSAIDs. It is available as tablets, soluble tablets, suppositories and capsules.
+▲ side-effects/warning: see under NSAID. It should not be used by women who are breast-feeding, or those with gout or certain bleeding disorders (eg haemophilia).
✪ Related entries: Actron; Alka-Seltzer Original; Anadin Analgesic Caplets; Anadin Analgesic Capsules, Maximum Strength; Anadin Extra; Anadin Extra Soluble Tablets; Angettes 75; Askit Capsules; Askit Powders; Aspav; Aspro Clear; Aspro Tablets; Beechams Powders; Beechams 75 mg Aspirin; Beechams Hot Lemon; Beechams Hot Lemon and Honey; Beechams Lemon Tablets; Beechams Powders Capsules; Benoral; Caprin; Codis 500; Cojene Tablets; Dispirin; Dispirin CV; Dispirin Direct; Dispirin Extra; Doloxene Compound; Dristan Decongestant Tablets; Equagesic; Femigraine; Fynnon Calcium Aspirin; Maximum Strength Aspro Clear; Migravess; Nu-Seals Aspirin; Nurse Sykes Powders; Paramax; Phensic; Platet; Powerin Analgesic Tablets; Robaxisal Forte; Veganin Tablets

Aspro Clear

(Roche) is a proprietary, non-prescription preparation of the (NSAID) NON-NARCOTIC ANALGESIC, ANTIRHEUMATIC and ANTIPYRETIC drug aspirin. It can be used to treat various aches and pains and fevers. It is available as effervescent, lemon-flavoured tablets and is not normally given to children under 12 years, except on medical advice.
+▲ side-effects/warning: SEE ASPIRIN

A

Aspro Tablets

(Roche) is a proprietary, non-prescription preparation of the (NSAID) NON-NARCOTIC ANALGESIC, ANTIRHEUMATIC and ANTIPYRETIC drug aspirin. It can be used to treat the symptoms of flu and feverish colds and mild to moderate pain (including muscular pain). It is available as tablets and is not normally given to children under 12 years, except on medical advice.

✚▲ side-effects/warning: see ASPIRIN

astemizole

is a recently developed ANTIHISTAMINE drug with less sedative side-effects than some of the older antihistamines. It can be used for the symptomatic relief of allergic symptoms such as hay fever and urticaria (itchy skin rash). Administration is oral in the form of tablets or a suspension.

✚▲ side-effects/warning: see under ANTIHISTAMINE; but the incidence of sedative and anticholinergic effects is low. Nevertheless, subjects should be made aware that drowsiness may impair the performance of skilled tasks such as driving. Do not use in patients who are pregnant and avoid pregnancy for several weeks after finishing treatment. Certain serious disturbances of heart rhythm have been observed after excessive dose. Occasionally, weight gain may occur.

○ Related entries: Hismanal; Pollon-eze

*astringent

agents precipitate proteins and are used in lotions to harden and protect skin where there are minor abrasions. They can also be used in lozenges, mouthwashes, eye-drops and antiperspirants. Examples include ZINC OXIDE and salts of aluminium (ALUMINIUM ACETATE, ALUMINIUM HYDROXIDE and ALUMINIUM CHLORIDE).

AT 10

(Sanofi Winthrop) is a proprietary, prescription-only preparation of dihydrotachysterol, which is a VITAMIN D analogue. It can be used in the treatment of vitamin D deficiency and is available as capsules and a solution.

✚▲ side-effects/warning: see DIHYDROTACHYSTEROL

Atarax

(Pfizer) is a proprietary, prescription-only preparation of the ANTIHISTAMINE drug hydroxyzine hydrochloride, which has some additional ANXIOLYTIC properties. It can be used for the relief of allergic symptoms such as itching and mild rashes and also for the short-term treatment of anxiety. It is available as tablets and as a syrup.

✚▲ side-effects/warning: see HYDROXYZINE HYDROCHLORIDE

Atenix

(Ashbourne) is is a proprietary, prescription-only preparation of the BETA-BLOCKER drug atenolol. It can be used as an ANTIHYPERTENSIVE treatment for raised blood pressure, as an ANTI-ANGINA treatment to relieve symptoms and improve exercise tolerance and as an ANTI-ARRHYTHMIC to regularize heartbeat and to treat myocardial infarction. It is available as tablets.

✚▲ side-effects/warning: see ATENOLOL

AtenixCo

(Ashbourne) is a proprietary, prescription-only COMPOUND PREPARATION of the BETA-BLOCKER drug atenolol and the DIURETIC chlorthalidone (a combination called co-tenidone). It can be used as an ANTIHYPERTENSIVE treatment for raised blood pressure and is available as tablets.

✚▲ side-effects/warning: see ATENOLOL: CHLORTHALIDONE

atenolol

is a BETA-BLOCKER drug. It can be used as an ANTIHYPERTENSIVE treatment for raised blood pressure, as ANTI-ANGINA treatment to relieve symptoms and to improve exercise tolerance and as an ANTI-

ARRHYTHMIC to regularize heartbeat and to treat myocardial infarction. Administration can oral as tablets, capsules or a syrup, or by injection. It is also available as an antihypertensive treatment in the form of COMPOUND PREPARATIONS with DIURETICS.

✚▲ side-effects/warning: see under PROPRANOLOL HYDROCHLORIDE

⊙ Related entries: Antipressan; Atenix; AtenixCo; Beta-Adalat, co-tenidone, Kalten; Tenchlor; Tenif; Tenoret 50; Tenoretic; Tenormin; Totamol

Atensine

(Berk) is a proprietary, prescription-only preparation of the BENZODIAZEPINE drug diazepam. It can be used as an ANXIOLYTIC drug to treat anxiety in the short term, as a HYPNOTIC to relieve insomnia and to assist in the treatment of alcohol withdrawal symptoms, as an ANTICONVULSANT and ANTI-EPILEPTIC for status epilepticus and as a SEDATIVE and SKELETAL MUSCLE RELAXANT in preoperative medication. It is available as tablets.

✚▲ side-effects/warning: see DIAZEPAM

Ativan

(Wyeth) is a proprietary, prescription-only preparation of the BENZODIAZEPINE drug lorazepam. It can be used as an ANXIOLYTIC drug in the short-term treatment of anxiety, as a HYPNOTIC for insomnia, as an ANTI-EPILEPTIC in status epilepticus and as a SEDATIVE, including in postoperative premedication because it also causes a degree of amnesia and so helps the patient to forget the procedure or operation. It is available as tablets or in a form for injection.

✚▲ side-effects/warning: see LORAZEPAM

atovaquone

is a recently introduced ANTIPROTOZOAL drug. It is used to treat pneumonia caused by the protozoan micro-organism *Pneumocystis carinii* in patients whose immune system has been suppressed (either following transplant surgery or

because of a disease such as AIDS). Administration is oral as tablets.

✚ side-effects: diarrhoea, nausea and vomiting, headache, insomnia, fever, rash, changes in liver and blood function and anaemia.

▲ warning: initial gastrointestinal upsets cause difficulties. Administer with care to patients with impaired kidney or liver function, or who are pregnant. Avoid its use in patients who are breast-feeding.

⊙ Related entry: Wellvone

atracurium besilate

See ATRACURIUM BESYLATE

atracurium besylate

(atracurium besilate) is a *non-depolarizing* SKELETAL MUSCLE RELAXANT drug. It can be used to induce muscle paralysis during surgery and is administered by injection.

✚▲ side-effects/warning: see under TUBOCURARINE CHLORIDE; histamine may be released; it causes little block of sympathetic or vagal nerves; and is relatively safe in patients with impaired liver or kidney function.

⊙ Related entry: Tracrium

Atromid-S

(Zeneca) is a proprietary, prescription-only preparation of the drug clofibrate. It can be used as a LIPID-LOWERING DRUG in hyperlipidaemia to reduce the levels, or change the proportions, of various lipids in the bloodstream. Generally, it is administered only to patients in whom a strict and regular dietary regime, alone, is not having the desired effect. It is available as capsules.

✚▲ side-effects/warning: see CLOFIBRATE

atropine sulphate

(hyoscyamine) is a powerful ANTICHOLINERGIC drug, sometimes referred to as a BELLADONNA ALKALOID because of its origin from the family of

A

plants that include *Atropa belladonna* (deadly nightshade). It is able to depress certain functions of the autonomic nervous system and is therefore a useful ANTISPASMODIC drug. It is commonly used during operations to dry up secretions and protect the heart.

It can also be used to cause a long-lasting dilation of the pupil of the eye for ophthalmic procedures. Atropine is able to decrease the secretion of gastric acid, but it has too many side-effects to make it suitable for routine treatment of peptic ulcers. Administration can be oral as tablets, as eye-drops, or by injection.

✚ side-effects: dry mouth, difficulty in swallowing and thirst, dilation of the pupils and loss of ability to focus, increase in intraocular pressure (pressure in the eye-ball), dry skin with flushing, slowing then speeding of the heart, difficulty in urination, constipation, palpitations and heart arrhythmias. Rarely, there may be high temperature accompanied by delirium or hallucinations.

▲ warning: it should not be administered to patients with closed-angle glaucoma; and used with caution in patients with prostate gland enlargement or urinary retention, ulcerative colitis, pyloric stenosis, or who are pregnant or breast-feeding. It may worsen gastro-oesophageal reflux.

⭕ Related entries: co-phenotrope; Diarphen; Isopto Atropine; Lomotil; Minims Atropine Sulphate

Atrovent

(Boehringer Ingelheim) is a proprietary, prescription-only preparation of the ANTICHOLINERGIC and BRONCHODILATOR drug ipratropium bromide. It can be used to treat the symptoms of reversible airways obstructive disease, particularly chronic bronchitis. It is available as an aerosol, a breath-actuated aerosol inhaler (*Autohaler*), a powder for inhalation (*Aerocaps*) *and* as a nebulizer solution.

✚▲ side-effects/warning: see
IPRATROPIUM BROMIDE

Audax Ear Drops

(Napp) is a proprietary, non-prescription COMPOUND PREPARATION of choline salicylate and glycerin. It can be used as a local pain-reliever in the outer or middle ear and as an aid to wax removal.

✚▲ side-effects/warning: see CHOLINE SALICYLATE; GLYCERIN

Audicort

(Lederle) is a proprietary, prescription-only COMPOUND PREPARATION of the ANTI-INFLAMMATORY and CORTICOSTEROID drug triamcinolone acetonide and the ANTIBACTERIAL and (AMINOGLYCOSIDE) ANTIBIOTIC drug neomycin (as undeconate). It can be used to treatment infections of the outer ear and is available as ear-drops.

✚▲ side-effects/warning: see NEOMYCIN SULPHATE; TRIAMCINOLONE ACETONIDE

Augmentin

(Beecham) is a proprietary, prescription-only COMPOUND PREPARATION of the broad-spectrum ANTIBACTERIAL and (PENICILLIN) ANTIBIOTIC drug amoxycillin and the ENZYME INHIBITOR clavulanic acid (a combination known as co-amoxclav). It can inhibit the enzymes (penicillinases) that are produced by some bacteria and which break down amoxycillin, so making it ineffective.

The combination is therefore active against many infections that would normally be resistant to amoxycillin alone and so extends the range and efficiency of amoxycillin as an antibiotic. It can be used to treat infections of the skin, ear, nose and throat and urinary tract. It is available in a number of forms: as tablets, dispersible tablets, an oral suspension and in a form for injection or infusion.

✚▲ side-effects/warning: see AMOXYCILLIN; CLAVULANIC ACID; CO-AMOXCLAV

auranofin

is a form in which the gold may be used as an ANTI-INFLAMMATORY and ANTIRHEUMATIC treatment. It is used to treat severe, progressive rheumatoid arthritis when NSAID treatment alone is not adequate. Administration is oral in the form of tablets.

✚ side-effects: see under SODIUM AUROTHIOMALATE; but with diarrhoea.

▲ warning: see under sodium aurothiomalate. Administer with caution to patients with inflammatory bowel disease.

✪ Related entry: Ridaura

Aureocort

(Lederle) is a proprietary, prescription-only COMPOUND PREPARATION of the CORTICOSTEROID drug triamcinolone acetonide and the ANTIBACTERIAL and (TETRACYCLINE) ANTIBIOTIC drug chlortetracycline (as hydrochloride). It can be used to treat severe inflammatory skin disorders, including forms of eczema that are resistant to less-powerful corticosteroids. It is available as an ointment and a cream.

✚▲ side-effects/warning: see CHLORTETRACYCLINE; TRIAMCINOLONE ACETONIDE

Aureomycin

(Lederle) is a proprietary, prescription-only preparation of the ANTIBACTERIAL and (TETRACYCLINE) ANTIBIOTIC drug chlortetracycline (as hydrochloride). It can be used to treat eye and skin infections and is available as an ophthalmic (eye) ointment and cream.

✚▲ side-effects/warning: see CHLORTETRACYCLINE

Aureomycin Topical

(Lederle) is a proprietary, prescription-only preparation of the ANTIBACTERIAL and (TETRACYCLINE) ANTIBIOTIC drug chlortetracycline (as hydrochloride). It can be used to treat skin infections and is available as an ointment for topical application.

✚▲ side-effects/warning: see CHLORTETRACYCLINE

Aveeno Cream

(Bioglan) is a proprietary, non-prescription preparation of colloidal oatmeal and an EMOLLIENT base. It can be used for eczema, itching and other skin complaints and is available as a cream and a bath oil.

Aveeno Oiliated

(Bioglan) is a proprietary, non-prescription preparation of colloidal oatmeal and an EMOLLIENT base. It can be used for eczema, itching and other skin complaints and is available as a bath additive.

Aveeno Regular

(Bioglan) is a proprietary, non-prescription preparation of colloidal oatmeal and an EMOLLIENT base. It can be used for eczema, itching and other skin complaints and is available as a bath oil and a bath additive.

Avloclor

(Zeneca) is a proprietary, prescription-only preparation of the ANTIMALARIAL drug chloroquine (as phosphate). It can be used to prevent or suppress certain forms of malaria and is also used as an ANTIRHEUMATIC to treat rheumatoid disease. It is available as tablets. (This product also appears in a non-prescription form labelled for use for the prevention of malaria.)

✚▲ side-effects/warning: see CHLOROQUINE

Avomine

(Rhône-Poulenc Rorer) is a proprietary, non-prescription preparation of the ANTIHISTAMINE drug promethazine theoclate. It can be used as an ANTINAUSEANT for nausea, motion sickness, vertigo and labyrinthine (ear) disorders.

It is available as tablets.

✚▲ side-effects/warning: see PROMETHAZINE THEOCLATE

A | ## Axid

(Lilly) is a proprietary, prescription-only preparation of the H_2-ANTAGONIST drug nizatidine. It can be used as an ULCER-HEALING DRUG for benign peptic ulcers (in the stomach or duodenum), gastro-oesophageal reflux, dyspepsia and associated conditions. It is available as capsules and in a form for injection.
✚▲ side-effects/warning: see NIZATIDINE

Axsain

(Euroderma) is a proprietary, non-prescription COMPOUND PREPARATION of capsicum oleoresin, which has a COUNTER-IRRITANT, or RUBEFACIENT, action. It can be applied to the skin for symptomatic relief of post-herpatic neuralgia and is available as a cream.
✚▲ side-effects/warning: see:
CAPSICUM OLEORESIN

Azactam

(Squibb) is a proprietary, prescription-only preparation of the ANTIBACTERIAL and (BETA-LACTAM) ANTIBIOTIC drug aztreonam. It can be used to treat severe infections caused by Gram-negative bacteria, including gonorrhoea and infections of the urinary tract. It is available in a form for injection.
✚▲ side-effects/warning: see AZTREONAM

Azamune

(Penn) is a proprietary, prescription-only preparation of the IMMUNOSUPPRESSANT drug azathioprine. It can be used to treat tissue rejection in transplant patients and for a variety of autoimmune diseases. It is available as tablets.
✚▲ side-effects/warning: see AZATHIOPRINE

azapropazone

is a (NSAID) NON-NARCOTIC ANALGESIC and ANTIRHEUMATIC drug. It is used to treat only serious cases of rheumatoid arthritis, acute gout and certain rheumatic diseases of the backbone (ankylosing spondylitis), because of its side-effects. Administration is oral in the form of capsules and tablets. It is not normally given to children, except on medical advice.
✚▲ side-effects/warning: see under NSAID; but there is a high incidence of gastrointestinal disturbances, so it is restricted to use where other drugs have proved ineffective in serious inflammatory conditions. It is not to be used if there is inflammatory bowel disease, or porphyria. There is also a seriously prolonged potentiation of the bleeding time when anticoagulants are being used. It should not be given to patients with gastric ulcers or kidney disease.

azatadine maleate

is an ANTIHISTAMINE drug. It can be used for the symptomatic relief of allergic symptoms such as hay fever and urticaria (itchy skin rash). Administration is oral in the form of tablets or a syrup.
✚▲ side-effects/warning: see under ANTIHISTAMINE. Because of its sedative side-effects, the performance of skilled tasks such as driving may be impaired.
❍ **Related entry: Optimine**

azathioprine

is a powerful CYTOTOXIC and IMMUNOSUPPRESSANT drug. It is mainly used to reduce tissue rejection in transplant patients, but it can also be used to treat myasthenia gravis, rheumatoid arthritis, ulcerative colitis and several autoimmune diseases. Administration is either oral as tablets or by injection.
✚ side-effects: hypersensitivity reactions including dizziness, malaise, vomiting, fever, muscular pains and shivering, joint pain, changes in liver function, jaundice, heart arrhythmias, low blood pressure (requiring withdrawal of treatment), symptoms of bone marrow suppression, which should be reported (eg bleeding or bruising), hair loss, increased susceptibility to infections, nausea, pneumonia and pancreatitis.
▲ warning: it is not to be given to patients with known sensitivity to azathioprine or

mercaptopurine; or who are pregnant; monitoring is required throughout treatment with blood count checks.
○ Related entries: Azamune; Berkaprine; Immunoprin; Imuran

azelaic acid

is a recently introduced drug that has mild ANTIBACTERIAL and KERATOLYTIC properties. It can be used to treat skin conditions such as acne and is available as a cream.
✚ side-effects: some patients experience skin irritation and sensitivity to light.
▲ warning: avoid the eyes when applying. Administer with caution to patients who are pregnant or breast-feeding.
○ Related entry: Skinoren

azelastine hydrochloride

is an ANTIHISTAMINE drug, which can be used for the symptomatic relief of allergic rhinitis (inflammation of the mucosal lining of the nose). Administration is topical in the form of a nasal spray.
✚▲ side-effects/warning: see under ANTIHISTAMINE; but any adverse effects are less severe when given locally. Local application to the nasal mucosa may cause irritation and taste disturbances.
○ Related entry: Rhinolast

azidothymidine

See ZIDOVUDINE

azithromycin

is a recently introduced ANTIBACTERIAL and ANTIBIOTIC drug of the MACROLIDE group. It has more activity against Gram-negative organisms compared to erythromycin (though less against Gram-positive) and is mainly used in patients allergic to penicillin. It has a long duration of action that usually means it can be taken once a day. It can be used to treat infections of the middle ear, the respiratory tract, the skin and soft tissues and genital chlamydia infections. Administration is oral as a suspension or as capsules.

✚▲ side-effects/warning: see under ERYTHROMYCIN. Administer with caution to patients who are pregnant or breast-feeding.
○ Related entry: Zithromax

azlocillin

is an ANTIBACTERIAL and (PENICILLIN) ANTIBIOTIC drug. It can be used primarily to treat infections by a type of Gram-negative bacteria called *Pseudomonas*, particularly in serious infections of the urinary and respiratory tracts and for septicaemia. Administration is by injection or infusion.
✚▲ side-effects/warning: see under BENZYLPENICILLIN
○ Related entry: Securopen

*azoles

including the IMIDAZOLES chemical group, are a family of ANTIMICROBIAL and ANTIPROTOZOAL drugs. The group includes METRONIDAZOLE and TINIDAZOLE (which also have ANTIBACTERIAL properties), FLUCONAZOLE, ITRACONAZOLE, CLOTRIMAZOLE and MICONAZOLE (which also have ANTIFUNGAL properties) and MEBENDAZOLE and THIABENDAZOLE (which are also used as ANTHELMINTIC drugs). Triazole drugs are also azoles and include the antifungal drugs FLUCYTOSINE and itraconazole. They are all synthetic drugs.

AZT

See ZIDOVUDINE

aztreonam

is an ANTIBACTERIAL and ANTIBIOTIC drug of the BETA-LACTAM group. It can be used to treat severe infections caused by Gram-negative bacteria, including *Pseudomonas aeruginosa*, *Haemophilus influenzae*, *Neisseria meningitidis*, lung infections in cystic fibrosis, gonorrhoea, cystitis and infections of the urinary tract. Administration is by injection or infusion.
✚ side-effects: vomiting, nausea, diarrhoea and abdominal pain; altered taste and mouth ulcers; skin rashes; hepatitis, jaundice and

aztreonam

A

blood disorders.

▲ warning: it should not be administered to patients known to be sensitive to aztreonam: who are pregnant or breast-feeding. Administer with caution in patients with certain liver or kidney disorders.

✪ Related entry: Azactam

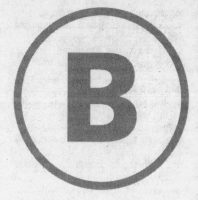

98

B

bacampicillin hydrochloride

is a broad-spectrum, penicillin-type ANTIBACTERIAL and ANTIBIOTIC drug, which is chemically an ester derivative of ampicillin and is converted to ampicillin in the body. However, it is better absorbed and has less gastrointestinal side-effects (eg diarrhoea) than ampicillin. It can be used to treat many infections, especially those of the urinogenital areas, upper respiratory tract, middle ear and gonorrhoea. Administration is oral in the form of tablets.

✚▲ side-effects/warning: see under AMPICILLIN

○ **Related entry: Ambaxin**

Bacillus Calmette-Guérin Vaccine, Dried

(District Health Authorities) (Dried Tub/Vac/BCG) is a non-proprietary, prescription-only preparation of BCG vaccine and is available in a form for injection.

✚▲ side-effects/warning: see BCG VACCINE

Bacillus Calmette-Guérin Vaccine, Percutaneous

(District Health Authorities) (Tub/Vac/BCG – Perc) is a non-proprietary, prescription-only preparation of BCG vaccine. It is administered percutaneously (multiple puncture through the skin).

✚▲ side-effects/warning: see BCG VACCINE

bacitracin zinc

is an ANTIBACTERIAL and ANTIBIOTIC drug (a polypeptide). It is commonly used for the treatment of infections of the skin and usually in combination with other antibiotics in the form of an ointment or spray for topical application.

○ **Related entries: Cicatrin; Polyfax; Tribiotic**

baclofen

is a SKELETAL MUSCLE RELAXANT drug. It is used for relaxing muscles that are in spasm, particularly when caused by an injury to or a disease of the central nervous system. It works by an action on the central nervous system. Administration is oral as tablets or an oral liquid.

✚ side-effects: sedation, drowsiness, nausea; sometimes light-headedness, fatigue, disturbances of gait, headache, hallucinations, euphoria, insomnia, depression, tremor, eye-flicker, loss of sensation in the extremities, convulsions, muscle weakness and pain, depression of respiration and blood pressure, gastrointestinal and urinary disturbances; rarely, taste alterations, visual disorders, sweating, rash, altered liver function, or paradoxical increase in muscle spasm.

▲ warning: it is not to be given to patients with peptic ulcer. Administer with caution to those with psychiatric disorders, impaired cerebrovascular, liver, or kidney function, epilepsy, porphyria, certain bladder dysfunction; or who are pregnant. Withdrawal of treatment should be gradual. It may affect the performance of skilled tasks such as driving.

○ **Related entries: Baclospas; Lioresal**

Baclospas

(Ashbourne) is a proprietary, prescription-only preparation of the SKELETAL MUSCLE RELAXANT drug baclofen. It can be used to treat muscle spasm caused by an injury to or a disease of the central nervous system. It is available as tablets.

✚▲ side-effects/warning: see BACLOFEN

Bactrim

(Roche) is a proprietary, prescription-only COMPOUND PREPARATION of the (SULPHONAMIDE) drug sulphamethoxazole and the antibacterial drug trimethoprim, which is a combination called co-trimoxazole. It can be used to treat bacterial infections, especially infections of the urinary tract, prostatitis and bronchitis. It is available as tablets and as a sugar-free paediatric syrup.

B

✚▲ side-effects/warning: see
CO-TRIMOXAZOLE

Bactroban

(Beecham) is a proprietary, prescription-only preparation of the ANTIBACTERIAL and ANTIBIOTIC drug mupirocin. It can be used to treat infections of the skin and is available as an ointment for topical application.

✚▲ side-effects/warning: see MUPIROCIN

Bactroban Nasal

(Beecham) is a proprietary, prescription-only preparation of the ANTIBACTERIAL and ANTIBIOTIC drug mupirocin. It can be used to treat staphylococcal infections (including methoxycillin-resistant *Staphylococcus aureus*) in and around the nostrils. It is available as an ointment for topical application.

✚▲ side-effects/warning: see MUPIROCIN

BAL (British Anti-Lewisite)

See DIMERCAPROL

Balanced Salt Solution

(Alcon; Ciba Vision) is a proprietary, non-prescription preparation of SODIUM CHLORIDE, sodium acetate, SODIUM CITRATE, calcium chloride, MAGNESIUM CHLORIDE and POTASSIUM CHLORIDE. It is a sterile solution that can be used as an eyewash for cleansing and washing out noxious substances.

Balmosa Cream

(Pharmax Healthcare) is a proprietary, non-prescription COMPOUND PREPARATION of capsicum oleoresin, camphor, menthol and methyl salicylate, which have COUNTER-IRRITANT, or RUBEFACIENT, actions. It can be applied to the skin for symptomatic relief of muscular rheumatism, fibrosis, lumbago and sciatica and also for pain associated with unbroken chilblains. It is available as a cream.

✚▲ side-effects/warning: see CAMPHOR;

CAPSICUM OLEORESIN; MENTHOL; METHYL SALICYLATE

Balneum with Tar

(Merck) is a proprietary, non-prescription preparation of coal tar. It can be used to treat psoriasis and eczema and is available as a bath oil.

✚▲ side-effects/warning: see COAL TAR

Baltar

(Merck) is a proprietary, non-prescription preparation of coal tar (as distillate). It can be used for conditions such as dandruff and psoriasis of the scalp and is available as a shampoo.

✚▲ side-effects/warning: see COAL TAR

Bambec

(Astra) is a proprietary, prescription-only preparation of the BETA-RECEPTOR STIMULANT bambuterol hydrochloride. It can be used as a BRONCHODILATOR in reversible obstructive airways disease, as an ANTI-ASTHMATIC treatment in severe acute asthma, or for the alleviation of symptoms of chronic bronchitis and emphysema. It is available as tablets.

✚▲ side-effects/warning: see BAMBUTEROL HYDROCHLORIDE

bambuterol hydrochloride

is a SYMPATHOMIMETIC and BETA-RECEPTOR STIMULANT that has good beta$\{2\}\{sub\}$-receptor selectivity. It is mainly used as a BRONCHODILATOR in reversible obstructive airways disease, as an ANTI-ASTHMATIC treatment in severe acute asthma and for the alleviation of symptoms of chronic bronchitis and emphysema.

It is a pro-drug of TERBUTALINE SULPHATE (that is, it is converted to terbutaline within the body) and is administered orally as tablets.

✚▲ side-effects/warning: see under SALBUTAMOL. It is not to be used by patients with certain liver disorders, or by pregnant women.

✪ Related entry: Bambec

Baratol

(Monmouth) is a proprietary, prescription-only preparation of the ALPHA-ADRENOCEPTOR BLOCKER drug indoramin hydrochloride. It can be used in ANTIHYPERTENSIVE treatment, often in conjunction with other antihypertensive drugs and is available as tablets.

+▲ side-effects/warning: see INDORAMIN

barbiturate

drugs are derived from barbituric acid and have a wide range of essentially depressant actions. They are used mostly as SEDATIVES, GENERAL ANAESTHETICS, ANTICONVULSANTS and as ANTI-EPILEPTICS. They work by a direct action on the brain, depressing specific areas and may be slow- or fast-acting, but are all extremely effective. However, they can rapidly cause tolerance and then both psychological and physical dependence (addiction) may result and so they are used as infrequently as possible.

Moreover, prolonged use even in small doses can have serious toxic side-effects and in overdose they are lethal. The best-known and most-used barbiturates include the HYPNOTIC drug AMYLOBARBITONE, the anticonvulsant and anti-epileptic drug PHENOBARBITONE and the general anaesthetic drugs THIOPENTONE SODIUM and METHOHEXITONE SODIUM.

+ side-effects: depending on the use, dose and type, there may be hangover with drowsiness, dizziness, unsteady gait, respiratory depression, headache, hypersensitivity reactions; in the elderly there may be paradoxical excitement and confusion.

▲ warning: depending on the use, dose and type; barbiturates should be avoided wherever possible; dependence can readily occur (with withdrawal syndrome including rebound insomnia, anxiety, tremor and convulsions). Administer with caution to patients with respiratory failure, or certain kidney or heart disorders.

*barrier creams

can be used to protect the skin against irritants, chapping, urine and faeces (nappy rash), bedsores and toxic substances. They are normally applied as an ointment or a cream (commonly in a WHITE SOFT PARAFFIN or LANOLIN oily base) and often incorporating a silicone (eg DIMETHICONE).

Baxan

(Bristol-Myers) is a proprietary, prescription-only preparation of the ANTIBACTERIAL and (CEPHALOSPORIN) ANTIBIOTIC drug cefadroxil. It can be used to treat many infections, especially those of the urinary tract and is available as capsules and an oral suspension.

+▲ side-effects/warning: see CEFADROXIL

Baycaron

(Bayer) is a proprietary, prescription-only preparation of the (THIAZIDE-like) DIURETIC drug mefruside. It can be used, either alone or in conjunction with other drugs, in the treatment of oedema and as an ANTIHYPERTENSIVE. It is available as tablets.

+▲ side-effects/warning: see MEFRUSIDE

BCG vaccine

(bacillus Calmette-Guérin vaccine) for IMMUNIZATION is a VACCINE produced from *live* attenuated strain of the tuberculosis bacillus *Mycobacterium bovis*, which no longer causes the disease in humans, but stimulates formation in the body of the specific antibodies that react with the tuberculosis bacillus *Mycobacterium tuberculosis* and so can be used as an ANTITUBERCULAR vaccine. It is used for routine vaccination of children and in those likely to come into contact with tuberculous individuals. It is available as Tub/Vac/BCG (Dried) for intradermal injection or as Tub/Vac/BCG (Perc) for percutaneous administration and as a number of other preparations.

+▲ side-effects/warning: see under VACCINE

B

✪ Related entries: Bacillus Calmette-Guérin Vaccine, Dried; Bacillus Calmette-Guérin Vaccine, Percutaneous

Beclazone

(Baker Norton) is a proprietary, prescription-only preparation of the CORTICOSTEROID and ANTI-ASTHMATIC drug beclomethasone dipropionate. It can be used to prevent asthmatic attacks and is available in an aerosol for inhalation.

✚▲ side-effects/warning: see BECLOMETHASONE DIPROPIONATE

Becloforte

(Allen & Hanburys) is a proprietary, prescription-only preparation of the CORTICOSTEROID and ANTI-ASTHMATIC drug beclomethasone dipropionate. It can be used to prevent asthmatic attacks. It is available in a range of aerosols for inhalation (one form, *Becloforte VM*, comes with a *Volumatic* inhaler) and as a dry powder for inhalation (in a *Diskhaler* blister pack).

✚▲ side-effects/warning: see BECLOMETHASONE DIPROPIONATE

beclometasone dipropionate

See BECLOMETHASONE DIPROPIONATE

beclomethasone dipropionate

(beclometasone dipropionate) is a CORTICOSTEROID drug, which is used primarily as an ANTI-ASTHMATIC treatment to prevent attacks and also as an ANTI-INFLAMMATORY drug for severe skin inflammation (eg eczema and psoriasis) and for inflammatory conditions of the nasal mucosa (eg rhinitis). Administration as an anti-inflammatory preparation is by topical application as a cream or an ointment; as an anti-asthmatic it is administered by inhalation from an aerosol, nasal spray, as a powder for insufflation, or as a suspension for nebulization.

✚▲ side-effects/warning: see under

CORTICOSTEROIDS; but systemic effects are unlikely with the low doses used. As a nasal spray it may cause sneezing and dryness and irritation of the nose and throat. As a cream or ointment, there may be local skin effects. When inhaled, it may cause hoarseness and Candidiasis of the throat and mouth.

✪ Related entries: AeroBec; AeroBec Forte; Beclazone; Becloforte; Becodisks; Beconase; Becotide Inhaler; Becotide Rotacaps; Filair Forte; Propaderm; Ventide

Becodisks

(Allen and Hanburys) is a proprietary, prescription-only preparation of the CORTICOSTEROID and ANTI-ASTHMATIC drug beclomethasone dipropionate. It can be used to prevent asthmatic attacks and is available as a powder in discs for inhalation from a *Diskhaler* device.

✚▲ side-effects/warning: see BECLOMETHASONE DIPROPIONATE.

Beconase

(Allen & Hanburys) is a proprietary, prescription-only preparation of the CORTICOSTEROID and ANTI-INFLAMMATORY drug beclomethasone dipropionate. It can be used to relieve the symptoms of conditions such as hay fever and rhinitis. It is available as *Beconase nasal spray (aerosol)* and as *Beconase aqueous nasal spray* (some versions for hayfever are available without a prescription).

✚▲ side-effects/warning: see BECLOMETHASONE DIPROPIONATE

Becotide Inhaler

(Allen & Hanburys) is a proprietary, prescription-only preparation of the CORTICOSTEROID and ANTI-ASTHMATIC drug beclomethasone dipropionate. It can be used to prevent asthmatic attacks and is available in an aerosol for inhalation in three forms: *Becotide-50*, *Becotide-100* and *Becotide-200*.

✚▲ side-effects/warning: see BECLOMETHASONE DIPROPIONATE

Becotide Rotacaps

(Allen & Hanburys) is a proprietary, prescription-only preparation of the CORTICOSTEROID and ANTI-ASTHMATIC drug beclomethasone dipropionate. It can be used to prevent asthmatic attacks and is available as a powder in cartridges (*Becotide Rotacaps*) and for inhalation from the *Becotide Rotahaler*.

✚▲ side-effects/warning. see BECLOMETHASONE DIPROPIONATE

Bedranol SR

(Lagap) is a proprietary, prescription-only preparation of the BETA-BLOCKER drug propranolol hydrochloride. It can be used as an ANTIHYPERTENSIVE treatment for raised blood pressure, as an ANTI-ANGINA treatment to relieve symptoms and improve exercise tolerance and as an ANTI-ARRHYTHMIC to regularize heartbeat and to treat myocardial infarction.

It can also be used as an ANTITHYROID drug for short-term treatment of thyrotoxicosis, as an ANTIMIGRAINE treatment to prevent attacks, as an ANXIOLYTIC treatment, particularly for symptomatic relief of tremor and palpitations and, with an ALPHA-ADRENOCEPTOR BLOCKER, in the acute treatment of phaeochromocytoma. It is available as modified-release capsules.

✚▲ side-effects/warning: see PROPRANOLOL HYDROCHLORIDE

Beecham Pills

(SmithKline Beecham) is a proprietary, non-prescription preparation of the (*stimulant*) LAXATIVE drug aloin. It can be used to relieve constipation and is available as tablets. It is not normally given to children, except on medical advice.

✚▲ side-effects/warning: see ALOIN

Beechams 75 mg Aspirin

(SmithKline Beecham) is a proprietary, non-prescription preparation of the (NSAID) NON-NARCOTIC ANALGESIC drug aspirin (at a lower analgesic dose than is usual). It can be used to treat mild to moderate pain and is available as tablets. It is not normally given to children under 12 years, except on medical advice.

✚▲ side-effects/warning: see ASPIRIN

Beechams Hot Blackcurrant

(SmithKline Beecham) is a proprietary, non-prescription COMPOUND PREPARATION of the NON-NARCOTIC ANALGESIC drug paracetamol, the SYMPATHOMIMETIC and DECONGESTANT drug phenylephrine hydrochloride and vitamin C. It can be used for the symptomatic relief of mild to moderate pain, colds and flu, aches and pains and nasal congestion. It is available as a powder and is not normally given to children, except on medical advice.

✚▲ side-effects/warning: see PARACETAMOL; PHENYLEPHRINE HYDROCHLORIDE

Beechams Hot Lemon

(SmithKline Beecham) is a proprietary, non-prescription COMPOUND PREPARATION of the NON-NARCOTIC ANALGESIC and ANTIRHEUMATIC drug paracetamol, the SYMPATHOMIMETIC and DECONGESTANT drug phenylephrine hydrochloride and vitamin C. It can be used for the symptomatic relief of mild to moderate pain, colds, flu, aches and pains and nasal congestion. It is available as a powder and is not normally given to children under 12 years, except on medical advice.

✚▲ side-effects/warning: see PARACETAMOL; PHENYLEPHRINE HYDROCHLORIDE

Beechams Hot Lemon and Honey

(SmithKline Beecham) is a proprietary, non-prescription COMPOUND PREPARATION of the NON-NARCOTIC ANALGESIC and ANTIRHEUMATIC drug paracetamol, the SYMPATHOMIMETIC and DECONGESTANT drug phenylephrine hydrochloride and vitamin C. It can be used for the symptomatic relief of mild to moderate pain, colds, flu, aches and pains and nasal congestion. It is available as a powder and is not normally

B

given to children under 12 years, except on medical advice.

✚▲ side-effects/warning: see PARACETAMOL; PHENYLEPHRINE HYDROCHLORIDE

Beechams Lemon Tablets

(SmithKline Beecham) is a proprietary, non-prescription preparation of the (NSAID) NON-NARCOTIC ANALGESIC and ANTIRHEUMATIC drug aspirin with glycine. It can be used for the symptomatic relief of mild to moderate pain, colds, flu, aches and pains (including the pain and inflammation of rheumatic disease), toothache and period pain. It is available as tablets and is not normally given to children under 12 years, except on medical advice.

✚▲ side-effects/warning: see ASPIRIN

Beechams Powders

(SmithKline Beecham) is a proprietary, non-prescription COMPOUND PREPARATION of the (NSAID) NON-NARCOTIC ANALGESIC and ANTIRHEUMATIC drug aspirin and the STIMULANT caffeine. It can be used for the symptomatic relief of mild to moderate pain, colds, flu, aches and pains (including the pain and inflammation of rheumatic disease) and period pain. It is available as tablets and is not normally given to children, except on medical advice.

✚▲ side-effects/warning: see ASPIRIN; CAFFEINE

Beechams Powders Capsules

(SmithKline Beecham) is a proprietary, non-prescription COMPOUND PREPARATION of the NON-NARCOTIC ANALGESIC and ANTIRHEUMATIC drug paracetamol, the SYMPATHOMIMETIC and DECONGESTANT drug phenylephrine hydrochloride and the STIMULANT caffeine. It can be used for the symptomatic relief of mild to moderate pain, colds, flu, aches and pains and nasal congestion.

It is available as capsules and is not

normally given to children under six years, except on medical advice.

✚▲ side-effects/warning: see CAFFEINE; PARACETAMOL; PHENYLEPHRINE HYDROCHLORIDE

belladonna alkaloids

are drugs derived from solanaceous plants such as *Atropa belladonna* (deadly nightshade) and which inlcude the drugs ATROPINE SULPHATE (hyoscyamine) and HYOSCINE HYDROBROMIDE (scopolamine). These drugs have ANTICHOLINERGIC properties and are used for a variety of medical purposes. Poisoning due to eating the berries of *Atropa belladonna* is not uncommon, particularly in children. Indeed, it has been one of the most popular poisons throughout history, from the time of Imperial Rome to the Borgias in fifteenth-century Italy. The name *belladonna* literally means 'beautiful lady' and is thought to refer to the use of the plant as a cosmetic in ancient times, when it was used as eye-drops to dilate the pupils.

✚▲ side-effects/warning: see under ATROPINE SULPHATE; HYOSCINE BUTYLBROMIDE; HYOSCINE HYDROBROMIDE

Bendogen

(Lagap) is a proprietary, prescription-only preparation of the ADRENERGIC NEURONE BLOCKER drug bethanidine sulphate. It can be used in ANTIHYPERTENSIVE treatment for moderate to severe high blood pressure and is available as tablets.

✚▲ side-effects/warning: see BETHANIDINE SULPHATE

bendrofluazide

(bendroflumethiazide) is a DIURETIC drug of the THIAZIDE class. It is used in ANTIHYPERTENSIVE treatment, either alone or in conjunction with other types of diuretic or other drugs. It can also be used in the treatment of oedema (accumulation of fluid in the tissues) associated with congestive heart failure.

Administration is oral in the form of tablets.

✚ side-effects: there may be mild gastrointestinal upsets, postural hypotension (low blood pressure on standing), reversible impotence; low blood potassium, sodium, magnesium and chloride; raised blood urea, glucose and lipids; rarely, gout, photosensitivity, blood disorders, skin reactions and pancreatitis.

▲ warning: it should not be administered to patients with certain severe kidney or liver disorders. It should be administered with caution to the elderly, or who are pregnant or breast-feeding. It may aggravate diabetes or gout. Blood potassium levels should be monitored in patients taking thiazide diuretics, because they may deplete the body of potassium. It should not be used where there are abnormal levels of sodium and potassium, or in Addison's disease.

✪ Related entries: Aprinox; Berkozide; Corgaretic 40; Corgaretic 80; Inderetic; Inderex; Neo-NaClex; Neo-NaClex-K; Prestim; Prestim Forte

bendroflumethiazide

See BENDROFLUAZIDE

Benemid

(Merck, Sharp & Dohme) is a proprietary, prescription-only preparation of the drug probenecid. It can be used to prevent gout and to reduce the excretion of certain ANTIBIOTICS by the kidney. It is available as tablets.

✚▲ side-effects/warning: see PROBENECID

Bengué's Balsam

(Bengué) is a proprietary, non-prescription COMPOUND PREPARATION of menthol and methyl salicylate, which both have COUNTER-IRRITANT, or RUBEFACIENT, actions. It can be applied to the skin for symptomatic relief of underlying muscle or joint pain. It is available as an ointment in a lanolin base.

✚▲ side-effects/warning: see LANOLIN; MENTHOL; METHYL SALICYLATE

Benoral

(Sanofi Winthrop) is a proprietary, non-prescription preparation of the (NSAID) NON-NARCOTIC ANALGESIC and ANTIRHEUMATIC drug benorylate, which is derived from both ASPIRIN and PARACETAMOL. It can be used to treat mild to moderate pain, especially the pain of rheumatic disease and other musculoskeletal disorders. It is available as tablets, as granules in sachets for oral solution and as a sugar-free suspension.

✚▲ side-effects/warning: see BENORYLATE

benorilate

See BENORYLATE

benorylate

is a (NSAID) NON-NARCOTIC ANALGESIC and ANTIRHEUMATIC drug with ANTIPYRETIC actions. It is chemically derived from both ASPIRIN and PARACETAMOL and these two pharmacologically active constituents are released into the bloodstream at different rates. It is used particularly to treat the pain of rheumatic disease and other musculoskeletal disorders and to lower a high temperature in fever. Administration is oral in the form of tablets, sachets for solution, or as a dilute suspension.

✚▲ side-effects/warning: see under NSAID; but it is better tolerated and causes less gastrointestinal disturbances than the majority of this class.

✪ **Related entry: Benoral**

benoxinate

is an alternative name for the LOCAL ANAESTHETIC drug OXYBUPROCAINE HYDROCHLORIDE.

Benoxyl 5 Cream

(Stiefel) is a proprietary, non-prescription COMPOUND PREPARATION of the ANTIFUNGAL drug miconazole (as nitrate) and the KERATOLYTIC and ANTIMICROBIAL drug benzoyl peroxide (5%). It can be used to treat acne and is available as a cream and a lotion for topical application.

B

✚▲ side-effects/warning: see BENZOYL
PEROXIDE; MICONAZOLE

Benoxyl 10 Lotion

(Stiefel) is a proprietary, non-prescription
COMPOUND PREPARATION of the ANTIFUNGAL
drug miconazole (as nitrate) and the
KERATOLYTIC and ANTIMICROBIAL drug
benzoyl peroxide (10%). It can be used to
treat acne and is available as a cream and
a lotion for topical application.
✚▲ side-effects/warning: see
BENZOYL PEROXIDE; MICONAZOLE

benperidol

is a powerful ANTIPSYCHOTIC drug and is
chemically a butyrophenone. It is used to
treat and tranquillize psychotics and is
especially suitable for treating antisocial
and deviant forms of sexual behaviour.
Administration is oral in the form of
tablets.
✚▲ side-effects/warning: see under
HALOPERIDOL
○ Related entry: Anquil

benserazide hydrochloride

is an ENZYME INHIBITOR, which is
administered therapeutically in
combination with the drug LEVODOPA to
treat parkinsonism, but not the
parkinsonian symptoms induced by drugs
(see ANTIPARKINSONISM). Benserazide
prevents levodopa being too rapidly
broken down in the body into dopamine
and so allowing more levodopa to reach
the brain to make up the deficiency of
dopamine, which is the major cause of
parkinsonian symptoms.

The combination of benserazide
hydrochloride with levodopa is known in
medicine by the simplified name of
CO-BENELDOPA. Administration of the
combination is oral in the form of
capsules or tablets.
○ Related entry: Madopar

bentonite

is an absorbent powder that is

administered therapeutically in
emergencies to absorb corrosive
substances like paraquat (the toxic
horticultural preparation) in cases of
accidental poisoning and to reduce further
absorption by the body.
See ANTIDOTE

Benylin Chesty Coughs Non-Drowsy

(Warner Wellcome) is a proprietary, non-
prescription preparation of the
EXPECTORANT drug guaiphenesin and
menthol. It can be used for the
symptomatic relief of cough and is
available as a syrup. It is not normally
given to children under six years, except
on medical advice.
✚▲ side-effects/warning: see GUAIPHENESIN

Benylin Chesty Coughs Original

(Warner Wellcome) is a proprietary, non-
prescription preparation of the
ANTIHISTAMINE drug diphenhydramine
hydrochloride. It can be used for the
symptomatic relief of cough and
associated congestive symptoms and is
available as a syrup. It is not normally
given to children under five years, except
on medical advice.
✚▲ side-effects/warning: see
DIPHENHYDRAMINE HYDROCHLORIDE

Benylin Children's Coughs Original

(Warner Wellcome) is a proprietary, non-
prescription preparation of the
ANTIHISTAMINE drug diphenhydramine
hydrochloride. It can be used for the
symptomatic relief of cough and its
congestive symptoms and for the
treatment of hay fever and other allergic
conditions. It is available in as a
syrup and is not normally given to
children under one year, except on
medical advice.
✚▲ side-effects/warning: see
DIPHENHYDRAMINE HYDROCHLORIDE

Benylin Children's Coughs Sugar Free/Colour Free

(Warner Wellcome) is a proprietary, non-prescription preparation of the ANTIHISTAMINE drug diphenhydramine hydrochloride and menthol. It can be used for the symptomatic relief of cough and congestion and in the treatment of hay fever and other allergic conditions affecting the upper respiratory tract in children. It is available as a syrup and is not normally given to children under one year, except on medical advice.

✚▲ side-effects/warning: see DIPHENHYDRAMINE HYDROCHLORIDE

Benylin Day and Night

(Warner Wellcome) is a proprietary, non-prescription preparation that can be used for the symptomatic relief of colds and flu. It is available in the form of two types of COMPOUND PREPARATIONS in the same pack: a yellow film-coated tablet (taken during the day) contains the NON-NARCOTIC ANALGESIC and ANTIPYRETIC drug paracetamol and the SYMPATHOMIMETIC drug phenylpropanolamine hydrochloride; a blue film-coated tablet (taken at night) contains paracetamol and the ANTIHISTAMINE diphenhydramine hydrochloride. It is not normally given to children, except on medical advice.

✚▲ side-effects/warning: see DIPHENHYDRAMINE HYDROCHLORIDE; PARACETAMOL; PHENYLPROPANOLAMINE HYDROCHLORIDE

Benylin Dry Coughs Non-Drowsy

(Warner Wellcome) is a proprietary, non-prescription preparation of the ANTITUSSIVE drug dextromethorphan hydrobromide. It can be used for the symptomatic relief of persistent, dry, irritating coughs. It is available as a syrup and is not normally given to children under six years, except on medical advice.

✚▲ side-effects/warning: see DEXTROMETHORPHAN HYDROBROMIDE

Benylin Dry Coughs Original

(Warner Wellcome) is a proprietary, non-prescription preparation of the ANTIHISTAMINE drug diphenhydramine hydrochloride, the ANTITUSSIVE drug dextromethorphan hydrobromide and menthol. It can be used for the symptomatic relief of persistent, dry, irritating coughs. It is available as a syrup and is not normally given to children under five years, except on medical advice.

✚▲ side-effects/warning: see DEXTROMETHORPHAN HYDROBROMIDE; DIPHENHYDRAMINE HYDROCHLORIDE

Benylin with Codeine

(Warner Wellcome) is a proprietary, non-prescription COMPOUND PREPARATION of the the ANTITUSSIVE drug codeine phosphate, the ANTIHISTAMINE diphenhydramine hydrochloride and menthol. It can be used for the symptomatic relief of persistent, dry cough and is available in the form of a syrup. It is not normally given to children under six years, except on medical advice.

✚▲ side-effects/warning: see CODEINE PHOSPHATE; DIPHENHYDRAMINE HYDROCHLORIDE

Benzagel

(Bioglan) is a proprietary, non-prescription COMPOUND PREPARATION of the ANTIFUNGAL drug miconazole (as nitrate) and the KERATOLYTIC and ANTIMICROBIAL drug benzoyl peroxide. It can be used to treat acne and is available as a cream and a lotion for topical application.

✚▲ side-effects/warning: see BENZOYL PEROXIDE; MICONAZOLE

benzalkonium chloride

is an ANTISEPTIC agent that has some KERATOLYTIC properties. It can be topically applied to remove hard, dead skin from around wounds or ulcers, or to dissolve

B

warts. It can also be used on minor abrasions and burns and (in the form of lozenges) for mouth ulcers, gum disease and sore throats. For other than oral purposes, administration is topical in the form of a cream or (combined with bromine) as a paint.

✚▲ side-effects/warning: avoid normal skin when using as a cream.

✿ Related entries: Bradosol Sugar Free Lozenges; Capitol; Conotrane; Drapolene Cream; Emulsiderm; Ionax Scrub; Ionil T; Roccal; Roccal Concentrate 10X

Benzamycin

(Bioglan) is a proprietary, non-prescription COMPOUND PREPARATION of the ANTIBACTERIAL and (MACROLIDE) ANTIBIOTIC drug erythromycin and the KERATOLYTIC and ANTIMICROBIAL drug benzoyl peroxide. It can be used to treat acne and is available as a gel for topical application.

✚▲ side-effects/warning: see benzoyl peroxide; erythromycin

benzatropine mesilate

See BENZTROPINE MESYLATE

benzhexol hydrochloride

(trihexyphenidyl hydrochloride) is an ANTICHOLINERGIC drug, which is used in the treatment of some types of parkinsonism (see ANTIPARKINSONISM). It increases mobility and decreases rigidity and tremor and the tendency to produce an excess of saliva is also reduced, but it has only a limited effect on bradykinesia. Additionally, the drug has the capacity to treat these symptoms, in some cases, where they are produced by drugs. It is thought to work by correcting the over-effectiveness of the NEUROTRANSMITTER ACETYLCHOLINE (cholinergic excess), which is caused by the deficiency of dopamine that occurs in parkinsonism. Administration, which may be in conjunction with other drugs used to

relieve parkinsonism, is oral in the form of tablets, modified-release capsules, or a syrup.

✚ side-effects: dry mouth, gastrointestinal disturbances, dizziness, blurred vision; less commonly there is urinary retention, speeding of the heart, sensitivity reactions, or nervousness. Rarely and only in susceptible patients, there may be confusion, excitement and psychological disturbance.

▲ warning: it should not be used in patients with urinary retention, closed-angle glaucoma, gastrointestinal obstruction. Administer with caution to those with impaired kidney or liver function, or cardiovascular disease. Withdrawal of treatment must be gradual.

✿ Related entries: Artane; Broflex

benzocaine

is a LOCAL ANAESTHETIC drug. It is used by topical application for the relief of pain in the skin surface or mucous membranes, particularly in or around the mouth and throat, or (in combination with other drugs) in the ears. Administration is topical and in various forms: as a gel, cream, lozenges, pastille, spray, ointment, or as ear-drops.

▲ warning: prolonged use should be avoided and some patients may experience sensitivity reactions.

✿ Related entries: Dequacaine Lozenges; Intralgin; Medilave; Merocaine Lozenges; Solarcaine; Tyrocane Throat Lozenges; Tyrozets

benzodiazepine

drugs are a large group of drugs that have a marked effect upon the central nervous system. The effect varies according to the level of dose, the frequency of dosage and which member of the group is used. They have, to varying degrees, SEDATIVE, ANXIOLYTIC, HYPNOTIC, ANTICONVULSANT, ANTI-EPILEPTIC and SKELETAL MUSCLE RELAXANT actions. They can also cause amnesia and may be used as a postoperative medication in order to allow patients to forget unpleasant procedures. Benzodiazepines that are used as hypnotics have virtually replaced earlier drugs, such as the BARBITURATES and CHLORAL HYDRATE, because they are just as effective but much safer in overdose.

There are now ANTAGONISTS, such as FLUMAZENIL, that can be used to reverse some of the central nervous system effects of benzodiazepines, for instance, at the end of operations. However, it is now realized that dependence may result from prolonged use and that there may be a paradoxical increase in hostility and aggression in patients having long-term treatment.

The best-known and most-used benzodiazepines include DIAZEPAM (which can be used for many purposes, including to control anxiety, skeletal muscle relaxation during operations, the convulsions of epilepsy, or for drug poisoning), NITRAZEPAM (a widely used hypnotic), CHLORDIAZEPOXIDE and LORAZEPAM (anxiolytic). See also: ALPRAZOLAM; BROMAZEPAM; CLONAZEPAM; FLUNITRAZEPAM; FLURAZEPAM; LORMETAZEPAM; NITRAZEPAM; OXAZEPAM; TEMAZEPAM

✚ side-effects: depending on use, dose and type, there may be drowsiness and light-headedness the day after treatment, confusion and impaired gait (particularly in the elderly), dependence, amnesia, aggression; occasionally, vertigo, headache, hypotension, salivation changes, rashes, visual disturbances, changes in libido, urinary retention, blood disorders, jaundice and gastrointestinal disorders.

▲ warning: depending on use, dose and type, they should not be given to patients with respiratory depression or acute pulmonary insufficiency, psychosis, or phobic or obsessional states. Administer with caution to those with respiratory disease, muscle weakness, history of alcohol or drug abuse, severe personality disorders, liver or kidney impairment; who are elderly or debilitated, or have porphyria, or who are pregnant or breast-feeding. Avoid prolonged use because of the risk of dependence.

benzoic acid
has ANTIFUNGAL and KERATOLYTIC activity and is incorporated into non-proprietary and proprietary ointments and creams.
✪ Related entries: Aserbine; benzoic acid ointment, compound, BP

benzoic acid ointment, compound, BP
is a COMPOUND PREPARATION of the ANTIFUNGAL and KERATOLYTIC agents salicylic acid and benzoic acid. It is commonly used to treat patches of ringworm infection on limbs, palms, soles of feet and chest. It is available in the form of an ointment, which is also known as *Whitfield's Ointment*.
✚▲ side-effects/warning: see BENZOIC ACID; SALICYLIC ACID

benzoin tincture, compound, BP
is a non-proprietary COMPOUND PREPARATION of balsam resin and balsamic acid. It is used as a base from which vapours may be inhaled (when added to boiling water) and can be used as a NASAL DECONGESTANT for blocked nose in sinusitis, rhinitis and bronchitis.

benzoyl peroxide
is a KERATOLYTIC and ANTIMICROBIAL drug. It is used in combination with other drugs to treat conditions like acne and skin infections such as athlete's foot. Administration is topical in the form of a cream, lotion, or gel.
✚ side-effects: some patients experience skin irritation.
▲ warning: it should not be used to treat the skin disease of the facial blood vessels, rosacea. When applying, avoid the eyes, mouth and mucous membranes. It may bleach fabrics.
✪ Related entries: Acetoxyl 25 Acne Gel; Acetoxyl 5 Acne Gel; Acnecide;

B

Acnegel; Acnegel Forte; Acnidazil; Benoxyl 5 Cream; Benoxyl 10 Lotion; Benzagel; Benzamycin; Mediclear 10 Acne Cream; Mediclear 5 Acne Cream; Mediclear Acne Lotion; Nericur; Oxy 5 Lotion; Oxy 10 Lotion; PanOxyl 5 Gel; PanOxyl 10 Gel; PanOxyl Aquagel 5; PanOxyl Aquagel 10; PanOxyl Aquagel 25; PanOxyl Wash; Quinoderm Cream; Quinoderm Cream 5; Quinoderm Lotio-Gel 5%; Quinoped; Ultra Clearasil Maximum Strength; Ultra Clearasil Regular Strength

benzthiazide

is a DIURETIC drug of the THIAZIDE class. It is used in ANTIHYPERTENSIVE treatment, in conjunction with other types of diuretics and in the treatment of oedema (accumulation of fluid in the tissues) associated with congestive heart failure. Administration is oral in the form of capsules.

+▲ side-effects/warning: see under BENDROFLUAZIDE

✪ Related entry: Dytide

benztropine mesylate

(benzatropine mesilate) is an ANTICHOLINERGIC drug, which is used in the treatment of some types of parkinsonism (see ANTIPARKINSONISM). It increases mobility and decreases rigidity and tremor and the tendency to produce an excess of saliva is also reduced, but it has only a limited effect on bradykinesia. Additionally, it has the capacity to treat these symptoms, in some cases, where they are produced by drugs.

It is thought to work by correcting the over-effectiveness of the NEUROTRANSMITTER ACETYLCHOLINE (cholinergic excess), which results from the deficiency of dopamine that occurs in parkinsonism. Because it also has some sedative properties, it is sometimes used in preference to the similar drug BENZHEXOL HYDROCHLORIDE. Administration, which may be in

conjunction with other drugs used to relieve parkinsonism, is either oral as tablets or by injection.

+▲ side-effects/warning: see under BENZHEXOL HYDROCHLORIDE; but it causes sedation rather than stimulation.

✪ Related entry: Cogentin

benzydamine hydrochloride

has COUNTER-IRRITANT, or RUBEFACIENT, action and can be used for the symptomatic relief of pain when applied to the skin, mouth ulcers and other sores or inflammation in the mouth and throat. It is available as a cream, for topical application, as a liquid mouthwash and a spray.

+ side-effects: stinging or numbness on initial application.

✪ Related entry: Difflam

benzyl benzoate

can be used either as a SCABICIDAL drug to treat infestation of the skin, chest and limbs by itch-mites (scabies) or as a PEDICULICIDAL drug to treat head lice infestation. Administration is in the form of a topical emulsion.

+ side-effects: there may be skin irritation, a burning sensation and occasionally a rash.

▲ warning: administer with caution to patients who are pregnant or breast-feeding; avoid contact with the eyes, mucous membranes and broken skin.

✪ Related entries; Anugesic-HC; Anusol-HC; Ascabiol Emulsion; Sudocrem Antiseptic Cream

benzylpenicillin

(penicillin G) is the chemical name for the ANTIBACTERIAL drug that was the first of the penicillins to be isolated and used as an ANTIBIOTIC. Despite the many hundreds of antibiotics introduced since, it still remains the drug of choice in treating many severe infections, including those caused by sensitive strains of meningococcus (eg meningitis and septicaemia.), pneumococcus (eg pneumonia and meningitis) and streptococcus (eg bacterial sore throat, scarlet fever and septicaemia), in serious conditions when the micro-organism causing the disease has not be identified for certain (eg endocarditis) and to prevent bacterial infection following limb amputation. In its long-acting form, PROCAINE PENICILLIN, it has an important role in treating syphilis.

It is usually injected because it is inactivated by digestive acids in the stomach. Its rapid excretion by the kidney also means frequent administration is necessary, unless long-acting preparations are used.

✚ side-effects: diarrhoea (after oral administration); more rarely, sensitivity reactions such as rashes, urticaria, angio-oedema. and blood changes; high temperature and joint pain. Allergic patients may suffer anaphylactic shock.

▲ warning: it should not be administered to patients with known allergy to penicillins; use with care in patients with impaired kidney function.

○ Related entry: Crystapen

Berkamil

(Berk) is a proprietary, prescription-only preparation of the (*potassium-sparing*) DIURETIC drug amiloride hydrochloride. It can be used to treat oedema, ascites in cirrhosis of the liver, congestive heart failure (in conjunction with other diuretics) and as an ANTIHYPERTENSIVE. It is available as tablets.

✚▲ side-effects/warning: see AMILORIDE HYDROCHLORIDE

Berkaprine

(Berk) is a proprietary, prescription-only preparation of the IMMUNOSUPPRESSANT drug azathioprine. It can be used to treat tissue rejection in transplant patients and for a variety of autoimmune diseases. It is available as tablets.

✚▲ side-effects/warning: see AZATHIOPRINE

Berkatens

(Berk) is a proprietary, prescription-only preparation of the CALCIUM-CHANNEL BLOCKER drug verapamil hydrochloride. It can be used as an ANTIHYPERTENSIVE treatment, as an ANTI-ANGINA drug in the prevention of attacks and as an ANTI-ARRHYTHMIC to correct heart irregularities. It is available as tablets.

✚▲ side-effects/warning: see VERAPAMIL HYDROCHLORIDE

Berkmycen

(Berk) is a proprietary, prescription-only preparation of the ANTIBACTERIAL and (TETRACYCLINE) ANTIBIOTIC drug oxytetracycline. It can be used to treat a wide range of infections and is available as tablets.

✚▲ side-effects/warning: see OXYTETRACYCLINE

Berkolol

(Berk) is a proprietary, prescription-only preparation of the BETA-BLOCKER drug propranolol hydrochloride. It can be used as an ANTIHYPERTENSIVE treatment for raised blood pressure, an ANTI-ANGINA treatment to relieve symptoms and improve exercise tolerance and as an ANTI-ARRHYTHMIC to regularize heartbeat and to treat myocardial infarction. It can also be used as an ANTITHYROID drug for short-term treatment of thyrotoxicosis, as an ANTIMIGRAINE treatment to prevent attacks, as an ANXIOLYTIC treatment, particularly for symptomatic relief of tremor and palpitations and, with an ALPHA-ADRENOCEPTOR BLOCKER, in the acute treatment of phaeochromocytoma. It is available as tablets.

✚▲ side-effects/warning: see PROPRANOLOL HYDROCHLORIDE

Berkozide

(Berk) is a proprietary, prescription-only preparation of the (THIAZIDE) DIURETIC drug bendrofluazide. It can be used, either alone or in conjunction with other drugs,

B

in the treatment of oedema with congestive heart failure and as an ANTIHYPERTENSIVE. It is available as tablets.

➕▲ side-effects/warning: see BENDROFLUAZIDE

Berotec

(Boehringer Ingelheim) is a proprietary, prescription-only preparation of the BETA-RECEPTOR STIMULANT fenoterol hydrobromide. It can be used as a BRONCHODILATOR in reversible obstructive airways disease, as an ANTI-ASTHMATIC treatment in severe acute asthma, or for the alleviation of symptoms of chronic bronchitis and emphysema. It is available as a metered aerosol inhalant.

➕▲ side-effects/warning: see FENOTEROL HYDROBROMIDE

Beta-Adalat

(Bayer) is a proprietary, prescription-only COMPOUND PREPARATION of the BETA-BLOCKER drug atenolol and the CALCIUM-CHANNEL BLOCKER drug nifedipine. It can be used as an ANTIHYPERTENSIVE treatment for raised blood pressure and is available as tablets.

➕▲ side-effects/warning: see ATENOLOL: NIFEDIPINE

beta-adrenoceptor blocking drugs

See BETA-BLOCKERS

beta-adrenoceptor stimulants

See BETA-RECEPTOR STIMULANTS

beta-agonists

SEE BETA-RECEPTOR STIMULANTS

*beta-blockers

(beta-adrenoceptor blocking drugs) are drugs that inhibit some actions of the sympathetic nervous system by preventing the action of ADRENALINE and NORADRENALINE (HORMONE and NEUROTRANSMITTER mediators,

respectively) by blocking the beta-adrenoceptors on which they act. Correspondingly, drugs called alpha-adrenoceptor blockers are drugs used to inhibit the remaining actions by occupying the other main class of adrenoceptor, alpha-adrenoceptors.

These two classes of adrenoceptor are responsible for the very widespread actions of adrenaline and noradrenaline in the body, both in normal physiology and in stress. For example, they speed the heart, constrict or dilate certain blood vessels (thereby increasing blood pressure) and suppress activity in the intestines. In general, they prepare the body for emergency action.

In disease, some of these actions may be inappropriate, exaggerated and detrimental to health, so beta-blockers may be used to restore a more healthy balance. Thus beta-blockers may be used as ANTIHYPERTENSIVES to lower blood pressure when it is abnormally raised in cardiovascular disease; as an ANTI-ARRHYTHMIC treatment to correct heartbeat irregularities; as an ANTI-ANGINA treatment to prevent the pain of angina pectoris during exercise and to treat myocardial infarction (damage to heart muscle) associated with heart attacks; as an ANTIMIGRAINE treatment (prophylaxis; to prevent migraine attacks); as an ANXIOLYTIC treatment to reduce anxiety, particularly its manifestations such as tremor; as an ANTITHYROID treatment, specifically, shortly before surgery to correct thyrotoxicosis; and, in the form of eye-drops, as a GLAUCOMA TREATMENT to lower raised intraocular pressure.

However, there may be a price to pay, in as much as they will also block beta-receptors elsewhere in the body, thereby reducing the normal, beneficial actions of adrenaline and noradrenaline and these effects may well be undesirable. For instance, they may precipitate asthma attacks and sufferers may require bigger doses of beta-receptor stimulant aerosols for their complaint. Similarly, the blood flow in the extremities will often be reduced, so patients may complain of cold feet or hands. The best-known and most-used beta-blockers include ACEBUTOLOL, OXPRENOLOL HYDROCHLORIDE, PROPRANOLOL HYDROCHLORIDE and SOTALOL HYDROCHLORIDE.

+▲ side-effects/warning: see under PROPRANOLOL HYDROCHLORIDE. Most beta blockers can cause tiredness, sleep disturbances and coldness in the extremities. They may cause asthma attacks in susceptible patients and, because they slow the heart, may cause heart failure, so they should only be used in patients where this is not a problem. These side-effects may occur when beta-blockers are used as eye-drops for glaucoma treatment. Some beta-blockers having fewer general side-effects are known as *cardioselective*.

Beta-Cardone

(Evans) is a proprietary, prescription-only preparation of the BETA-BLOCKER drug sotalol hydrochloride. It can be used as an ANTIHYPERTENSIVE treatment for raised blood pressure, as an ANTI-ANGINA treatment to relieve symptoms and improve exercise tolerance and as an ANTI-ARRHYTHMIC to regularize heartbeat and to treat myocardial infarction. It can also be used as an ANTITHYROID drug for short-term treatment of thyrotoxicosis. It is available as tablets.

+▲ side-effects/warning: see SOTALOL HYDROCHLORIDE

Betadine

(Seton Healthcare) is a proprietary, non-prescription range of preparations of the ANTISEPTIC agent povidone-iodine. It is available as a vaginal cleansing kit containing pessaries, a gel and a solution for the treatment of bacterial infections in the vagina and cervix. A more dilute solution may also be used as a mouthwash and gargle for the mouth and throat. For the treatment of skin infections it is available in solutions of differing concentrations as a paint, a lotion, a scalp and skin cleanser, a shampoo, a skin cleanser solution and a mouthwash or gargle. It is also available as a dry powder and an ointment that can be used to dress minor cuts and abrasions.

+▲ side-effects/warning: see POVIDONE-IODINE

Betadur CR

(Monmouth) is a proprietary, prescription-only preparation of the BETA-BLOCKER drug propranolol hydrochloride. It can be used as an ANTIHYPERTENSIVE treatment for raised blood pressure, as an ANTI-ANGINA treatment to relieve symptoms and improve exercise tolerance and as an ANTI-ARRHYTHMIC to regularize heartbeat and to treat myocardial infarction. It can also be used as an ANTITHYROID drug for short-term treatment of thyrotoxicosis, as an ANTIMIGRAINE treatment to prevent attacks, as an ANXIOLYTIC treatment, particularly for symptomatic relief of tremor and palpitations and, with an ALPHA-ADRENOCEPTOR BLOCKER, in the acute treatment of phaeochromocytoma. It is available as modified-release capsules.

+▲ side-effects/warning: see PROPRANOLOL HYDROCHLORIDE

Betagan

(Allergan) is a proprietary, prescription-only preparation of the BETA-BLOCKER drug levobunolol hydrochloride. It can be used for GLAUCOMA TREATMENT and is available as eye-drops.

+▲ side-effects/warning: see LEVOBUNOLOL HYDROCHLORIDE

betahistine hydrochloride

is an ANTINAUSEANT drug. It is used to treat the vertigo, hearing loss and tinnitus (ringing in the ears) associated with Ménière's disease. Administration is oral in the form of tablets.

+ side-effects: gastrointestinal disturbances, headache, rash.

B

▲ warning: it is not to be given to patients with phaeochromocytoma; administer with caution to those with peptic ulcer or asthma.
○ Related entry: Serc

*beta-lactam
is the chemical name for ANTIBIOTICS that have a chemical ring structure – a lactam ring. This extensive family includes the PENICILLINS (whose generic names usually end *-cillin*) and the CEPHALOSPORINS (whose names often include *cef* or *ceph*).

Betaloc
(Astra) is a proprietary, prescription-only preparation of the BETA-BLOCKER drug metoprolol tartrate. It can be used as an ANTIHYPERTENSIVE treatment for raised blood pressure, as an ANTI-ANGINA treatment to relieve symptoms and improve exercise tolerance and as an ANTI-ARRHYTHMIC to regularize heartbeat and to treat myocardial infarction. It can also be used as an ANTITHYROID drug for short-term treatment of thyrotoxicosis and as an ANTIMIGRAINE treatment to prevent attacks. It is available as tablets and in a form for injection.
+▲ side-effects/warning: see METOPROLOL TARTRATE

Betaloc-SA
(Astra) is a proprietary, prescription-only preparation of the BETA-BLOCKER drug metoprolol tartrate. It can be used as an ANTIHYPERTENSIVE treatment for raised blood pressure, as an ANTI-ANGINA treatment to relieve symptoms and improve exercise tolerance and as an ANTI-ARRHYTHMIC to regularize heartbeat and to treat myocardial infarction. It can also be used as an ANTIMIGRAINE treatment to prevent attacks. It is available as modified-release tablets.
+▲ side-effects/warning: see METOPROLOL TARTRATE

betamethasone
is a CORTICOSTEROID with ANTI-INFLAMMATORY properties. It is used in the treatment of many kinds of inflammation, particularly inflammation associated with skin conditions such as eczema and psoriasis and of the eyes, ears, or nose.

It is also used to treat cerebral oedema (fluid retention in the brain) and congenital adrenal hyperplasia (abnormal growth of a part of the adrenal gland called the adrenal cortex). It is administered in several forms by different methods, depending on the form of the drug. Administration as *betamethasone* is either oral as tablets, or by injection; as *betamethasone dipropionate* by topical application as a cream, ointment, or a scalp lotion; as *betamethasone sodium phosphate* by topical application as eye-, ear-, or nose-drops; and as *betamethasone valerate* also by topical application as a cream, ointment, lotion, or a rectal ointment. Betamethasone is also available in several COMPOUND PREPARATIONS with ANTIMICROBIAL and LOCAL ANAESTHETIC drugs.
+▲ side-effects/warning: see under CORTICOSTEROIDS. Systemic side-effects are unlikely with topical application, but there may be local skin reactions.
○ Related entry: Betnelan; Betnesol; Betnesol-N; Betnovate; Betnovate-C; Betnovate-N; Betnovate-RD; Diprosalic; Diprosone; Fucibet; Lotriderm; Vista-Methasone; Vista-Methasone-N

betamethasone dipropionate
See BETAMETHASONE

betamethasone sodium phosphate
See BETAMETHASONE

betamethasone valerate
See BETAMETHASONE

Beta-Prograne
(Tillomed) is a proprietary, prescription-

only preparation of the BETA-BLOCKER drug propranolol hydrochloride. It can be used as an ANTIHYPERTENSIVE treatment for raised blood pressure, as an ANTI-ANGINA treatment to relieve symptoms and improve exercise tolerance and as an ANTI-ARRHYTHMIC to regularize heartbeat and to treat myocardial infarction. It can also be used as an ANTITHYROID drug for the short-term treatment of thyrotoxicosis, as an ANTIMIGRAINE treatment to prevent attacks, as an ANXIOLYTIC treatment, particularly for symptomatic relief of tremor and palpitations and, with an ALPHA-ADRENOCEPTOR BLOCKER, in the acute treatment of phaeochromocytoma. It is available as modified-release capsules.
+▲ side-effects/warning: see PROPRANOLOL HYDROCHLORIDE

*beta-receptor stimulants

(beta-adrenoceptor stimulants; beta-agonists) are a class of drugs that act at beta-receptors, which, along with alpha-adrenoceptors, are the sites that recognize and respond to the natural hormones and neurotransmitters (adrenaline and noradrenaline) of the sympathetic nervous system. Drugs that activate this system, by whatever mechanism, are called SYMPATHOMIMETICS. Notable actions of beta-receptor stimulants include bronchodilation, speeding and strengthening of the heartbeat and relaxation of contraction of the uterus and intestine. Importantly, differences in receptors at different sites allow selectivity of action.

For example, $beta_2$sub-receptor stimulant drugs are normally used as BRONCHODILATORS in the treatment of asthma, since they can do this without significant and potentially dangerous, parallel stimulation of the heart (which is a $beta_1$sub-receptor site). Examples of $beta_2$sub-stimulant drugs used to cause bronchodilation are SALBUTAMOL and TERBUTALINE SULPHATE. In contrast, $beta_1$sub-receptor stimulants, such as

XAMOTEROL, may be used to stimulate the failing heart.

betaxolol hydrochloride

is a BETA-BLOCKER that can be used as an ANTIHYPERTENSIVE treatment for raised blood pressure. Administration can be oral as tablets, or in a form for injection. It can also be used, in the form of eye-drops, as a GLAUCOMA TREATMENT for chronic simple glaucoma.
+▲ side-effect/warning: see under PROPRANOLOL HYDROCHLORIDE. When given as eye-drops, it may cause dry eyes and eyelids and allergic reactions (conjunctivitis). In view of possible absorption, systemic side-effects should be considered, particularly the danger of bronchospasm in asthmatics and interactions with calcium-channel blockers.
○ Related entries: Betoptic; Kerlone

bethanechol chloride

is a PARASYMPATHOMIMETIC drug. It is used to stimulate motility in the intestines and to treat urinary retention (particularly following surgery). Administration is oral in the form of tablets.
+ side-effects: there may be sweating, blurred vision, nausea and vomiting, intestinal colic and a slow heart rate.
▲ warning: it should not be administered to patients who suffer from urinary or intestinal obstruction, asthma, epilepsy, parkinsonism, thyroid or certain heart disorders, who have peptic ulceration, or are pregnant.
○ Related entry: Myotonine

bethanidine sulphate

is an ADRENERGIC NEURONE BLOCKER, which is an ANTISYMPATHETIC class of drug. It prevents release of noradrenaline from sympathetic nerves. It can be used in ANTIHYPERTENSIVE treatment for moderate to severe high blood pressure, especially when other forms of treatment have failed and usually with other antihypertensive drugs (eg DIURETICS or BETA-BLOCKERS). Administration is oral in the form of tablets.

B

+▲ side-effects/warning: see under
GUANETHIDINE MONOSULPHATE, except it does
not cause diarrhoea.
○ **Related entry: Bendogen**

Betim

(Leo) is a proprietary, prescription-only
preparation of the BETA-BLOCKER drug
timolol maleate. It can be used as an
ANTIHYPERTENSIVE treatment for raised
blood pressure, as an ANTI-ANGINA
treatment to relieve symptoms and
improve exercise tolerance and as an
ANTI-ARRHYTHMIC to regularize heartbeat
and to treat myocardial infarction. It can
also be used as an ANTIMIGRAINE treatment
to prevent attacks. It is available as tablets.
+▲ side-effects/warning: see
TIMOLOL MALEATE

Betnelan

(Evans) is a proprietary, prescription-only
preparation of the CORTICOSTEROID and
ANTI-INFLAMMATORY drug betamethasone.
It can be used to treat inflammation,
especially in rheumatic or allergic
conditions, cerebral oedema and
congenital adrenal hyperplasia. It is
available as tablets.
+▲ side-effects/warning: see
BETAMETHASONE

Betnesol

(Evans) is a proprietary, prescription-only
preparation of the CORTICOSTEROID and
ANTI-INFLAMMATORY drug betamethasone
(as sodium phosphate). It can be used to
treat local inflammations (eg of ear, eye,
or nose) as well as more widespread
rheumatic or allergic conditions,
including severe asthma. It is available as
tablets, as ear-, eye- and nose-drops, an
eye ointment and in a form for injection.
+▲ side-effects/warning: see
BETAMETHASONE

Betnesol-N

(Evans) is a proprietary, prescription-only
COMPOUND PREPARATION of the ANTI-
INFLAMMATORY and CORTICOSTEROID drug
betamethasone (as sodium phosphate)
and the ANTIBACTERIAL and ANTIBIOTIC
drug neomycin sulphate. It can be used to
treat local inflammations and is available
as ear-, eye- and nose-drops and an eye
ointment.
+▲ side-effects/warning: see
BETAMETHASONE; NEOMYCIN SULPHATE

Betnovate

(Glaxo) is a proprietary, prescription-only
preparation of the ANTI-INFLAMMATORY and
CORTICOSTEROID drug betamethasone (as
valerate). It can be used topically to treat
severe non-infective inflammation of the
skin, rectum and scalp. It is available as a
cream, ointment, lotion and a scalp
preparation. A rectal ointment is also
available as a COMPOUND PREPARATION of
betamethasone (as valerate), the LOCAL
ANAESTHETIC drug lignocaine
hydrochloride and the SYMPATHOMIMETIC
and VASOCONSTRICTOR drug phenylephrine
hydrochloride.
+▲ side-effects/warning: see
BETAMETHASONE; LIGNOCAINE
HYDROCHLORIDE; PHENYLEPHRINE
HYDROCHLORIDE

Betnovate-C

(Glaxo) is a proprietary, prescription-only
COMPOUND PREPARATION of the ANTI-
INFLAMMATORY and CORTICOSTEROID drug
betamethasone (as valerate) and the
ANTIMICROBIAL drug clioquinol. It can be
used topically to treat severe, non-infective
inflammation such as skin eczema. It is
available as a cream.
+▲ side-effects/warning: see
BETAMETHASONE; CLIQUINOL

Betnovate-N

(Glaxo) is a proprietary, prescription-only
COMPOUND PREPARATION of the ANTI-
INFLAMMATORY and CORTICOSTEROID drug
betamethasone (as valerate) and the
ANTIBACTERIAL and ANTIBIOTIC drug
neomycin sulphate. It can be used

topically to treat severe inflammation such as skin psoriasis and eczema and is available as a cream and an ointment.
+▲ side-effects/warning: see BETAMETHASONE; NEOMYCIN SULPHATE

Betnovate-RD

(Glaxo) is a proprietary, prescription-only, preparation of the CORTICOSTEROID and ANTI INFLAMMATORY drug betamethasone (as valerate). It can be used to treat severe, non-infective inflammation of the skin and scalp. It is available as a cream and an ointment for topical application.
+▲ side-effects/warning: see BETAMETHASONE

Betoptic

(Alcon) is a proprietary, prescription-only preparation of the BETA-BLOCKER drug betaxolol hydrochloride. It can be used, in the form of eye-drops, for GLAUCOMA TREATMENT.
+▲ side-effects/warning: see BETAXOLOL HYDROCHLORIDE

bezafibrate

is used as a LIPID-LOWERING DRUG in hyperlipidaemia to reduce the levels, or change the proportions, of various lipids (eg cholesterol and LDL) in the bloodstream.

Generally, it is administered only to patients in whom a strict and regular dietary regime, alone, is not having the desired effect. Administration is oral in the form of tablets.
+ side-effects: there may be nausea, abdominal pain, loss of appetite; skin complaints, including rashes and itching; and impotence. Occasionally, dizziness and vertigo; fatigue and headache; hair loss; muscle weakness.
▲ warning: avoid administering to patients who have severely impaired kidney or liver function, disease of the gall bladder, or who are pregnant or breast-feeding.
○ Related entries: Bezalip; Bezalip-Mono

Bezalip

(Boehringer Mannheim) is a proprietary, prescription-only preparation of the LIPID-LOWERING DRUG bezafibrate. It can be used in hyperlipidaemia to reduce the levels, or change the proportions, of various lipids (eg cholesterol and LDL) in the bloodstream. It is available as capsules.
+▲ side-effects/warning: see BEZAFIBRATE

Bezalip-Mono

(Boehringer Mannheim) is a proprietary, prescription-only preparation of the LIPID-LOWERING DRUG bezafibrate. It can be used in hyperlipidaemia to reduce the levels, or change the proportions, of various lipids (eg cholesterol and LDL) in the bloodstream. It is available as tablets.
+▲ side-effects/warning: see BEZAFIBRATE

Bicillin

(Yamanouchi) is proprietary, prescription-only preparation of the ANTIBACTERIAL and (PENICILLIN) ANTIBIOTIC drug procaine penicillin. It can be used in long-lasting intramuscular (depot) injections to treat conditions such as syphilis and gonorrhoea. It is released slowly into the blood, therefore avoiding the need for frequent injections.
+▲ side-effects/warning: see PROCAINE PENICILLIN

BiCNU

(Bristol-Myers) is a proprietary, prescription-only preparation of the (CYTOTOXIC) ANTICANCER drug carmustine. It can be used in the treatment of certain myelomas, lymphomas and brain tumours. It is available in a form for injection.
+▲ side-effects/warning: see CARMUSTINE

biguanide

is the chemical name for the HYPOGLYCAEMIC drugs, such as metformin hydrochloride, which are used in DIABETIC TREATMENT for Type II diabetes (non-insulin-dependent diabetes mellitus; NIDDM; maturity-onset diabetes).

B

BiNovum

(Ortho) is a proprietary, prescription-only COMPOUND PREPARATION that can be used as a (*biphasic*) ORAL CONTRACEPTIVE (and also for certain menstrual problems) of the type that combines an OESTROGEN and a PROGESTOGEN, in this case ethinyloestradiol and norethisterone. It is available in the form of tablets in a calendar pack.

+▲ side-effects/warning: see ETHINYLOESTRADIOL; NORETHISTERONE

Bioplex

(Thames) is a proprietary, prescription-only preparation of the CYTOPROTECTANT drug carbenoxolone sodium. It can be used to treat mouth ulcers and is available as granules to make up into a mouthwash.

+▲ side-effects/warning: see CARBENOXOLONE SODIUM

Bioral Gel

(Sterling Health) is a proprietary, prescription-only preparation of the ANTI-INFLAMMATORY drug carbenoxolone sodium. It can be used to treat mouth ulcers and is available as a gel.

+▲ side-effects/warning: see CARBENOXOLONE SODIUM

Biorphen

(Bioglan) is a proprietary, prescription-only preparation of the ANTICHOLINERGIC drug orphenadrine hydrochloride. It can be used to relieve some of the symptoms of parkinsonism, especially muscle rigidity and the tendency to produce an excess of saliva (see ANTIPARKINSONISM). The drug also has the capacity to treat these symptoms, in some cases, where they are produced by drugs. It is available as an elixir.

+▲ side-effects/warning: see ORPHENADRINE HYDROCHLORIDE

biosynthetic human growth hormone

See SOMATROPIN

biperiden

is an ANTICHOLINERGENIC drug. It is used in the treatment of some types of parkinsonism (see ANTIPARKINSONISM). It increases mobility and decreases rigidity and the tendency to produce an excess of saliva is also reduced, but it has only a limited effect on bradykinesia. Additionally, it has the capacity to treat these symptoms, in some cases, where they are produced by drugs. It is thought to work by correcting the over-effectiveness of the NEUROTRANSMITTER ACETYLCHOLINE (cholinergic excess), which results from the deficiency of dopamine that occurs in parkinsonism. Because it also has some sedative properties, it is sometimes used in preference to the similar drug BENZHEXOL HYDROCHLORIDE. Administration, which may be in conjunction with other drugs used to relieve parkinsonism, is either oral as tablets or by injection.

+▲ side-effects/warning: see under BENZHEXOL HYDROCHLORIDE; but may cause sedation; when administered by injection it may cause hypotension.

۞ Related entry: Akineton

biphasic insulin

is a form of purified insulin, which is prepared as a sterile suspension of bovine insulin crystals in a solution of porcine insulin. It is used in DIABETIC TREATMENT to treat and maintain diabetic patients. It is available in vials for injection and has an intermediate duration of action.

+▲ side-effects/warning: see under INSULIN

۞ Related entry: Rapitard MC

biphasic isophane insulin

is a form of purified insulin, which is prepared as a sterile buffered suspension of porcine insulin complexed with protamine in a solution of porcine insulin, or human insulin complex in a solution of human insulin. It is used in DIABETIC TREATMENT to maintain diabetic patients. It is available in vials for injection and has an intermediate duration of action.

+▲ side-effects/warning: see under INSULIN

✪ Related entries: Human Actraphane 30/70; Human Initard 50/50; Human Mixtard 30/70; Humulin M1; Humulin M2; Humulin M3; Humulin M4; Mixtard 30/70; PenMix 10/90; PenMix 20/80; PenMix 30/70; PemMix 40/60; PemMix 50/50; Pur-In Mix 15/85; Pur-In Mix 25/75; Pur In Mix 50/50

bisacodyl

is a (*stimulant*) LAXATIVE. It is used to promote defecation and relieve constipation and seems to work by stimulating motility in the intestine, but some medical authorities do not approve of the frequent use of *stimulant laxatives* (as compared to the relatively benign *bulking agent laxatives*, which help establish good bowel habit). Medically, bisacodyl can be used to evacuate the colon prior to rectal examination or surgery. Administration is either oral in the form of tablets (full effects are achieved after several hours) or topical as suppositories (with effects achieved within an hour).

+ side-effects: there may be abdominal cramps, griping, nausea, or vomiting. Suppositories sometimes cause local irritation.

▲ warning: it should not be administered to patients with intestinal obstruction.

✪ Related entries: Dulco-lax Suppositories; Dulco-lax Suppositories for Children; Dulco-lax Tablets; Nylax Tablets

Bismag Tablets

(Whitehall Laboratories) is a proprietary, non-prescription COMPOUND PREPARATION of the ANTACIDS sodium bicarbonate, calcium carbonate and mixed magnesium carbonates.

It can be used for the symptomatic relief of hyperacidity, indigestion, heartburn, dyspepsia and flatulence. It is available as tablets and is not normally given to children, except on medical advice.

+▲ side-effects/warning: see CALCIUM CARBONATE; MAGNESIUM CARBONATE; SODIUM BICARBONATE

bismuth chelate

See TRIPOTASSIUM DICITRATOBISMUTHATE

bismuth oxide

is a mild ASTRINGENT agent, which is used in the treatment of haemorrhoids and is available as suppositories.

✪ Related entries: Anugesic-HC; Anusol; Anusol HC

bismuth subgallate

is a mild ASTRINGENT agent, which is used in the treatment of haemorrhoids and is available as suppositories.

✪ Related entry: Anusol-HC

bismuth subnitrate

is a mild ASTRINGENT agent, which is used as a dusting powder in certain skin disorders and as suppositories in the treatment of haemorrhoids.

✪ Related entry: Caved-S

Bisodol Antacid Powder

(Whitehall Laboratories) is a proprietary, non-prescription COMPOUND PREPARATION of the ANTACIDS sodium bicarbonate and magnesium carbonate. It can be used for the relief of indigestion, heartburn, dyspepsia, acidity and flatulence. It is available as a powder and is not normally given to children, except on medical advice.

+▲ side-effects/warning: see MAGNESIUM CARBONATE; SODIUM BICARBONATE

Bisodol Antacid Tablets

(Whitehall Laboratories) is a proprietary, non-prescription COMPOUND PREPARATION of the ANTACIDS sodium bicarbonate, calcium carbonate and mixed magnesium carbonates. It can be used for the relief of indigestion, heartburn, dyspepsia, acidity and flatulence. It is available as tablets and is not normally given to children, except on medical advice.

+▲ side-effects/warning: see CALCIUM CARBONATE; MAGNESIUM CARBONATE; SODIUM BICARBONATE

Bisodol Extra Tablets

(Whitehall Laboratories) is a proprietary, non-prescription COMPOUND PREPARATION of the ANTACIDS sodium bicarbonate, calcium carbonate and magnesium carbonate and the ANTIFOAMING AGENT dimethicone (as simethicone). It can be used for the relief of indigestion, heartburn, dyspepsia, acidity and flatulence and is available as tablets.

+▲ side-effects/warning: see CALCIUM . CARBONATE; DIMETHICONE; MAGNESIUM CARBONATE; SODIUM BICARBONATE

Bisodol Heartburn

(Whitehall Laboratories) is a proprietary, non-prescription COMPOUND PREPARATION of the ANTACIDS sodium bicarbonate and magaldrate and the DEMULCENT alginic acid. It can be used for the relief of indigestion, heartburn, dyspepsia, acidity and flatulence. It is available as tablets and is not normally given to children under six years, except on medical advice.

+▲ side-effects/warning: see ALGINIC ACID; MAGALDRATE; SODIUM BICARBONATE

bisoprolol fumarate

is a BETA-BLOCKER that can be used as an ANTIHYPERTENSIVE treatment for raised blood pressure and as an ANTI-ANGINA treatment to relieve symptoms and to improve exercise tolerance It is also available as an ANTIHYPERTENSIVE treatment in the form of a COMPOUND PREPARATION with a DIURETIC. Administration is oral in the form of tablets.

+▲ side-effects/warning: see under PROPRANOLOL HYDROCHLORIDE

○ Related entries: Emcor; Monocor; Monozide 10

Blemix

(Ashbourne) is a proprietary, prescription-only preparation of the ANTIBACTERIAL and (TETRACYCLINE) ANTIBIOTIC drug minocycline. It can be used to treat a wide range of infections and is available as tablets.

+▲ side-effects/warning: see MINOCYCLINE

Bleomycin

(Lundbeck) is a proprietary, prescription-only preparation of the (CYTOTOXIC) ANTICANCER drug bleomycin. It can be used in the treatment of certain cancers and is available in a form for injection.

+▲ side-effects/warning: see BLEOMYCIN

bleomycin

is a CYTOTOXIC DRUG (an ANTIBIOTIC in origin) that is used as an ANTICANCER drug. Administration is by injection.

+▲ side-effects/warning: see under CYTOTOXIC DRUGS; causes little bone marrow depression. Hypersensitivity reactions (chills and fevers) and effects on the lung and skin.

○ Related entry: Bleomycin

Blisteze

(DDD) is a proprietary, non-prescription preparation of the ANTISEPTIC agent phenol (with ammonia solution). It can be used for cold sores and chapped cracked lips and is available as a cream.

+▲ side-effects/warning: see PHENOL

Blocadren

(Merck, Sharp & Dohme) is a proprietary, prescription-only preparation of the BETA-BLOCKER drug timolol maleate. It can be used as an ANTIHYPERTENSIVE treatment for raised blood pressure, as an ANTI-ANGINA treatment to relieve symptoms and improve exercise tolerance and as an ANTI-ARRHYTHMIC to regularize heartbeat and to treat myocardial infarction. It may also be used as an ANTIMIGRAINE treatment to prevent attacks. It is available as tablets.

+▲ side-effects/warning: see TIMOLOL MALEATE

BN Liniment

(3M Health Care) is a proprietary, non-prescription COMPOUND PREPARATION of turpentine oil, ammonia and ammonium chloride, which have COUNTER-IRRITANT, or RUBEFACIENT, actions. It can be applied to the skin for the symptomatic relief of pain associated with rheumatism, neuralgia, fibrosis, sprains and stiffness of joints. It is available as an emulsion for topical application and is not normally used for children under six years, except on medical advice.

✚▲ side-effects/warning: see
AMMONIUM CHLORIDE; TURPENTINE OIL

Bocasan

(Oral-B Lab) is a proprietary, non-prescription preparation of the ANTISEPTIC agent sodium perborate. It can be used to cleanse and disinfect the mouth and is available in a form for making up into a mouthwash.

✚▲ side-effects/warning: see
SODIUM PERBORATE

Bolvidon

(Organon) is a proprietary, prescription-only preparation of the (TRICYCLIC-related) ANTIDEPRESSANT drug mianserin hydrochloride. It can be used to treat depressive illness, especially where sedation is required. It is available as tablets.

✚▲ side-effects/warning: see
MIANSERIN HYDROCHLORIDE

Bonefos

(Boehringer Ingelheim) is a recently introduced, proprietary, prescription-only preparation of the drug sodium chlodronate. It is used to treat high calcium levels associated with malignant tumours and bone lesions. It is available as capsules and in a form for infusion.

✚▲ side-effects/warning: see
SODIUM CHLODRONATE

Bonjela Antiseptic Pain-Relieving Pastilles

(Reckitt & Colman) is a proprietary, non-prescription COMPOUND PREPARATION of the LOCAL ANAESTHETIC drug lignocaine hydrochloride and the ANTISEPTIC agent aminacrine hydrochloride. It can be used to treat the pain of mouth ulcers.

✚▲ side-effects/warning: see AMINACRINE
HYDROCHLORIDE; LIGNOCAINE
HYDROCHLORIDE

Bonjela Oral Pain-Relieving Gel

(Reckitt & Colman) is a proprietary, non-prescription COMPOUND PREPARATION of the ANTISEPTIC agent cetalkonium chloride and choline salicylate, which has COUNTER-IRRITANT, or RUBEFACIENT, action. It can be applied to the mouth for symptomatic relief of pain from mouth ulcers, cold sores, denture irritation, inflammation of the tongue and teething in infants.

It is available as a gel to be massaged in gently. It should not be given to children under four months, except on medical advice.

✚▲ side-effects/warning: see
CHOLINE SALICYLATE

Bonomint

(Intercare Products) is a proprietary, non-prescription preparation of the (*stimulant*) LAXATIVE phenolphthalein. It can be used to relieve constipation and is available as a coated tablet with a chewing gum centre. It is not normally given to children under six years, except on medical advice.

✚▲ side-effects/warning: see
PHENOLPHTHALEIN

Boots Covering Cream

(Boots) is a proprietary, non-prescription preparation that is used to mask scars and other skin disfigurements. It is available as a cream and a powder and may be obtained on prescription under certain circumstances.

B

Boots Travel Calm Tablets

(Boots) is a proprietary, non-prescription preparation of the ANTICHOLINERGIC drug hyoscine hydrobromide. It can be used as an ANTINAUSEANT in the treatment of motion sickness and is available as chewable tablets. It is not normally given to children under three years, except on medical advice.

✚▲ side-effects/warning: see HYOSCINE HYDROBROMIDE

Botox

(Allergan) is a proprietary, prescription-only preparation of botulinum A toxin-haemagglutin complex. It can be used for treating blepharospasm (a tight contraction of the eyelids) and one-sided facial spasm and is available in a form for injection.

✚▲ side-effects/warning: see BOTULINUM A TOXIN-HAEMAGGLUTIN COMPLEX

botulinum A toxin-haemagglutin complex

is used for treating blepharospasm (a tight contraction of the eyelids) and one-sided facial spasm. Administration is by local injection.

▲ warning: avoid it is use in patients who are pregnant, breast-feeding, oe with certain muscle disorders (eg myasthenia gravis). It may have many effects on the eye such as bruising and swelling.

Botulism Antitoxin

(Department of Health) is a non-proprietary, prescription-only preparation of botulism antitoxin. It can be used to immunize people at risk from the disease following exposure to an infected patient and also as a treatment for those already infected. It is available in a form for injection or intravenous infusion.

✚▲ side-effects/warning: see BOTULISM ANTITOXIN

botulism antitoxin

is a preparation that neutralizes the toxins produced by botulism bacteria (*Clostridium bolulinum* types A, B and E). It can therefore be used in IMMUNIZATION to provide *passive immunity* to people who have been exposed to botulism in order to prevent them from developing the disease. It is also given to the infected patient as a means of treatment. Hypersensitivity reactions are common and it is not effective against some strains of botulism. Administration is by injection or intravenous infusion.

✚▲ side-effects/warning: see IMMUNIZATION
♻ Related entries: Botulism Antitoxin

bowel-cleansing solutions

are used prior to colonic surgery, colonoscopy, or barium enema to ensure that the bowel is free of solid contents. They are available in sachets for making up with water.

✚ side-effects: nausea and occasionally vomiting, transient abdominal cramps, bloated feeling, running nose, skin and anal irritations.

▲ warning: administer with care to patients who are pregnant, who have ulcerative colitis, or reflux oesophagitis. Bowel-cleansing solutions should not be used for patients suffering from certain gastrointestinal conditions, eg perforated bowel or obstruction.

♻ Related entry: Klean-Prep

Bradosol Plus

(Zyma Healthcare) is a proprietary, non-prescription COMPOUND PREPARATION of the ANTISEPTIC agent domiphen bromide and the LOCAL ANAESTHETIC drug lignocaine hydrochloride. It can be used for the symptomatic relief of a painful sore throat and is available as lozenges. It is not normally given to children under 12 years, except on medical advice.

✚▲ side-effects/warning: see DOMIPHEN BROMIDE; LIGNOCAINE HYDROCHLORIDE

Bradosol Sugar-Free Lozenges

(Zyma Healthcare) is a proprietary, non-prescription preparation of the ANTISEPTIC agent benzalkonium chloride. It can be used for the symptomatic relief of a painful sore throat.

✚▲ side-effects/warning: see BENZALKONIUM CHLORIDE

bran

is a natural *bulking agent* LAXATIVE, which is commonly used to keep people 'regular' and to treat constipation. It works by increasing the overall mass of faeces (by retaining a lot of water) and so stimulating bowel movement (the full effect may not be achieved for many hours). As an excellent source of dietary fibre, bran is thought to reduce the risk of diverticular disease while actively assisting digestion. It is useful in managing patients with colostomy, ileostomy, haemorrhoids, chronic diverticular disease, irritable bowel syndrome and ulcerative colitis.

✚ side-effects: some patients cannot tolerate bran, particularly patients sensitive to the compound gluten.

▲ warning: it should not be consumed if there is intestinal blockage or coeliac disease. Adequate fluid intake must be maintained to avoid faecal impaction.

✪ **Related entries: Procotofibe; Trifyba**

Brasivol

(Stiefel) is a proprietary, non-prescription preparation of particles of aluminium oxide, which has abrasive properties that can be used to cleanse skin with acne. It is available as a paste in three grades – fine, medium and coarse – within a soap base.

Brelomax

(Abbott) is a proprietary, prescription-only preparation of the BETA-RECEPTOR STIMULANT tulobuterol hydrochloride. It can be used as a BRONCHODILATOR in reversible obstructive airways disease, as an ANTI-ASTHMATIC treatment in severe acute asthma, or for the alleviation of symptoms of chronic bronchitis and emphysema. It is available in the form of tablets.

✚▲ side-effects/warning: see TULOBUTEROL HYDROCHLORIDE

Bretylate

(Wellcome) is a proprietary, prescription-only preparation of the ADRENERGIC NEURONE BLOCKER drug bretylium tosylate. It can be used in ANTI-ARRHYTHMIC treatment to treat abnormal heart rhythms in resuscitation and where other treatments have not been successful. Administration is by injection.

✚▲ side-effects/warning: see BRETYLIUM TOSYLATE

bretylium tosilate

See BRETYLIUM TOSYLATE

bretylium tosylate

(bretylium tosilate) is an ADRENERGIC NEURONE BLOCKER, which is an ANTISYMPATHETIC class of drug that prevents release of noradrenaline from sympathetic nerves. It can be used in ANTI-ARRHYTHMIC treatment of abnormal heart rhythms in resuscitation, where other therapies have not been successful. Administration is by injection.

✚ side-effects: hypotension; nausea and vomiting; tissue damage at the site of injection.

▲ warning: it should not be used in patients with phaeochromocytoma.

✪ **Related entries: Bretylate; Min-I-Jet Bretylate Tosylate**

Brevibloc

(Du Pont) is a proprietary, prescription-only preparation of the BETA-BLOCKER drug esmolol hydrochloride. It can be used as an ANTIHYPERTENSIVE treatment for raised blood pressure during operations and as an ANTI-ARRHYTHMIC, in the short term, to regularize heartbeat and to treat myocardial infarction. It is available in a

B

form for injection.
+▲ side-effects/warning: see ESMOLOL
HYDROCHLORIDE

Brevinor

(Syntex) is a proprietary, prescription-only COMPOUND PREPARATION that can be used as a (*monophasic*) ORAL CONTRACEPTIVE (and also for certain menstrual problems) of the type that combines an OESTROGEN and a PROGESTOGEN, in this case ethinyloestradiol and norethisterone. It is available in the form of tablets in a calendar pack.
+▲ side-effects/warning: see
ETHINYLOESTRADIOL; NORETHISTERONE

Bricanyl

(Astra) is a proprietary, prescription-only preparation of the BETA-RECEPTOR STIMULANT terbutaline sulphate. It can be used as a BRONCHODILATOR in reversible obstructive airways disease, as an ANTI-ASTHMATIC treatment in severe acute asthma, or for the alleviation of symptoms of chronic bronchitis and emphysema. It is available as tablets and modified-release tablets (*Bricanyl SA*), in a form for injection or infusion, as a metered aerosol used with a device called a *Spacer inhaler* or a *Nebuhaler*, as a breath-actuated dry powder with an inhaler called a *Turbohaler*, in single-dose nebulization solution called *Respules* and as a respirator solution (for use with a nebulizer or a ventilator). It can also be used as a means of slowing premature labour.
+▲ side-effects/warning: see TERBUTALINE
SULPHATE

Brietal Sodium

(Lilly) is a proprietary, prescription-only preparation of the GENERAL ANAESTHETIC drug methohexitone sodium. It can be used for the induction and maintainance of anaesthesia and is available in a form for injection.

+▲ side-effects/warning: see
METHOHEXITONE SODIUM

Britaject

(Britannia) is a prescription-only preparation of the ANTIPARKINSONISM drug apomorphine hydrochloride. It is available in a form for injection.
+▲ side-effects/warning: see APOMORPHINE
HYDROCHLORIDE

Britiazim

(Thames) is a proprietary, prescription-only preparation of the CALCIUM-CHANNEL BLOCKER drug diltiazem hydrochloride. It can be used as an ANTIHYPERTENSIVE treatment and as an ANTI-ANGINA drug in the prevention of attacks. It is available as modified-release tablets.
+▲ side-effects/warning: see DILTIAZEM
HYDROCHLORIDE

BritLofex

(Britannia) is a proprietary, prescription-only preparation of the recently introduced drug lofexidine hydrochloride. It can be used to alleviate the symptoms of OPIOID withdrawal and is available as tablets.
+▲ side-effects/warning: see LOFEXIDINE
HYDROCHLORIDE

Brocadopa

(Yamanouchi) is a proprietary, prescription-only preparation of the ANTIPARKINSONISM drug levodopa. It can be used to treat parkinsonism and is available as capsules.
+▲ side-effects/warning: see LEVODOPA

Broflex

(Bioglan) is a proprietary, prescription-only preparation of the ANTICHOLINERGIC drug benzhexol hydrochloride. It can be used in the treatment of parkinsonism to control tremors and involuntary movement. It is available as a syrup.
+▲ side-effects/warning: see BENZHEXOL
HYDROCHLORIDE

Brolene Eye Drops

(Rhône-Poulenc Rorer) is a proprietary, non-prescription preparation of the ANTIBACTERIAL drug propamidine isethionate. It can be used to treat infections of the eyelids or conjunctiva (including acanthamoeba keratitis) and is available as eye-drops.

✚▲ side effects/warnings: see PROPAMIDINE ISETHIONATE

Brolene Eye Ointment

(Rhône-Poulenc Rorer) is a proprietary, non-prescription preparation of the ANTIBACTERIAL drug dibromopropamidine isethionate. It can be used to treat infections of the eyelids or conjunctiva (including acanthamoeba keratitis) and is available as an eye ointment.

✚▲ side effects/warnings: see DIBROMOPROPAMIDINE ISETHIONATE

Brol-eze Eye Drops

(Rhône-Poulenc Rorer) is a proprietary, non-prescription preparation of the ANTI-ALLERGIC drug sodium cromoglycate. It can be used to treat allergic conjunctivitis, including when it is associated with hay fever and is avaialble as eye-drops.

✚▲ side-effects/warning: see SODIUM CROMOGLYCATE

bromazepam

is a BENZODIAZEPINE drug, which is used as an ANXIOLYTIC in the short-term treatment of anxiety. Administration is oral in the form of tablets.

✚▲ side-effects/warning: see under BENZODIAZEPINE

◎ Related entry: Lexotan

bromocriptine

is an ergot ALKALOID drug that is used primarily to treat parkinsonism (but not the parkinsonian symptoms caused by certain drug therapies: see ANTIPARKINSONISM). It works by stimulating the DOPAMINE receptors in the brain and so is slightly different from the more commonly used treatment with levodopa, which is converted to dopamine in the body. It is therefore particularly useful in the treatment of patients who, for one reason or another, cannot tolerate levodopa. Occasionally, the two drugs are combined. Bromocriptine has alternative uses (some related to its ability to inhibit prolactin secretion by the pituitary gland): to treat delayed puberty caused by hormonal insufficiency; to relieve certain menstrual disorders, or to reduce or halt lactation (in galactorrhoea), prolactinoma (tumour of the pituitary gland, leading to excess prolactin secretion) and to treat cyclical benign breast disease; and sometimes for treating acromegaly (over-secretion of the anterior pituitary gland due to a tumour). Administration is oral as tablets and capsules.

✚ side-effects: there may be nausea, vomiting, headache, dizziness (especially on rising from sitting or lying down – postural hypotension), spasm in the blood vessels of the extremities and drowsiness. High dosage may cause hallucinations, a state of confusion, leg cramps and a variety of rare disorders.

▲ warning: do not use in hypertension or in the toxaemia of pregnancy; and in certain liver or kidney disorders. Full, regular monitoring of various body systems is essential during treatment. If the drug fails to stop lactation, women should nevertheless stop breast-feeding.

◎ Related entry: Parlodel

brompheniramine maleate

is an ANTIHISTAMINE drug. It is used to treat the symptoms of allergic conditions such as hay fever and urticaria (itchy skin rash) and is also used, in combination with other drugs, in the treatment of coughs. Administration is oral in the form of tablets, a syrup, or an elixir.

✚▲ side-effects/warning: see under ANTIHISTAMINE. Because of its sedative side-effects, the performance of skilled tasks such as driving may be impaired.

B

✪ Related entries: Dimotane Expectorant; Dimotane with Codeine; Dimotane with Codeine Paediatric; Dimotapp Elixir; Dimotapp Elixir Paediatric; Dimotapp LA Tablets

Bronalin Dry Cough Elixir

(Seton Healthcare) is a proprietary, non-prescription preparation of the ANTITUSSIVE drug dextromethorphan hydrobromide, the SYMPATHOMIMETIC and DECONGESTANT drug pseudoephedrine hydrochloride and alcohol. It can be used for the symptomatic relief of dry, ticklish coughs and colds and is available as an oral solution. It is not normally given to children under six years, except on medical advice.

✚▲ side-effects/warning: see ALCOHOL; DEXTROMETHORPHAN HYDROBROMIDE; PSEUDOEPHEDRINE HYDROCHLORIDE

Bronchodil

(ASTA Medica) is a proprietary, prescription-only preparation of the BETA-RECEPTOR STIMULANT reproterol hydrochloride. It can be used as a BRONCHODILATOR in reversible obstructive airways disease, as an ANTI-ASTHMATIC treatment in severe acute asthma, or for the alleviation of symptoms of chronic bronchitis and emphysema. It is available as a metered aerosol inhalant.

✚▲ side-effects/warning: see REPROTEROL HYDROCHLORIDE

*bronchodilator

is any drug that relaxes the smooth muscle of the bronchioles (air passages in the lungs), so allowing air to flow more easily in or out (the latter being the major problem in obstructive airways disease). There are a number of conditions that cause bronchospasm (spasm in the bronchial muscles) and increased secretion of mucus and hence blockage, but the most common are asthma and bronchitis. The type of drug mainly used to treat bronchospasm is a BETA-RECEPTOR

STIMULANT and SYMPATHOMIMETIC drug. These drugs (eg.SALBUTAMOL and TERBUTALINE SULPHATE) work by stimulating beta-adrenoceptors on the smooth muscle of the airways, which normally respond to adrenal hormones and sympathetic nerve neurotransmitters (adrenaline and noradrenaline). Other types of bronchodilator, such as the xanthine compounds AMINOPHYLLINE and THEOPHYLLINE, act directly on the smooth muscle of the bronchioles. All these drugs are best administered directly to the airways (except in an emergency) in the form of aerosols, ventilator sprays, or nebulizing mists, because this minimizes side-effects.

Brooklax

(Intercare Products) is a proprietary, non-prescription preparation of the *stimulant* LAXATIVE phenolphthalein. It can be used to relieve constipation and is available as a chocolate bar. It is not normally used for children under six years, except on medical advice.

✚▲ side-effects/warning: see PHENOLPHTHALEIN

Brufen

(Boots) is a proprietary, prescription-only preparation of the (NSAID) NON-NARCOTIC ANALGESIC and ANTIRHEUMATIC drug ibuprofen. It can be used to relieve pain, particularly the pain of rheumatic disease and other musculoskeletal disorders. It is available as tablets, a syrup for dilution and effervescent granules.

✚▲ side-effects/warning: see IBUPROFEN

Brufen Retard

(Boots) is a proprietary, prescription-only preparation of the (NSAID) NON-NARCOTIC ANALGESIC and ANTIRHEUMATIC drug ibuprofen. It can be used to relieve pain and inflammation, particularly the pain of rheumatic disease and other musculoskeletal disorders. It is available

as modified-release tablets.
+▲ side-effects/warning: see IBUPROFEN

Brulidine

(Rhône-Poulenc Rorer) is a proprietary, non-prescription preparation of the ANTISEPTIC agent dibromopropamidine isethionate. It can be used to treat minor burns and abrasions and is available as a cream for topical application.
+▲ side-effects/warning: see DIBROMOPROPAMIDINE ISETHIONATE

Brush Off Cold Sore Lotion

(Seton Healthcare) is a proprietary, non-prescription preparation of the ANTISEPTIC agent povidone-iodine. It can be used for the treatment of cold sores and is available as a quick-drying paint.
+▲ side-effects/warning: see POVIDONE-IODINE

Buccastem

(Reckitt & Coleman) is a proprietary, prescription-only preparation of the drug prochlorperazine (as maleate). It can be used as an ANTINAUSEANT to relieve symptoms of nausea caused by the vertigo and loss of balance experienced due to infections of the inner and middle ears, or by cytotoxic drugs in the treatment of cancer. It can also be used as an ANTIPSYCHOTIC to treat schizophrenia and other psychoses and for the short-term treatment of acute anxiety. It is available as buccal tablets (placed between the upper lip and gum and left to dissolve).
+▲ side-effects/warning: see PROCHLORPERAZINE

buclizine hydrochloride

is an ANTIHISTAMINE drug that is included in a proprietary ANTIMIGRAINE treatment.
+▲ side-effects/warning: see under ANTIHISTAMINE
○ Related entry: Migraleve

budesonide

is a CORTICOSTEROID drug with ANTI-INFLAMMATORY, ANTI-ALLERGIC and ANTI-ASTHMATIC properties, which is used to prevent attacks of asthma, rhinitis (inflammation of the nasal lining) and severe inflammatory skin disorders (eg.psoriasis and eczema). Administration is by inhalation or a nasal spray, or topically as a cream or ointment.
+▲ side-effects/warning: see under BECLOMETHASONE DIPROPIONATE
○ Related entries: Preferid; Pulmicort Inhaler; Pulmicort Respules; Pulmicort Turbohaler; Rhinocort

bumetanide

is a powerful DIURETIC drug, one of the class of *loop diuretics*. It can be used to treat oedema (accumulation of fluid in the tissues), particularly pulmonary (lung) oedema in patients with left ventricular or chronic heart failure and low urine production due to kidney failure (oliguria). Administration can be oral as tablets or oral solutions, or by injection or infusion.
+▲ side-effects/warning: see under FRUSEMIDE; there may also be muscle pain.
○ Related entries: Burinex; Burinex K

bupivacaine hydrochloride

is a LOCAL ANAESTHETIC drug with a long duration of action. It is an amide and is chemically related to lignocaine hydrochloride, but is particularly long lasting. It is commonly used for spinal anaesthesia, including epidural injection (especially during labour) and also for nerve block and by local infiltration. Administration is by injection.
+▲ side-effects/warning: see under LIGNOCAINE HYDROCHLORIDE. Heart depression may be more severe.
○ Related entries: Marcain; Marcain with Adrenaline

buprenorphine

is a NARCOTIC ANALGESIC, an OPIOID, that is long-acting (its effects last longer than morphine) and used to treat moderate to

B

severe pain, including during surgical operations. Preparations of buprenorphine are on the Controlled Drugs List, because it can cause dependence (addiction). It has some OPIOID ANTAGONIST properties and so may be dangerous to use in combination with other narcotic analgesics and can precipitate withdrawal symptoms in those habituated to, for instance, morphine or diamorphine. Administration is oral as tablets placed sublingually (under the tongue), or by intramuscular or slow intravenous injection.

✚▲ side-effect/warning: see under OPIOID. It may cause vomiting.

⊕ Related entry: Temgesic

Burinex

(Leo) is a proprietary, prescription only preparation of the (*loop*) DIURETIC drug bumetanide. It can be used to treat oedema, particularly pulmonary (lung) oedema in patients with left ventricular or chronic heart failure and low urine production due to kidney failure (oliguria). It is available as tablets, an oral liquid and in a form for injection.

✚▲ side-effects/warning see BUMETANIDE

Burinex K

(Leo) is a proprietary, prescription-only COMPOUND PREPARATION of the (*loop*) DIURETIC drug bumetanide and the potassium supplement potassium chloride. It can be used to treat oedema, for instance in congestive heart failure and low urine production due to kidney failure (oliguria). It is available as tablets, which should be swallowed whole with plenty of fluid at meals or when in an upright posture.

✚▲ side-effects/warning: see BUMETANIDE; POTASSIUM CHLORIDE

Buscopan

(Boehringer Ingelheim) is a proprietary, prescription-only preparation of the ANTICHOLINERGIC drug hyoscine

butylbromide, which can be used as an ANTISPASMODIC drug. It is available as tablets and in a form for injection. (The tablets are also available without a prescription under certain conditions.)

✚▲ side-effects/warning: HYOSCINE BUTYLBROMIDE

buserelin

is an analogue of the hypothalamic HORMONE GONADORELIN (gonadothrophin-releasing hormone; GnRH). It reduces secretion of gonadotrophin by the pituitary gland, which results in reduced secretion of sex hormones by the ovaries or testes. Buserelin is used to treat endometriosis (a growth of the lining of the uterus in inappropriate sites) and as an ANTICANCER drug to treat cancer of the prostate gland. It is also used prior to *in vitro* fertilization. Administration (as buserelin acetate) is by injection or a nasal spray.

✚ side-effects: in women: there may be menstruation-like and breakthrough bleeding and symptoms similar to the menopause (sweating, hot flushes, palpitations, vaginal dryness). There may be mood changes; back, muscle and abdominal pain; changes to breast size and tenderness; acne and dry skin; nervousness, tiredness and sleep disturbances; ovarian cysts; skin disturbances (eg.rashes); constipation; blurred vision; vaginal discharge; tingling and sensitivity in fingers and toes; and changes in body hair. In men: there may be bone pain; hot flushes; nausea and diarrhoea; occasional increase in breast size. In men and women: there may be changes in libido; dizziness; vomiting; headache. There may be irritation on using the nasal spray.

▲ warning: do not use in pregnancy or when breast-feeding, or where there is vaginal bleeding of unknown origin. Some men initially experience increased tumour growth, to the extent even of compressing the spinal cord and additional drugs may be necessary to counteract this.

⊕ Related entries: Suprecur; Suprefact

B

Buspar

(Bristol-Myers) is a proprietary, prescription-only preparation of the recently introduced ANXIOLYTIC drug buspirone hydrochloride. It can be used for the short-term treatment of anxiety and is available as tablets.

✚▲ side-effects/warning: see BUSPIRONE HYDROCHLORIDE

buspirone hydrochloride

is a recently introduced ANXIOLYTIC drug, which is thought to work by stimulating SEROTONIN receptors in the brain. It can be used for the short-term treatment of anxiety and is administered orally as tablets.

✚ side-effects: nausea, dizziness, headache, nervousness, excitement, light-headedness; rarely, increase in heart rate, palpitations, chest pain, drowsiness, dry mouth, confusion, fatigue, or sweating.

▲ warning: it should not be given to patients with epilepsy, severe liver or kidney impairment; or who are pregnant or breast-feeding. It may impair the performance of skilled tasks such as driving; avoid alcohol because its effects are enhanced.

❂ Related entry: Buspar

busulphan

is a CYTOTOXIC DRUG that is used as an ANTICANCER treatment, particularly for chronic myeloid leukaemia. It works by direct interference with the DNA and is administered orally in the form of tablets.

✚▲ side-effects/warning: see under CYTOTOXIC DRUGS. Avoid its use in patients with porphyria.

❂ Related entry: Myleran

Butacote

(Geigy) is a proprietary, prescription-only preparation of the (NSAID) NON-NARCOTIC ANALGESIC and ANTIRHEUMATIC drug phenylbutazone. Because of its sometimes severe side-effects, it is used solely in the treatment of ankylosing spondylitis under medical supervision in hospitals.

Administration is oral in the form of tablets.

✚▲ side-effects/warning: see PHENYLBUTAZONE

butobarbitone

is a BARBITURATE drug, which is used only when absolutely necessary as a HYPNOTIC to treat severe and intractable insomnia. Administration is oral in the form of tablets. Preparations containing butobarbitone are on the Controlled Drugs List.

✚▲ side-efects/warning: see under BARBITURATE

❂ Related entry: Soneryl

C

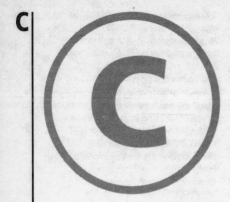

cabergoline

is a recently introduced drug with properties similar to bromocriptine, for which it may be substituted if one or the other is not tolerated. There are more established drugs for ANTIPARKINSONISM, but for uses in hormonal disorders see bromocriptine. Administration is oral in the form of tablets.

✚▲ side-effects/warning: see under BROMOCRIPTINE. The side-effects are somewhat different and there may be gastrointestinal and epigastric pain and other side-effects. Do not use in pregnancy.

✪ Related entry: Dostinex

Cafergot

(Sandoz) is a proprietary, prescription-only COMPOUND PREPARATION of the VASOCONSTRICTOR drug ergotamine tartrate and the STIMULANT caffeine. It can be used as an ANTIMIGRAINE treatment for acute attacks and is available as tablets and suppositories.

✚▲ side-effects/warning: see CAFFEINE; ERGOTAMINE TARTRATE

caffeine

is a weak STIMULANT, which is present in tea, coffee and some soft drinks. It is also included in many analgesic preparations, partly in the belief that it speeds absorption.

✚ side-effects: excessive doses may cause headache either directly or on withdrawal and also anxiety.

✪ Related articles: Actron; Anadin Analgesic Caplets; Anadin Analgesic Capsules, Maximum Strength; Anadin Extra; Anadin Extra Soluble Tablets; Askit Capsules; Askit Powders; Beechams Hot Lemon; Beechams Powders; Beechams Powders Capsules; Cafergot; Catarrh-Ex; Cojene Tablets; Cold Relief Capsules; Do-Do Tablets; Doloxene Compound; Dristan Decongestant Tablets; Feminax; Flurex Tablets; Hedex Extra Tablets; Lemsip Cold Relief Capsules; Migril; Nurse

Sykes Powders; Panadol Extra Soluble Tablets; Panadol Extra Tablets; Paraclear Extra Strength; Phensic; Powerin Analgesic Tablets; Propain Tablets; Solpadeine Capsules; Solpadeine Soluble Tablets; Solpadeine Tablets; Syndol

Calabren

(Berk) is a proprietary, prescription-only preparation of the SULPHONYLUREA drug glibenclamide. It can be used in DIABETIC TREATMENT of Type II diabetes (non-insulin-dependent diabetes mellitus; maturity-onset diabetes) and works by augmenting what remains of INSULIN production in the pancreas. It is available as tablets.

✚▲ side-effects/warning: see GLIBENCLAMIDE

Caladryl Cream

(Warner-Wellcome) is a proprietary, non-prescription COMPOUND PREPARATION of the ANTIHISTAMINE drug diphenhydramine hydrochloride, camphor and zinc oxide. It can be used for the relief of skin irritation associated with urticaria, herpes, minor skin afflictions, insect bites, nettle sting and sunburn.

✚▲ side-effects/warning: see CAMPHOR; DIPHENHYDRAMINE HYDROCHLORIDE; ZINC OXIDE

Caladryl Lotion

(Warner-Wellcome) is a proprietary, non-prescription COMPOUND PREPARATION of the ANTIHISTAMINE drug diphenhydramine hydrochloride, camphor and zinc oxide. It can be used for the relief of skin irritation associated with urticaria, herpes, minor skin afflictions, insect bites, nettle sting and sunburn.

✚▲ side-effects/warning: see CAMPHOR; DIPHENHYDRAMINE HYDROCHLORIDE; ZINC OXIDE

calamine

is a suspension containing mainly (basic) zinc carbonate (with added ferric oxide), which has a mild ASTRINGENT action. It is incorporated into several preparations that are used to cool and soothe itching skin in conditions such as pruritus, eczema and psoriasis and is also used in some EMOLLIENT preparations. Adminsitration is in the form of a lotion, cream, or an ointment.

○ Related entries: calamine and coal tar ointment, BP; calamine cream, aqueous, BP; calamine lotion, aqueous, BP; Hydrocal; Vasogen Cream

calamine and coal tar ointment, BP

is a non-proprietary preparation of calamine and coal tar. It can be used by topical application to treat chronic eczema and psoriasis and to relieve itching. It is available as an ointment.

✚▲ side-effects/warning: see COAL TAR; CALAMINE

calamine cream, aqueous, BP

is a preparation consisting of a suspension of zinc carbonate, zinc oxide, liquid paraffin and other constituents. It is used to cool and soothe itching skin and is available as a cream.

✚▲ side-effects/warning: see CALAMINE

calamine lotion, aqueous, BP

is a preparation consisting of a suspension of zinc carbonate, zinc oxide, liquid paraffin and other constituents. It is used to cool and soothe itching skin and is available as a lotion.

✚▲ side-effects/warning: see CALAMINE

calciferol

See ERGOCALCIFEROL

Calcijex

(Abbott) is a proprietary, prescription-only preparation of calcitriol, which is a VITAMIN D analogue that can be used in

vitamin D deficiency. It is available in a
form for injection.
✚▲ side-effects/warning: see CALCITRIOL

Calcilat

(Eastern) is a proprietary, prescription-
only preparation of the CALCIUM-CHANNEL
BLOCKER drug nifedipine. It can be used as
an ANTI-ANGINA drug in the prevention of
attacks, as an ANTIHYPERTENSIVE treatment
and as a VASODILATOR in peripheral
vascular disease (Raynaud's
phenomenon). It is available as capsules.
✚▲ side-effects/warning: see NIFEDIPINE

Calciparine

(Sanofi Winthrop) is a proprietary,
prescription-only preparation of the
ANTICOAGULANT drug heparin calcium. It
can be used to treat various forms of
thrombosis and is available in a form for
injection.
✚▲ side-effects/warning: see HEPARIN

calcipotriol

is used to treat chronic or milder forms of
psoriasis by topical application. It is
available as a cream ointment and a scalp
solution.
✚ side-effects: local irritation, various skin
irritations (itching, dermatitis, reddening,
photosensitivity); raised blood calcium.
▲ warning: do not use in patients with
disorders of calcium metabolism. Administer
with caution during pregnancy; avoid contact
with the face.
✪ Related entry: Dovonex

Calcisorb

(3M Health Care) is a proprietary, non-
prescription preparation of sodium
cellulose phosphate. It can be used to help
reduce high calcium levels in the
bloodstream by inhibiting calcium
absorption from food. It is available as
sachets of powder for solution in water or
to sprinkle over food.
✚▲ side-effects/warning: see SODIUM
CELLULOSE PHOSPHATE

Calcitare

(Rhône-Poulenc Rorer) is a proprietary,
prescription-only preparation of the
THYROID HORMONE calcitonin. It can be
used to lower blood levels of calcium
when they are abnormally high
(hypercalaemia) and to treat Paget's
disease of the bone. It is available in a
form for injection.
✚▲ side-effects/warning: see CALCITONIN

calcitonin

is a THYROID HORMONE produced and
secreted by the thyroid gland at the base of
the neck. Its function is to lower the levels
of calcium and phosphate in the blood
and together with the correspondingly
opposite action of a parathyroid hormone
(parathormone) regulates these levels.
Therapeutically, calcitonin is used to lower
blood levels of calcium when they are
abnormally high (hypercalaemia), to treat
Paget's disease of the bone and when there
is cancer. Administration is by injection. It
is available in the porcine form and the
salmon form (referred to as SALCATONIN).
✚ side-effects: there may be nausea, vomiting
and flushing; there may also be a tingling
sensation in the hands and a peculiar taste in
the mouth and inflammation at the site of
injection.
▲ warning: prolonged use of calcitonin
derived from animals may eventually lead to
the body producing antibodies against it and
consequent neutralization of its effect. Some
patients may become hypersensitive to animal
calcitonin. It should be used with caution in
pregnant women and not at all by those who
are breast-feeding.
✪ Related entry: Calcitare

calcitriol

(1,25-dihydroxycholecalciferol) is a
synthesized form of VITAMIN D that is used
to make up vitamin D deficiency in the
body, particularly in the treatment of
certain forms of hypoparathyroidism and
rickets. Administration is oral in the form
of capsules or solution.

✚▲ side-effects/warning: see under VITAMIN D

❍ Related entries: Calcijex, Rocaltrol

calcium

is a metallic element essential for the normal growth and development of the body, especially (in the form of calcium phosphate) of the bones and teeth. Its level in blood is regulated by the opposing actions of the thyroid hormone CALCITONIN and the parathyroid HORMONE parathormone. Its uptake from food is enhanced by vitamin D (CALCIFEROL). Good food sources include most dairy products. Salts of calcium used therapeutically include the ANTACID calcium carbonate, the folinic acid supplement calcium folinate, the MINERAL SUPPLEMENTS calcium gluconate and calcium lactate.

▲ warning: deficiency of vitamin D leads to calcium deficiency and corresponding bone, blood and nerve and muscle disorders. Conversely, excess calcium in the body may cause the formation of stones (calculi, generally composed of calcium oxalate), particularly in the kidney or gall bladder.

❍ Related entries: Calcium-500; calcium and ergocalciferol tablets; calcium carbonate; calcium folinate; calcium lactate; Calcium-Sandoz; Ossopan; Sandocal

calcium and ergocalciferol tablets

is a non-proprietary, non-prescription COMPOUND PREPARATION of the VITAMIN ergocalciferol (vitamin D_2) and CALCIUM (in the form of calcium lactate and calcium phosphate).

It can be used as a MINERAL SUPPLEMENT in the treatment of nutritional or absorptive deficiencies.

✚▲ side-effects/warning: see CALCIUM; ERGOCALCIFEROL

calcium antagonists

See CALCIUM-CHANNEL BLOCKER

calcium carbonate

or chalk, is used therapeutically as an ANTACID. It is incorporated into many proprietary preparations that are used to relieve hyperacidity, dyspepsia and for the symptomatic relief of heartburn and symptoms of peptic ulcer in the treatment of peptic ulcers. It is also used by mouth in the treatment of hyperphosphataemia (abnormally raised levels of phosphates in the blood). Administration is oral as tablets, chewable tablets, or a liquid suspension.

✚ side-effects: treatment with calcium carbonate as an antacid may cause belching (due to carbon dioxide).

▲ warning: its prolonged use as an antacid can induce tolerance and eventually cause renewed acid secretion. There may also be abnormally high levels of calcium in the blood. Antacids may impair the absorption of other drugs.

❍ Related entries: Andrews Antacid; Bismag Tablets; Bisodol Antacid Tablets; Bisodol Extra Tablets; Calcium-500; Calcium-Sandoz; Didronel; Didronel PMO; Eno; Fynnon Calcium Aspirin; Gaviscon Liquid; ❍ Collis Browne's Tablets; Maclean Indigestion Tablets; Moorland Tablets; Nulacin Tablets; Ossopan; Remegel Original; Rennie Gold (Minty); Rennie Rap-Eze; Rennie Tablets, Digestif; Sandocal; Setlers Tablets Peppermint Flavour; Setlers Tums-Assorted Fruit Flavour; Titralac

*calcium-channel blockers

(calcium antagonists; calcium-entry blockers) are a type of drug that has been introduced fairly recently and which are being increasingly used in therapeutics. They work by blocking entry of calcium through channels (specialized 'pores' in a cell's membrane) that admit calcium ions from the fluid surrounding cells to the interior of the cell. Since calcium has very profound activities within cells (such as increasing muscle contraction and electrical excitability), these drugs have

C

powerful effects on cell function. Their main uses include: a direct SMOOTH MUSCLE RELAXANT action causing dilation of blood vessels and effects on heart muscle, which has led to their widespread use in ANTIHYPERTENSIVE treatment (eg.AMLOPIDINE, ISRADIPINE, NICARDIPINE HYDROCHLORIDE, NIFEDIPINE and VERAPAMIL HYDROCHLORIDE); as ANTI-ANGINA treatment (eg.amlopidine, DILTIAZEM HYDROCHLORIDE, nicardipine hydrochloride, nifedipine and verapamil); as ANTI-ARRHYTHMIC agents (eg. verapamil); as VASODILATORS to treat peripheral vascular disease – Raynaud's phenomenon (eg.nifedipine); in the prevention of damage to the brain due to ischaemia (lack of blood supply) following subarachnoid haemorrhage (bleeding from blood vessels supplying the outer surface of the brain) (eg.nimodipine); and as an ANTIMIGRAINE treatment to prevent attacks (eg. nifedipine and verapamil).

calcium-entry blocker

See CALCIUM-CHANNEL BLOCKER

calcium folinate

is the usual form in which folinic acid (a derivative of folic acid, which is a vitamin of the VITAMIN B complex) is administered as a supplement to patients who are susceptible to some of the toxic effects caused by the folate-antagonist activity of certain anticancer drugs, especially METHOTREXATE. Administration is oral in the form of tablets.

+▲ side-effects/warning: see under FOLINIC ACID

Calcium-500

(Renacare) is a proprietary, non-prescription preparation of calcium carbonate. It can be used as a MINERAL SUPPLEMENT for calcium in cases of deficiency. It is available as tablets.

+▲ side-effects/warning: see CALCIUM CARBONATE

Calcium Leucovorin

(Lederle) is a proprietary, prescription-only preparation of folinic acid, which can be used to counteract the toxic effects of certain anticancer drugs, especially METHOTREXATE. It is available as tablets and in a form for injection.

+▲ side-effects/warning: see FOLINIC ACID

Calcium Resonium

(Sanofi Winthrop) is a proprietary, non-prescription preparation of calcium polystyrene sulphonate, which is a resin that can be used to treat high blood potassium levels, particularly in patients who suffer from fluid retention or undergo kidney dialysis. It is available in the form of a powdered resin for se as a rectal enema or by mouth.

+▲ side-effects/warning: see under POLYSTYRENE SULPHONATE RESINS

Calcium-Sandoz

(Sandoz) is a proprietary, non-prescription preparation of calcium glubionate and calcium lactobionate. It can be used as a MINERAL SUPPLEMENT for calcium in cases of calcium deficiency. It is available as a syrup and in a form for injection.

+▲ side-effects/warning: see CALCIUM CARBONATE

Calfig California Syrup of Figs

(Sterling Health) is a proprietary, non-prescription preparation of the (*stimulant*) LAXATIVE senna. It can be used for the relief of constipation and is available as a viscous liquid. It is not normally given to children under one year, except on medical advice.

+▲ side-effects/warning: see SENNA

Calmurid

(Novex) is a proprietary, non-prescription COMPOUND PREPARATION of lactic acid and the HYDRATING AGENT urea. It can be used

for dry, scaly, or hard skin and is available
as a cream.

Calmurid HC

(Novex) is a proprietary, prescription-only
COMPOUND PREPARATION of the
CORTICOSTEROID and ANTI-INFLAMMATORY
drug hydrocortisone and the HYDRATING
AGENT urea (with lactic acid). It can be
used as a treatment for mild inflammation
of the skin caused by conditions such as
eczema. It is available as a cream for
topical application.
✚▲ side-effects/warning: see
HYDROCORTISONE; UREA

Calpol Infant Suspension

(Wellcome) is a proprietary, non-
prescription preparation of the NON-
NARCOTIC ANALGESIC drug paracetamol. It
can be used to treat mild to moderate pain
(including teething pain) and as an
ANTIPYRETIC (for instance, to reduce fever
after vaccination, when it can be used in
two-month-old babies). It is available as a
liquid suspension and is not normally
given to infants under three months,
except on medical advice.
✚▲ side-effects/warning: see PARACETAMOL

Calpol Infant Suspension, Sugar-Free

(Wellcome) is a proprietary, non-
prescription preparation of the NON-
NARCOTIC ANALGESIC drug paracetamol. It
can be used to treat mild to moderate pain
(including teething pain) and as an
ANTIPYRETIC (for instance, to reduce fever
after vaccination, when it can be used in
two-months-old babies). It is available as
a liquid suspension and is not normally
given to infants under three months,
except on medical advice.
✚▲ side-effects/warning: see PARACETAMOL

Calpol Six Plus

(Wellcome) is a proprietary, non-
prescription preparation of the NON-
NARCOTIC ANALGESIC and ANTIPYRETIC drug

paracetamol. It can be used to treat mild
to moderate pain and to reduce fever in
children. However, it is not normally given
to children under six years, except on
medical advice. It is available in the form
of a liquid suspension.
✚▲ side-effects/warning: see
PARACETAMOL

Calsynar

(Rhône-Poulenc Rorer) is a proprietary,
prescription-only preparation of the
THYROID HORMONE calcitonin, in the form
of salcatonin. It can be used to lower
blood levels of calcium when they are
abnormally high (hypercalaemia) and to
treat Paget's disease of the bone. It is
available in a form for injection.
✚▲ side-effects/warning: see SALCATONIN

CAM

(Rybar) is a proprietary, prescription-only
preparation of the BETA-RECEPTOR
STIMULANT ephedrine hydrochloride. It
can be used as a BRONCHODILATOR in
reversible obstructive airways disease and
as an ANTI-ASTHMATIC treatment in severe
acute asthma. It is available as a sugar-free
mixture.
✚▲ side-effects/warning: see
EPHEDRINE HYDROCHLORIDE

Camcolit 250

(Norgine) is a proprietary, prescription-
only preparation of the ANTIMANIA drug
lithium (as lithium carbonate). It can be
used to prevent and treat mania and
manic-depressive bouts and is available as
tablets.
✚▲ side-effects/warning: see LITHIUM

Camcolit 400

(Norgine) is a proprietary, prescription-
only preparation of the ANTIMANIA drug
lithium (as lithium carbonate). It can be
used to prevent and treat mania and
manic-depressive bouts and is available as
tablets.
✚▲ side-effects/warning: see LITHIUM

C **camphor**
is an aromatic substance with mild
COUNTER-IRRITANT, or RUBEFACIENT,
properties. It is incorporated into a
number of topical preparations that used
to help relieve itchiness and for the
symptomatic relief of muscular
rheumatism, fibrosis, lumbago, sciatica,
and skin irritation.
**O Related articles: Aspellin; Balmosa
Cream; Caladryl Cream; Caladryl Lotion;
Nicobrevin; Radian B Heat Spray;
Radian B Muscle Lotion; Radian B
Muscle Rub**

Camsilon
(Cambridge) is a proprietary,
prescription-only preparation of the
ANTICHOLINESTERASE drug edrophonium
chloride. It can be used in the diagnosis of
myasthenia gravis and at the termination
of operations to reverse the actions of
neuromuscular blocking agents (when it
is often administered with atropine
sulphate). It is available in a form for
injection. (This drug was formerly known
as *Tensilon*.)
+▲ side-effects/warning: see
EDROPHONIUM CHLORIDE

Canesten
(Bayer) is the name of several proprietary
preparations of the ANTIFUNGAL drug
clotrimazole. They can be used to treat
fungal infections, particularly vaginal
candiasis (thrush) and skin infections
such as nappy rash and balanitis
(infection of the glans penis). The
preparations are available in several forms
and strengths, including a skin cream, a
dusting powder, a vaginal cream, vaginal
tablets (pessaries) and a *Duopak*
containing vaginal tablets and a cream.
Most of these products are now
available on a non-prescription basis for
stated conditions, though their use will
generally follow medical diagnosis, but
Caneston-HC is available only on
prescription. The various preparations

are detailed under separate headings.
+▲ side-effects/warning: see CLOTRIMAZOLE

Canesten 1 VT
(Bayer) is a proprietary, non-prescription
preparation of the ANTIFUNGAL drug
clotrimazole. It can be used particularly to
treat vaginal candiasis (thrush) and is
available as vaginal tablets (pessaries). It
is not normally given to children, except
on medical advice.
+▲ side-effects/warning: see CLOTRIMAZOLE

Canesten 1%
(Bayer) is a proprietary, non-prescription
preparation of the ANTIFUNGAL drug
clotrimazole. It can be used to treat fungal
and *Candida* skin infections, including
Candida nappy rash, vulvitis and balanitis
(infection of the glans penis). It is
available as a cream for topical
application.
+▲ side-effects/warning: see CLOTRIMAZOLE

Canesten 10% VC
(Bayer) is a proprietary, non-prescription
preparation of the ANTIFUNGAL drug
clotrimazole. It can be used particularly to
treat vaginal candiasis (thrush) and is
available as a vaginal cream to be inserted
through a special applicator. It is not
normally given to children, except on
medical advice.
+▲ side-effects/warning: see CLOTRIMAZOLE

Canesten-HC
(Baypharm) is a proprietary, prescription-
only COMPOUND PREPARATION of the
CORTICOSTEROID drug hydrocortisone and
the ANTIFUNGAL drug clotrimazole. It can
be used to treat fungal infections,
particularly those associated with
inflammation. It is available as a cream for
topical application.
+▲ side-effects/warning: see CLOTRIMAZOLE;
HYDROCORTISONE

Cantil
(Boehringer Mannheim) is a proprietary,

prescription-only preparation of the ANTICHOLINERGIC drug mepenzolate bromide. It can be used as an ANTISPASMODIC for the symptomatic relief of smooth muscle spasm in the gastro-intestinal tract. It is available as tablets.

+▲ side-effects/warning: see MEPENZOLATE BROMIDE

Capasal

(Dermal) is a proprietary, non-prescription COMPOUND PREPARATION of coal tar and salicylic acid (with coconut oil). It can be used for conditions such as dandruff and psoriasis of the scalp and is available as a shampoo.

+▲ side-effects/warning: see COAL TAR; SALICYLIC ACID

Capastat

(Dista) is a proprietary, prescription-only preparation of the ANTIBIOTIC and ANTITUBERCULAR drug capreomycin (as sulphate). It can be used to treat tuberculosis that is resistant to other drugs and is available in a form for injection.

+▲ side-effects/warning: see CAPREOMYCIN

Capitol

(Dermal) is a proprietary, non-prescription preparation of the ANTISEPTIC agent benzalkonium chloride. It can be used to treat dandruff and other scalp conditions and is available as a shampoo.

+▲ side-effects/warning: see BENZALKONIUM CHLORIDE

Caplenal

(Berk) is a proprietary, prescription-only preparation of the ENZYME INHIBITOR allopurinol, which is a XANTHINE OXIDASE INHIBITOR. It can be used to treat excess uric acid in the blood and to prevent renal stones and attacks of gout. It is available as tablets.

+▲ side-effects/warning: see ALLOPURINOL

Capoten

(Squibb) is a proprietary, prescription-

only preparation of the ACE INHIBITOR captopril. It can be used as an ANTIHYPERTENSIVE and in HEART FAILURE TREATMENT, usually in conjunction with other classes of drug. It is available as tablets.

+▲ side-effects/warning: see CAPTOPRIL

Capozide

(Squibb) is a proprietary, prescription-only COMPOUND PREPARATION of the ACE INHIBITOR captopril and the DIURETIC drug hydrochlorothiazide. It can be used as an ANTIHYPERTENSIVE treatment and is available as tablets.

+▲ side-effects/warning: see CAPTOPRIL; HYDROCHLOROTHIAZIDE

capreomycin

is an ANTIBACTERIAL and ANTIBIOTIC drug. It is used specifically in the treatment of tuberculosis that proves to be resistant to the first-line drugs (see ANTITUBERCULAR), or in cases where those drugs are not tolerated. Administration is by injection in combination with other drugs.

+ side-effects: there may be kidney toxicity and impaired hearing with or without tinnitus or vertigo; sometimes there are sensitivity reactions such as rashes or urticaria and blood changes.

▲ warning: it should not be administere to patients who are pregnant; administer with caution to those who have impaired liver or kidney function or sense of hearing (functions that should be monitored during treatment), or who are already taking other ototoxic antibiotics, or who are breast-feeding.

○ Related entry: Capastat

Caprin

(Sinclair) is a proprietary, non-prescription preparation of the (NSAID) NON-NARCOTIC ANALGESIC and ANTIRHEUMATIC drug aspirin. It can be used to treat headache and rheumatic conditions and is available as modified-release tablets. It is not normally given to

children, except on medical advice.
✚▲ side-effects/warning: see ASPIRIN

capsaicin

is the active principle of capsicum, which
is often used medically in the form of the
resin called CAPSICUM OLEORESIN and is a
pungent extract from capsicum peppers.
Both capsicum resin and capsaicin are
incorporated into medicines with
RUBEFACIENT, or COUNTER-IRRITANT, action
and when rubbed in topically to the skin
cause a feeling of warmth that offsets the
pain from underlying muscles, joints, or
internal organs.

capsicum oleoresin

or capsicum resin, is a pungent extract
from capsicum peppers. The active
principle of these 'hot' peppers, which are
also used for culinary purposes as chilli
and cayenne pepper, is CAPSAICIN. Both
capsicum resin and capsaicin are
incorporated into medicines with
RUBEFACIENT, or COUNTER-IRRITANT, action
and when rubbed in topically to the skin,
cause a feeling of warmth that offsets the
pain from underlying muscles, joints, or
internal organs.
✚ side-effects: there may be local irritation.
▲ warning: it should not be used on
inflamed or broken skin, or on mucous
membranes. Keep away from the eyes.
❂ Related entries: **Algipan Rub; Axsain;
Balmosa Cream; Cremalgin Balm;
Radian B Muscle Rub; Ralgex Cream;
Ralgex Stick**

captopril

is an ACE INHIBITOR. It is a powerful
VASODILATOR that can be used as an
ANTIHYPERTENSIVE and in HEART FAILURE
TREATMENT. It is often used in conjunction
with other classes of drug, particularly
(THIAZIDE) DIURETICS. Additionally, it can
be used following myocardial infarction
(damage to heart muscle, usually after a
heart attack) and in diabetic nephropathy
(kidney disease) in insulin-dependent

diabetes. Administration is oral in the
form of tablets.
✚ side-effects: hypotension; headache and
fatigue; nausea and vomiting; diarrhoea or
constipation, abdominal pain and dyspepsia;
muscle cramps; dry cough and sore throat
with voice changes; loss of taste and body
weight; skin rash and itching; impaired
kidney function with high blood potassium;
blood disorders. A number of other, rarer,
side-effects have been reported.
▲ warning: there may be a rapid initial drop
in blood pressure. It should not be given to
patients who are breast-feeding, or have
porphyria or renovascular disease.
❂ Related entries: **Acepril; Capoten;
Capozide**

Carace

(Du Pont) is a proprietary,
prescription-only preparation of the ACE
INHIBITOR lisinopril. It can be used as an
ANTIHYPERTENSIVE and in HEART FAILURE
TREATMENT. It is available as tablets.
✚▲ side-effects/warning: see
LISINOPRIL

Carace Plus

(Du Pont) is a proprietary, prescription-
only COMPOUND PREPARATION of the ACE
INHIBITOR lisinopril and the DIURETIC drug
hydrochlorothiazide. It can be used as an
ANTIHYPERTENSIVE treatment and is
available as tablets (*Carace 10 Plus* and
Carace 20 Plus).
✚▲ side-effects/warning: see
HYDROCHLOROTHIAZIDE; LISINOPRIL

carbachol

is a PARASYMPATHOMIMETIC drug. It is
used in GLAUCOMA TREATMENT to lower
pressure in the eyeball (while constricting
the pupil) and to treat urinary retention
(particularly following surgery).
Administration can be oral in the form of
tablets or by eye-drops or injection.
✚▲ side-effects/warning: see under
BETHANECHOL CHLORIDE
❂ Related entry: **Isopto Carbachol**

Carbalax

(Pharmax) is a proprietary, non-prescription preparation of the (*osmotic*) LAXATIVE sodium acid phosphate. It can be used to relieve constipation and to evacuate the rectum prior to abdominal procedures. It is available as an effervescent suppository.

+▲ side-effects/warning: see SODIUM ACID PHOSPHATE

carbamazepine

is an ANTICONVULSANT and ANTI-EPILEPTIC drug. It is used in the preventive treatment of most forms of epilepsy (except absence seizures), to relieve the pain of trigeminal neuralgia (a searing pain from the trigeminal nerve in the face), in the management of manic-depressive illness resistant to lithium and in the treatment of diabetes insipidus. Administration is either oral as a liquid or by suppositories.

+ side-effects: there are many and include blood, liver and skin disorders, nausea and vomiting, dizziness, drowsiness, headache, unsteady gait, confusion and agitation (particularly in the elderly), visual disturbances, constipation or diarrhoea, anorexia, kidney failure, hair loss, effect on the heart, growth of breasts in man, impotence, aggression and depression.

▲ warning: it should not be administered to patients who suffer from certain heart defects, porphyria, or bone marrow depression. Use with caution in those with impaired liver, kidney, or heart function, a history of blood reactions to other drugs, glaucoma, or who are pregnant or breast-feeding. Seek medical advice if fever, bruising, sore throat, rash, or mouth ulcers occur.

✪ Related entry: Tegretol

carbaryl

is a PEDICULICIDAL drug that is used in the treatment of head lice and crab lice. Administration, as an aqueous or alcohol solution, is either as a lotion or a shampoo.

+ side-effects: skin irritation.

▲ warning: avoid contact with the eyes and broken or infected skin. It should not be used by asthmatics.

✪ Related entries: Carylderm; Clinicide; Derbac-C ; Suleo-C

carbenicillin

is an ANTIBACTERIAL and ANTIBIOTIC drug of the penicillin family. It is used to treat serious infections caused by sensitive Gram-negative organisms and sometimes in combination with AMINOGLYCOSIDE antibiotics. However, it has now largely been superseded by more potent drugs such as TICARCILLIN. Administration is by injection or infusion.

+▲ side-effects/warning: see under BENZYLPENICILLIN. There may also be lowered blood potassium and altered blood platelet function.

✪ Related entry: Pyopen

carbenoxolone sodium

is derived from LIQUORICE and is a synthetic derivative of glycyrrhizinic acid. It can be used as an ULCER-HEALING DRUG for benign gastric ulcers, because it promotes healing of the stomach lining when this has been eroded by acid and enzymes (in a way that is not well understood) and is used for oesophageal ulceration and inflammation. Oral administration can be in the form of chewable tablets or as a liquid and in both cases with incorporated antacids. It may also be used locally to soothe mouth ulcers in the form of a gel or mouthwash.

+ side-effects: there may be oedema (accumulation of fluid in the tissues, potentially leading to hypertension and heart problems), raised blood potassium levels (leading to muscle damage and other problems).

▲ warning: it should not be administered to patients with cardiac failure, certain liver or kidney disorders, with hyperkalaemia (raised blood potassium), or who are pregnant. Use with caution in patients with hypertension or heart disease.

C

○ Related entries: Bioplex; Bioral Gel; Pyrogastrone

carbidopa

is a drug that is administered in combination with levodopa to treat parkinsonism, but not the parkinsonian symptoms induced by other drugs (see ANTIPARKINSONISM). It is levodopa that actually has the major effect, but carbidopa inhibits the break down of levodopa to dopamine in the body before it reaches the brain where it carries out its function. The presence of carbidopa allows the dose of levodopa to be at a minimum and so minimizes potentially severe side-effects and speeds the therapeutic response. However, it is also responsible for producing some involuntary body movements.
Administration of carbidopa and levodopa is oral as single-compound tablets called CO-CARELDOPA.
✚▲ side-effects/warning: see under LEVODOPA
○ Related entries: Half Sinemet CR; Sinemet; Sinemet CR; Sinemet LS; Sinemet-Plus

carbimazole

is a drug that acts as an indirect HORMONE ANTAGONIST, by inhibiting the production of the THYROID HORMONES by the thyroid gland, therefore treating an excess in the blood of thyroid hormones and the symptoms that it causes (thyrotoxicosis). Treatment may be on a maintenance basis over a long period (with dosage adjusted to optimum effect) or prior to surgical removal of the thyroid gland.
Administration is oral in the form of tablets.
✚ side-effects: there may be rash; nausea and headache; occasionally, jaundice; hair loss; blood disorders; joint pain.
▲ warning: it should be administered with caution to patients who are pregnant, breast-feeding, or who have large goitre.
○ Related entry: Neo-Mercazole

carbocisteine

is a MUCOLYTIC drug used to reduce the viscosity of sputum and thus acts as an EXPECTORANT in patients with disorders of the upper respiratory tract, such as chronic asthma and bronchitis. Administration is oral as capsules or a syrup.
✚▲ side-effects/warning: see under ACETYLCYSTEINE
○ Related entry: Mucodyne

Carbo-Cort

(Lagap) is a proprietary, prescription-only COMPOUND PREPARATION of the CORTICOSTEROID and ANTI-INFLAMMATORY drug hydrocortisone and coal tar. It can be used to treat eczema and psoriasis and is available as a cream for topical application.
✚▲ side-effects/warning: see COAL TAR; HYDROCORTISONE

Carbo-Dome

(Lagap) is a proprietary, prescription-only preparation of coal tar. It can be used by topical application to treat eczema and psoriasis and is available as a cream.
✚▲ side-effects/warning: see COAL TAR

carbomer

(CIBA Vision) is a synthetic agent that can be used in artificial tears where there is dryness of the eye due to a disease such as keratoconjunctivitis. It is available as a liquid gel for application to the eye.
○ Related entry: Viscotears

Carbomix

(Penn) is a proprietary, non-prescription preparation of activated charcoal. It can be used to treat patients suffering from poisoning or a drug overdose and is available as a granulated powder.

*carbonic anhydrase inhibitor

drugs have ENZYME-INHIBITOR actions against the enzyme carbonic anhydrase,

C

which is widely distributed throughout the body and has a fundamental role in the control of acid-base balance (pH). Medical application of carbonic anhydrase inhibitor drugs include as a weak DIURETIC to treat systemic oedema (accumulation of fluid in the tissues), as a GLAUCOMA TREATMENT in reducing fluid (aqueous humour) and intraocular pressure in the eye (the pressure in the eyeball) and as a preventive measure against motion sickness.

carboplatin

is a CYTOTOXIC DRUG (derived from cisplatin) that is used as an ANTICANCER treatment specifically for cancer of the ovary. Administration is by injection.
+▲ side-effects/warning: see under CYTOTOXIC DRUGS
۞ Related entry: Paraplatin

carboprost

is a drug used to treat haemorrhage following childbirth, which is caused by the muscles of the uterus losing their tone. It is an analogue of PROSTAGLANDIN (a synthetic form related to $PGF_2\alpha$), which is a LOCAL HORMONE naturally involved in controlling the muscles of the uterus. It is generally used in patients who are unresponsive to ERGOMETRINE MALEATE and OXYTOCIN. It is available in a form for injection.
+ side-effects: there may be nausea, headache and dizziness, vomiting and diarrhoea; flushing, chills and hyperthermia. There may be raised blood pressure, oedema of the lungs, shortness of breath and sweating. There may be pain at the site of injection.
▲ warning: use with caution in patients with a history of glaucoma, anaemia, jaundice, epilepsy, asthma, abnormal blood pressure (high or low) and uterine scars or any other predisposition to uterine rupture. It should not be used in patients with certain acute inflammatory disease; heart, kidney, lung, or liver disorders.
۞ Related entry: Hemabate

Cardene

(Syntex) is a proprietary, prescription-only preparation of the CALCIUM-CHANNEL BLOCKER drug nicardipine hydrochloride. It can be used as an ANTIHYPERTENSIVE treatment and as an ANTI-ANGINA drug in the prevention and treatment of attacks. It is available as capsules.
+▲ side-effects/warning: see NICARDIPINE HYDROCHLORIDE

Cardene SR

(Syntex) is a proprietary, prescription-only preparation of the CALCIUM-CHANNEL BLOCKER drug nicardipine hydrochloride. It can be used as an ANTIHYPERTENSIVE treatment and as an ANTI-ANGINA drug in the prevention and treatment of attacks. It is available as modified-release capsules.
+▲ side-effects/warning: see NICARDIPINE HYDROCHLORIDE

cardiac glycosides

are a class of drugs derived from the leaf of the *Digitalis* foxgloves. These drugs have a pronounced effect on the failing heart by increasing the force of contraction and so have been commonly used for their CARDIAC STIMULANT actions to increase the force in congestive HEART FAILURE TREATMENT. They can also correct certain abnormal heart rhythms and are therefore used as an ANTI-ARRHYTHMIC treatment. However, today, these drugs are no longer used, because doses that are useful therapeutically are close to those that are toxic, so dose must be carefully adjusted in the individual. A digitalis antidote for use in overdose, DIGIBIND, is available. Examples of cardiac glycosides include DIGOXIN and DIGITOXIN.

*cardiac stimulant

drugs are used in medicine to stimulate the rate or the force of the heartbeat, but only when it is weak as a result of some disease state, or in medical emergencies. CARDIAC GLYCOSIDES have a pronounced effect on the failing heart, increasing the

C

force of contraction and so have been widely prescribed in the treatment of congestive HEART FAILURE TREATMENT. A number of SYMPATHOMIMETIC drugs can be used directly to stimulate the heart through their BETA-RECEPTOR STIMULANT properties, for example DOPEXAMINE HYDROCHLORIDE, DOBUTAMINE HYDROCHLORIDE, ISOPRENALINE and ADRENALINE. Most of these drugs tend to be reserved for acute emergencies such as cardiogenic shock, septic shock, during heart surgery and in cardiac infarction and cardiac arrest.

Cardilate MR

(Norton) is a proprietary, prescription-only preparation of the CALCIUM-CHANNEL BLOCKER drug nifedipine. It can be used as an ANTI-ANGINA drug in the prevention of attacks and as an ANTIHYPERTENSIVE treatment. It is available as tablets.
+▲ side-effects/warning: see NIFEDIPINE

Cardinol

(CP) is a proprietary, prescription-only preparation of the BETA-BLOCKER drug propranolol hydrochloride. It can be used as an ANTIHYPERTENSIVE treatment for raised blood pressure, as an ANTI-ANGINA treatment to relieve symptoms and improve exercise tolerance and as an ANTI-ARRHYTHMIC to regularize heartbeat and to treat myocardial infarction. It can also be used as an ANTITHYROID drug for short-term treatment of thyrotoxicosis, as an ANTIMIGRAINE treatment to prevent attacks, as an ANXIOLYTIC treatment, particularly for symptomatic relief of tremor and palpitations, and, with an ALPHA-ADRENOCEPTOR BLOCKER, in the acute treatment of phaeochromocytoma. It is available as tablets.
+▲ side-effects/warning: see PROPRANOLOL HYDROCHLORIDE

Cardura

(Invicta) is a proprietary, prescription-only preparation of the ALPHA-ADRENOCEPTOR BLOCKER drug doxazosin. It can be used in ANTIHYPERTENSIVE treatment, often in conjunction with other antihypertensive drugs and is available as tablets.
+▲ side-effects/warning: see DOXAZOSIN

Carisoma

(Pharmax) is a proprietary, prescription-only preparation of the SKELETAL MUSCLE RELAXANT drug carisoprodol. It can be used to treat muscle spasm caused by an injury to or a disease of the central nervous system. It is available as tablets.
+▲ side-effects/warning: see CARISOPRODOL

carisoprodol

is a SKELETAL MUSCLE RELAXANT drug. It can be used for relaxing muscles that are in spasm, particularly when caused by an injury to or a disease of the central nervous system. It works by an action on the central nervous system and is administered orally as tablets.
+▲ side-effects/warning: see under MEPROBAMATE; but drowsiness is less common. Avoid its use in patients with porphyria.
○ Related entry: Carisoma

carmellose sodium

is a substance that is used as the basis for a paste or a powder, which is spread or sprinkled over lesions in or around the mouth in order to provide a protective barrier and relieve some of the discomfort while the lesions heal.
○ Related entries: artificial saliva; Glandosane; Luborant; Orabase; Orahesive; Salivace

carmustine

is a CYTOTOXIC DRUG that works by direct interference with DNA and so prevents normal cell replication. It is used as an ANTICANCER drug to treat some myelomas, lymphatic cancer and brain tumours. Administration is by injection.

+▲ side-effects/warning: see under
CYTOTOXIC DRUGS
○ Related entry: BiCNU

carteolol hydrochloride

is a BETA-BLOCKER that can be used as a
GLAUCOMA TREATMENT for chronic simple
glaucoma. It is thought to work by slowing
the rate of production of the aqueous
humour in the eye and is available as eye
drops.
+ side-effects: there may be some systemic
absorption into the body, so some of the side-
effects listed under PROPRANOLOL
HYDROCHLORIDE may be seen. Dry eyes and
some local allergic reactions of the eye-lids,
including conjunctivitis, may also occur.
▲ warning: in view of possible systemic
absorption, dangerous side-effects should be
borne in mind; in particular the danger of
bronchospasm in asthmatics and interactions
with calcium-channel blockers.
○ Related entry: Teoptic

carvedilol

is a BETA-BLOCKER drug, which can be
used as an ANTIHYPERTENSIVE.
Administration is oral in the form of
tablets.
+▲ side-effects/warning: see under
PROPRANOLOL HYDROCHLORIDE. It should not
be given to patients with kidney impairment.
○ Related entry: Eucardic

Carylderm

(Napp) is a proprietary, non-prescription
preparation of the PEDICULICIDAL drug
carbaryl. It can be used to treat
infestations of lice in the scalp and pubic
hair. It is available as a lotion a shampoo.
+▲ side-effects/warning: see CARBARYL

castor oil

has both (*stimulant*) LAXATIVE and
EMOLLIENT properties and is found in
some skin preparations and BARRIER
CREAMS.
**○ Related entries: Panda Baby Cream &
Castor Oil Cream with Lanolin**

Catapres

(Boehringer Ingelheim) is a proprietary,
prescription-only preparation of the
ANTISYMPATHETIC drug clonidine
hydrochloride. It can be used in
ANTIHYPERTENSIVE and ANTIMIGRAINE
treatment and is available as tablets and in
a form for injection.
+▲ side-effects/warning: see CLONIDINE
HYDROCHLORIDE

Catapres Perlongets

(Boehringer Ingelheim) is a proprietary,
prescription-only preparation of the
ANTISYMPATHETIC drug clonidine
hydrochloride. It can be used in
ANTIHYPERTENSIVE treatment and is
available as modified-release capsules.
+▲ side-effects/warning: see
CLONIDINE HYDROCHLORIDE

Catarrh-Ex

(Thompson) is a proprietary, non-
prescription COMPOUND PREPARATION of
the NON-NARCOTIC ANALGESIC drug
paracetamol, the SYMPATHOMIMETIC and
DECONGESTANT drug phenylephrine
hydochloride and the STIMULANT caffeine.
It can be used for the relief of cold and flu
symptoms and sinusitis. It is available as
tablets and is not normally given to
children, except on medical advice.
+▲ side-effects/warning: see
CAFFEINE; PARACETAMOL; PHENYLEPHRINE
HYDOCHLORIDE

Caved-S

(Pharmacia) is a proprietary, non-
prescription COMPOUND PREPARATION of
the ANTACIDS aluminium hydroxide,
magnesium carbonate and sodium
bicarbonate and the CYTOPROTECTANTS
bismuth subnitrate and deglycyrrhizinised
liquorice. It can be used to treat peptic
ulcers and is available as tablets.
+▲ side-effects/warning: see ALUMINIUM
HYDROXIDE; BISMUTH SUBNITRATE;
LIQUORICE, DEGLYCYRRHIZINISED; MAGNESIUM
CARBONATE; SODIUM BICARBONATE

C

Caverject

(Upjohn) is a PROSTAGLANDIN, alprostadil
(PGE₁). It is a recently introduced,
prescription-only treatment for men to
manage penile erectile dysfunction. It is
administered by intracavernosal injection
into the penis and is available in a form
for injection.

✚▲ side-effects/warning: see ALPROSTADIL

CCNU

(Lundbeck) is a proprietary, prescription-
only preparation of the (CYTOTOXIC)
ANTICANCER drug lomustine. It can be used
in the treatment of Hodgkin's disease and
some solid tumours. It is available in a
form for injection.

✚▲ side-effects/warning: see LOMUSTINE

Ceanel Concentrate

(Quinoderm) is a proprietary, non-
prescription COMPOUND PREPARATION of
the ANTISEPTIC agent cetrimide and the
ANTIFUNGAL drug undecenoic acid (with
phenylethyl alcohol). It can be used to
treat psoriasis and other non-infective
scalp conditions and is available as a
shampoo.

✚▲ side-effects/warning: see CETRIMIDE;
UNDECENOIC ACID

Cedax

(Schering-Plough) is a proprietary,
prescription-only preparation of the
ANTIBACTERIAL and (CEPHALOSPORIN)
ANTIBIOTIC drug ceftibuten. It can be used
to treat acute bacterial infections of the
urinary and respiratory tracts by Gram-
positive and Gram-negative organisms. It
is available as capsules and an oral
suspension.

✚▲ side-effects/warning: see CEFTIBUTEN

Cedocard

(Pharmacia) is a proprietary, non-
prescription preparation of the
VASODILATOR and ANTI-ANGINA drug
isosorbide dinitrate. It can be used to treat
and prevent angina pectoris and in HEART
FAILURE TREATMENT. It is available as short-
acting, sublingual, or oral tablets in three
doses: *Cedocard-5*, *Cedocard-10* and
Cedocard-20.

✚▲ side-effects/warning: see
ISOSORBIDE DINITRATE

Cedocard-Retard

(Pharmacia) is a proprietary, non-
prescription preparation of the
VASODILATOR and ANTI-ANGINA drug
isosorbide dinitrate. It can be used to
prevent angina pectoris and is available as
modified-release tablets.

✚▲ side-effects/warning: see
ISOSORBIDE DINITRATE

cefaclor

is a broad-spectrum ANTIBACTERIAL and
ANTIBIOTIC drug, which is one of the
second-generation CEPHALOSPORINS. It is
now primarily used to treat Gram-positive
and Gram-negative bacterial infections of
the respiratory and urinary tracts. It is
used particularly for urinary tract
infections that do not respond to other
drugs, or which occur during pregnancy
and pneumonia. Administration is oral in
the form of capsules or a dilute
suspension.

✚ side-effects: nausea, vomiting, diarrhoea,
headache, colitis (more likely at high doses);
sensitivity reactions that may be serious (from
rashes to anaphylaxis); blood and liver
disturbances, behavioural and nervous
disturbances.

▲ warning: it should not be administered to
patients who are sensitive to penicillins and
cephalosporins. Do not use in patients with
porphyria and with caution in those who are
pregnant or breast-feeding.

❂ **Related entries: Distaclor;
Distaclor MR**

cefadroxil

is a broad-spectrum ANTIBACTERIAL and
ANTIBIOTIC drug, which is one of the first-
generation CEPHALOSPORINS. It is now
primarily used to treat bacterial infections

of the urinary tract that do not respond to other drugs, or which occur during pregnancy. Administration is oral in the form of capsules or a dilute suspension.
✚▲ side-effects/warning: see under CEFACLOR
✪ Related entry: Baxan

cefalexin
See CEPHALEXIN

cefamandole
See CEPHAMANDOLE

cefazolin
See CEPHAZOLIN

cefibuten
is a broad-spectrum ANTIBACTERIAL and (CEPHALOSPORIN) ANTIBIOTIC drug. It can be used to treat acute bacterial infections by Gram-positive and Gram-negative organisms, particularly of the urinary and respiratory tracts. Administration is oral in the form of capsules or a suspension.
✚▲ side-effects/warning: see under CEFACLOR
✪ Related entry: Cedax

cefixime
is a broad-spectrum ANTIBACTERIAL and (CEPHALOSPORIN) ANTIBIOTIC drug. It is used to treat acute bacterial infections by Gram-positive and Gram-negative organisms, particularly of the urinary tract. It has a longer duration of action than any other cephalosporin taken by mouth. Administration is oral in the form of capsules or a paediatric suspension.
✚▲ side-effects/warning: see under CEFACLOR
✪ Related entry: Suprax

Cefizox
(Wellcome) is a proprietary, prescription-only preparation of the ANTIBACTERIAL and (CEPHALOSPORIN) ANTIBIOTIC drug ceftizoxime. It can be used used to treat many infections, particularly of the upper

respiratory and urinary tracts and gonorrhoea. It is available in a form for injection.
✚▲ side-effects/warning: see CEFTIZOXIME

cefodizime
is a broad-spectrum ANTIBACTERIAL and ANTIBIOTIC drug, which is one of the third-generation CEPHALOSPORINS. It can be used to treat infections of the lower respiratory tract, including pneumonia and bronchopneumonia and of the urinary tract, including cystitis and pyelonephritis. Administration is by intramuscular or intravenous injection or infusion.
✚▲ side-effects/warning: see under CEFACLOR
✪ Related entry: Timecef

cefotaxime
is a broad-spectrum ANTIBACTERIAL and ANTIBIOTIC drug, which is one of the third-generation CEPHALOSPORINS. It can be used to treat a wide range of bacterial infections, particularly of the skin and soft tissues, the urinary tract, the meninges of the brain (in meningitis) and gonorrhoea. It can also be used to prevent infection during surgery. Administration is by intravenous or intramuscular injection or infusion.
✚▲ side-effects/warning: see under CEFACLOR
✪ Related entry: Claforan

cefoxitin
is a broad-spectrum ANTIBACTERIAL and ANTIBIOTIC drug, which is one of the second-generation CEPHALOSPORINS. It can be used to treat a wide range of bacterial infections, particularly Gram-negative infections of the skin and soft tissues, the urinary and respiratory tracts and the peritoneum (in peritonitis). Administration is by intramuscular injection or intravenous infusion.
✚▲ side-effects/warning: see under CEFACLOR
✪ Related entry: Mefoxin

C

cefpodoxime

is a broad-spectrum ANTIBACTERIAL and (CEPHALOSPORIN) ANTIBIOTIC drug. It can be used to treat bacterial infections of the respiratory tract, including bronchitis and pneumonia and tonsillitis infections that are recurrent, chronic, or resistant to other drugs. Administration is oral in the form of tablets.

+▲ side-effects/warning: see under CEFACLOR

✪ Related entry: Orelox

cefradine

See CEPHRADINE

ceftazidime

is a broad-spectrum ANTIBACTERIAL and ANTIBIOTIC drug, which is one of the third-generation CEPHALOSPORINS. It is among the most effective of the cephalosporins against bacterial infections and can be used particularly to treat infections of the skin and soft tissues, the urinary and respiratory tracts, the ear, nose and throat (eg.*Pseudomonal* lung infections in cystic fibrosis) and to prevent infection following surgery. It can also be used to treat infection in patients whose immune systems are defective. Administration is by intravenous or intramuscular injection.

+▲ side-effects/warning: see under CEFACLOR

✪ Related entries: Fortum; Kefadim

ceftizoxime

is a broad-spectrum ANTIBACTERIAL and ANTIBIOTIC drug, which is one of the third-generation CEPHALOSPORINS. It can be used to treat a wide range of Gram-negative bacterial infections, particularly of the skin and soft tissues, the urinary tract, the genital organs (eg.gonorrhoea), the lower respiratory tract, the meninges of the brain (in meningitis) and the blood (in septicaemia). Administration is by intravenous or intramuscular injection.

+▲ side-effects/warning: see under CEFACLOR

✪ Related entry: Cefizox

ceftriaxone

is a broad-spectrum ANTIBACTERIAL and ANTIBIOTIC drug, which is a recently introduced, third-generation CEPHALOSPORIN. It can be used to treat a wide range of Gram-negative bacterial infections, including septicaemia, pneumonia and gonorrhoea and to prevent meningococcal meningitis. It can also be used to prevent infections during surgery. It has a much longer duration of action than others of this class and so only needs to be taken once a day. Administration is by intravenous or intramuscular injection.

+▲ side-effects/warning: see under CEFACLOR. Administer with caution to patients with certain liver disorders; the calcium salt form of the drug may precipitate or form gallstones to be passed in the urine.

✪ Related entry: Rocephin

cefuroxime

is a broad-spectrum ANTIBACTERIAL and ANTIBIOTIC drug, which is one of the second-generation CEPHALOSPORINS. It can be used to treat a wide range of bacterial infections, particularly Gram-negative infections of the urinary, respiratory and genital tracts and the meninges (in meningitis). It can also be used to prevent infection during surgery. Administration is by intravenous or intramuscular injection.

+▲ side-effects/warning: see under CEFACLOR

✪ Related entries: Zinacef; Zinnat

Celance

(Lilly) is a proprietary, prescription-only preparation of pergolide, which can be used as an ANTIPARKINSONISM drug. It is available in the form of tablets.

+▲ side-effects/warning: see PERGOLIDE

Celectol

(Rhône-Poulenc Rorer) is a proprietary, prescription-only preparation of the BETA-BLOCKER drug celiprolol hydrochloride. It can be used as an ANTIHYPERTENSIVE treatment for raised blood pressure and is available as tablets.

+▲ side-effects/warning: see CELIPROLOL HYDROCHLORIDE

Celevac

(Monmouth) is a proprietary, non-prescription preparation of the (*bulking agent*) LAXATIVE methylcellulose. It can be used to treat a number of gastrointestinal disorders and is available as tablets.

+▲ side-effects/warning: see METHYLCELLULOSE

celiprolol hydrochloride

is a BETA-BLOCKER that can be used as an ANTIHYPERTENSIVE treatment for raised blood pressure. It is available as tablets.

+▲ side-effects/warning: see under PROPRANOLOL HYDROCHLORIDE. There may also be headache, sleepiness, fatigue, nausea, bronchospasm and slowing of the heart. It should be prescribed with caution to those who are breast-feeding or pregnant, or who have certain liver or kidney disorders. Withdrawal of treatment should be gradual.

✪ Related entry: Celectol

cephalexin

(cefalexin) is a broad-spectrum ANTIBACTERIAL and ANTIBIOTIC drug, which is one of the orally active CEPHALOSPORINS. It can be used to treat a wide range of bacterial infections, particularly of the urinary tract. Administration is oral in the form of capsules, tablets, liquid suspensions, syrups, or paediatric drops.

+▲ side-effects/warning: see under CEFACLOR

✪ Related entries: Ceporex; Keflex

cephalosporins

are broad-spectrum ANTIBACTERIAL and ANTIBIOTICS drugs that act against both Gram-positive and Gram-negative bacteria. Their chemical structure bears a strong resemblance to that of the penicillins as they both contain a beta-lactam ring, hence their classification as *beta-lactam antibiotics*. The similarity in structure extends to their mechanism of action: both classes inhibit the synthesis of the bacterial cell wall, so killing growing bacteria – they are *bactericidal*.

As a group, the cephalosporins are generally active against streptococci, staphylococci and a number of Gram-negative bacteria, including many coliforms. Examples of the original, first-generation cephalosporins are CEPHRADINE and CEFADROXIL. Some second-generation cephalosporins (eg.CEFUROXIME and CEPHAMANDOLE) are resistant to inactivation by bacterial PENCILLINASE enzymes, which widens their range of action to include treating sensitive Gram-negative organisms, including *Haemophilus influenzae*.

Some of the latest, third-generation, cephalosporins (eg.CEFOTAXIME, CEFTAZIDIME, CEFTIZOXIME and CEFODIZIME) act as antibacterials against certain Gram-negative bacteria (eg.*Haemophilus influenzae*) and pseudomonal infections (eg.*Pseudomonas aeruginosa*). Many cephalosporins are actively excreted by the kidney and therefore reach considerably higher concentrations in the urine than in the blood. For this reason, they may be used to treat infections of the urinary tract during their own excretion. In general, cephalosporins are rarely the drug of first choice, but provide a useful alternative, or reserve option, in particular situations.

The cephalosporins currently used are relatively non-toxic and only occasional blood-clotting problems, superinfections and hypersensitivity reactions occur (only 10% of patients allergic to penicillin show sensitivity to cephalosporins).

C

cephamandole
(cefamandole) is a broad-spectrum
ANTIBACTERIAL and ANTIBIOTIC drug, which
is one of the second-generation
CEPHALOSPORINS. It is less susceptible to
inactivation by bacterial penicillinases
than others in its class and for this reason
is effective against a greater range of
Gram-negative bacteria, for example,
penicillin-resistant *Neisseria gonorrhoeae*
and *Haemophilus influenzae*. It can be
used to treat a wide range of bacterial
infections, particularly of the skin and soft
tissues, the genito-urinary and upper
respiratory tracts and middle ear. It is also
used to prevent infection during surgery.
Administration is by injection.
+▲ side-effects/warning: see under
CEFACLOR
◯ Related entry: Kefadol

cephazolin
(cefazolin) is a broad-spectrum
ANTIBACTERIAL and ANTIBIOTIC drug, which
is one of the first-generation
CEPHALOSPORINS. It can be used to treat a
wide range of bacterial infections,
particularly of the skin and soft tissues,
urinary and upper respiratory tracts and
middle ear. It can also be used to prevent
infection during surgery. Administration is
by injection.
+▲ side-effects/warning: see under
CEFACLOR
◯ Related entry: Kefzol

cephradine
(cefradine) is a broad-spectrum
ANTIBACTERIAL and ANTIBIOTIC drug, which
is one of the first-generation
CEPHALOSPORINS. It can be used to treat a
wide range of bacterial infections,
particularly streptococcal infections of the
skin and soft tissues, the urinary and
upper respiratory tracts and middle ear.
It is also used to prevent infection during
surgery. Administration can be oral as
capsules or a dilute syrup, or
by injection.

+▲ side-effects/warning: see under
CEFACLOR
◯ Related entry: Velosef

Ceporex
(Glaxo) is a proprietary, prescription-only
preparation of the ANTIBACTERIAL and
(CEPHALOSPORIN) ANTIBIOTIC drug
cephalexin. It can be used to treat many
infections, including of the urinogenital
tract. It is available as capsules, tablets,
paediatric drops, an oral suspension and
as a syrup.
+▲ side-effects/warning: see CEPHALEXIN

Cerumol
(LAB) is a proprietary, non-prescription
COMPOUND PREPARATION of the ANTISEPTIC
agent chlorbutol and arachis oil (with
paradichlorobenzene). It can be used to
remove earwax and is available as ear-
drops.
+▲ side-effects/warning: see CHLORBUTOL;
ARACHIS OIL

Cesamet
(Lilly) is a proprietary, prescription-only
preparation of the ANTINAUSEANT and ANTI-
EMETIC drug nabilone. It can be used to
treat nausea in patients undergoing
chemotherapy and is available as capsules.
+▲ side-effects/warning: see NABILONE

Cetavlex
(Zeneca) is a proprietary, non-
prescription COMPOUND PREPARATION of
the ANTISEPTIC agent chlorbutol and
arachis oil (with paradichlorobenzene). It
can be used to treat cuts and abrasions
and is available as a water-based cream.
+▲ side-effects/warning: see ARACHIS OIL;
CETRIMIDE

cetirizine
is a recently developed ANTIHISTAMINE
drug with less side-effects (such as
sedation) than some of the older members
of this class. It can be used for the
symptomatic relief of allergic symptoms

such as hay fever and urticaria (itchy skin rash). Administration is oral in the form of tablets or a solution.

✚▲ side-effects/warning: see under ANTIHISTAMINE. Administer with caution to patients with kidney impairment. The incidence of sedation and anticholinergic effects is low.

⊙ **Related entry:** Zirtek

cetrimide

is an ANTISEPTIC and DISINFECTANT agent. It is used therapeutically (often in combination with CHLORHEXIDINE) for cleansing the skin and scalp, burns and wounds, and, as a cream, as a soap-substitute for conditions such as acne and seborrhoea.

✚ side-effects: there may be skin irritation.
▲ warning: avoid contact with eyes and body cavities.

⊙ **Related entries:** Ceanel Concentrate; Cetavlex; Drapolene Cream; Hibicet Hospital Concentrate; Savlon Antiseptic Cream; Siopel; Tisept; Travasept 100

cetylpyridinium chloride

in an ANTISEPTIC agent that is used as a mouthwash or gargle for oral hygiene. It is available as a gel, lozenges and an oral solution.

⊙ **Related entries:** Anbesol Liquid; Anbesol Teething Gel; Medilave; Meltus Junior Expectorant Linctus; Merocaine Lozenges; Merocets Gargle/Mouthwash; Merothol Lozenges; Merovit Lozenges; Tyrocane Junior Antiseptic Lozenges; Tyrocane Throat Lozenges; Vicks Original Formula Cough Syrup

C-Film

(FP) is a proprietary, non-prescription SPERMICIDAL CONTRACEPTIVE for use in combination with barrier methods of contraception (such as a condom). It is available as a film containing nonoxinol.

✚▲ side-effects/warning: see NONOXINOL.

chalk
See CALCIUM CARBONATE

*chelating agent

is a drug that is an ANTIDOTE to metal poisoning. It works by chemically binding to certain metallic ions and other substances, making them less toxic and allowing their excretion. They are used to reduce unacceptably high levels of metals of external origin (accidental or environmental) and due to abnormal metabolism (eg.of copper in Wilson's disease) and to treat disease states (eg.PENICILLAMINE in rheumatoid arthritis).

See: DESFERRIOXAMINE MESYLATE; DICOBALT EDETATE; DIMERCAPROL; SODIUM CALCIUMEDETATE.

Chemotrim

(RP Drugs) is a proprietary, prescription-only COMPOUND PREPARATION of the (SULPHONAMIDE) ANTIBACTERIAL drug sulphamethoxazole and the antibacterial drug trimethoprim, which is a combination known as co-trimoxazole. It can be used to treat bacterial infections, particularly infections of the urinary tract, prostatitis and bronchitis.

It is available as a paediatric oral suspension.

✚▲ side effects/warning: see CO-TRIMOXAZOLE

Chendol

(CP Pharmaceuticals) is a proprietary, prescription-only preparation of chenodeoxycholic acid. It can be used to dissolve gallstones and is available as tablets.

✚▲ side-effects/warning: see CHENODEOXYCHOLIC ACID

chenodeoxycholic acid

(a bile acid) is a drug that can dissolve gallstones *in situ*. Administration is oral in the form of capsules or tablets.

✚ side-effects: there is diarrhoea and

C

itching, mild liver dysfunction and changes in blood enzymes.

▲ warning: it should not be used in patients with impaired gall bladder, chronic liver disease, inflammatory disorders of the intestines, or who are pregnant.

○ Related entries: Chendol; Chenofalk; Combidol

Chenofalk

(Thames) is a proprietary, prescription-only preparation of chenodeoxycholic acid. It can be used to dissolve gallstones and is available as capsules.

✚▲ side-effects/warning: see CHENODEOXYCHOLIC ACID

Children's Vitamin Drops

(Hough) is a proprietary, non-prescription MULTIVITAMIN preparation of vitamins A, C and D. It is recommended by the Department of Health for routine supplement to the diet of young children from 6 months to 2-5 years and in some cases from as early as 1 month. It is available direct to families under the Welfare Food Scheme.

✚▲ side-effects/warning: see ASCORBIC ACID; RETINOL; VITAMIN D

Chloractil

(DDSA Pharmaceuticals) is a proprietary, prescription-only preparation of the (PHENOTHIAZINE) ANTIPSYCHOTIC drug chlorpromazine hydrochloride. It can be used in patients undergoing behavioural disturbances, or who are psychotic (especially schizophrenics) or showing severe anxiety where a degree of sedation is useful. It can also be used as an ANTINAUSEANT and ANTI-EMETIC drug to relieve nausea and vomiting, particularly in terminal illness and in preoperative medication. It is available as tablets.

✚▲ side-effects/warning: see CHLORPROMAZINE HYDROCHLORIDE

chloral elixir, paediatric, BP

is a non-proprietary, prescription-only

preparation of the HYPNOTIC drug chloral hydrate, which is used to treat insomnia. It is available as an elixir for children.

✚▲ side-effects/warning: see CHLORAL HYDRATE

chloral hydrate

is a short-term SEDATIVE and HYPNOTIC drug. It is considered to be particularly useful in inducing sleep in children or elderly patients. Administration is usually oral as capsules, tablets, an elixir, or a liquid mixture.

✚ side-effects: stomach irritation, abdominal distension and flatulence; occasionally, rashes, headache, blood changes and excitement. Dependence can occur with prolonged use.

▲ warning: it should not be administered to patients with severe heart disease, inflammation of the stomach, or severely impaired function of the liver or kidneys. It should be administered with caution to those with respiratory disorders; who are pregnant or breast-feeding, or elderly or debilitated, or who have a history of drug abuse. Avoid contact with the skin or mucous membranes.

○ Related entries: Noctec; Welldorm

chloral mixture, BP

is a non-proprietary, prescription-only preparation of the HYPNOTIC drug chloral hydrate, which is used to treat insomnia. It is available as a mixture.

✚▲ side-effects/warning: see CHLORAL HYDRATE

chlorambucil

is a CYTOTOXIC DRUG that is used as an ANTICANCER treatment, particularly for chronic lymphocytic leukaemia, lymphomas and solid tumours. It works by interfering with the DNA and so preventing normal cell replication. It can also be used as an IMMUNOSUPPRESSANT drug in the treatment of rheumatoid arthritis. Administration is oral in the form of tablets.

✚▲ side-effects/warning: see under

CYTOTOXIC DRUGS; but there may also be haemorrhagic cystitis (though this is rare); avoid its use in patients with porphyria and administer with care to those with renal impairment.

○ Related entry: Leukeran

chloramphenicol

is a broad-spectrum ANTIBACTERIAL and ANTIBIOTIC drug, which can be used to treat many forms of infection. However, the serious side-effects caused by its systemic use mean that it is normally restricted to certain severe infections, such as typhoid fever (*Haemophilus meningitis*) and, in particular, infections caused by *Haemophilus influenzae*. It is useful in treating conditions such as bacterial conjunctivitis, otitis externa, or many types of skin infection, because it is applied topically to the eyes, ears, or skin and therefore its toxicity is not encountered. Topical administration is by eye-drops, ear-drops, or a cream. Systemic administration is by capsules, a dilute suspension, or by injection or infusion.

✚ side-effects: depending on the route of administration, there may be nausea, vomiting, diarrhoea; certain types of neuritis. Systemic treatment may cause serious damage to the bone marrow, which results in blood disorders.

▲ warning: it should not be administered to patients who are pregnant or breast-feeding, or have porphyria. Administer with caution to those with impaired liver or kidney function. Topical treatment may cause stinging and it should be kept away from open wounds. Prolonged or repeated use should be avoided. Regular blood counts are essential.

○ Related entries: Actinac; Chloromycetin; Chloromycetin Hydrocortisone; Kemicetine; Minims Chloramphenicol; Sno Phenicol

Chlorasept 2000

(Baxter) is a proprietary, non-prescription preparation of the ANTISEPTIC agent chlorhexidine (as acetate). It can be used to cleanse and disinfect skin, wounds and burns and is available as a solution.

✚▲ side-effects/warning: see CHLORHEXIDINE

Chloraseptic

(Procter & Gamble) is a proprietary, non-prescription preparation of the ANTISEPTIC agent phenol. It can be used to treat minor mouth and gum disorders, sore throats and mouth ulcers. It is available as a solution for use as a mouthwash or gargle. It is not usually given to children, except on medical advice.

✚▲ side-effects/warning: see PHENOL

Chlorasol

(Seton Healthcare) is a proprietary, non-prescription preparation of the ANTISEPTIC agent sodium hypochlorite. It can be used as a cleanser to treat skin infections and particularly for cleansing wounds and ulcers. It is available as a solution.

✚▲ side-effects/warning: see SODIUM HYPOCHLORITE

chlorbutanol

See CHLORBUTOL

chlorbutol

(chlorbutanol) is used as a preservative in some drug preparations for removing earwax.

○ Related entry: CERUMOL; ELUDRIL MOUTHWASH

chlordiazepoxide

is a BENZODIAZEPINE drug. It can be used as an ANXIOLYTIC in the short-term treatment of anxiety and in conjunction with other drugs in the treatment of acute alcohol withdrawal symptoms. Administration is oral in the form of capsules or tablets.

✚▲ side-effects/warning: see under BENZODIAZEPINE

○ Related entries: Librium; Tropium

C

chlorhexidine

is an ANTISEPTIC and DISINFECTANT agent that is a constituent in many preparations. It can be used prior to surgery and in obstetrics, but is used mainly (as chlorhexidine gluconate, chlorhexidine acetate, or chlorhexidine hydrochloride) either as a mouthwash for oral hygiene or as a dressing for minor skin wounds and infections. It can also be used for instillation in the bladder to relieve minor infections.

✚ side-effects: some patients experience sensitivity reactions. It may cause irritation, burning and blood in the urine when used to irrigate the bladder.

▲ warning: avoid contact with the eyes and delicate body tissues.

○ Related entries: Chlorasept 2000; Corsodyl; CX Antiseptic Dusting Powder; Eludril Mouthwash; Eludril Spray; Germoline Cream; Hibicet Hospital Concentrate; Hibisol; Hibitane; Instillagel; Mycil Powder; Naseptin; Nystaform; Phiso-med; Savlon Antiseptic Cream; Steripod Chlorhexidine; Tisept; Travasept 100; Unisept

chlormethiazole

(clomethiazole) is a drug with a number of uses. It is a useful HYPNOTIC for treating severe insomnia (especially in elderly patients because it is relatively free of a 'hangover' effect), as an ANTICONVULSANT and ANTI-EPILEPTIC to treat status epilepticus, eclampsia, and, under strict medical supervision, to reduce the symptoms of withdrawal from alcohol and also for maintaining unconsciousness under regional anaesthesia with LOCAL ANAESTHETICS. Administration is either oral as capsules or a syrup, or by intravenous infusion.

✚ side-effects: nasal congestion, sneezing, irritation of the conjunctiva of the eyes and nose, headache; when given by injection or infusion, there is rarely an increase in heart rate and decrease in blood pressure and

thrombophlebitis excitement, confusion, gastrointestinal upsets, rashes and urticaria (itchy skin rash), anaphylaxis, blood and liver changes, or dependence.

▲ warning: it should not be given to patients with acute pulmonary insufficiency, or who are alcoholics who continue to drink. Use with care in patients with heart or respiratory disease, or impaired liver or kidney function, or who have a history of alcohol or drug abuse. Withdrawal of treatment should be gradual. It may cause drowsiness the next day, which can impair the performance of skilled tasks such as driving. The effects of alcohol may be enhanced.

○ Related entry: Heminevrin

chlormethine hydrochloride

See MUSTINE HYDROCHLORIDE

chlormezanone

is an ANXIOLYTIC and HYPNOTIC drug that also has SKELETAL MUSCLE RELAXANT properties. It is used in the short-term treatment of anxiety and tension and to induce sleep. It is not of proven value as a muscle relaxant, though it is available as a COMPOUND ANALGESIC preparation with paracetamol (called *Lobak*) that is intended for the relief of muscle spasm. Administration is oral in the form of tablets.

✚ side-effects: concentration and speed of thought and movement may be affected; the effects of alcohol may be enhanced. There may be drowsiness, dizziness, nausea, headache, dry mouth and shallow breathing; hypersensitivity reactions or jaundice may occur.

▲ warning: it should not be administered to patients with certain lung disorders; and only with caution to those who have muscle weakness, a history of drug or alcohol abuse, or with porphyria. Prolonged use or abrupt withdrawal of treatment should be avoided. The sedative effects may persist and impair

the performance of skilled tasks such as driving.
○ **Related entries: Lobak; Trancopal**

Chloromycetin

(Parke-Davis) is a proprietary, prescription-only preparation of the broad-spectrum ANTIBACTERIAL and ANTIBIOTIC drug chloramphenicol. When injected, it can be used to treat potentially dangerous bacterial infections, such as typhoid fever. When applied topically, as creams or drops, it can be used to treat eye infections. It is available as capsules, a suspension for dilution, as an eye ointment (*Redidrops*), eye-drops and in a form for injection.
+▲ side-effects/warning: see CHLORAMPHENICOL

Chloromycetin Hydrocortisone

(Parke-Davis) is a proprietary, prescription-only COMPOUND PREPARATION of the ANTI-INFLAMMATORY and CORTICOSTEROID drug hydrocortisone (as acetate) and the broad-spectrum ANTIBACTERIAL and ANTIBIOTIC drug chloramphenicol. It can be used to treat eye infections with inflammation and is available as an eye ointment.
+▲ side-effects/warning: see CHLORAMPHENICOL; HYDROCORTISONE

chloroquine

is an ANTIMALARIAL drug that is used as an AMOEBICIDAL to treat and to prevent contraction of malaria. In certain areas of the world strains of *Plasmodium falciparum* have recently exhibited resistance to chloroquine, so an alternative therapy is now advised. Chloroquine is also used as an ANTIRHEUMATIC to slow the progress of rheumatic disease (eg.rheumatoid arthritis and lupus erythematosus). Administration can be oral as tablets or a dilute syrup, or by injection or infusion.
+ side-effects: there may be nausea and

vomiting, headache; gastrointestinal disturbance; some patients itch and break out in a rash. Susceptible patients may suffer psychotic episodes, blood disorders, damage to the the eyes and effects to the hair.
▲ warning: administer with caution to those with porphyria, G6PD deficiency, psoriasis, or who have certain kidney, liver or gastrointestinal disorders, or neurological disorders. Ophthalmic checks should be made for long-term patients.
○ **Related entries: Avloclor; Nivaquine**

chlorothiazide

is a DIURETIC of the THIAZIDE class. It is used in ANTIHYPERTENSIVE treatment, either alone or in conjunction with other drugs and can also be used in the treatment of oedema (accumulation of fluid in the tissues) associated with congestive heart failure. Administration is oral in the form of tablets.
+▲ side-effects/warning: see under BENDROFLUAZIDE
○ **Related entries: Co-Betaloc; Co-Betaloc SA; Saluric**

chlorphenamine maleate

See CHLORPHENIRAMINE MALEATE

chlorpheniramine maleate

(chlorphenamine maleate) is an ANTIHISTAMINE drug. It is used to treat the symptoms of allergic conditions such as hay fever and urticaria (itchy skin rash) and is also occasionally used in emergencies to treat anaphylactic shock. Administration is either oral as tablets or a syrup, or by injection.
+▲ side-effects/warning: see under ANTIHISTAMINE. Because of its sedative side-effects, the performance of skilled tasks such as driving may be impaired. Injections may be irritant and cause short-lasting hypotension and stimulation of the central nervous system.
○ **Related entries: Contac 400; Dristan Decongestant Tablets; Expulin Children's Cough Linctus – Sugar Free; Expulin Cough Linctus – Sugar Free;**

C

Expulin Decongestant For Babies And Children (Linctus); Haymine; Piriton; Tixylix Cough and Cold; Lemsip Night-Time; Expulin Decongestant for Babies and Children (Linctus)

chlorpromazine hydrochloride

is chemically an important member of the PHENOTHIAZINE group and has a number actions and uses. It is used as an ANTIPSYCHOTIC and has marked sedative effects that make it a useful treatment for schizophrenia and other psychoses, particularly during violent behavioural disturbances. It can also be used as an ANXIOLYTIC in the short-term treatment of severe anxiety, to soothe the terminally ill, sometimes as a premedication prior to surgery to induce hypothermia and reduce shivering and to remedy an intractable hiccup. Additionally, it has an important use as an ANTINAUSEANT and ANTI-EMETIC to relieve nausea and vomiting, particularly in terminal illness. Administration can be oral as tablets, a suspension or an elixir, or topical as suppositories, or by injection.

✚ side-effects: extrapyramidal symptoms (muscle tremor and rigidity), drowsiness, apathy, pallor, insomnia, nightmares, depression (or, rarely, agitation), changes in heart rate and rhythm, dry mouth, nasal constriction, difficulty in urination, constipation, blurred vision, changes in hormone function (irregular menstruation, growth of breasts, abnormal milk production, impotence, weight gain), sensitivity reactions, blood changes, photosensitization, contact sensitization, rashes, jaundice and alterations in liver function, lupus-like syndrome and effects on the eye and skin. Intramuscular injection may be painful.

▲ warning: it should not be given to patients with bone marrow depression, or phaeochromocytoma. Administer with care to those with vascular disease states, respiratory disease, parkinsonism and epilepsy, liver and kidney impairment, a history of jaundice, blood disorders, myasthenia gravis, hypothyroidism, hypertrophy of the prostate gland, closed-angle glaucoma, hypothyroidism; or who are pregnant or breast-feeding. Withdrawal of treatment should be gradual. Because of its sedative effects, the performance of skilled tasks may be impaired.

✪ Related entries: Chloractil; Largactil

chlorpropamide

is a SULPHONYLUREA drug used in DIABETIC TREATMENT of Type II diabetes mellitus (non-insulin-dependent diabetes mellitus; maturity-onset diabetes). It works by augmenting what remains of INSULIN production in the pancreas and its effect lasts longer than that of most similar drugs. Unusually for a sulphonylurea, chlorpropamide can also be used to treat diabetes insipidus, though only mild forms caused by pituitary or thalamic malfunction, because it also reduces frequency of urination. Administration is oral in the form of tablets.

✚▲ side-effects/warning: see under GLIBENCLAMIDE; but has more side-effects. The consumption of alcohol may cause flushing.

✪ Related entry: Diabinese

chlorquinaldol

is an ANTIMICROBIAL drug that is included in some preparations incorporating a CORTICOSTEROID and which are used for treatment of inflammatory skin conditions.

✪ Related entry: Locoid C

chlortalidone

See CHLORTHALIDONE

chlortetracycline

is a broad-spectrum ANTIBACTERIAL and (TETRACYCLINE) ANTIBIOTIC drug. It can be used to treat many forms of infection, especially of the eye and skin (such as acne and impetigo). Administration (as chlortetracycline hydrochloride) is

topical as a cream, an ointment, or an
eye ointment.
+▲ side-effects/warning: see under
TETRACYCLINE. Topical application would not
usually cause most of these side-effects,
though local sensitivity reactions may occur.
**☉ Related entries: Aureocort;
Aureomycin; Aureomycin Topical;
Deteclo**

chlorthalidone
(chlortalidone) is a DIURETIC related to
the THIAZIDES. It is used to treat oedema
(accumulation of fluid in the tissues),
hypertension and diabetes insipidus.
Administration is oral in the form of
tablets.
+▲ side-effects/warning: see under
BENDROFLUAZIDE
**☉ Related entries: AtenixCo;
co-tenidone; Hygroton; Kalspare;
Tenchlor; Tenoret 50; Tenoretic**

Cho/Vac
is an abbreviation for CHOLERA VACCINE.

Cholera Vaccine
(Evans) (Cho/Vac) is a prescription-only
preparation of cholera VACCINE, which is
available in a form for injection.

cholera vaccine
is a VACCINE for IMMUNIZATION that
contains heat-killed strains of the bacteria
that causes cholera, *Vibrio cholerae* and
is effective for about six months. However,
it provides only a limited degree of
protection and travellers should still take
great care over the food and drink they
consume. Administration is by
subcutaneous or intramuscular injection.
+▲ side-effects/warning: see VACCINE

cholestyramine
(colestyramine) is a resin that binds bile
acids in the gut and is used as a LIPID-
LOWERING DRUG in hyperlipidaemia to
reduce the levels, or change the
proportions, of various lipids in the

bloodstream. It has various other uses,
including as an ANTIDIARRHOEAL and in
certain biliary disturbances (including
pruritus in biliary obstruction, or biliary
cirrhosis). Generally, it is administered
only to patients in whom a strict and
regular dietary regime, alone, is not
having the desired effect. Administration is
oral in the form of a powder taken with
liquids.
+ side-effects: nausea and vomiting;
flatulence with abdominal discomfort,
constipation or diarrhoea; and heartburn.
(Prolonged use may lead to vitamin K
deficiency with increased bleeding.)
▲ warning: it should not be administered to
patients who suffer from complete blockage of
the bile ducts; use with caution in those who
are pregnant or breast-feeding. High dosage
may require simultaneous administration of
fat-soluble vitamins and folic acid.
**☉ Related entries: Questran;
Questran A**

choline salicylate
is a drug with mild, local pain-relieving
properties, which are principally due to a
COUNTER-IRRITANT, or RUBEFACIENT, action.
It can be used by topical application in the
mouth or ears to relieve, for example, the
pain of teething, ulcers, or of minor
scratches. Administration is in the form of
an oral gel or ear-drops.
+▲ side-effects/warning: see under
METHYL SALICYLATE
**☉ Related entries: Audax Ear Drops;
Bonjela Oral Pain-Relieving Gel;
Teejel Gel**

chorionic gonadotrophin
(human chorionic gonadotrophin; HCG) is
secreted by the placenta and so is
obtained from the urine of pregnant
women. Its main actions are the same as
those of LUTEINIZING HORMONE (LH). It can
be used as an infertility treatment. It can
also be used to correct deficiencies in
prepubertal males, including aiding
decent of testicles and to treat delayed

C

puberty (though use of testosterone for this purpose may be preferred). It is administered by intramuscular injection.

✚ side-effects: oedema (accumulation of fluid in the tissues), tiredness and mood changes, headache; breast enlargement in males; sexual precocity, over-stimulation of the ovary; reactions at site of injection.

▲ warning: it should be given with caution to patients with certain heart or kidney disorders, asthma, epilepsy, or migraine.

⭘ Related entries: see
Gonadotraphon LH; Pregnyl; Profasi

chymotrypsin

is an enzyme that can be used to dissolve a suspensory ligament of the lens of the eye (zonulysin) to aid surgical removal of the lens because of cataract. Administration is by injection.

⭘ Related entry: Zonulysin

Cicatrin

(Wellcome) is a proprietary, prescription-only preparation of the (AMINOGLYCOSIDE) ANTIBIOTIC drugs neomycin sulphate and bacitracin zinc. It can be used to treat skin infections and is available as a cream, a dusting-powder and an aerosol powder-spray.

✚▲ side-effects/warning: see BACITRACIN ZINC; NEOMYCIN SULPHATE

ciclosporin

See CYCLOSPORIN

Cidomycin

(Roussel) is a proprietary, prescription-only preparation of the ANTIBACTERIAL and (AMINOGLYCOSIDE) ANTIBIOTIC drug gentamicin (as sulphate). It can be used to treat many forms of infection, particularly serious infections by Gram-negative bacteria. It is available in various forms for intravenous and intramuscular injection, as ear- or eye-drops and as an eye ointment.

✚▲ side-effects/warning: see GENTAMICIN

Cidomycin Topical

(Roussel) is a proprietary, prescription-only preparation of the ANTIBACTERIAL and (AMINOGLYCOSIDE) ANTIBIOTIC drug gentamicin (as sulphate). It can be used to treat skin infections, particularly by Gram-negative bacteria. It is available as a cream and an ointment for topical application.

✚▲ side-effects/warning: see
GENTAMICIN

cilastin

is an ENZYME INHIBITOR that inhibits an enzyme in the kidney which breaks down the ANTIBACTERIAL and (BETA-LACTAM) ANTIBIOTIC drug imipenem and so prolongs and enhances the antibiotic's effects. Cilastin and imipenemare are administered together in a preparation called impenem with cilastin. Administration is by injection or intravenous infusion.

✚▲ side-effects/warning: see under
IMIPENEM WITH CILASTIN

⭘ Related entry: Primaxin

cilazapril

is an ACE INHIBITOR. It is a powerful VASODILATOR that can be used in ANTIHYPERTENSIVE treatment, often in conjunction with other classes of drug, particularly (THIAZIDE) DIURETICS. Administration is oral in the form of tablets.

✚▲ side-effects/warning: see under
CAPTOPRIL

⭘ Related entry: Vascase

Ciloxan

(Alcon) is a proprietary, prescription-only preparation of the ANTIBACTERIAL and (QUINOLONE) ANTIBIOTIC drug ciprofloxacin. It can be used to treat a variety of infections, especially ones that are resistant to more conventional drugs and also corneal ulcers. It is available as eye-drops.

✚▲ side-effects/warning: see CIPROFLOXACIN

cimetidine

is an effective and much-prescribed, H$_2$-ANTAGONIST, ULCER-HEALING DRUG. It is used to assist in the treatment of benign peptic (gastric and duodenal) ulcers, to relieve heartburn in cases of reflux oesophagitis (caused by regurgitation of acid and enzymes into the oesophagus), Zollinger-Ellison syndrome and a variety of conditions where reduction of acidity is beneficial. It is now also available without prescription – in a limited amount and for short-term uses only – for the relief of heartburn, dyspepsia and hyperacidity. It works by reducing the secretion of gastric acid (by acting as a histamine receptor H$_2$-receptor antagonist), so reducing erosion and bleeding from peptic ulcers and allowing them a chance to heal. However, treatment with cimetidine should not be given before full diagnosis of gastric bleeding or serious pain has been carried out, because its action in restricting gastric secretions may possibly mask the presence of other serious disorders such as stomach cancer. Cimetidine can also be used to treat ulceration induced by NSAID treatment. Administration can be oral as tablets, effervescent tablets or a syrup, or by infusion or injection.

✚ side-effects: there are effects on bowel function, tiredness, rash, dizziness, headache or confusion (especially in the elderly) and reversible liver damage. Rarely, there may be blood disorders, muscle or joint pain, changes in heart, kidney and pancreas function. In men, high doses may cause reversible and temporary feminization (growth of breasts) and impotence.

▲ warning: it should be administered with caution to patients with impaired liver or kidney function, who are pregnant or breast-feeding. Treatment of undiagnosed dyspepsia may potentially mask the onset of stomach or duodenal cancer and is therefore undesirable. Cimetidine (but not the other available H$_2$-antagonists) inhibits microsomal metabolic enzymes (such as the microsomal oxidative system of the liver), so it interacts with a number of other drugs: this is of special importance in patients stabilized on the drugs warfarin, theophylline, aminophylline and phenytoin.

❂ Related entries: Algitec; Dyspamet; Galenamet; Peptimax; Phimetin; Tagamet; Ultec; Zita

cinchocaine

is a LOCAL ANAESTHETIC drug. It is used to relieve pain, particularly in dental surgery but also in the skin or mucous membranes. Administration is by topical application as an ointment.

✚▲ side-effects/warning: see under LIGNOCAINE HYDROCHLORIDE

❂ Related entries: Proctosedyl; Scheriproct; Ultraproct; Uniroid-HC

cinchona alkaloids

are chemically complex substances extracted from the bark of the cinchona tree (it is also known as Peruvian, Jesuit's, or Cardinal's bark). The best-known and most-used cinchona alkaloid is QUININE, which has been used for many centuries to treat fevers and is still an important drug in the treatment of malaria. It has a bitter taste and is incorporated into non-medicinal drinks to mask its flavour and those who are sensitive to it or who consume large quantities of 'tonic water' may experience one of its more marked side-effects, which is tinnitus (a ringing in the ears). The other main cinchona alkaloid is QUINIDINE (which is chemically similar to quinine, but is its isomer) and is used as an ANTI-ARRHYTHMIC drug to treat heartbeat irregularities.

cineole

is a TERPENE drug, which is a class of drugs that are chemically unsaturated hydrocarbons and are found in terpene plant oils and resins. Cineole is included, as a NASAL DECONGESTANT, in a number of preparations used for the relief of cold

C

symptoms.
○ Related entries: Copholco; Merothol Lozenges; Vicks Sinex Decongestant Nasal Spray

cinnarizine

is drug with ANTIHISTAMINE properties and is used for a number of purposes. It is mainly used as an ANTINAUSEANT (and thus an ANTI-EMETIC), for example, in the treatment of vestibular balance disorders (especially vertigo, tinnitus, nausea and vomiting in Ménière's diseases) and motion sickness. Quite separately, it has VASODILATOR properties that affect the blood vessels of the hands and feet and so may be used to improve the circulation in peripheral vascular disease (Raynaud's phenomenon). Administration is oral in the form of tablets.
✚▲ side-effects/warning: see under CYCLIZINE. It may also cause fatigue and skin reactions. Rarely, extrapyramidal symptoms (muscle tremor and rigidity) in the elderly and hypotension at high doses. Do not administer to those with porphyria.
○ Related entries: Stugeron; Stugeron Forte

Cinobac

(Lilly) is a proprietary, prescription-only preparation of the ANTIBACTERIAL and (QUINOLONE) ANTIBIOTIC drug cinoxacin. It can be used to treat various infections, particularly of the urinary tract and is available as capsules.
✚▲ side-effects/warning: see CINOXACIN

cinoxacin

is an ANTIBACTERIAL and (QUINOLONE) ANTIBIOTIC drug. It is used primarily to treat infections of the urinary tract. Administration is oral in the form of capsules.
✚▲ side-effects/warning: see under ACROSOXACIN. Avoid its use in patients with severe kidney impairment. Other side-effects include oedema (accumulation of fluid in the tissues) and tinnitus (ringing in the ears).

○ Related entry: Cinobac

ciprofibrate

is used as a LIPID-LOWERING DRUG in hyperlipidaemia to reduce the levels, or change the proportions, of various lipids in the bloodstream. It is usually administered only to patients in whom a strict and regular dietary regime, alone, is not having the desired effect. Administration is oral in the form of tablets.
✚▲ side-effects/warning: see under BEZAFIBRATE
○ Related entry: Modalim

ciprofloxacin

is an ANTIBACTERIAL and ANTIBIOTIC drug, which is one of the QUINOLONE family. It can be used to treat infections in patients who are allergic to penicillin or whose strain of bacterium is resistant to standard antibiotics. It is active against Gram-negative bacteria including Salmonella, Shigella, Campylobacter, Neisseria and Pseudomonas; and to a lesser extent against Gram-positive bacteria of the Streptococcal family. It is used to treat infections of the urinary, gastrointestinal and respiratory tracts, gonorrhoea and septicaemia. But usually only when these cases are resistant to more conventional agents. It can also be used to prevent meningococcal meningitis and infection during surgical procedures.
Administration can be oral in the form of tablets or as eye-drops, or by intravenous infusion.
✚▲ side-effects/warning: see under ACROSOXACIN. Other side-effects include dyspepsia, flatulence, liver and kidney impairment, difficulty in swallowing. An adequate fluid intake should be maintained. Use with caution in patients with G6PD deficiency.
○ Related entries: Ciloxan; Ciproxin

Ciproxin

(Baypharm) is a proprietary, prescription-

only preparation of the ANTIBACTERIAL and (QUINOLONE) ANTIBIOTIC drug ciprofloxacin. It can be used to treat a variety of infections, for example of the urinary tract and gonorrhoea. It is available as tablets and in a form for intravenous infusion.
✚▲ side-effects/warning: see CIPROFLOXACIN

cisapride
is a recently introduced MOTILITY STIMULANT. It acts within the stomach and small intestine and can be used to treat oesophageal reflux (regurgitation of acid and enzymes into the oesophagus), for short-term management of non-ulcer dyspepsia, for symptomatic relief of delayed gastric emptying associated with diabetes and systemic sclerosis and autonomic neuropathy. It is thought to act by releasing the NEUROTRANSMITTER acetylcholine from the nerves of the stomach and intestine. Administration is oral in the form of tablets.
✚ side-effects: there may be abdominal cramps, diarrhoea; sometimes headache and light-headedness. Extrapyramidal motor disturbances (muscle tremor and rigidity) have been reported.
▲ warning: it should not be administered to patients who are pregnant, or where stimulation of the intestine may be dangerous. Use with care in those with impaired liver or kidney function.
❍ Related entries: Alimix; Prepulsid

cisplatin
is a CYTOTOXIC DRUG (an organic complex of platinum) that works by damaging the DNA of replicating cells and so can be used as an ANTICANCER drug in the treatment of certain solid tumours, including ovarian cancer and testicular teratoma. Administration is by injection.
✚▲ side-effects/warning: see under CYTOTOXIC DRUGS; but also severe nausea and vomiting, kidney damage, ototoxicity (toxic to the ears, causing loss of hearing and ringing

in the ears) and peripheral nerve effects.

Citanest
(Astra) is a proprietary, prescription-only preparation of the LOCAL ANAESTHETIC drug prilocaine hydrochloride. It can be used for various types of anaesthesia and is available in a form for injection.
✚▲ side-effects/warning: see PRILOCAINE HYDROCHLORIDE

Citanest with Octapressin
(Astra) is a proprietary, prescription-only COMPOUND PREPARATION of the LOCAL ANAESTHETIC drug prilocaine hydrochloride and the VASOCONSTRICTOR drug felypressin. It can be used in dental surgery and is available in a form for injection.
✚▲ side-effects/warning: see FELYPRESSIN; PRILOCAINE HYDROCHLORIDE

Citramag
(Bioglan) is a proprietary, non-prescription preparation of the (*osmotic*) LAXATIVE magnesium citrate. It can be used to relieve constipation and is available as an effervescent powder.

Claforan
(Roussel) is a proprietary, prescription-only preparation of the ANTIBACTERIAL and (CEPHALOSPORIN) ANTIBIOTIC drug cefotaxime. It can be used to treat many infections, including meningitis and is available in a form for injection.
✚▲ side-effects/warning: see CEFOTAXIME

clarithromycin
is an ANTIBACTERIAL and (MACROLIDE) ANTIBIOTIC drug. It is a derivative of erythromycin and is usually given to patients who are allergic to penicillin. It can be used to treat skin, soft tissue and respiratory tract infections. Administration can be oral as tablets or an oral suspension, or by intravenous infusion.
✚▲ side-effects/warning: see under ERYTHROMYCIN. Adminster with caution to patients who are pregnant or breast-feeding.

C

Blood disorders have been reported. There may be headache, effects on taste and inflammation of the tongue and mouth.
○ Related entry: Klaricid

Clarityn

(Schering-Plough) is a proprietary, prescription-only preparation of the ANTIHISTAMINE drug loratadine. It can be used to treat the symptoms of allergic disorders such as hay fever and urticaria and is available as tablets and a syrup.
✚▲ side-effects/warning: see LORATADINE

clavulanic acid

is an ANTIBIOTIC drug that is only weakly ANTIBACTERIAL, but which prevents bacterial resistance. It works as an ENZYME INHIBITOR by inhibiting penicillinase enzymes that are produced by some bacteria. These enzymes can inactivate many antibiotics of the penicillin family, such as amoxycillin and ticarcillin and so prevent the antibiotics from working. Clavulanic acid is therefore used in combination with amoxycillin or ticarcillin.
○ Related entries: Augmentin; Timentin

Clearine Eye Drops

(Crookes Healthcare) is a non-prescription preparation of the SYMPATHOMIMETIC and VASOCONSTRICTOR drug naphazoline hydrochloride. It can be used to treat redness in the eyes due to minor infections and is available as eye-drops. It is not normally given to children, except on medical advice.
✚▲ side-effects/warning: see NAPHAZOLINE HYDROCHLORIDE

clemastine

is an ANTIHISTAMINE drug. It can be used for the symptomatic relief of allergic symptoms such as hay fever and urticaria (itchy skin rash). Administration is oral in the form of tablets or a liquid.
✚▲ side-effects/warning: see under ANTIHISTAMINE. Because of its sedative side-effects, the performance of skilled tasks such as driving may be impaired.
○ Related entries: Aller-eze; Aller-eze Plus; Tavegil

Clexane

(Rhône-Poulenc Rorer) is a proprietary, prescription-only preparation of the ANTICOAGULANT drug enoxaparin, which is a low molecular weight version of heparin. It can be used for long-duration prevention of venous thrombo-embolism, particularly in orthopaedic use. It is available in a form for injection.
✚▲ side-effects/warning: see ENOXAPARIN

Climagest

(Sandoz) is a proprietary, prescription-only COMPOUND PREPARATION of the female SEX HORMONES oestradiol (as valerate; an OESTROGEN) and norethisterone (a PROGESTOGEN). It can be used to treat menopausal problems, including in HRT (hormone replacement therapy) and is available as tablets.
✚▲ side-effects/warning: see NORETHISTERONE; OESTRADIOL

Climaval

(Sandoz) is a proprietary, prescription-only preparation of the OESTROGEN oestradiol (as valerate). It can be used in HRT (hormone replacement therapy) and is available in the form of a calendar pack of tablets.
✚▲ side-effects/warning: see OESTRADIOL

clindamycin

is an ANTIBACTERIAL and ANTIBIOTIC drug. It is used to treat infections of bones and joints, peritonitis (inflammation of the peritoneal lining of the abdominal cavity) and to assist in the prevention of endocarditis (inflammation of the lining of the heart). It is active against many anaerobic bacteria (including *Bacteroides fragilis* and Gram-positive cocci (including penicillin-resistant *Staphylocci*). It can also be used topically to treat acne and vaginal infections. However, it is not widely used because of its serious side-effects. Administration can be oral as capsules or a suspension, as a vaginal cream, by injection or infusion, or as a topical solution and lotion.

✚ side-effects: if diarrhoea or colitis appear during treatment, administration must be halted (see below). There may be nausea and vomiting; abdominal discomfort; jaundice, liver dysfunction; blood disorders.

▲ warning: it should not be administered to patients suffering from diarrhoea; and if diarrhoea or other symptoms of colitis appear during treatment, administration must be stopped. This is because clindamycin greatly alters the normal balance of bacteria in the gut and in a few cases this allows a superinfection by the anaerobe *Clostridium difficile*, which causes a form of colitis that can be serious. It should be administered with caution to those with certain liver or kidney disorders, or who are pregnant or breast-feeding.

⊙ Related entries: Dalacin; Dalacin C; Dalacin T

Clinicide

(De Witt) is a proprietary, non-prescription preparation of the PEDICULICIDAL drug carbaryl. It can be used to treat infestations of the scalp and pubic hair by lice. It is available as a lotion and a shampoo and is not normally given to infants under six months, except on medical advice.

✚▲ side-effects/warning: see CARBARYL

Clinitar

(Shire) is a proprietary, prescription-only preparation of coal tar. It can be used by topical application to treat eczema and psoriasis and is available as a cream and a shampoo.

✚▲ side-effects/warning: see COAL TAR

Clinoril

(Merck, Sharp & Dohme) is a proprietary, prescription-only preparation of the

(NSAID) NON-NARCOTIC ANALGESIC and ANTIRHEUMATIC drug sulindac. It can be used to treat rheumatic conditions and other musculoskeletal disorders and acute gout. It is available as tablets.

✚▲ side-effects/warning: see SULINDAC

clioquinol

is an ANTIMICROBIAL drug, which is chemically an iodine-containing member of the 8-hydroxyquinoline group. It can be used as an ANTIFUNGAL and AMOEBICIDAL drug and its primary use is to treat *Candida* fungal infections of the skin and the outer ear. Administration is topical as drops, creams, ointments and anal suppositories.

✚ side-effects: some patients experience sensitivity reactions.

⊙ Related entries: Betnovate-C; Haelan-C; Locorten-Vioform; Oralcer; Synalar C; Vioform-Hydrocortisone

clobazam

is a BENZODIAZEPINE drug, which is used as an ANXIOLYTIC in the short-term treatment of anxiety. It can also be used, in conjunction with other drugs, in ANTI-EPILEPTIC therapy. Administration is oral in the form of capsules.

✚▲ side-effects/warning: see under BENZODIAZEPINE

⊙ Related entry: Frisium

clobetasol propionate

is an extremely powerful CORTICOSTEROID drug with ANTI-INFLAMMATORY properties. It is used to treat severe, non-infective inflammation of the skin caused by conditions such as eczema and psoriasis, especially in cases where less-powerful steroid treatments have failed. Administration is by topical application in the form of an aqueous cream, an ointment, or a scalp lotion.

✚▲ side-effects/warning: see under CORTICOSTEROIDS; though systemic side-effects are unlikely with topical application,

C

but there may be local skin reactions. The amount applied to the skin each week should be below a certain maximum amount.
❂ Related entries: Dermovate; Dermovate-NN

clobetasone butyrate
is a CORTICOSTEROID drug with ANTI-INFLAMMATORY properties. It is used in the treatment of severe inflammation of the skin caused by conditions such as eczema and certain types of dermatitis, especially as a maintenance treatment between courses of more potent corticosteroids. Administration is by topical application in the form of a cream or an ointment.
✚▲ side-effects/warning: see under CORTICOSTEROIDS; though systemic effects are unlikely with topical application, but there may be local skin reactions.
❂ Related entries: Eumovate; Eumovate-N; Trimovate

clofazimine
is an ANTIBACTERIAL drug that is used, in combination with dapsone and rifampicin, in the treatment of the major form of leprosy. The fact that the treatment requires no fewer than three drugs is due to the increasing resistance shown by the leprosy bacterium. Administration is oral in the form of capsules.
✚ side-effects: there may be nausea and giddiness, diarrhoea and headache. The skin and urine may have a reddish tinge and skin lesions may be discoloured.
▲ warning: it should be administered with caution to patients with impaired kidney or liver function. Regular tests on both functions are essential.
❂ Related entry: Lamprene

clofibrate
is used as a LIPID-LOWERING DRUG in hyperlipidaemia to reduce the levels, or change the proportions, of various lipids in the bloodstream. It is usually administered only to patients in whom a

strict and regular dietary regime, alone, is not having the desired effect. Administration is oral in the form of capsules.
✚▲ side-effects/warning: see under BEZAFIBRATE
❂ Related entry: Atromid-S

clomethiazole
See CHLORMETHIAZOLE

Clomid
(Merrell) is a proprietary, prescription-only preparation of the HORMONE ANTAGONIST clomiphene citrate, which is an ANTI-OESTROGEN. It can be used to treat infertility due to ovulatory failure and is available as tablets.
✚▲ side-effects/warning: see CLOMIPHENE CITRATE

clomiphene citrate
is a sex HORMONE ANTAGONIST (an ANTI-OESTROGEN) that is used as a fertility treatment in women whose condition is linked to the persistent presence of oestrogens and a consequent failure to ovulate (characterized by sparse or infrequent periods). Clomiphene prevents the action of oestrogens and this increases secretion of GONADOTROPHINS, which cause ovulation. Administration is oral in the form of tablets.
✚ side-effects: multiple births may result. Hot flushes; nausea; vomiting; visual disturbances; dizziness and insomnia; breast tenderness; weight gain; rashes; and hair loss may occur.
▲ warning: it should not be administered to patients with ovarian cysts; cancer of the womb lining; certain liver disorders; abnormal uterine bleeding; or who are pregnant.
❂ Related entries: Clomid; Serophene

clomipramine hydrochloride
is a (TRICYCLIC) ANTIDEPRESSANT drug that also has SEDATIVE properties. It is used primarily to treat depressive illness, but

can also be used to assist in treating phobic or obsessional states and to try to reduce the incidence of catalepsy in narcoleptic patients (those who fall asleep in quiet or monotonous periods). Administration is by capsules, modified-release tablets, a syrup, or by injection.

+▲ side-effects/warning: see under AMITRIPTYLINE HYDROCHLORIDE

☉ Related entry: Anafranil

clonazepam

is a BENZODIAZEPINE drug, which is used as an ANTICONVULSANT and ANTI-EPILEPTIC for all forms of epilepsy, especially myoclonus and status epilepticus. Administration is either oral as tablets or by injection or infusion.

+▲ side-effects/warning: see under BENZODIAZEPINE; but is not to be used in patients with certain lung disorders.

☉ Related entry: Rivotril

clonidine hydrochloride

is an ANTISYMPATHETIC drug that decreases the release of NORADRENALINE from sympathetic nerves. It can be used in ANTIHYPERTENSIVE treatment, ANTIMIGRAINE treatment (for reducing the incidence of attacks), for vascular headaches and menopausal flushing (however, authorities are not convinced of its efficacy for this purpose). Additionally, there is some use for it in treating the symptoms (tics) of Giles de la Tourette syndrome. Administration is either oral in the form of tablets and modified-release capsules, or by injection.

+ side-effects: sedation, drowsiness, headache, depression or euphoria; dry mouth; fluid retention; rashes; nausea and constipation; blood disorders; slow heart rate, poor circulation in the extremities; rarely, there may be a failure to ejaculate and sleep disturbances.

▲ warning: it should not be administered to patients who have a history of depression. It must be given with caution to those with porphyria or peripheral vascular disease. The drug may cause drowsiness and impair the ability to drive or operate machinery. Withdrawal of treatment should be gradual.

☉ Related entries: Catapres; Catapres Perlongets; Dixarit

clopamide

is a DIURETIC of the THIAZIDE class. It can be used in ANTIHYPERTENSIVE treatment in conjunction with BETA-BLOCKERS. Administration is oral in the form of tablets.

+▲ side-effects/warning: see under BENDROFLUAZIDE

☉ Related entry: Viskaldix

Clopixol

(Lundbeck) is a proprietary, prescription-only preparation of the ANTIPSYCHOTIC drug zuclopenthixol dihydrochloride. It can be used for the long-term maintenance of schizophrenia and other psychoses. It is available as tablets (as zuclopenthixol dihydrochloride) and a depot deep intramuscular injection called (as zuclopenthixol decanoate). There is a range of *Clopixol* preparations and they differ in their duration of action and may be used according to the length of treatment intended.

+▲ side-effects/warning: see ZUCLOPENTHIXOL DECANOATE; ZUCLOPENTHIXOL DIHYDROCHLORIDE

Clopixol Acuphase

(Lundbeck) is a proprietary, prescription-only preparation of the ANTIPSYCHOTIC drug zuclopenthixol acetate. It can be used for short-term management of acute psychosis and mania or exacerbation of a chronic psychotic disorder. It is available in a form for depot deep intramuscular injection.

+▲ side-effects/warning: see ZUCLOPENTHIXOL ACETATE

Clopixol Conc.

(Lundbeck) is a proprietary, prescription-only preparation of the ANTIPSYCHOTIC

C

drug zuclopenthixol decanoate. It can be used for long-term maintenance of schizophrenia and other psychoses. It is available in a form for depot deep intramuscular injection.
+▲ side-effects/warning: see
ZUCLOPENTHIXOL DECANOATE

clorazepate dipotassium

is a BENZODIAZEPINE drug, which is used as an ANXIOLYTIC in the short-term treatment of anxiety. Administration is oral in the form of capsules.
+▲ side-effects/warning: see under
BENZODIAZEPINE
✪ Related entry: Tranxene

Clostet

(Evans) is a proprietary, prescription-only VACCINE preparation of adsorbed tetanus vaccine. It can be used for active IMMUNIZATION against tetanus and is available in a form for injection.

clotrimazole

is an (AZOLE) ANTIMICROBIAL and ANTIFUNGAL drug. It can be used in topical application to treat fungal infections of the skin and mucous membranes (especially the vagina, the outer ear and the toes). Administration is in the form of a cream, a dusting-powder, a spray, vaginal inserts (pessaries), or a lotion (solution).
+ side-effects: rarely, there may be a burning sensation or irritation; a very few patients experience sensitivity reactions.
✪ Related entries: Canesten; Canesten 1%; Canesten 1 VT; Canesten 10% VC; Canesten-HC; Lotriderm; Masnoderm

cloxacillin

is an ANTIBACTERIAL and ANTIBIOTIC drug of the PENICILLIN family. It is *penicillinase-resistant*, which means that it is not inactivated by the penicillinase enzymes produced by bacteria such as *Staphylococci* and is therefore primarily used to treat infections that other penicillins are incapable of countering

due to the presence of this enzyme. Administration is either oral in the form of capsules or by injection.
+▲ side-effects/warning: see under
BENZYLPENICILLIN
✪ Related entries: Ampiclox; Ampiclox Neonatal; Orbenin

clozapine

is an ANTIPSYCHOTIC drug, which can be used for the treatment of schizophrenia in patients who do not respond to, or who can not tolerate, conventional antipsychotic drugs. Because clozapine can cause serious blood disorders, its use is restricted to patients registered with the Sandoz Clozaril Patient Monitoring Service. Administration is oral in the form of tablets.
+ side-effects: see under CHLORPROMAZINE HYDROCHLORIDE. But it is less sedating and with a higher incidence of anticholinergic symptoms. Extrapyramidal symptoms (muscle tremor and rigidity) are less frequent. There are potentially very serious effects on the blood (agranulocytosis and neutropenia). Headache and dizziness, salivation, urinary incontinence, persistent erection, heart dysfunction, delirium, nausea and vomiting.
▲ warning: because of its effects on the blood (especially to depress the white cell count) this drug can only be used on registration with and concurrent monitoring by, the special patient monitoring service. It should not be given to patients who are pregnant or breast-feeding.
✪ Related entry: Clozaril

Clozaril

(Sandoz) is a proprietary, prescription-only preparation of the ANTIPSYCHOTIC drug clozapine. It can be used to treat schizophrenics who are unresponsive to other drugs. It is subject to special monitoring because of its potentially severe effects on the blood. It is available as tablets.

+▲ side-effects/warning: see CLOZAPINE

coal tar

is a black, viscous liquid obtained
by the distillation of coal. It is used on the
skin to reduce inflammation and itching
and also has some KERATOLYTIC properties.
Therapeutically, it is used to treat
psoriasis and eczema, where it is used in
solution at a concentration determined by
a patient's condition and response.
It is a constituent in many non-proprietary
and proprietary preparations, especially
pastes.

+ side-effects: skin irritation, an acne-like
rash and sensitivity to light.

▲ warning: avoid contact with broken or
inflamed skin and the eyes. Coal tar stains
skin, hair and fabric.

**◐ Related entries: Alphosyl;
Alphosyl 2 in 1 Shampoo;
Alphosyl HC; Balneum with Tar; Baltar;
calamine and coal tar ointment, BP;
Capasal; Carbo-Cort; Carbo-Dome;
Clinitar; coal tar and salicylic acid
ointment, BP; Cocois; Gelcosal;
Gelcotar; Genisol; Ionil T; Pentrax;
Polytar Emollient; Pragmatar;
Psoriderm; PsoriGel; Psorin; T/Gel;
Tarcortin**

coal tar and salicylic acid ointment, BP

is a non-proprietary preparation of coal
tar and salicylic acid. It can be used by
topical application to treat chronic eczema
and psoriasis and is available as an
ointment.

+▲ side-effects/warning: see COAL TAR;
SALICYLIC ACID

co-amilofruse 5/40

is a simplified name for the COMPOUND
PREPARATION of the (*potassium-sparing*)
DIURETIC drug amiloride hydrochloride
and the (*loop*) diuretic frusemide, in the
ratio of 5:40 (mg).

+▲ side-effects/warning: see
AMILORIDE HYDROCHLORIDE; FRUSEMIDE

◐ Related entries: Fru-Co; Frumil;

Lasoride

co-amilofruse 10/80

is a simplified name for the COMPOUND
PREPARATION of the (*potassium-sparing*)
DIURETIC drug amiloride hydrochloride
and the (*loop*) diuretic frusemide, in the
ratio of 10:80 (mg).

+▲ side-effects/warning: see AMILORIDE
HYDROCHLORIDE; FRUSEMIDE

◐ Related entry: Frumil Forte

co-amilozide 2.5/25

is a simplified name for the COMPOUND
PREPARATION of the (*potassium-sparing*)
DIURETIC drug amiloride hydrochloride
and the (THIAZIDE) diuretic
hydrochlorothiazide, in the ratio 2.5:25
(mg).

+▲ side-effects/warning: see AMILORIDE
HYDROCHLORIDE; HYDROCHLORITHIAZIDE

◐ Related entry: Moduret-25

co-amilozide 5/50

is a simplified name for the COMPOUND
PREPARATION of the (*potassium-sparing*)
DIURETIC drug amiloride hydrochloride
and the (THIAZIDE) diuretic
hydrochlorothiazide, in the ratio 5:50
(mg).

+▲ side-effects/warning: see AMILORIDE
HYDROCHLORIDE; HYDROCHLOROTHIAZIDE

**◐ Related entries: Amil-Co; Delvas;
Moduretic**

co-amoxclav

is a simplified name for the COMPOUND
PREPARATION of the broad-spectrum
ANTIBACTERIAL and (PENICILLIN)
ANTIBIOTIC drug amoxycillin and the
ENZYME INHIBITOR clavulanic acid (in the
form of its potassium salt). Clavulanic acid
interferes with the action of beta-
lactamase and so makes amoxycillin
penicillinase-resistant when it is used
against *Staphylococcus aureus,
Haemophilus influenzae* and certain
other bacteria that would otherwise
inactivate the antibiotic. Co-amoxclav can
be used to treat many infections including

C

C

those of the upper respiratory tract, of the ear, nose and throat and of the urinogenital tracts. Administration is either oral as tablets, dispersible tablets or suspensions, or by injection.

+▲ side-effects/warning: see AMOXYCILLIN; CLAVULANIC ACID. Administer with caution to patients with liver impairment, jaundice, certain blood disorders; or who are pregnant or breast-feeding.

☉ Related entry: Augmentin

Cobadex

(Cox) is a proprietary, prescription-only COMPOUND PREPARATION of the CORTICOSTEROID and ANTI-INFLAMMATORY drug hydrocortisone and the ANTIFOAMING AGENT dimethicone. It can be used to treat mild inflammatory skin conditions (such as eczema) and is available as a cream.

+▲ side-effects/warning: see DIMETHICONE; HYDROCORTISONE

Cobalin-H

(Link) is a proprietary, prescription-only preparation of the VITAMIN hydroxocobalamin. It can be used to correct deficiency of vitamin B_{12}, including pernicious anaemia and is available in a form for injection.

+▲ side-effects/warning: see HYDROXOCOBALAMIN

co-beneldopa

is a simplified name for the COMPOUND PREPARATION of the ANTIPARKINSONISM drug levodopa and the ENZYME INHIBITOR benserazide hydrochloride (in a ratio of benzeride/levodopa 1:4). It is used to treat parkinsonism, but not the parkinsonian symptoms induced by drugs. Benserazide prevents levodopa from being broken down too rapidly in the body (into dopamine) and so allowing more of it to reach the brain to make up the deficiency of dopamine, which is the cause of

parkinsonian symptoms. Administration is oral as capsules, tablets, or dispersible tablets.

+▲ side-effects/warning: see LEVODOPA

☉ Related entry: Madopar

Co-Betaloc

(Astra) is a proprietary, prescription-only COMPOUND PREPARATION of the BETA-BLOCKER drug metoprolol tartrate and the DIURETIC drug chlorothiazide. It can be used as an ANTIHYPERTENSIVE treatment for raised blood pressure and is available as tablets.

+▲ side-effects/warning: see CHLOROTHIAZIDE; METOPROLOL TARTRATE

Co-Betaloc SA

(Astra) is a proprietary, prescription-only COMPOUND PREPARATION of the BETA-BLOCKER drug metoprolol tartrate and the DIURETIC drug chlorothiazide. It can be used as an ANTIHYPERTENSIVE treatment for raised blood pressure and is available as modified-release tablets.

+▲ side-effects/warning: see CHLOROTHIAZIDE; METOPROLOL TARTRATE

cocaine

is a central nervous system STIMULANT that rapidly causes dependence (addiction). Therapeutically, it is used as a LOCAL ANAESTHETIC for topical application to the throat, nose, or eyes. It is available as a solution, a paste to apply to the nasal mucosa and as eye-drops.

+ side-effects: stimulation of the central nervous system, sympathomimetic effects and heart arrythmias.

▲ warning: avoid its use in patients with porphyria.

co-careldopa

is a simplified name for the COMPOUND PREPARATION of the ANTIPARKINSONISM drug levodopa and the ENZYME INHIBITOR carbidopa (the proportion of carbidopa to levodopa varies). It is used to treat parkinsonism, but not the parkinsonian

symptoms induced by drugs. Carbidopa prevents levodopa from being broken down too rapidly in the body (into dopamine) and so allowing more of it to reach the brain to make up the deficiency of dopamine, which is the cause of parkinsonian symptoms. Administration is oral in the form of capsules.
✚▲ side-effects/warning: see LEVODOPA
❍ Related entries: Half Sinemet; Half Sinemet CR; Sinemet; Sinemet CR; Sinemet LS; Sinemet-Plus

Cocois

(Bioglan) is a proprietary, non-prescription COMPOUND PREPARATION of salicylic acid, coal tar and sulphur (in coconut oil). It is used to treat eczema and psoriasis and is available as a scalp ointment.
✚▲ side-effects/warning: see COAL TAR; SALICYLIC ACID; SULPHUR

co-codamol

is a COMPOUND ANALGESIC preparation of the (OPIOID) NARCOTIC ANALGESIC drug codeine phosphate and the NON-NARCOTIC drug paracetamol; in either a ratio of 8:500 (mg) – *co-codamol 8/500*, or the stronger and more recently introduced 30:500 (mg) – *co-codamol 30/500*. The 8/500 preparation is available on a non-prescription basis (as it has a lower codeine content) either as one of an extensive range of generic preparations or in proprietary forms that cannot be prescribed under the National Health Service. The 30/500 preparation is available only on prescription and should be used with caution, especially in the elderly.
✚▲ side-effects/warning: see CODEINE PHOSPHATE; PARACETAMOL
❍ Related entries: Kapake; Panadeine Tablets; Paracodol Capsules; Paracodol Tablets; Parake; Solpadol; Tylex

co-codaprin

(8/400) is a COMPOUND ANALGESIC

preparation of the (OPIOID) NARCOTIC ANALGESIC drug codeine phosphate and the (NSAID) NON-NARCOTIC ANALGESIC and ANTIRHEUMATIC drug aspirin; in a ratio of 8:400 (mg). It is available as tablets and soluble tablets.
✚▲ side-effects/warning: see ASPIRIN; CODEINE PHOSPHATE

Codafen Continus

(Napp) is a proprietary, prescription-only COMPOUND ANALGESIC preparation of the (NSAID) NON-NARCOTIC ANALGESIC and ANTIRHEUMATIC drug ibuprofen and the (OPIOID) NARCOTIC ANALGESIC drug codeine phosphate (in higher amounts than in proprietary, non-prescription compound analgesics). It can be used particularly for treating the pain of musculoskeletal disorders and is available as tablets.
✚▲ side-effects/warning: see CODEINE PHOSPHATE; IBUPROFEN

Codalax

(Napp) is a proprietary, prescription-only preparation of co-danthramer 25/200, which is a (*stimulant*) LAXATIVE based on danthron. It can be used to treat constipation and to prepare patients for abdominal procedures. It is available as an oral suspension.
✚▲ side-effects/warning: see DANTHRON

Codalax Forte

(Napp) is a proprietary, prescription-only preparation of co-danthramer 75/1000, which is a (*stimulant*) LAXATIVE based on danthron. It can be used to treat constipation and to prepare patients for abdominal procedures. It is available as an oral suspension.
✚▲ side-effects/warning: see DANTHRON

Coda-Med

(Thompson Medical) is a proprietary, non-prescription COMPOUND PREPARATION of the NARCOTIC ANALGESIC drug codeine phosphate, the NON-NARCOTIC ANALGESIC

C

and ANTIPYRETIC drug paracetamol and the STIMULANT caffeine. It can be used for the symptomatic relief of pain (including rheumatic pain, toothache, period pain and neuralgia), headache and raised body temperature (eg.in flu). It is available as tablets and is not normally given to children under eight years, except on medical advice.

+▲ side-effects/warning: see CAFFEINE; CODEINE PHOSPHATE; PARACETAMOL

Codanin Tablets

(Whitehall Laboratories) is a proprietary, non-prescription COMPOUND ANALGESIC preparation of the NON-NARCOTIC ANALGESIC and ANTIPYRETIC drug paracetamol and the (OPIOID) NARCOTIC ANALGESIC codeine phosphate. It can be used for the symptomatic relief of mild to moderate pain and raised body temperature. It is available as tablets and is not normally given to children under six years, except on medical advice.

+▲ side-effects/warning: see CODEINE PHOSPHATE; PARACETAMOL

co-danthramer 25/200

is a non-proprietary, prescription-only COMPOUND PREPARATION of the (*stimulant*) LAXATIVE danthron and poloxamer '188'. It is available as an oral suspension.

+▲ side-effects/warning: see DANTHRON
○ Related entry: Codalax

co-danthramer 75/1000

is a non-proprietary, prescription-only COMPOUND PREPARATION of the (*stimulant*) LAXATIVE danthron and poloxamer '188'. It is available as an oral suspension.

+▲ side-effects/warning: see DANTHRON
○ Related entry: Codalax Forte

co-danthrusate 50/60

is a non-proprietary, prescription-only COMPOUND PREPARATION of the

(*stimulant*) LAXATIVES danthron and docusate sodium. It is available as an oral suspension.

+▲ side-effects/warning: see DANTHRON; DOCUSATE SODIUM
○ Related entry: Normax

codeine phosphate

is an (OPIOID) NARCOTIC ANALGESIC that also has the properties of an ANTITUSSIVE. As an analgesic, codeine is a common but often minor constituent of non-proprietary and proprietary preparations for the relief of mild to moderate pain. The drug also has the capacity to reduce intestinal motility and so can be used as an ANTIDIARRHOEAL and antimotility treatment. Administration can be oral as tablets or a syrup, or by injection.

+▲ side-effects/warning: see under OPIOID. Tolerance occurs readily, though dependence (addiction) is relatively unusual.

○ Related entries: Aspav; Benylin with Codeine; co-codamol; co-codaprin; Coda-Med; Codafen Continus; Codanin Tablets; Codis 500; Cojene Tablets; Diarrest; Dimotane with Codeine; Dimotane with Codiene Pediatric; Famel Original; Feminax; Galcodine; Galcodine Paediatric; Kaodene; Kapake; Migraleve; Panadeine Tablets; Panadol Ultra; Papaveretum; Paracodol Capsules; Paracodol Tablets; Parake; Propain Tablets; Solpadeine Capsules; Solpadeine Soluble Tablets; Solpadeine Tablets; Solpadol; Syndol; Tylex; Veganin Tablets

co-dergocrine mesylate

is a VASODILATOR drug that affects the blood vessels of the brain. It consists of a mixture of dihydroergocornine mesylate, dihydroergocristine mesylate and alpha- and beta-dihydroergocryptine mesylates. It has on occasion been claimed to improve brain function, but clinical results of psychological tests during and following treatment have neither proved nor disproved such a claim. It is for the treatment of senile dementia that the drug is most frequently used. Administration is oral as tablets.

✚ side-effects: there may be gastrointestinal disturbances, flushing, a blocked nose and a rash. Postural hypotension (low blood pressure on standing up from a lying or sitting position, causing dizziness).

▲ warning: it should be administered with caution to patients who have a particularly slow heart rate.

⊘ Related entry: Hydergine

cod-liver oil

has EMOLLIENT properties and is one of the constituents of a proprietary COMPOUND PREPARATION that is administered by topical application to the skin in the form of a cream. At one time cod-liver oil was commonly used as a source of VITAMIN A and VITAMIN D, but now HALIBUT-LIVER OIL is preferred.

⊘ Related entry: Morhulin Ointment

Codis 500

(Reckitt & Colman) is a proprietary, non-prescription COMPOUND ANALGESIC preparation of the (NSAID) NON-NARCOTIC ANALGESIC and ANTIRHEUMATIC drug aspirin and the (OPIOID) NARCOTIC ANALGESIC codeine phosphate. It can be used to relieve mild to moderate pain and high body temperature. It is available as soluble tablets and is not normally given to children under 12 years, except on medical advice.

✚▲ side-effects/warning: see ASPIRIN; CODEINE PHOSPHATE

co-dydramol

is a prescription-only COMPOUND ANALGESIC preparation of the (OPIOID) NARCOTIC ANALGESIC drug dihydrocodeine and the NON-NARCOTIC ANALGESIC drug paracetamol; in a ratio of 10:500 (mg) — although some non-prescription preparations have different ratios. It is available in many generic and some proprietary preparations. There are

further prescription-only versions that are similar, but have a higher proportion of dihydocodeine (see REMEDEINE). This compound analgesic has the advantages and disadvantages of both drugs. It is particularly dangerous in overdose because of the opioid dihydrocodeine tartrate component. It is available as tablets.

✚▲ side-effects/warning: see DIHYDROCODEINE TARTRATE; PARACETAMOL

⊘ Related entries: Galake; Paramol

co-fluampicil

is a simplified name for the COMPOUND PREPARATION of the broad-spectrum, penicillin-like ANTIBACTERIAL and ANTIBIOTIC drug ampicillin and the *penicillinase-resistant*, penicillin-like antibacterial and antibiotic drug flucloxacillin. It can be used to treat severe infection where the causative organism has not been identified, but Gram-positive staphylococcal infection is suspected, or where penicillin-resistant bacterial infection is probable. It is available as capsules, a syrup and in a form for injection.

✚▲ side-effects/warning: see AMPICILLIN; FLUCLOXACILLIN

⊘ Related entries: Flu-Amp; Magnapen

co-flumactone 25/25

is a simplified name for the COMPOUND PREPARATION of the (*aldosterone-antagonist* and *potassium-sparing*) DIURETIC drug spironolactone and the (*potassium-depleting* THIAZIDE) diuretic hydroflumethiazide, in the ratio 25:25 (mg).

✚▲ side-effects/warning: see HYDROFLUMETHIAZIDE; SPIRONOLACTONE

⊘ Related entries: Aldactide 25; Spiro-Co

co-flumactone 50/50

is a simplified name for the COMPOUND PREPARATION of the (*aldosterone-antagonist* and *potassium-sparing*)

C

DIURETIC drug spironolactone and the (*potassium-depleting* THIAZIDE) diuretic hydroflumethiazide, in the ratio of 50:50 (mg).

✚▲ side-effects/warning: see HYDROFLUMETHIAZIDE; SPIRONOLACTONE

⊕ **Related entries: Aldactide 50; Spiro-Co 50**

Cogentin

(Merck, Sharp & Dohme) is a proprietary, prescription-only preparation of the ANTICHOLINERGIC drug benztropine mesylate. It can be used in the treatment of parkinsonism and is available as tablets and in a form for injection.

✚▲ side-effects/warning: see BENZTROPINE MESYLATE

Cojene Tablets

(Roche) is a proprietary, non-prescription COMPOUND PREPARATION of the (NSAID) NON-NARCOTIC ANALGESIC and ANTIRHEUMATIC drug aspirin, the (OPIOID) NARCOTIC ANALGESIC codeine phosphate and the STIMULANT caffeine. It can be used to relieve pain (especially rheumatic pain), fever and flu and cold symptoms. It is available as tablets and is not normally given to children under 12 years, except on medical advice.

✚▲ side-effects/warning: see ASPIRIN; CODEINE PHOSPHATE; CAFFEINE

colchicine

is a drug derived from the autumn crocus *Colchicum autnale*. It is used in the treatment of gout, particularly as a short-term, introductory measure to prevent acute attacks during initial treatment with other drugs that reduce uric acid levels in the blood. Administration is oral in the form of tablets.

✚ side-effects: nausea, vomiting and abdominal pain. High or excessive dosage may lead to gastrointestinal bleeding and diarrhoea, rashes and even kidney damage. Rarely, peripheral nerve disorders, loss of hair, or blood disorders.

▲ warning: administer with caution to patients with gastrointestinal disease, impaired kidney function; or who are pregnant or breast-feeding.

Cold Relief Capsules

(Sussex Pharmaceuticals) is a proprietary, non-prescription COMPOUND PREPARATION of the NON-NARCOTIC ANALGESIC drug paracetamol and the STIMULANT caffeine. It can be used to relieve cold and flu symptoms and is available as capsules. It is not normally given to children, except on medical advice.

✚▲ side-effects/warning: see CAFFEINE; PARACETAMOL

Coldrex Powders, Blackcurrant

(Sterling Health) is a proprietary, non-prescription COMPOUND PREPARATION of the NON-NARCOTIC ANALGESIC drug paracetamol, the SYMPATHOMIMETIC and DECONGESTANT drug phenylephrine hydochloride and vitamin C. It can be used to relieve cold and flu symptoms and is available as a powder. It is not normally given to children, except on medical advice.

✚▲ side-effects/warning: see PARACETAMOL; PHENYLEPHRINE HYDROCHLORIDE

Coldrex Tablets

(Sterling Health) is a proprietary, non-prescription COMPOUND PREPARATION of the NON-NARCOTIC ANALGESIC drug paracetamol, the SYMPATHOMIMETIC and DECONGESTANT drug phenylephrine hydochloride, the STIMULANT caffeine and vitamin C. It can be used to relieve cold and flu symptoms and is available as tablets. It is not normally given to children, except on medical advice.

✚▲ side-effects/warning: see CAFFEINE; PARACETAMOL; PHENYLEPHRINE HYDROCHLORIDE

Colestid

(Upjohn) is a proprietary, prescription-

only preparation of the LIPID-LOWERING DRUG colestipol hydrochloride. It can be used in hyperlipidaemia to reduce the levels, or change the proportions, of lipids in the bloodstream. It is available as granules to be taken with liquids.
✚▲ side-effects/warning: see COLESTIPOL HYDROCHLORIDE

colestipol hydrochloride

is a resin that binds bile acids and lowers LDL-cholesterol. It is used as a LIPID-LOWERING DRUG in hyperlipidaemia to reduce the levels, or change the proportions, of various lipids in the bloodstream. It is usually administered only to patients in whom a strict and regular dietary regime, alone, is not having the desired effect. Administration is oral in the form of a granules taken with liquids.
✚▲ side-effects/warning: see under CHOLESTYRAMINE
○ Related entry: Colestid

colestyramine

See CHOLESTYRAMINE

Colifoam

(Stafford-Miller) is a proprietary prescription-only preparation of the CORTICOSTEROID drug hydrocortisone (as acetate). It can be used to treat inflammation with colitis and proctitis and is available as a foam and applied with an aerosol.
✚▲ side-effects/warning: see HYDROCORTISONE

colistin

is an ANTIBACTERIAL and ANTIBIOTIC drug, which is a comparatively toxic member of the POLYMIXIN family. It is active against Gram-negative bacteria, including *Pseudomonas aeruginosa* and can be used in topical application (as colistin sulphate) to treat infections of the skin. However, in certain conditions and under strict supervision, the drug may be administered orally (primarily to sterilize the bowel and is not absorbed) or by injection, infusion, or inhalation (as an adjunct to standard antibiotic treatment). Administration can be by tablets, a syrup, by injection, or as a topical solution.
✚ side-effects: there may be breathlessness, vertigo, numbness round the mouth and muscular weakness and a tingling sensation. Rarely, slurred speech, confusion and visual disturbances.
▲ warning: it should not be administered to patients who suffer from the neuromuscular disease myasthenia gravis, or who are pregnant or breast-feeding. It should be administered with caution to those who suffer from impaired kidney function or porphyria.
○ Related entry: Colomycin

Colofac

(Duphar) is a proprietary, prescription-only preparation of the ANTISPASMODIC drug mebeverine hydrochloride. It can be used to treat gastrointestinal spasm and is available as tablets and an oral suspension.
✚▲ side-effects/warning: see MEBEVERINE HYDROCHLORIDE

Colomycin

(Pharmax) is a proprietary, prescription-only preparation of the ANTIBACTERIAL and (POLYMIXIN) ANTIBIOTIC drug colistin. It can be used by topical application to treat skin infections, burns and wounds; and also by mouth and by injection. It is available as a sterile powder (to make up into a topical solution), tablets, as a syrup and in a form for injection.
✚▲ side-effects/warning: see COLISTIN

Colpermin

(Pharmacia) is a proprietary, non-prescription preparation of the ANTISPASMODIC drug peppermint oil. It can be used to relieve the discomfort of abdominal colic and distension,

C

particularly in irritable bowel syndrome. It is available as capsules.
+▲ side-effects/warning: see
PEPPERMINT OIL

Combantrin

(Pfizer) is a proprietary, prescription-only preparation of the ANTHELMINTIC drug pyrantel. It can be used to treat infestations by roundworm, threadworm and hookworm. It is available as tablets.
+▲ side-effects/warning: see
PYRANTEL

Combidol

(CP Pharmaceuticals) is a proprietary, prescription-only COMPOUND PREPARATION of chenodeoxycholic acid and ursodeoxycholic acid. It can be used to dissolve gallstones and is available as tablets.
+▲ side-effects/warning: see
CHENODEOXYCHOLIC ACID;
URSODEOXYCHOLIC ACID

Comixco

(Ashbourne) is a proprietary, prescription-only COMPOUND PREPARATION of the (SULPHONAMIDE) ANTIBACTERIAL drug sulphamethoxazole and the antibacterial drug trimethoprim, which is a combination called co-trimoxazole. It can be used to treat bacterial infections, particularly infections of the urinary tract, prostatitis and bronchitis. It is available as soluble tablets.
+▲ side-effects/warning: see
CO-TRIMOXAZOLE

Comox

(Norton) is a proprietary, prescription-only COMPOUND PREPARATION of the (SULPHONAMIDE) ANTIBACTERIAL drug sulphamethoxazole and the antibacterial drug trimethoprim, which is a combination called co-trimoxazole. It can be used to treat bacterial infections, particularly infections of the urinary tract,

prostatitis and bronchitis. It is available as soluble tablets.
+▲ side-effects/warning: see
CO-TRIMOXAZOLE

*compound analgesic

drugs combine two or more ANALGESICS in one preparation. There are a number of proprietary preparations with some combination of the NON-NARCOTIC ANALGESIC drug PARACETAMOL, the NSAID analgesics ASPIRIN and IBUPROFEN and the (OPIOID) NARCOTIC ANALGESICS CODEINE PHOSPHATE, DEXTROPROPOXYPHENE HYDROCHLORIDE and DIHYDROCODEINE TARTRATE. There are also several 'official', non-proprietary compound analgesics that contain specified amounts of various analgesics: see CO-CODAMOL, CO-CODAPRIN, CO-DYDRAMOL and CO-PROXAMOL.

*compound preparation

is a term that is used to describe a combination of two or more pharmacologically active constituents in a single preparation. Many proprietary preparations contain a number of active constituents with differing actions (especially in cough and cold remedies). However, medical attitudes to compound preparations are mixed. The main criticism is that in certain circumstances it may be necessary to adjust the dose of one or all of the constituents independently, in order to achieve a reliable and safe response, but this is impossible in a compound preparation. For instance, POTASSIUM CHLORIDE is now rarely included in preparations containing DIURETICS that cause potassium loss from the body, because the amount of potassium required is very variable and best controlled independently of the (critical) dose of the diuretic. On the other hand, certain combinations of drugs (in a standard ratio of doses) have gained an established place in both prescription-only and non-prescription applications. Most examples of these compound preparations have a *CO-* prefix, which means compound. For example, CO-CODAMOL 8/500 is a compound preparation of CODEINE PHOSPHATE and PARACETAMOL, in a ratio of 8 mg of codeine phosphate to 500 mg of paracetamol.

compound thymol glycerin, BP

is a non-proprietary preparation of GLYCEROL and THYMOL (with colour and flavouring). It can be used as a mouthwash for oral hygiene.

Concordin

(Merck, Sharp & Dohme) is a proprietary, prescription-only preparation of the (TRICYCLIC) ANTIDEPRESSANT drug protriptyline hydrochloride. It can be used to treat depressive illness, especially in apathetic or withdrawn patients and is available as tablets.
+▲ side-effects/warning: see PROTRIPTYLINE HYDROCHLORIDE

Condyline

(Yamanouchi) is a proprietary, prescription-only COMPOUND PREPARATION of the KERATOLYTIC agent podophyllum. It can be used in men to treat and remove penile warts, or in women on the external genitalia. It is available as a solution for topical application.
+▲ side-effects/warning: see POPOPHYLLIN

conjugated oestrogens

are naturally obtained OESTROGENs obtained from the urine of pregnant mares, which are used in HRT (hormone replacement therapy). Administration is oral in the form of tablets.
+▲ side-effects/warning: see under OESTROGEN
☉ Related entries: Premarin; Prempak-C

Conotrane

(Yamanouchi) is a proprietary, non-prescription preparation of the ANTISEPTIC

agent benzalkonium chloride (with dimethicone '350'). It can be used for the relief of nappy rash and skin sores and is available as a cream.
+▲ side-effects/warning: see BENZALKONIUM CHLORIDE

Conova 30

(Searle) is a proprietary, prescription-only COMPOUND PREPARATION that can be used as a (*monophasic*) ORAL CONTRACEPTIVE (and also for certain menstrual problems) of the type that combines an OESTROGEN and a PROGESTOGEN, in this case ethinyloestradiol and ethynodiol diacetate. It is available in the form of tablets.
+▲ side-effects/warning: see ETHINYLOESTRADIOL; ETHYNODIOL DIACETATE

Contac 400

(SmithKline Beecham) is a proprietary, non-prescription COMPOUND PREPARATION of the SYMPATHOMIMETIC and DECONGESTANT drug phenylpropanolamine hydrochloride and the ANTIHISTAMINE drug chlorpheniramine maleate. It can be used for symptomatic relief of nasal over-secretion and is available as capsules.
+▲ side-effects/warning: see CHLORPHENIRAMINE MALEATE; PHENYLPROPANOLAMINE HYDROCHLORIDE

Contac Coughcaps

(SmithKline Beecham) is a proprietary, non-prescription preparation of the ANTITUSSIVE and (OPIOID) NARCOTIC ANALGESIC drug dextromethorphan hydrobromide. It can be used for the symptomatic relief of unproductive coughs. It is available as controlled-release beads in capsules and is not normally given to children, except on medical advice.
+▲ side-effects/warning: see DEXTROMETHORPHAN HYDROBROMIDE

*contraceptive

is a drug, method, or device that prevents

C

conception. Contraceptive drugs include ORAL CONTRACEPTIVES (most notably the Pill), which contain either a hormonal combination of a PROGESTOGEN plus an OESTROGEN (combined oral contraceptive pill; COC), just a progestogen (progesterone-only contraceptive pill; POP), or parenteral contraceptives (progesterone-only preparations given by injection or implantation and renewable every three months). SPERMICIDAL preparations contain drugs that kill sperm and/or prevent sperm motility within the vagina or cervix and should only be used in combination with barrier methods of contraception (such as a condom or diaphragm). Post-coital emergency contraception consists of a high dose of a combined preparation of oestrogen and progestogen (known as the *morning-after pill*). Intra-uterine contraceptive devices are not normally regarded as drugs (and are not within the scope of this book), but have a copper wire or ring incorporated which is thought to be pharmacologically active in changing production of local mediators (especially PROSTAGLANDINS), which effect implantation. All contraceptives that involve the use of drugs produce side-effects and requires expert advice to identify the form ideally suited to a patient's circumstances.

Contraflam

(Berk) is a proprietary, prescription-only preparation of the (NSAID) NON-NARCOTIC ANALGESIC and ANTIRHEUMATIC drug mefenamic acid. It can be used to treat pain in rheumatoid arthritis, osteoarthritis and other musculoskeletal disorders and also period pain. It is available as capsules.

+▲ side-effects/warning: see MEFENAMIC ACID

Convulex

(Pharmacia) is a proprietary, prescription-only preparation of the ANTICONVULSANT and ANTI-EPILEPTIC drug valproic acid. It is a valuable drug in the treatment of all forms of epilepsy and is available as capsules.

+▲ side-effects/warning: see under SODIUM VALPROATE

co-phenotrope

is an ANTIDIARRHOEAL COMPOUND PREPARATION of the OPIOID drug diphenoxylate hydrochloride and the ANTICHOLINERGIC drug atropine sulphate. It can be used to treat chronic diarrhoea (eg in mild chronic ulcerative colitis), but dependency may occur with prolonged use. It is available as tablets and a sugar-free liquid.

+▲ side effects/warning: see ATROPINE SULPHATE; DIPHENOXYLATE HYDROCHLORIDE

✪ Related entries: Diarphen: Lomotil

Copholco

(Roche) is a proprietary, non-prescription preparation of the ANTITUSSIVE and EXPECTORANT drug pholcodine, along with terpin, cineole and menthol. It can be used for the symptomatic relief of ticklish cough and is available as a linctus.

+▲ side-effects/warning: see PHOLCODINE

Copholcoids Cough Pastilles

(Roche) is a proprietary, non-prescription preparation of the ANTITUSSIVE and EXPECTORANT drug pholcodine, along with menthol and terpin hydrate. It can be used for the symptomatic relief of ticklish coughs.

+▲ side-effects/warning: see PHOLCODINE

Coppertone Ultrashade 23 Lotion

(Scholl) is a proprietary, non-prescription SUNSCREEN preparation, which protects against UVA and UVB ultraviolet radiation (UVB-SPF 23). It contains several agents used to help protect the skin, such as ethylhexyl-methoxycinnamate, oxybenzone and padimate-O. A patient whose skin condition requires this sort of protection may be prescribed it at the discretion of their doctor.

co-praxamol

is a COMPOUND ANALGESIC preparation of the (OPIOID) NARCOTIC ANALGESIC drug dextropropoxyphene hydrochloride and the NON-NARCOTIC ANALGESIC drug paracetamol; in a ratio of 32.5:325 (mg) It is available in many generic and some proprietary preparations and has the advantages and disadvantages of both drugs. It is particularly dangerous to overdose because of the opioid dextropropoxyphene component. It is available as tablets.

+▲ side effects/warning: see
DEXTROPROPOXYPHENE HYDROCHLORIDE;
PARACETAMOL
**O Related entries: Cosalgesic;
Distagesic**

Coracten

(Evans) is a proprietary, prescription-only preparation of the CALCIUM-CHANNEL BLOCKER nifedipine. It can be used as an ANTI-ANGINA drug in the prevention of attacks and as an ANTIHYPERTENSIVE treatment. It is available as capsules.

+▲ side-effects/warning: see NIFEDIPINE

Cordarone X

(Sanofi Winthrop) is a proprietary, prescription-only preparation of the ANTI-ARRHYTHMIC drug amiodarone hydrochloride. It can be used to treat heartbeat irregularities and is available as tablets and in a form for injection.

+▲ side-effects/warning: see
AMIODARONE HYDROCHLORIDE

Cordilox

(Baker Norton) is a proprietary, prescription-only preparation of the CALCIUM-CHANNEL BLOCKER verapamil hydrochloride. It can be used as an ANTIHYPERTENSIVE treatment, as an ANTI-ANGINA drug in the prevention of attacks

and as an ANTI-ARRHYTHMIC to correct heart irregularities. It is available as tablets and in a form for injection.

+▲ side-effects/warning: see
VERAPAMIL HYDROCHLORIDE

Corgard

(Sanofi Winthrop) is a proprietary, prescription-only preparation of the BETA-BLOCKER drug nadolol. It can be used as an ANTIHYPERTENSIVE treatment for raised blood pressure, as an ANTI-ANGINA treatment to relieve symptoms and improve exercise tolerance and as an ANTI-ARRHYTHMIC to regularize heartbeat and to treat myocardial infarction. It can also be used as an ANTIMIGRAINE treatment to prevent attacks and as an ANTITHYROID for short-term treatment of thyrotoxicosis. It is available as tablets.

+▲ side-effects/warning: see
NADOLOL

Corgaretic 40

(Sanofi Winthrop) is a proprietary, prescription-only COMPOUND PREPARATION of the BETA-BLOCKER drug nadolol and the DIURETIC drug bendrofluazide. It can be used as an ANTIHYPERTENSIVE treatment for raised blood pressure and is available as tablets.

+▲ side-effects/warning: see
BENDROFLUAZIDE; NADOLOL

Corgaretic 80

(Sanofi Winthrop) is a proprietary, prescription-only COMPOUND PREPARATION of the BETA-BLOCKER drug nadolol hydrochloride and the DIURETIC bendrofluazide. It can be used as an ANTIHYPERTENSIVE treatment for raised blood pressure and is available as tablets.

+▲ side-effects/warning: see
BENDROFLUAZIDE; NADOLOL

Corlan

(Evans) is a proprietary, non-prescription preparation of the CORTICOSTEROID and ANTI-INFLAMMATORY drug hydrocortisone

C

175

C

(as sodium succinate). It can be used treat ulcers and sores in the mouth and is available as lozenges.

✚▲ side-effects/warning: see HYDROCORTISONE

Coro-nitro Spray

(Boehringer Mannheim) is a proprietary, non-prescription preparation of the VASODILATOR and ANTI-ANGINA drug glyceryl trinitrate. It can be used to treat and prevent angina pectoris and in HEART FAILURE TREATMENT. It is available in the form of an aerosol spray in metered doses.

✚▲ side-effects/warning: see GLYCERYL TRINITRATE

Correctol

(Schering-Plough) is a proprietary, non-prescription COMPOUND PREPARATION of the (*stimulant*) LAXATIVES docusate sodium and phenolphthalein. It can be used to relieve constipation and is available as tablets. It is not normally given to children, except on medical advice.

✚▲ side-effects/warning: see DOCUSATE SODIUM; PHENOLPHTHALEIN

Corsodyl

(SmithKline Beecham) is a proprietary, non-prescription preparation of the ANTISEPTIC agent chlorhexidine (as gluconate). It can be used by topical application to treat inflammations and infections of the mouth. It is available as a dental gel, a mouthwash and an oral spray.

✚▲ side-effects/warning: see CHLORHEXIDINE

*corticosteroids

are steroid hormones secreted by the cortex (outer part) of the adrenal glands, or are synthetic substances that closely resemble the natural forms. There are two main types, *glucocorticoids* and *mineralocorticoids*. The latter assist in maintaining the salt-and-water balance of the body. Corticosteroids such as the glucocorticoid HYDROCORTISONE and the mineralocorticoid FLUDROCORTISONE ACETATE can be given to patients for replacement therapy where there is a deficiency, or in Addison's disease, or following adrenalectomy or hypopituitarism. The glucocorticoids are potent ANTI-INFLAMMATORY and ANTI-ALLERGIC drugs and are frequently used to treat inflammatory and/or allergic reactions of the skin, airways and elsewhere. COMPOUND PREPARATIONS are available that contain both an ANTIBACTERIAL or ANTIFUNGAL drug with an anti-inflammatory corticosteroid and can be used in conditions where an infection is also present. However, these preparations must be used with caution because the corticosteroid component diminishes the patient's natural immune response to the infective agent. Absorption of a high dose of corticosteroid over a period of time may also cause undesirable, systemic side-effects.

✚ side-effects: *mineralocorticoid* adverse effects include hypertension, sodium and water retention and potassium loss. *Glucocorticoid* adverse effects include diabetes, osteoporosis, avascular necrosis, mental disturbances, euphoria, muscle wasting and possibly peptic ulceration. Corticosteroids may also cause Cushing's syndrome, suppressed growth in children and adrenal atrophy. If administered during pregnancy, they may affect adrenal gland development in the child. Suppression of the symptoms of infection may occur.

▲ warning: withdrawal of treatment must be gradual (patients are given a *steroid card* with general advice).

corticotrophin

or adrenocorticotrophic hormone (ACTH), is a HORMONE produced and secreted by the pituitary gland in order to control the production and secretion of other hormones – CORTICOSTEROIDS – in the adrenal glands, generally as a response to stress. Therapeutically, synthetic corticotrophin analogues (eg.TETRACOSACTRIN) can be administered to make up for hormonal deficiency in the pituitary gland, to cause the production of extra corticosteroids in the treatment of inflammatory conditions such as rheumatoid arthritis and Crohn's disease, or to test the function of the adrenal glands.

cortisol
See HYDROCORTISONE

cortisone acetate
is a CORTICOSTEROID hormone with ANTI-INFLAMMATORY properties and has both *glucocorticoid* and *mineralocorticoid* activity. It can therefore be used to make up for hormonal deficiency (especially relating to the salt-and-water balance in the body), for instance, following surgical removal of the adrenal glands. Administration is oral in the form of tablets.
+▲ side-effects/warning: see under CORTICOSTEROIDS
✪ Related entries: Cortistab; Cortisyl

Cortistab
(Boots) is a proprietary, prescription-only preparation of the CORTICOSTEROID and ANTI-INFLAMMATORY drug cortisone acetate. It can be used in replacement therapy to make up hormonal deficiency, for instance, following surgical removal of one or both of the adrenal glands. It is available as tablets.
+▲ side-effects/warning: see CORTISONE ACETATE

Cortisyl
(Roussel) is a proprietary, prescription-only preparation of the CORTICOSTEROID and ANTI-INFLAMMATORY drug cortisone acetate. It can be used in replacement therapy to make up hormonal deficiency, for instance,

following surgical removal of one or both of the adrenal glands. It is available as tablets.
+▲ side-effects/warning: see CORTISONE ACETATE

Corwin
(Stuart) is a proprietary, prescription-only preparation of the SYMPATHOMIMETIC and CARDIAC STIMULANT drug xamoterol (as xamoterol fumarate). It can be used for the treatment of heart conditions where moderate stimulation of the force of heartbeat is required, such as chronic moderate heart failure. It is available as tablets.
+▲ side-effects/warning: see XAMOTEROL

Cosalgesic
(Cox) is a proprietary, prescription-only COMPOUND ANALGESIC preparation of the (OPIOID) NARCOTIC ANALGESIC drug dextropropoxyphene hydrochloride and the NON-NARCOTIC ANALGESIC paracetamol (a combination called co-proxamol). It can be used to treat many types of pain and is available as tablets. It is not normally given to children, except on medical advice.
+▲ side-effects/warning: see DEXTROPROPOXYPHENE HYDROCHLORIDE; PARACETAMOL

Cosmegen Lyovac
(Merck, Sharp & Dohme) is a proprietary, prescription-only preparation of the (CYTOTOXIC) ANTICANCER drug dactinomycin. It is used particularly to treat cancer in children and is available in form for injection.
+▲ side-effects/warning: see DACTINOMYCIN

Cosuric
(DDSA Pharmaceuticals) is a proprietary, prescription-only preparation of the ENZYME INHIBITOR allopurinol, which is a XANTHINE OXIDASE INHIBITOR. It can be

C

used to treat excess uric acid in the blood and to prevent renal stones and attacks of gout. It is available as tablets.
✚▲ side-effects/warning: see ALLOPURINOL

co-tenidone
is a COMPOUND PREPARATION of the BETA-BLOCKER atenolol and the DIURETIC chlorthalidone. It can be used as an ANTIHYPERTENSIVE treatment for raised blood pressure and is avalable as tablets.
✚▲ side effects/warning: see ATENOLOL; CHLORTHALIDONE
◯ Related entries: AtenixCo; Tenchlor

co-triamterzide 50/25
is a simplified name for the COMPOUND PREPARATION of the (*potassium-sparing*) DIURETIC drug triamterine and the (THIAZIDE) diuretic hydrochlorothiazide, in the ratio 50:25 (mg).
✚▲ side effects/warning: see HYDROCHLOROTHIAZIDE; TRIAMTERINE
◯ Related entries: Dyazide; Triam-Co; TrimazCo

co-trimoxazole
is a simplified name for the COMPOUND PREPARATION of the (SULPHONAMIDE) ANTIBACTERIAL drug sulphamethoxazole and the similar, but not related, antibacterial drug trimethoprim (a folic acid inhibitor); in the ratio of 5:1. It is thought that each drug enhances the action of the other, giving a combined effect greater than the sum of the two. Although there is little evidence to support this, the combination remains a very useful antibacterial preparation. It is used to treat and prevent the spread of infections of the urinary tract, chronic bronchitis, the prostate and salmonella infections (particularly in patients allergic to penicillin). Administration is either oral as tablets, a pediatric syrup or a suspension, or by injection or infusion.
✚ side effects: these are largely due to the sulphonamide and may include nausea and vomiting; diarrhoea and rashes. Blood

disorders may occur.
▲ warning: it should not be administered to patients who are pregnant; who have certain blood, liver or kidney disorders, or jaundice. It should be administered with caution to patients who are elderly or breast-feeding. Adequate fluid intake must be maintained. Prolonged treatment requires regular blood counts.
◯ Related entries: Bactrim; Chemotrim; Comixco; Comox; Fectrim; Laratrim; Septrim

*counter-irritants
also called RUBEFACIENTS, are preparations that cause a feeling of warmth and offset the pain from underlying muscle and joints or viscera when rubbed in topically to the skin. A number of them are aromatic or volatile oils. How these agents act is uncertain, but the reddening of the skin (denoted by the name *rube*facient) indicates a dilatation of the blood vessels which gives a soothing feeling of warmth. The term counter-irritant refers to the idea that irritation of the sensory nerve endings alters or offsets pain in the underlying muscle or joints that are served by the same nerves. See: CAPSAICIN; CAPSICUM OLEORESIN; CHOLINE SALICYLATE; ETHYL SALICYLATE; GLYCOL SALICYLATE; METHYL SALICYLATE; MENTHOL; SALICYLIC ACID; TURPENTINE OIL.

Coversyl
(Servier) is a proprietary, prescription-only preparation of the ACE INHIBITOR perindopril. It can be used as an ANTIHYPERTENSIVE and in HEART FAILURE TREATMENT and is available as tablets.
✚▲ side-effects/warning: see PERINDOPRIL

Covonia Bronchial Balsam
(Thornton & Ross) is a proprietary, non-prescription COMPOUND PREPARATION of the ANTITUSSIVE and (OPIOID) NARCOTIC ANALGESIC drug dextromethorphan hydrobromide, the EXPECTORANT guaiphenesin and menthol. It can be used

for the symptomatic relief of non-productive coughs, such as those associated with colds and bronchitis. It is available as a linctus and is not normally given to children under six years, except on medical advice.

+▲ side-effects/warning: see DEXTROMETHORPHAN HYDROBROMIDE; GUAIPHENESIN; MENTHOL

Covonia for Children

(Thornton & Ross) is a proprietary, non-prescription preparation of the ANTITUSSIVE and (OPIOID) NARCOTIC ANALGESIC drug dextromethorphan hydrobromide. It can be used for the symptomatic relief of non-productive coughs, including those associated with the common cold. It is available as a sugar-free linctus and is not normally given to children under two years, except on medical advice.

+▲ side-effects/warning: see DEXTROMETHORPHAN HYDROBROMIDE

Cremalgin Balm

(Rhône-Poulenc Rorer) is a proprietary, non-prescription COMPOUND PREPARATION of capsicum oleoresin, methyl nicotinate and glycol salicylate, which all have COUNTER-IRRITANT, or RUBEFACIENT, actions. It can be applied to the skin for symptomatic relief of underlying muscle or joint pain and is available as a balm.

+▲ side-effects/warning: see CAPSICUM OLEORESIN; GLYCOL SALICYLATE; METHYL NICOTINATE

Creon

(Duphar) is a proprietary, non-prescription preparation of the digestive enzyme pancreatin. It can be used to treat deficiencies of digestive juices that are normally supplied by the pancreas. It is available as capsules and granules.

+▲ side-effects/warning: see PANCREATIN

Creon 25 000

(Duphar) is a proprietary, non-

prescription preparation of the digestive enzyme pancreatin. It can be used to treat deficiencies of digestive juices that are normally supplied by the pancreas. It is available as capsules (in a higher strength than *Creon*).

+▲ side-effects/warning: see PANCREATIN

cristantaspase

is an enzyme called asparaginase and is used as a ANTICANCER treatment almost exclusively for acute lymphoblastic leukaemia. Administration is by injection.

+ side-effects: there may be nausea, vomiting, central nervous system depression and changes in liver function and blood lipids (requiring careful monitoring, including of the urine for glucose) and anaphylaxis.

◉ Related entry: Erwinase

crotamiton

is a drug that is used to relieve pruritus (itching) of the skin, for example, with scabies. It is available as a lotion or a cream.

▲ warning: it should not be used on broken skin or near the eyes.

◉ Related entry: Eurax

crystal violet

(gentian violet; methyl violet; methylrosanilium chloride) is a dye with astringent and oxidizing properties that is used as an ANTISEPTIC agent. It is occasionally administered to treat certain bacterial and fungal skin infections or abrasions and minor wounds. Administration is usually as an ointment, paint, or lotion. A a non-proprietary, antiseptic paint preparation is used specifically to prepare skin for surgery.

+ side-effects: it may cause mucosal ulcerations.

▲ warning: it should not be applied to mucous membranes or broken skin. It stains clothes as well as skin.

Crystapen

(Britannia) is a proprietary, prescription-

C

only preparation of the ANTIBACTERIAL and (PENICILLIN) ANTIBIOTIC drug benzylpenicillin (as sodium). It can be used to treat infections of the skin, middle ear, throat, the respiratory tract (such as tonsillitis) and certain severe systemic infections (such as meningitis). It is available in a form for injection or infusion.

+▲ side-effects/warning: see BENZYLPENICILLIN

Cultivate

(Glaxo) is a proprietary, prescription-only preparation of the CORTICOSTEROID and ANTI-INFLAMMATORY drug fluticasone propionate. It can be used to treat inflammatory skin disorders such as dermatitis, eczema and psoriasis. It is available as a cream for topical application.

+▲ side-effects/warning: see FLUTICASONE PROPIONATE

Cupanol Over 6 Paracetamol Oral Suspension

(Seton Healthcare) is a proprietary, non-prescription preparation of the NON-NARCOTIC ANALGESIC and ANTIPYRETIC drug paracetamol. It can be used to treat mild to moderate pain, migraine, toothache, headache and feverish conditions. It is available as a liquid suspension and is not normally given to children under six years, except on medical advice.

+▲ side-effects/warning: see PARACETAMOL

Cupanol Under 6 Paracetamol Oral Suspension

(Seton Healthcare) is a proprietary, non-prescription preparation of the NON-NARCOTIC ANALGESIC and ANTIPYRETIC drug paracetamol. It can be used to treat mild to moderate pain, such as teething and feverish conditions (including after vaccination, when it may be given to two-month-old babies). It is available as a

liquid suspension and is not normally given to infants under three months, except on medical advice.

+▲ side-effects/warning: see PARACETAMOL

Cuplex

(Smith & Nephew) is a proprietary, non-prescription preparation of the KERATOLYTIC agent salicylic acid (together with lactic acid and copper acetate). It can be used to remove warts and hard skin and is available as a gel.

+▲ side-effects/warning: see SALICYLIC ACID

Cuprofen Ibuprofen Tablets

(Seton Healthcare) is a proprietary, non-prescription preparation of the (NSAID) NON-NARCOTIC ANALGESIC and ANTIRHEUMATIC drug ibuprofen. It can be used for the relief of headache, period pain, muscular pain, dental pain, feverishness and cold and flu symptoms. It is available as tablets and is not normally given to children under 12 years, except on medical advice.

+▲ side-effects/warning: see IBUPROFEN

CX Antiseptic Dusting Powder

(Bio-Medical) is a proprietary, non-prescription preparation of the ANTISEPTIC agent chlorhexidine (as acetate). It can be used by topical application for disinfection and antisepsis.

+▲ side-effects/warning: see CHLORHEXIDINE

cyanocobalamin

is a form of vitamin B_{12} that is readily found in most normal, well-balanced diets (for example, in fish, eggs, liver and red meat). Vegans, who eat no animal products at all, may eventually suffer from deficiency of this vitamin. A deficiency of vitamin B_{12} eventually causes *megaloblastic anaemia*, degeneration of nerves in the central and peripheral nervous systems and abnormalities of epithelia (particularly the lining of the mouth and gut). Apart from poor diet, deficiency can also be caused by the lack of an *intrinsic factor* necessary for absorption in the stomach (*pernicious anaemia*) and by various malabsorption syndromes in the gut (sometimes due to drugs). Deficiency may be rectified by giving HYDROXOCOBALAMIN (a form of vitamin B_{12}) and supplements of vitamin B_{12} are administered by injection. There is no beneficial effect to include vitamin B_{12} (as cyanocobalamin) in proprietary multivitamin 'tonics'.

Cyclimorph

(Wellcome) is a proprietary, prescription-only preparation of the (OPIOID) NARCOTIC ANALGESIC drug morphine tartrate and the ANTI-EMETIC drug cyclizine tartrate. It can be used to treat moderate to severe pain, especially in serious conditions of fluid within the lungs. It is available, in two strengths (*Cyclimorph-10* and *Cyclimorph-15*) for injection and is on the Controlled Drugs List.
+▲ side-effects/warning: see CYCLIZINE; OPIOID

cyclizine

is an ANTIHISTAMINE and ANTINAUSEANT drug. It can be used to treat nausea, vomiting, vertigo, motion sickness and disorders of the balance function of the inner ear. Administration can be oral in the form of tablets or by injection.
+ side-effects: see under ANTIHISTAMINE; there may also be drowsiness, occasional dry mouth and blurred vision.
▲ warning: it may aggravate severe heart failure. Drowsiness may impair the performance of skilled tasks such as driving; avoid alcohol as its effects may be enhanced.
✪ Related entries: Cyclimorph; Diconal; dipipanone; Femigraine; Migril; Valoid

Cyclodox

(Berk) is a proprietary, prescription-only preparation of the ANTIBACTERIAL and (TETRACYCLINE) ANTIBIOTIC drug

doxycycline. It can be used to treat a wide variety of infections and is available as capsules.
+▲ side-effects/warning: see DOXYCYCLINE

Cyclogest

(Hoechst) is a proprietary, prescription-only preparation of the PROGESTOGEN progesterone. It can be used to treat many conditions of hormonal deficiency in women, including menstrual difficulty and premenstrual syndrome. It is available as (vaginal or anal) pessaries.
+▲ side-effects/warning: see PROGESTERONE

cyclopenthiazide

is a DIURETIC of the THIAZIDE class. It can be used as an ANTIHYPERTENSIVE treatment (either alone or in conjunction with other types of diuretic or other drugs) and in the treatment of oedema (accumulation of fluid in the tissues). Administration is oral in the form of tablets.
+▲ side-effects/warning: see under BENDROFLUAZIDE
✪ Related entries: Navidrex; Navispare; Trasidrex

cyclopentolate hydrochloride

is an ANTICHOLINERGIC drug, which can be used to dilate the pupil and paralyse the focusing of the eye for ophthalmic examination. It is available as eye-drops.
+▲ side-effects/warning: see under ATROPINE SULPHATE. When applied locally it has few side-effects, but it should not be used in patients with raised intraocular pressure (it may precipitate glaucoma).
✪ Related entries: Minims Cyclopentolate; Mydrilate

cyclophosphamide

is a CYTOTOXIC DRUG, which is used as an ANTICANCER treatment of chronic lymphatic leukaemia, lymphomas and some solid tumours. It works by interfering with DNA and so preventing normal cell replication.

C

It can also be used as an IMMUNOSUPPRESSANT drug in the treatment of complicated rheumatoid arthritis (unlicensed use). Administration is either oral as tablets or by injection.
+▲ side-effects/warning: see under CYTOTOXIC DRUGS. Avoid its use in patients with porphyria; rarely, it may cause haemorrhagic cystitis.
۞ Related entry: Endoxana.

Cyclo-Progynova

(Schering Health) is a proprietary, prescription-only COMPOUND PREPARATION of female SEX HORMONES oestradiol (as valerate; an OESTROGEN) and norgestrel (a PROGESTOGEN). It can be used in HRT and is available as tablets.
+▲ side-effects/warning: see NORGESTREL; OESTRADIOL

cyclopropane

is a gas that is used as an inhalant GENERAL ANAESTHETIC for rapid induction and maintenance of general anaesthesia. Administration is by inhalation.

Cycloserine

(Lilly) is a proprietary, prescription-only preparation of the ANTIBACTERIAL drug cycloserine. It can be used specifically as an ANTITUBERCULAR treatment for tuberculosis that is resistant to the powerful drugs ordinarily used first, or in cases where those drugs are not tolerated. It is available as capsules.
+▲ side-effects/warning: see CYCLOSERINE

cycloserine

is an ANTIBACTERIAL drug that is used specifically as an ANTITUBERCULAR treatment for tuberculosis that is resistant to the powerful drugs ordinarily used first, or in cases where those drugs are not tolerated. Administration is oral in the form of capsules.
+ side-effects: there may be headache, dizziness, drowsiness, depression, convulsions, tremor and allergic dermatitis.

▲ warning: it should not be administered to patients with epilepsy, alcoholism, depressive illness, anxiety or psychosis, porphyria or severe kidney impairment; it should be administered with caution to those with impaired kidney function, or who are pregnant or breast-feeding. Blood, kidney and liver function should be monitored.
۞ Related entry: Cycloserine

cyclosporin

(ciclosporin) is an IMMUNOSUPPRESSANT drug, which is used particularly to limit tissue rejection during and following organ transplant surgery. It can also be used to treat severe, active rheumatoid arthritis and some skin conditions such as severe, resistant atopic dermatitis and (under special supervision) psoriasis. It has very little effect on the blood-cell producing capacity of the bone marrow, but does have liver toxicity. Administration is oral or by intravenous infusion.
+ side-effects: these include changes in blood enzymes, disturbances in liver, kidney and cardiovascular function, excessive hair growth, gastrointestinal disturbances, tremor, gum growth, oedema (accumulation of fluid in the tissues), fatigue and burning sensations in the hands and feet.
▲ warning: treatment with cyclosporin inevitably leaves the body vulnerable to infection. Administer with caution to patients who are pregnant or breast-feeding, or with porphyria. Body functions (liver, kidney and cardiovascular system) should be monitored. When used for rheumatoid arthritis, it should not be given to patients with abnormal kidney function, uncontrolled hypertension, infections, or malignancy.
۞ Related entry: Sandimmun

Cyklokapron

(Pharmacia) is a proprietary, prescription-only preparation of the antifibrinolytic drug tranexamic acid. It can be used to stop bleeding in circumstances such as dental extraction in a haemophiliac patient or menorrhagia (excessive period bleeding). It is available as tablets, a dilute syrup and in a form for injection.

✚▲ side-effects/warning: see
TRANEXAMIC ACID

Cymevene

(Syntex) is a proprietary, prescription-only preparation of the ANTIVIRAL drug ganciclovir. It can be used to treat life-threatening or sight-threatening viral infections and in immunocompromised patients. It is available in a form for intravenous infusion.

✚▲ side-effects/warning: see GANCICLOVIR

cyproheptadine hydrochloride

is an ANTIHISTAMINE drug. It can be used for the symptomatic relief of allergic symptoms such as hay fever and urticaria (itchy skin rash). It differs from other antihistamines in having additional actions as an antagonist of SEROTONIN and as a CALCIUM-CHANNEL BLOCKER and is useful in a wider range of conditions, such as the prevention of migraine attacks. Administration is oral in the form of tablets or as a syrup.

✚▲ side-effects/warning: see under ANTIHISTAMINE. It may cause weight gain. Because of its sedative side-effects, the performance of skilled tasks such as driving may be impaired.

✪ Related entry: Periactin

Cyprostat

(Schering Health) is a proprietary, prescription-only preparation of the sex HORMONE ANTAGONIST drug cyproterone acetate, which is an ANTI-ANDROGEN. It can be used as an ANTICANCER drug for cancer of the prostate gland. It works by neutralizing the effects of the male sex hormones (androgens) that contribute to the cancer. It is available as tablets.

✚▲ side-effects/warning: see

CYPROTERONE ACETATE
cyproterone acetate

is a sex HORMONE ANTAGONIST, an ANTI-ANDROGEN, that reduces the effects of male sex hormones (androgens) in the body. It is used as an ANTICANCER treatment for cancer of the prostate gland. It can also be used for the treatment of hypersexuality or sexual deviation in men, in whom the drug causes a condition of reversible sterility through a reduction in the production of sperm. Additionally, it can be used (in a preparation containing oestrogen) to treat acne and excess body hair (hirsutism) in women. Administration is oral in the form of tablets.

✚ side-effects: concentration and speed of thought and movement may be affected; breathlessness; weight gain; fatigue and lethargy. Hormonal effects include changes in hair-growth patterns and enlargement of the breasts and inhibition of sperm production in men. Rarely, there is osteoporosis ('brittle bones'); and liver abnormalities.

▲ warning: except for use in prostate cancer, it should not be administered to patients who have sickle-cell anaemia, severe diabetes, liver disease, or severe depression; who have a history of thrombosis; who are pregnant; or who are adolescent boys (in whom bone growth and testicular development may be arrested). It should be administered with caution to those with diabetes or insufficient secretion of adrenal hormones, or who are breast-feeding. Regular checks on liver function, adrenal gland function, blood counts and determination of levels of glucose are needed.

✪ Related entries: Androcur; Cyprostat; Dianette

Cystrin

(Pharmacia) is a proprietary, prescription-only preparation of the ANTICHOLINERGIC drug oxybutynin hydrochloride. It can be used as an

C ANTISPASMODIC in the treatment of urinary frequency and incontinence. It is available as tablets.

➕▲ side-effects/warning: see OXYBUTYNIN HYDROCHLORIDE

cytarabine

is a CYTOTOXIC DRUG, which is used as an ANTICANCER treatment primarily of acute leukaemia. It works by by interfering with pyrimidine synthesis (a chemical needed for cell replication/DNA) and so prevents normal cell replication. Administration is by injection.

➕▲ side-effects/warning: see under CYTOTOXIC DRUGS

○ Related entries: Alexan; Alexan 100; Cytosar

*cytoprotectant

is the term used to describe the capacity of some drugs to protect the gastric mucosa (the lining of the stomach) from the normal stomach contents of acid and enzymes, which can cause erosion and pain in peptic ulcers (gastric and duodenal ulcers). They may have some long-term ULCER-HEALING properties as well as affording short-term relief from discomfort. Examples of cytoprotectant drugs include: *liquorice extracts*, LIQUORICE, DEGLYCYRRHIZINISED and CARBENOXOLONE SODIUM; *bismuth salts*, bismuth chelate and TRIPOTASSIUM DICITRATOBISMUTHATE; and SUCRALFATE.

Cytosar

(Upjohn) is a proprietary, prescription-only preparation of the (CYTOTOXIC) ANTICANCER drug cytarabine. It can be used to treat acute leukaemia and is available in a form for injection.

➕▲ side-effects/warning: see CYTARABINE

Cytotec

(Searle) is a proprietary, prescription-only preparation of the synthetic PROSTAGLANDIN analogue misoprostol. It can be used to treat gastric and duodenal ulcers and is available as tablets.

➕▲ side-effects/warning: see MISOPROSTOL

*cytotoxic drugs

are used mainly in the treatment of cancer and are an important group of ANTICANCERS drugs. They have the essential property of preventing normal cell replication and so inhibiting the growth of tumours or of excess cells in body fluids.

There are several mechanisms by which they do this, but in every case they inevitably also affect the growth of normal healthy cells and cause toxic side-effects, generally nausea and vomiting, with hair loss. The most-used cytotoxic drugs are the *alkylating agents*, which work by interfering with the action of DNA in cell replication (eg.BUSULPHAN, CHLORAMBUCIL, CISPLATIN, CYCLOPHOSPHAMIDE, LOMUSTINE, MELPHALAN and THIOTEPA). The VINCA ALKALOIDS are also effective cytotoxic drugs and work by damaging part of the metabolic features of new-forming cells, however, they have severe side-effect (such as damage to peripheral nerves) which limits their use. A number of cytotoxic drugs are ANTIBIOTICS in origin, but ANTIMICROBIAL actions do not contribute an important part of their action (eg.BLEOMYCIN, DACTINOMYCIN, DOXORUBICIN HYDROCHLORIDE and EPIRUBICIN HYDROCHLORIDE). There are some cytotoxic drugs that are not primarily administered in anticancer treatment, some are used as IMMUNOSUPPRESSANTS to limit tissue rejection during and following transplant surgery and in the treatment of autoimmune diseases such as rheumatoid arthritis and lupus erythematosus (eg.AZATHIOPRINE; chlorambucil, cyclophosphamide, CYCLOSPORIN and METHOTREXATE).

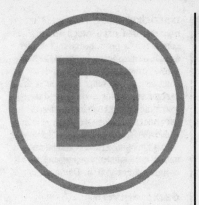

D

✚ side-effects: vomiting and nausea, bone-marrow suppression, hair loss, teratogenetic (damage to the foetus).
▲ warning: under no circumstances are they to be administered in the period before conception or during pregnancy.

D

dacarbazine
is a CYTOTOXIC DRUG, which is used
comparatively rarely because of its high
toxicity. It may be used to treat the skin
(mole) cancer melanoma and, in
combination with other ANTICANCER drugs,
in some soft-tissue sarcomas and the
lymphatic cancer Hodgkin's disease.
Administration is by injection.
+▲ side-effects/warning: see under
CYTOTOXIC DRUGS. There is also intense
nausea and vomiting; myelosuppression.
✪ Related entry: DTIC-Dome

dactinomycin
(actinomycin D) is a CYTOTOXIC DRUG (an
ANTIBIOTIC in origin) that is used as an
ANTICANCER drug, particularly to treat
cancer in children. Administration is by
injection.
+▲ side-effects/warning: see under
CYTOTOXIC DRUGS; similar side-effects to
DOXORUBICIN but with less heart toxicity.
✪ Related entry: Cosmegen Lyovac

Daktacort
(Janssen) is a proprietary,
prescription-only COMPOUND PREPARATION
of the CORTICOSTEROID drug
hydrocortisone and the (IMIDAZOLE)
ANTIFUNGAL drug miconazole (as nitrate).
It can be used to treat skin infections
with inflammation and is available as a
cream and an ointment for topical
application.
+▲ side-effects/warning: see
HYDROCORTISONE; MICONAZOLE

Daktarin
(Janssen) is a proprietary, prescription-
only preparation of the (IMIDAZOLE)
ANTIFUNGAL drug miconazole. It can be
used to treat both systemic and skin-
surface fungal infections. It is available as
tablets, an oral gel and as a solution for
infusion. (There are other forms for
topical application that are available
without prescription.)
+▲ side-effects/warning: see MICONAZOLE

Daktarin Cream
(Janssen) is a proprietary, non-
prescription preparation of the
(IMIDAZOLE) ANTIFUNGAL drug miconazole
(as nitrate). It can be used for the
prevention and treatment of fungal (and
associated bacterial) infections of the
skin, such as athlete's foot, intertrigo and
infected nappy rash. It is available as a
cream for topical application.
+▲ side-effects/warning: see MICONAZOLE

Daktarin Oral Gel
(Janssen) is a proprietary, non-
prescription preparation of the
(IMIDAZOLE) ANTIFUNGAL drug miconazole
(as base). It can be used for the
prevention and treatment of fungal
infections of the mouth and is available as
an oral gel for use by adults and children.
+▲ side-effects/warning: see MICONAZOLE

Daktarin Powder
(Janssen) is a proprietary, non-
prescription preparation of the
(IMIDAZOLE) ANTIFUNGAL drug miconazole
(as nitrate). It can be used for the
prevention and treatment of fungal (and
associated bacterial) infections of the
skin, such as athlete's foot, intertrigo and
infected nappy rash. It is available as a
powder for application to the skin and
clothes.
+▲ side-effects/warning: see MICONAZOLE

Daktarin Spray Powder
(Janssen) is a proprietary, non-
prescription preparation of the
(IMIDAZOLE) ANTIFUNGAL drug miconazole
(as nitrate). It can be used for the
prevention and treatment of fungal
infections of the mouth and is available as
a powder spray for application to the skin,
clothes and shoes.
+▲ side-effects/warning: see MICONAZOLE

Dalacin
(Upjohn) is a proprietary, prescription-
only preparation of the ANTIBACTERIAL and

ANTIBIOTIC drug clindamycin. It can be used to treat vaginal infections and is available as a cream.
+▲ side-effects/warning: see CLINDAMYCIN; the vaginal cream may damage latex condoms and diaphragms.

Dalacin C

(Upjohn) is a proprietary, prescription-only, preparation of the ANTIBACTERIAL and ANTIBIOTIC drug clindamycin. It can be used to treat infections of the bones and joints and peritonitis (inflammation of the peritoneal lining of the abdominal cavity). It is available as capsules, a paediatric suspension and in a form for injection.
+▲ side-effects/warning: see CLINDAMYCIN

Dalacin T

(Upjohn) is a proprietary, prescription-only preparation of the ANTIBACTERIAL and ANTIBIOTIC drug clindamycin. It can be used to treat acne and is available as a lotion and a solution for topical application.
+▲ side-effects/warning: see CLINDAMYCIN

Dalmane

(Roche) is a proprietary, prescription-only preparation of the BENZODIAZEPINE drug flurazepam. It can be used as a relatively long-acting HYPNOTIC for the short-term treatment of insomnia, where a degree of sedation during the daytime is acceptable. It is available as capsules.
+▲ side-effects/warning: see FLURAZEPAM

dalteparin

is a low molecular weight version of heparin that is used as an ANTICOAGULANT. It has some advantages over heparin when used in the long-duration prevention of venous thrombo-embolism, particularly in orthopaedic use. Administration is by injection.
+▲ side-effects/warning: see under HEPARIN
✪ Related entry: Fragmin

danaparoid sodium

(Org 10172) is a version of heparin (called a heparinoid) that is used as an ANTICOAGULANT. It has some advantages over heparin when used for prevention of deep-vein thrombosis, particularly in orthopaedic surgery. Administration is by injection.
+▲ side-effects/warning: see under HEPARIN. There may also be thrombocytopenia, liver changes, hypersensitivity, osteoporosis and pain or tissue damage at injection site. Administer with care to pateints who are pregnant, breast-feeding, or have certain liver or kidney disorders.
✪ Related entry: Orgaran

danazol

is a drug with weak androgen activity, plus HORMONE ANTAGONIST actions as an ANTI-OESTROGEN and antiprogesterone. It inhibits the release of pituitary hormones, GONADOTROPHINS. It can be used to treat endometriosis (the presence of areas of uterus-lining, endometrium, outside the uterus); gynaecomastia (the development of breasts on a male); menorrhagia (excessive menstrual flow) and other menstrual disorders; benign breast cysts and breast pain. It can also be used to treat hereditary angio-oedema. Administration is oral in the form of capsules.
+ side-effects: backache, dizziness, flushing, weight gain, menstrual disorders, nervousness, rash, flushing, reduction in breast size, muscle spasm, hair loss, masculinization in women (oily skin, acne, hair growth, voice changes, enlarged clitoris), blood disorders, visual disturbances, jaundice and insulin resistance.
▲ warning: it should not be administered to patients who are pregnant or breast-feeding; non-hormonal contraceptive methods should be used where applicable. Use with caution in patients with certain heart, liver, or kidney disorders; diabetes, epilepsy, migraine, hypertension, thrombosis, blood disorders, have thrombo-embolitic diseases,

D

androgen-dependent tumours, or porphyria.
○ Related entry: Danol

Daneral SA

(Hoechst) is a proprietary, prescription-
only preparation of the ANTIHISTAMINE
drug pheniramine maleate. It can be used
to treat the symptoms of allergic disorders
such as hay fever and urticaria and is
available as tablets.
✚▲ side-effects/warning: see
PHENIRAMINE MALEATE

Danol

(Sanofi Winthrop) is a proprietary,
prescription-only preparation of the drug
danazol, which inhibits the release of the
pituitary HORMONES gonadotrophins,
which in turn prevents the release of sex
hormones. It is used to treat conditions
such as inflammation of the endometrial
lining of the uterus, gynaecomastia
(development of breasts in the male) and
menstrual disorders. It is available as
capsules.
✚▲ side-effects/warning: see DANAZOL

danthron

(dantron) is a (*stimulant*) LAXATIVE. It is
used to promote defecation and so relieve
constipation and seems to work by
stimulating motility in the intestine.
Therapeutically, it is used for constipation
in geriatric practice (particularly
analgesic-induced constipation in the
terminally ill) and in cardiac failure and
coronary thrombosis (to avoid strain). It
is also available in COMPOUND
PREPARATIONS with DOCUSATE SODIUM
(CO-DANTHRUSATE 50/60) or
poloxamer '188'.
✚ side-effects: there may be abdominal pain,
griping, nausea, or vomiting. The urine may
be coloured red. Prolonged contact with the
skin may cause irritation.
▲ warning: it should not be taken when
pregnant or breast-feeding.
○ Related entries: co-danthramer
25/200; co-danthramer 75/1000;

co-danthrusate 50/60; Codalax; Codalax
Forte; Normax

Dantrium

(Procter & Gamble) is a proprietary,
prescription-only preparation of the
SKELETAL MUSCLE RELAXANT drug
dantrolene sodium. It can be used for
relieving severe spasticity of muscles in
spasm and is available as capsules and in
a form for injection.
✚▲ side-effects/warning: see
DANTROLENE SODIUM

dantrolene sodium

is a SKELETAL MUSCLE RELAXANT drug. It
acts directly on skeletal muscle and can be
used for relieving severe spasticity of
muscles in spasm. Administration is either
oral as capsules or by injection.
✚ side-effects: transient drowsiness, dizziness,
weakness, general malaise, fatigue, diarrhoea
(if severe, stop treatment), nausea, anorexia,
headache, rash; sometimes constipation,
difficulty in swallowing, visual and speech
disturbances, confusion, nervousness,
depression, insomnia, seizures, chills, urinary
frequency; rarely, speeding of the heart,
irregular blood pressure, difficulty in
breathing, various urinary problems, liver
toxicity.
▲ warning: do not administer to patients
with liver impairment or acute muscle spasm.
Administer with caution to those with
impaired heart and liver function (liver
function should be checked regularly); effect
is slow to develop. Drowsiness may impair the
performance of skilled tasks such as driving.
○ Related entry: Dantrium

dantron

See DANTHRON

Daonil

(Hoechst) is a proprietary, prescription-
only preparation of the SULPHONYLUREA
drug glibenclamide. It can be used in
DIABETIC TREATMENT of Type II diabetes
(non-insulin-dependent diabetes mellitus;

NIDDM; maturity-onset diabetes) and is available as tablets at twice the strength of SEMI-DAONIL tablets.
+▲ side-effects/warning: see
GLIBENCLAMIDE

dapsone
is an ANTIBACTERIAL drug (a SULPHONE), which is used as an ANTITUBERCULAR treatment against leprosy in both lepromatous and tuberculoid forms. It is also sometimes used to treat severe forms of dermatitis (dermatitis herpetiformis) or, in combination with the enzyme inhibitor pyrimethamine (under the name *Maloprim*), to prevent travellers in tropical regions from contracting malaria. Administration is either oral as tablets or by injection.
+ side-effects: side-effects are rare at low doses (when used for leprosy), but with higher dosage there may be nausea, vomiting and headache, insomnia and increased heart rate, severe weight loss, anaemia, hepatitis, peripheral nerve disease and blood changes.
▲ warning: it should be administered with caution to patients with anaemia, porphyria, G6PH deficiency, certain heart or lung diseases, or who are pregnant or breast-feeding.
۞ Related entry: Maloprim

Daranide
(Merck, Sharp & Dohme) is a proprietary, prescription-only preparation of the weak DIURETIC drug dichlorphenamide. It can be used in GLAUCOMA TREATMENT because it reduces the amount of aqueous humour in the eyeball. It is available as tablets.
+▲ side-effects/warning: see
DICHLORPHENAMIDE

Daraprim
(Wellcome) is a proprietary, non-prescription preparation of the ANTIMALARIAL drug pyrimethamine. It can be used to prevent or treat malaria in combination with other drugs, but is not administered as the sole agent of

prevention. It is available as tablets.
+▲ side-effects/warning: see
PYRIMETHAMINE

Day Cold Comfort Capsules
(Boots) is a proprietary, non-prescription COMPOUND PREPARATION of the NON-NARCOTIC ANALGESIC drug paracetamol, the SYMPATHOMIMETIC and DECONGESTANT drug pseudoephedrine hydrochloride and the ANTITUSSIVE pholcodine. It can be used for the relief of cold and flu symptoms and is available as capsules. It is not normally given to children under six years, except on medical advice.
+▲ side-effects/warning: see PARACETAMOL; PHOLCODINE; PSEUDOEPHEDRINE HYDROCHLORIDE

Day Nurse Capsules
(SmithKline Beecham) is a proprietary, non-prescription COMPOUND PREPARATION of the NON-NARCOTIC ANALGESIC drug paracetamol, the SYMPATHOMIMETIC and DECONGESTANT drug phenylpropanolamine hydrochloride and the ANTITUSSIVE dextromethorphan hydrobromide. It can be used for the relief of cold and flu symptoms and is available as capsules. It is not normally given to children under six years, except on medical advice.
+▲ side-effects/warning: see
DEXTROMETHORPHAN HYDROBROMIDE; PARACETAMOL; PHENYLPROPANOLAMINE HYDROCHLORIDE

Day Nurse Liquid
(SmithKline Beecham) is a proprietary, non-prescription COMPOUND PREPARATION of the NON-NARCOTIC ANALGESIC drug paracetamol, the SYMPATHOMIMETIC and DECONGESTANT drug phenylpropanolamine hydrochloride and the ANTITUSSIVE dextromethorphan hydrobromide. It can be used for the relief of cold and flu symptoms and is available as a liquid. It is not normally given to children under six years, except on medical advice.
+▲ side-effects/warning: see

D DEXTROMETHORPHAN HYDROBROMIDE;
PARACETAMOL; PHENYLPROPANOLAMINE
HYDROCHLORIDE

DDAVP

(Ferring) is a proprietary, prescription-only preparation of desmopressin, which is an analogue of the pituitary HORMONE vasopressin (ADH). It is administered primarily to diagnose or to treat pituitary-originated diabetes insipidus. It can be used for some other diagnostic tests, to boost the blood concentration of blood-clotting factors in haemophiliac patients and to treat bed-wetting. It is available as tablets (as the acetate), as nose-drops and in a form for injection.

+▲ side-effects/warning: see DESMOPRESSIN

DDC

See ZALCITABINE

DDI

See DIDANOSINE

debrisoquine

is an ADRENERGIC NEURONE BLOCKER, which is an ANTISYMPATHETIC class of drug that prevents the release of noradrenaline from sympathetic nerves. It can be used, usually in combination with other drugs (such as a DIURETIC or BETA-BLOCKER), in ANTIHYPERTENSIVE treatment of moderate to severe high blood pressure, especially when other forms of treatment have failed. Administration is oral in the form of tablets.

+▲ side-effects/warning: see under GUANETHIDINE MONOSULPHATE; except it does not cause diarrhoea.

○ Related entry: Declinax

Decadron

(Merck, Sharp & Dohme) is a proprietary, prescription-only preparation of the CORTICOSTEROID and ANTI-INFLAMMATORY drug dexamethasone. It can be used in the suppression of allergic and inflammatory conditions in shock, diagnosis of

Cushing's disease, congenital adrenal hyperplasia and cerebral oedema. It is available as tablets and in a form for injection.

+▲ side-effects/warning: see DEXAMETHASONE

Decadron Shock-Pak

(Merck, Sharp & Dohme) is a proprietary, prescription-only preparation of the CORTICOSTEROID and ANTI-INFLAMMATORY drug dexamethasone (as sodium phosphate). It can be used in the treatment of shock and is available in a form for intravenous injection.

+▲ side-effects/warning: see DEXAMETHASONE

Deca-Durabolin

(Organon) is a proprietary, prescription-only preparation of the (*anabolic*) STEROID nandrolone (as decanoate). It can be used to treat osteoporosis in postmenopausal women and aplastic anaemia. It is available in a form for injection and also in a higher-dose preparation, *Deca-Durabolin 100*.

+▲ side-effects/warning: see NANDROLONE

Decazate

(Berk) is a proprietary, prescription-only preparation of the ANTIPSYCHOTIC drug fluphenazine decanoate. It can be used in the long-term maintenance of the tranquillization of patients suffering from psychotic disorders (including schizophrenia). It is available in forms for depot deep intramuscular injection.

+▲ side-effects/warning: see FLUPHENAZINE DECANOATE

Declinax

(Roche) is a proprietary, prescription-only preparation of the ADRENERGIC NEURONE BLOCKER drug debrisoquine. It can be used in ANTIHYPERTENSIVE treatment of moderate to severe high blood pressure and is available as tablets.

+▲ side-effects/warning: see DEBRISOQUINE

*decongestants

are drugs administered to relieve or
reduce the symptoms of congestion
of the airways and/or nose. NASAL
DECONGESTANTS are generally applied
in the form of nose-drops or as a nasal
spray, which avoids the tendency of such
drugs to have side-effects, such as raising
the blood pressure, though some are
administered orally.

Most decongestants are
SYMPATHOMIMETIC drugs, which work
by constricting blood vessels in the
mucous membranes of the airways and
nasal cavity, so reducing the membranes'
thickness, improving drainage and
possibly decreasing mucous and fluid
secretions. However, rhinitis (nasal
congestion), especially when caused
by an allergy (eg.hay fever), is usually
dealt with by using ANTIHISTAMINES,
which inhibit the detrimental and
congestive effects of histamine released
by an allergic response, or by drugs
which inhibit the allergic response
itself and so effectively reduce
inflammation (eg. CORTICOSTEROIDS or
SODIUM CROMOGLYCATE).

Decongestant drugs are often
included in COMPOUND PREPARATIONS
that are used to treat colds and which
may contain a number of other
constituents.

However, most people are unaware
of this, but it is important to realize
that the vasoconstriction, speeding of
the heart and hypertension often caused
by sympathomimetic drugs are
detrimental and potentially dangerous
in a number of cardiovascular disorders.
Further, sympathomimetics can have
serious interactions with a number of
other drug classes, especially (MAOI)
ANTIDEPRESSANTS.

Decortisyl

(Roussel) is a proprietary, prescription-
only preparation of the CORTICOSTEROID
and ANTI-INFLAMMATORY drug prednisone.

It can be used to treat a variety of
inflammatory and allergic disorders and is
available as tablets.
+▲ side-effects/warning: see
PREDNISONE

Delfen

(Ortho) is a proprietary, non-prescription
SPERMICIDAL CONTRACEPTIVE for use in
combination with barrier methods of
contraception (such as a condom).
It is available as a foam containing
nonoxinol.
+▲ side-effects/warning: see NONOXINOL

Deltacortril Enteric

(Pfizer) is a proprietary,
prescription-only preparation of the
CORTICOSTEROID and ANTI-INFLAMMATORY
drug prednisolone. It can be used to
treat allergic and rheumatic conditions,
particularly those affecting the joints and
soft tissues. It is available as tablets.
+▲ side-effects/warning: see
PREDNISOLONE

Deltastab

(Boots) is a proprietary, prescription-only
preparation of the CORTICOSTEROID and
ANTI-INFLAMMATORY drug prednisolone. It
can be used to treat allergic and
rheumatic conditions, particularly those
affecting the joints and soft tissues. It is
available as tablets and in a form for
injection.
+▲ side-effects/warning: see
PREDNISOLONE

Delvas

(Berk) is a proprietary, prescription-only
COMPOUND PREPARATION of the
(*potassium-sparing*) DIURETIC drug
amiloride hydrochloride and the
(THIAZIDE) diuretic drug
hydrochlorothiazide (a combination
called co-amilozide 5/50). It can be used
to treat oedema, congestive heart failure
and as an ANTIHYPERTENSIVE. It is available
as tablets.

D

＋▲ side-effects/warning: see
AMILORIDE HYDROCHLORIDE;
HYDROCHLOROTHIAZIDE

demeclocycline hydrochloride

is a broad-spectrum ANTIBACTERIAL and
ANTIBIOTIC drug, which is one of the
TETRACYCLINES. It can be used to treat
many kinds of infection, but particularly
those of the respiratory tract, the ear, nose
and throat, the gastrointestinal and
genitourinary tracts and a wide variety of
soft-tissue infections. Administration is
oral as tablets or capsules. It is also used,
quite separately to its use as an antibiotic,
as a HORMONE ANTAGONIST to treat over-
secretion of antidiuretic hormone (ADH)
through an action on the kidney.
＋▲ side-effects/warning: see under
TETRACYCLINE; but the incidence of
photosensitivity is greater.
⊕ Related entries: Deteclo; Ledermycin

Demix

(Ashbourne) is a proprietary,
prescription-only preparation of the
ANTIBACTERIAL and (TETRACYCLINE)
ANTIBIOTIC drug doxycycline. It can be
used to treat infections of many kinds and
is available as capsules.
＋▲ side-effects/warning: see DOXYCYCLINE

Demser

(Merck, Sharp & Dohme) is a proprietary,
prescription-only preparation of the
ANTISYMPATHETIC drug metirosine. It can
be used in the preoperative treatment of
phaeochromocytoma and is available as
capsules.
＋▲ side-effects/warning: see METIROSINE

*demulcent

agents or preparations protect the mucous
membranes and relieve pain and
irritation. They work by forming a
protective film and are incorporated into
ANTACID preparations for protecting the
gastric mucosa (stomach lining) and into

mouthwashes, gargles, etc, to soothe the
membranes of the mouth. The most
commonly used demulcent agent is
ALGINIC ACID or one of its alginate salts.

De-Nol

(Yamanouchi) is a proprietary, non-
prescription preparation of the
CYTOPROTECTANT drug tripotassium
dicitratobismuthate. It can be used as an
ULCER-HEALING DRUG for benign peptic
ulcers in the stomach and duodenum and
is available as an oral liquid.
＋▲ side-effects/warning: see TRIPOTASSIUM
DICITRATOBISMUTHATE

De-Noltab

(Yamanouchi) is a proprietary, non-
prescription preparation of the
CYTOPROTECTANT drug tripotassium
dicitratobismuthate. It can be used as an
ULCER-HEALING DRUG for benign peptic
ulcers in the stomach and duodenum and
is available as tablets.
＋▲ side-effects/warning: see TRIPOTASSIUM
DICITRATOBISMUTHATE

Dentomycin

(Lederle) is a proprietary, prescription-
only preparation of the ANTIMICROBIAL
drug metronidazole, which has
ANTIBACTERIAL and ANTIPROTOZOAL
actions. It can be used for the treatment of
local infections in dental surgery and is
available as a gel.
＋▲ side-effects/warning: see
METRONIDAZOLE

Depixol

(Lundbeck) is a proprietary, prescription-
only preparation of the ANTIPSYCHOTIC
drug flupenthixol. It can be used to treat
patients suffering from psychotic disorders
(including schizophrenia), especially
those with a type of psychosis that renders
them apathetic and withdrawn. It can also
be used for short-term treatment of
depressive illness. It is available as tablets
(as flupenthixol) and in a forms for depot

Jeep intramuscular injection (as flupenthixol decanoate).

+▲ side-effects/warning: see FLUPENTHIXOL; FLUPENTHIXOL DECANOATE

Depixol Conc.

(Lundbeck) is a proprietary, prescription-only preparation of the ANTIPSYCHOTIC drug flupenthixol decanoate. It can be used in the maintenance of patients suffering from schizophrenia and other psychotic disorders. It is available in a form for depot deep intramuscular injection.

+▲ side-effects/warning: see FLUPENTHIXOL DECANOATE

Depixol Low Volume

(Lundbeck) is a proprietary, prescription-only preparation of the ANTIPSYCHOTIC drug flupenthixol decanoate. It can be used in the maintenance of patients suffering from schizophrenia and other psychotic disorders. It is available in a form for depot deep intramuscular injection.

+▲ side-effects/warning: see FLUPENTHIXOL DECANOATE

Depo-Medrone

(Upjohn) is a proprietary, prescription-only preparation of the CORTICOSTEROID and ANTI-INFLAMMATORY drug methylprednisolone (as acetate). It can be used to relieve allergic and inflammatory disorders, particularly of the joints and soft tissues and also to treat shock and cerebral oedema. It is available in a form for injection.

+▲ side-effects/warning: see METHYLPREDNISOLONE

Depo-Medrone with Lidocaine

(Upjohn) is a proprietary, prescription-only COMPOUND PREPARATION of the CORTICOSTEROID and ANTI-INFLAMMATORY drug methylprednisolone (as acetate) and the LOCAL ANAESTHETIC drug lignocaine

hydrochloride. It can be used to treat inflammation in the joints (for example, in rheumatic disease) or soft tissue. It is available in a form for injection.

+▲ side-effects/warning: see LIGNOCAINE HYDROCHLORIDE; METHYLPREDNISOLONE

Deponit

(Schwarz) is a proprietary, non-prescription preparation of the VASODILATOR and ANTI-ANGINA drug glyceryl trinitrate. It can be used to treat and prevent angina pectoris. It is available as a self-adhesive dressing (patch), which, when placed on the chest wall, is absorbed through the skin and helps to give lasting relief.

+▲ side-effects/warning: see GLYCERYL TRINITRATE

Depo-Provera

(Upjohn) is a proprietary, prescription-only preparation of the SEX HORMONE medroxyprogesterone acetate (a PROGESTOGEN). It can be used as an ANTICANCER treatment for cancer of the uterus, breast, or prostate, as a hormonal supplement in women whose progestogen level requires boosting (eg.in endometriosis or dysfunctional uterine bleeding) and as a long-lasting *progesterone-only* CONTRACEPTIVE preparation (administered by intramuscular injection every three months). It is available as tablets and in a form for injection.

+▲ side-effects/warning: see MEDROXYPROGESTERONE ACETATE

Depostat

(Schering Health) is a proprietary, prescription-only preparation of gestronol hexanoate, which is a synthetic SEX HORMONE (PROGESTOGEN). It is used in women to treat cancer of the endometrium and in men to treat benign enlargement of the prostate gland and malignant enlargement of the kidneys. It is available

D

D

in a form for injection.
+▲ side-effects/warning: see
GESTRONOL HEXANOATE

Dequacaine Lozenges

(Crookes Healthcare) is a proprietary,
non-prescription COMPOUND PREPARATION
of the ANTISEPTIC agent dequalinium
chloride and the LOCAL ANAESTHETIC drug
benzocaine. It can be used relieve the
discomfort of a severe sore throat.
It is not normally given to children
under 12 years, except on medical
advice.
+▲ side-effects/warning: see BENZOCAINE;
DEQUALINIUM CHLORIDE

Dequadin Lozenge

(Crookes Healthcare) is a proprietary,
non-prescription preparation of the
ANTISEPTIC agent DEQUALINIUM CHLORIDE.
It can be used to treat common infections
of the mouth and throat. It is not normally
given to children under ten years, except
on medical advice.

dequalinium chloride

is a mild ANTISEPTIC agent with some weak
ANTIFUNGAL properties. It can be used to
treat infections of the mouth and throat
and administration is oral as lozenges.
It is also available in some COMPOUND
PREPARATIONS combined with LOCAL
ANAESTHETIC drugs.
**✪ Related entries: DEQUACAINE
LOZENGES; DEQUADIN LOZENGE;
LABOSEPT PASTILLES**

Derbac-C

(Napp) is a proprietary, non-prescription
preparation of the PEDICULICIDAL drug
carbaryl. It can be used to treat
infestations of the scalp and pubic hair by
lice (pediculosis). It is available as a
liquid and a shampoo. It is not normally
used for infants under six months, except
on medical advice.
+▲ side-effects/warning: see
CARBARYL

Derbac-M

(Napp) is a proprietary, non-prescription
preparation of the SCABICIDAL and
PEDICULICIDAL drug malathion. It can be
used to treat infestations of the scalp and
pubic hair by lice (pediculosis) or of the
skin by the itch-mite (scabies). It is
available as a liquid and is not normally
used for infants under six months, except
on medical advice.
+▲ side-effects/warning: see MALATHION

Dermalex

(Sanofi Winthrop) is a proprietary,
non-prescription preparation of the
ANTISEPTIC agent hexachlorophane. It
can be used to treat urinary rash and to
prevent bedsores. It is available as a
skin lotion and is not normally used for
children under two years, except on
medical advice.
+▲ side-effects/warning: see
HEXACHLOROPHANE

Dermovate

(Glaxo) is a proprietary,
prescription-only preparation of the
CORTICOSTEROID and ANTI-INFLAMMATORY
drug clobetasol propionate. It can be
used for the
short-term treatment of severe,
inflammatory skin disorders, such as
eczema and psoriasis, that are resistant
to weaker corticosteroids. It is available
as a cream, an ointment and a scalp
application for topical application.
+▲ side-effects/warning: see
CLOBETASOL PROPIONATE

Dermovate-NN

(Glaxo) is a proprietary, prescription-only
COMPOUND PREPARATION of the
CORTICOSTEROID drug clobetasol
propionate, the ANTIBACTERIAL and
(AMINOGLYCOSIDE) ANTIBIOTIC drug
neomycin sulphate and the ANTIFUNGAL
and antibiotic drug nystatin. It can be
used, in the short term, to treat
inflammation of the skin in which

infection is also present. It is available as an ointment and a cream for topical application.

✚▲ side-effects/warning: see CLOBETASOL PROPIONATE; NEOMYCIN SULPHATE; NYSTATIN

*desensitizing vaccines

are preparations of particular allergens (substances to which a patient has an allergic reaction) that are administered, in progressive doses, to reduce the degree of allergic reaction the patient suffers when exposed to the allergen. For example, preparations of grass pollens are administered for the treatment of hay fever, or bee venom or wasp venom to protect against the effects of subsequent stings. The mechanism by which they work is not clear.

✚ side-effects: allergic reactions, especially in small children.

▲ warning: they are not to be used in patients who are pregnant, who have acute asthma, or febrile conditions. A heavy meal must not be eaten before treatment. Injections should be administered under close medical supervision and in locations where emergency facilities for full cardio-respiratory resuscitation are immediately available.

◐ Related entry: Pharmalgen

Deseril

(Sandoz) is a proprietary, prescription-only preparation of the drug methysergide. It can be used as an ANTIMIGRAINE treatment to prevent severe, recurrent migraine and similar headaches in patients for whom other forms of treatment have failed. It is available as tablets.

✚▲ side-effects/warning: see METHYSERGIDE

Desferal

(Ciba) is a proprietary, prescription-only preparation of the CHELATING AGENT desferrioxamine mesylate. It can be used as an ANTIDOTE to treat iron poisoning and iron overload. It is available as an oral solution or in a form for injection.

✚▲ side-effects/warning: see DESFERRIOXAMINE MESYLATE

desferrioxamine mesylate

is a CHELATING AGENT, which is used as an ANTIDOTE to treat iron poisoning and iron overload (eg.in aplastic anaemia due to repeated blood transfusion).
Administration is either oral as a solution or by injection.

✚ side-effects: there may be pain at the site of injection, gastrointestinal disturbances, hypotension, heart rate changes, anaphylaxis, convulsions, dizziness, disturbances in vision and hearing and skin disorders.

▲ warning: avoid its use in patients with kidney impairment; or who are pregnant or breast-feeding.

◐ Related entry: Desferal

desflurane

is a recently introduced inhalant GENERAL ANAESTHETIC drug. It can be used along with nitrous oxide-oxygen mixtures for the induction and maintenance of anaesthesia during surgery. Administration is by inhalation.

✚ side-effects: coughing, laryngospasm and increased airways secretions and breath-holding.

◐ Related entry: Enflurane

desipramine hydrochloride

is an ANTIDEPRESSANT drug of the TRICYCLIC group. It can be used to treat depressive illness and has less sedative properties than many tricyclics, which makes it more suitable for the treatment of withdrawn and apathetic patients. Administration is oral in the form of tablets.

✚▲ side-effects/warning: see under AMITRYPTYLINE HYDROCHLORIDE; but with a less sedative effect.

◐ Related entry: Pertofran

desmopressin

is one of two major analogues of the antidiuretic HORMONE vasopressin (ADH),

D

which naturally reduces urine production. It is used to diagnose or to treat certain (pituitary-originated) types of diabetes insipidus, to test renal function and to prevent bed-wetting. It is also used to boost blood concentrations of some blood-clotting factors in haemophiliac patients. Administration can be oral as tablets, topical in the form of nose-drops or a nasal spary, or by injection.

+▲ side-effects/warning: see under VASOPRESSIN. There is less rise in blood pressure, but nevertheless care is needed in patients with certain cardiovascular or kidney disorders, or hypertension. Fluid retention and raised sodium levels may occur unless fluid intake is restricted. There may be vomiting, headache and nosebleeds.

○ Related entries: DDAVP; Desmospray; Desmotabs

Desmospray

(Ferring) is a proprietary, prescription-only preparation of desmopressin, which is an analogue of the pituitary HORMONE vasopressin (ADH). It is administered primarily to diagnose or to treat pituitary-originated diabetes insipidus. It can be used for some other diagnostic tests, to boost the blood concentration of blood-clotting factors in haemophiliac patients and to prevent bed-wetting. It is available as a nasal spray.

+▲ side-effects/warning: see DESMOPRESSIN

Desmotabs

(Ferring) is a proprietary, prescription-only preparation of desmopressin, which is an analogue of the pituitary HORMONE vasopressin (ADH). It is used primarily to diagnose or to treat pituitary-originated diabetes insipidus. It can also be used for some other diagnostic tests, to boost the blood concentration of blood-clotting factors in haemophiliac patients and to prevent bed-wetting. It is available (as desmopressin acetate) as tablets.

196 **+▲** side-effects/warning: see DESMOPRESSIN

desogestrel

is a PROGESTOGEN that is used as a constituent of the *combined* ORAL CONTRACEPTIVES that contain an OESTROGEN and a PROGESTOGEN. Administration is oral as tablets.

+▲ side-effects/warning: see under PROGESTOGEN

○ Related entries: Marvelon; Mercilon

desoximetasone

See DESOXYMETHASONE

desoxymethasone

(desoximetasone) is a CORTICOSTEROID with ANTI-INFLAMMATORY properties. It is used in the treatment of severe, acute inflammation of the skin and chronic skin disorders such as psoriasis. Administration is by topical application as a cream or lotion.

+▲ side-effects/warning: see under CORTICOSTEROIDS; though systemic effects are unlikely with topical application, but there may be local skin reactions.

○ Related entry: Stiedex

desquamating agents

See KERATOLYTICS

Destolit

(Merrell) is a proprietary, prescription-only preparation of ursodeoxycholic acid. It is used to dissolve gallstones and is available as tablets.

+▲ side-effects/warning: see URSODEOXYCHOLIC ACID

Deteclo

(Lederle) is a proprietary, prescription-only COMPOUND PREPARATION of the ANTIBACTERIAL and (TETRACYCLINE) ANTIBIOTIC drugs chlortetracycline (as hydrochloride), tetracycline (as hydrochloride) and demeclocycline hydrochloride. It can be used to treat many kinds of infection and is available as tablets.

+▲ side-effects/warning: see

CHLORTETRACYCLINE; DEMECLOCYCLINE HYDROCHLORIDE; TETRACYCLINE

De Witt's Worm Syrup

(De Witt) is a proprietary, non-prescription preparation of the ANTHELMINTIC drug piperazine (as citrate). It can be used to treat infections by threadworm and roundworm and is available as an oral powder. It is not normally given to children under four years, except on medical advice.

+▲ side-effects/warning: see PIPERAZINE

Dexamethasone

(Organon) is a proprietary, prescription-only preparation of the CORTICOSTEROID and ANTI-INFLAMMATORY drug dexamethasone. It can be used in the suppression of allergic and inflammatory conditions, in the treatment of shock, congenital adrenal hyperplasia, cerebral oedema and in the diagnosis of Cushing's disease. It is available as tablets and in a form for injection.

+▲ side-effects/warning: see DEXAMETHASONE

dexamethasone

is a CORTICOSTEROID with ANTI-INFLAMMATORY properties. It is used for a variety of purposes, including the suppression of inflammatory and allergic disorders, in the treatment of shock, in the diagnosis of Cushing's disease, to treat congenital adrenal hyperplasia, cerebral oedema and in rheumatic disease to relieve pain and to increase mobility and decrease deformity of joints. It is used in several forms: dexamethasone, dexamethasone sodium phosphate and dexamethasone isonicotinate. Administration is either by topical application in the form of tablets, eye-drops or an ointment, or by injection.

+▲ side-effects/warning: see under CORTICOSTEROIDS; though systemic effects are unlikely with topical application, but there may be local skin reactions.

○ Related entries: Decadron; Decadron Shock-Pak; Dexa-Rhinaspray; Dexamethasone; Maxidex; Maxitrol; Sofradex

dexamphetamine sulphate

is a drug that, in adults, works directly on the brain as a STIMULANT and can be used to treat narcolepsy (a condition involving irresistible attacks of sleep during the daytime). Paradoxically, in children it has more of a sedative action and can be used in the treatment of hyperactivity. It is on the Controlled Drugs List because of its addictive potential. Administration is oral in the form of tablets.

+ side-effects: insomnia, irritability, restlessness, night terrors, euphoria, tremor, dizziness, headache, dependence, tolerance, psychosis, gastrointestinal symptoms, anorexia, growth retardation in children, dry mouth, sweating and effects on the cardiovascular system.

▲ warning: it should not be administered to patients with heart disease, hypertension, hyperexcitability states, hyperthyroidism, history of drug abuse, glaucoma, extrapyramidal disorders, or who are pregnant or breast-feeding. Avoid its use in those with porphyria; and avoid alcohol because of the potential of unpredictable reactions. It may impair the performance of skilled tasks such as driving. Withdrawal of treatment should be gradual.

○ Related entry: Dexedrine

Dexa-Rhinaspray

(Boehringer Ingelheim) is a proprietary, prescription-only COMPOUND PREPARATION of the ANTI-INFLAMMATORY and CORTICOSTEROID drug dexamethasone (as isonicotinate), the (AMINOGLYCOSIDE) ANTIBIOTIC drug neomycin sulphate and the SYMPATHOMIMETIC and VASOCONSTRICTOR drug tramazoline hydrochloride. It can be used to treat allergic rhinitis

D

and is available as an aerosol for nasal inhalation.

✚▲ side-effects/warning: see DEXAMETHASONE; NEOMYCIN SULPHATE; TRAMAZOLINE HYDROCHLORIDE

Dexedrine

(Evans) is a proprietary, prescription-only preparation of the powerful STIMULANT drug dexamphetamine sulphate and is on the Controlled Drugs List. It can be used to treat narcolepsy in adults and medically diagnosed hyperactivity in children. It is available as tablets.

✚▲ side-effects/warning: see DEXAMPHETAMINE SULPHATE

dexfenfluramine hydrochloride

is an APPETITE SUPPRESSANT that is used for the treatment of obesity. It is the dextro-isomer of the powerful appetite suppressant drug fenfluramine hydrochloride. Dexfenfluramine is a sedative rather than a stimulant, which is the case with most other appetite suppressants and may affect a patient's thought and movement and is potentially addictive (though this is rare). It is available in the form of capsules.

✚▲ side-effects/warning: see under FENFLURAMINE HYDROCHLORIDE. It should not be used in patients with certain liver or kidney disorders.

⭘ Related entry: Adifax

dextromethorphan hydrobromide

is an (OPIOID) ANTITUSSIVE drug that is used alone or in combination with other drugs in linctuses, syrups and lozenges to relieve dry or painful coughs.

✚▲ side-effects/warning: see under OPIOID; but side-effects are rare.

⭘ Related entries: Actifed Compound Linctus; Actifed Junior Cough Relief; Benylin Dry Coughs Non-Drowsy; Benylin Dry Coughs Original; Bronalin Dry Cough Elixir; Contac Coughcaps;

Covonia Bronchial Balsam; Covonia for Children; Day Nurse Capsules; Day Nurse Liquid; Flurex Cold/Flu Capsules with Cough Suppressant; Franolyn for Dry Cough; Lemsip Night-Time; Meltus Dry Cough Elixir, Adult; Meltus Junior Dry Cough Elixir; Night Nurse Capsules; Night Nurse Liquid; Nirolex Lozenges; Owbridge's for Dry Tickly and Allergic Coughs; Robitussin Chesty Cough with Congestion; Robitussin Dry Cough; Robitussin Junior Persistent Cough Medicine; Sudafed; Sudafed Linctus; Tancolin; Vicks Children's Vaposyrup; Vicks Coldcare Capsules; Vicks Vaposyrup for Dry Coughs and Nasal Congestion

dextromoramide

is an (OPIOID) NARCOTIC ANALGESIC drug that is a synthetic derivative of morphine. It can be used to treat severe and intractable pain, particularly in the final stages of terminal illness. It is less sedating and shorter acting than morphine. Its proprietary forms are on the Controlled Drugs List because, as with morphine, it is potentially addictive. Administration can be oral as tablets or as suppositories.

✚▲ side-effects/warning: see under OPIOID. It is not used in obstetrics because it may affect the unborn child.

⭘ Related entry: Palfium

dextropropoxyphene hydrochloride

is an (OPIOID) NARCOTIC ANALGESIC drug that is used to treat pain anywhere in the body. It is usually combined with other analgesics (especially paracetamol or aspirin) as a COMPOUND ANALGESIC. Administration of the drug on its own is oral as capsules.

✚▲ side-effects/warning: see under OPIOID. There may be occasional liver toxicity, porphyria in susceptible individuals and convulsions in overdose. It is not to be used in patients with suicidal tendencies or with a history of addiction.

D

O Related entries: co-proxamol;
Cosalgesic; Distalgesic; Doloxene;
Doloxene Compound

dextrose
or dextrose monohydrate, is another term
for glucose.

DF118
(Napp) is a proprietary, prescription-only
preparation of the (OPIOID) NARCOTIC
ANALGESIC drug dihydrocodeine tartrate,
which is on the Controlled Drugs List. It
can be used to treat moderate to severe
pain and is available in a form for
injection (the proprietary name was
previously used for a tablet form).
+▲ side-effects/warning: see
DIHYDROCODEINE TARTRATE

DF118 Forte
(Napp) is a proprietary, prescription-only
preparation of the (OPIOID) NARCOTIC
ANALGESIC drug dihydrocodeine tartrate. It
can be used to treat acute and chronic
severe pain and is available as tablets.
+▲ side-effects/warning: see
DIHYDROCODEINE TARTRATE

DHC Continus
(Napp) is a proprietary, prescription-only
preparation of the (OPIOID) NARCOTIC
ANALGESIC drug dihydrocodeine tartrate. It
can be used to treat moderate to severe
pain and is available as modified-release
tablets.
+▲ side-effects/warning: see
DIHYDROCODEINE TARTRATE

Diabetamide
(Ashbourne) is a proprietary,
prescription-only preparation of the
SULPHONYLUREA drug glibenclamide. It is
used in DIABETIC TREATMENT of Type II
diabetes (non-insulin-dependent diabetes
mellitus; NIDDM; maturity-onset diabetes)
and is available as tablets.
+▲ side-effects/warning: see
GLIBENCLAMIDE

*diabetes insipidus treatment
involves the administration of drugs to
counteract the under-production of
ANTIDIURETIC HORMONE (ADH; also called
VASOPRESSIN) by the pituitary gland, which
is a characteristic of diabetes insipidus.
Vasopressin itself may be used or the
analogue LYPRESSIN and they can both
administered topically in the form of a
nasal spray (because the hormone is a
peptide it cannot be given by mouth).
Diabetes insipidus is a rare disease and
has no connection at all with diabetes
mellitus, which is also a HORMONE
disorder, but due to the under-production
of INSULIN by the pancreas. However, in
both conditions there is thirst and a
production of large quantities of dilute
urine.

*diabetic treatment
consists of the administration of one of
two types of treatment. The first treatment
involves the use of ORAL HYPOGLYCAEMIC
drugs, which are synthetic agents taken by
mouth to reduce the levels of glucose
(sugar) in the bloodstream and are used
primarily in the treatment of Type II
diabetes (non-insulin-dependent diabetes
mellitus; NIDDM; maturity-onset diabetes)
when there is still some residual capacity
in the pancreas for the production of the
HORMONE insulin. The main oral
hypoglycaemics used are the
SULPHONYLUREAS and BIGUANIDES.
  The second treatment involves the
administration of INSULIN, which is mainly
used in Type I diabetes (insulin-dependent
diabetes mellitus; IDDM; juvenile-onset
diabetes) and must be injected. There are
many insulin preparations available and
the difference between them is mainly
their duration of action.

Diabinese
(Pfizer) is a proprietary, prescription-only
preparation of the SULPHONYLUREA drug
chlorpropamide. It is used in DIABETIC

D

TREATMENT of Type II diabetes (non-insulin-dependent diabetes mellitus; NIDDM; maturity-onset diabetes) and is available as tablets.

+▲ side-effects/warning: see CHLORPROPAMIDE

Diagesil

(Berk) is a proprietary, prescription-only preparation of the (OPIOID) NARCOTIC ANALGESIC and ANTITUSSIVE drug diamorphine hydrochloride (heroin hydrochloride), which is on the Controlled Drugs List. It can be used primarily to relieve intractable pain, especially during the final stages of terminal malignant disease. It is available in a form for injection.

+▲ side-effects/warning: see DIAMORPHINE HYDROCHLORIDE

Dialar

(Lagap) is a proprietary, prescription-only preparation of the BENZODIAZEPINE drug diazepam. It can be used as an ANXIOLYTIC in the short-term treatment of anxiety, as a HYPNOTIC to relieve insomnia, as an ANTICONVULSANT and ANTI-EPILEPTIC for status epilepticus, as a SEDATIVE in preoperative medication, as a SKELETAL MUSCLE RELAXANT and to assist in the treatment of alcohol withdrawal symptoms. It is available as an oral solution.

+▲ side-effects/warning: see DIAZEPAM

Diamicron

(Servier) is a proprietary, prescription-only preparation of the SULPHONYLUREA drug gliclazide. It is used in DIABETIC TREATMENT of Type II diabetes (non-insulin-dependent diabetes mellitus; NIDDM; maturity-onset diabetes) and is available as tablets.

+▲ side-effects/warning: see GLICLAZIDE

diamorphine hydrochloride

is the chemical name of heroin

hydrochloride (a chemical derivative of morphine) and is a powerful (OPIOID) NARCOTIC ANALGESIC. It can be used in the treatment of moderate to severe pain (though it has a shorter duration of action than morphine). It is also occasionally used as an ANTITUSSIVE to treat severe and painful cough and for acute airways oedema (especially in the treatment of terminal lung cancer). Its use quickly tends to tolerance and then dependence (addiction). Administration can be oral as tablets or an elixir, or by injection. All preparations are on the Controlled Drugs List.

+▲ side-effects/warning: see under OPIOID; but may cause less nausea and hypotension.

○ Related entries: Diagesil; Diaphine

Diamox

(Storz) is a proprietary, prescription-only preparation of the CARBONIC ANHYDRASE INHIBITOR drug acetazolamide. It is mainly used in GLAUCOMA TREATMENT, but also has DIURETIC properties. It is available as tablets and as a modified-release capsules (*Diamox SR*).

+▲ side-effects/warning: see ACETAZOLAMIDE

Dianette

(Schering Health) is a proprietary, prescription-only COMPOUND PREPARATION of the OESTROGEN HORMONE ethinyloestradiol and the ANTI-ANDROGEN cyproterone. It can be used in women, in certain circumstances, to treat acne and is available as tablets.

+▲ side-effects/warning: see CYPROTERONE ACETATE; ETHINYLOESTRADIOL

Diaphine

(Napp) is a proprietary, prescription-only preparation of the (OPIOID) NARCOTIC ANALGESIC and ANTITUSSIVE drug diamorphine hydrochloride (heroin hydrochloride), which is on the Controlled Drugs List. It is used primarily to relieve intractable pain, especially during the final stages of terminal malignant disease. It is available in a form for injection.

+▲ side-effects/warning: see DIAMORPHINE HYDROCHLORIDE

Diarphen

(Mepra-pharm) is a proprietary, prescription-only COMPOUND PREPARATION of the (OPIOID) ANTIDIARRHOEAL drug diphenoxylate hydrochloride and the ANTICHOLINERGIC drug atropine sulphate (a combination called co-phenotrope). It can be used to treat chronic diarrhoea, for example in mild chronic ulcerative colitis. Dependence may occur with prolonged use. It is available as tablets and is not normally given to young children, except on medical advice.

+▲ side-effects/warning: see ATROPINE SULPHATE; DIPHENOXYLATE HYDROCHLORIDE

Diarrest

(Galen) is a proprietary, prescription-only preparation of the (OPIOID) ANTIDIARRHOEAL drug codeine phosphate with sodium and potassium salts. It can be used to supplement or replace minerals lost through vomiting or diarrhoea. It should be used only for short-term treatment of diarrhoea and cramps and is available as an oral liquid.

+▲ side-effects/warning: see CODEINE PHOSPHATE

Diazemuls

(Dumex) is a proprietary, prescription-only preparation of the BENZODIAZEPINE drug diazepam. It can be used as an ANXIOLYTIC in the short-term treatment of anxiety, as a HYPNOTIC to relieve insomnia, as an ANTICONVULSANT and ANTI-EPILEPTIC for status epilepticus, as a SEDATIVE in preoperative medication, as a SKELETAL MUSCLE RELAXANT and to assist in the treatment of alcohol withdrawal symptoms. It is available in a form for injection.

+▲ side-effects/warning: see DIAZEPAM

diazepam

is chemically a BENZODIAZEPINE. It can be used as an ANXIOLYTIC in the short-term treatment of anxiety, as a HYPNOTIC to relieve insomnia, as an ANTICONVULSANT and ANTI-EPILEPTIC for status epilepticus and convulsions due to poisoning, as a SEDATIVE in preoperative medication, as a SKELETAL MUSCLE RELAXANT and to assist in the treatment of alcohol withdrawal symptoms. Administration can be oral as tablets or a solution, or as suppositories or a rectal solution, or by injection.

+▲ side effects/warning see under BENZODIAZEPINES. When injected, there may be pain, inflammation and swelling at the injection site.

✪ Related entries: Atensine; Dialar; Diazemuls; Diazepam Rectubes; Rimapam; Stesolid; Tensium; Valclair; Valium

Diazepam Rectubes

(CP Pharmaceuticals) is a proprietary, prescription-only preparation of the BENZODIAZEPINE drug diazepam. It can be used as an ANXIOLYTIC in the short-term treatment of anxiety, as a HYPNOTIC to relieve insomnia, as an ANTICONVULSANT and ANTI-EPILEPTIC for status epilepticus, as a SEDATIVE in preoperative medication, as a SKELETAL MUSCLE RELAXANT and to assist in the treatment of alcohol withdrawal symptoms. It is available as a rectal solution.

+▲ side-effects/warning: see DIAZEPAM

diazoxide

is a drug that has two separate actions and uses. It lowers blood pressure rapidly on injection and can therefore be used as an ANTIHYPERTENSIVE in treating acute hypertensive crisis. It is also a hyperglycaemic drug and can be used by mouth to treat chronic hypoglycaemia (abnormally low levels of glucose in the bloostream), for example, where a pancreatic tumour causes excessive secretion of INSULIN. It is available as

D

D

tablets and in a form for injection.

✚ side-effects: there may be nausea and vomiting, an increased heart rate with hypotension, loss of appetite, oedema (accumulation of fluid in the tissues), heart arrhythmias and increased heart rate and hyperglycaemia; excessive growth of hair with chronic treatment.

▲ warning: administer with caution to patients with reduced blood supply to the heart, certain kidney disorders, who are pregnant, or in labour. During prolonged treatment, regular monitoring of blood constituents and blood pressure is required.

**۞ Related entries:
Eudemine (injection);
Eudemine (tablets)**

Dibenyline

(Forley) is a proprietary, prescription-only preparation of the ALPHA-ADRENOCEPTOR BLOCKER drug phenoxybenzamine hydrochloride. It can be used, in conjunction with a BETA-BLOCKER, as an ANTIHYPERTENSIVE treatment, in hypertensive crises in phaeochromocytoma and in severe shock. It is available as capsules and in a form for injection.

✚▲ side-effects/warning: see PHENOXYBENZAMINE HYDROCHLORIDE

dibromopropamidine isethionate

is an ANTIBACTERIAL drug, which is used specifically to treat infections of the eyelids or conjunctiva, including the amoebic infection acanthamoeba keratitis (sometimes with additional drugs). Administration is topical in the form of an eye ointment.

**۞ Related entries:
Brolene Eye Ointment; Brulidine;
Golden Eye Ointment**

dichlorphenamide

is a CARBONIC ANHYDRASE INHIBITOR drug that has the effect of a DIURETIC. It is used as a GLAUCOMA TREATMENT because it

reduces the aqueous humour (fluid) in the eyeball. Administration is oral in the form of tablets.

✚▲ side-effects/warning: see under ACETAZOLAMIDE

۞ Related entry: Daranide

diclofenac sodium

is a (NSAID) NON-NARCOTIC ANALGESIC and ANTIRHEUMATIC drug. It is used to treat pain and inflammation in rheumatic disease and other musculoskeletal disorders (such as juvenile arthritis and gout). Administration can be oral as tablets, topical as suppositories, or in a form for injection.

✚▲ side-effects/warning: see under NSAID. Avoid its use in patients with porphyria. There may be local irritation if using suppositories, or pain at the site of injection.

۞ Related entries: Arthrotec; Diclomax Retard; Diclozip; Flamrase SR; Isclofen; Motifene 75 mg; Rhumalgan; Valenac; Volraman; Voltarol; Voltarol Emulgel; Voltarol Optha

Diclomax Retard

(Parke-Davis) is a proprietary, prescription-only preparation of the (NSAID) NON-NARCOTIC ANALGESIC and ANTIRHEUMATIC drug diclofenac sodium. It can be used to treat arthritic and rheumatic pain and inflammation and other musculoskeletal disorders. It is available as modified-release capsules.

✚▲ side-effects/warning: see DICLOFENAC SODIUM

Diclozip

(Ashbourne) is a proprietary, prescription-only preparation of the (NSAID) NON-NARCOTIC ANALGESIC and ANTIRHEUMATIC drug diclofenac sodium. It can be used to treat arthritic and rheumatic pain and inflammation and other musculoskeletal disorders. It is available as tablets.

✚▲ side-effects/warning: see DICLOFENAC SODIUM

dicobalt edetate

is used as an ANTIDOTE to acute cyanide poisoning. It acts as a CHELATING AGENT by binding to cyanide to form a compound that can be excreted from the body. Administration is by injection.

✚ side-effects: vomiting, transient hypotension and tachycardia.

▲ warning: because of its toxicity, it is normally used only when the patient is losing, or has lost, consciousness.

○ Related entry: Kelocyanor

Diconal

(Wellcome) is a proprietary, prescription-only COMPOUND PREPARATION of the (OPIOID) NARCOTIC ANALGESIC drug dipipanone hydrochloride and the ANTIHISTAMINE and ANTINAUSEANT drug cyclizine hydrochloride. It can be used to treat moderate to severe pain and is available as tablets. It is on the Controlled Drugs List and is not normally given to children, except on medical advice.

✚▲ side-effects/warning: see CYCLIZINE; DIPIPANONE

dicyclomine hydrochloride

(dicyloverine hydrochloride) is an ANTICHOLINERGIC drug that can be used as an ANTISPASMODIC for the symptomatic relief of muscle spasm in the gastrointestinal tract. It is available as tablets, a syrup and a gel.

✚▲ side-effects/warning: see under ATROPINE SULPHATE

○ Related entries: Kolanticon Gel; Merbentyl; Merbentyl 20

dicyloverine hydrochloride

See DICYCLOMINE HYDROCHLORIDE

Dicynene

(Delandale) is a proprietary, prescription-only preparation of ethamsylate, which is a drug that can be used in certain situations where antifibrinolytic drugs might be administered It can be used for a variety of purposes, including bleeding in premature infants and in menorrhagia (excessive periods bleeding). It is available as tablets and in a form for injection.

✚▲ side-effects/warning: see ETHAMSYLATE

didanosine

(DDI) is an ANTIVIRAL drug that can be used in the treatment of AIDS. It is administered to patients who are intolerant to, or have not benefited from, zidovudine. It is available as tablets.

✚ side-effects: pancreatitis, peripheral neuropathy or raised urea levels in the blood (monitoring is necessary). Other possible side-effects include nausea, vomiting, confusion, fever and headache.

▲ warning: it should not be given to patients with peripheral neuropathy, who are pregnant, or breast-feeding. Administer with caution where there is a history of pancreatitis or impaired liver or kidney function.

○ Related entry: Videx

Didronal PMO

(Procter & Gamble) is a proprietary, prescription-only COMPOUND PREPARATION of the drugs disodium etidronate and calcium carbonate. It can be used to reduce the rate of bone turnover in treating the condition known as Paget's disease of the bone and also to treat high calcium levels associated with malignant tumours. It is available as tablets.

✚▲ side-effects/warning: see CALCIUM CARBONATE; DISODIUM ETIDRONATE

Didronel

(Procter & Gamble) is a proprietary, prescription-only preparation of the drug disodium etidronate. It can be used to reduce the rate of bone turnover in treating the condition known as Paget's disease of the bone and also to treat high calcium levels associated with malignant tumours. It is available as tablets.

✚▲ side-effects/warning: see DISODIUM ETIDRONATE

D

Didronel IV

(Procter & Gamble) is a proprietary,
prescription-only preparation of the drug
disodium etidronate. It can be used to
reduce the rate of bone turnover in
treating the condition known as Paget's
disease of the bone and also to treat high
calcium levels associated with malignant
tumours. It is available as tablets.

✚▲ side-effects/warning: see
DISODIUM ETIDRONATE

dienoestrol

is a synthetic OESTROGEN, a SEX HORMONE,
that can be used as part of HRT (hormone
replacement therapy). Administration is by
topical application in the form of a vaginal
cream.

✚▲ side effects/warning: see under
OESTROGEN

○ Related entry: Ortho Dienoestrol

diethylamine salicylate

is a constituent with a COUNTER-IRRITANT,
or RUBEFACIENT, action. It can be applied
to the skin for symptomatic relief of
underlying muscle or joint pain.

✚▲ side-effects/warning: see under METHYL
SALICYLATE. It should not be used on inflamed
or broken skin, or on mucous membranes.

○ Related entries: Algesal;
Lloyd's Cream

diethyl ether

is an inhalant GENERAL ANAESTHETIC drug,
which is more familiarly known as ether. It
is now obsolete in developed countries,
but is still used elsewhere in the world
because it is cheap, requires only simple
apparatus to administer and is suitable for
single-handed use.

✚ side-effects: it is irritant to the upper
airways and tends to cause nausea and
vomiting.

diethylpropion hydrochloride

is an APPETITE SUPPRESSANT drug related to
amphetamine. It is used occasionally

under medical supervision and on a short-
term basis to aid weight loss in severe
obesity. It is a STIMULANT potentially
subject to abuse and is therefore on the
Controlled Drugs List. There is growing
doubt among experts over the medical
value of such treatment. Administration is
oral as modified-release tablets.

✚ side-effects: there is commonly rapid heart
rate, nervous agitation and insomnia,
depression, rashes, constipation, dry mouth,
dizziness and headache. Tolerance and
dependence may occur. Susceptible patients
may undergo psychotic episodes. It may cause
enlargement of the breasts in men.

▲ warning: it should not be administered to
patients who suffer from glaucoma or any
medical condition (such as thyrotoxicosis)
that disposes towards excitability; administer
with caution to those with heart disease,
diabetes, epilepsy, peptic ulcer, depression or
unstable personality and to those with a
history of alcohol or drug abuse.

○ Related entries: Apisate; Tenuate
Dospan

diethylstilbestrol

See STILBOESTROL

Difflam

(3M Health Care) is a proprietary, non-
prescription preparation of benzydamine
hydrochloride, which has a COUNTER-
IRRITANT, or RUBEFACIENT, action. It can be
used for symptomatic relief of pain on the
skin, mouth ulcers and other sores or
inflammation in the mouth and throat. It is
available as a cream for topical
application and as a liquid mouthwash or
spray.

✚▲ side-effects/warning: see
BENZYDAMINE HYDROCHLORIDE

Diflucan

(Pfizer) is a proprietary, prescription-only
preparation of the ANTIFUNGAL drug
fluconazole. It can be used to treat
candidiasis (thrush) of the vagina, mouth
and other tissue areas. It is available as

capsules and in a form for intravenous infusion.

+▲ side-effects/warning: see FLUCONAZOLE

diflucortolone valerate

is a CORTICOSTEROID with ANTI-INFLAMMATORY properties. It is used in the treatment of severe, acute inflammatory skin disorders, such as eczema and psoriasis, that are unresponsive to less potent corticosteroids. Administration is by topical application in the form of a cream or ointment.

+▲ side-effects/warning: see under CORTICOSTEROIDS; though systemic effects are unlikely with topical application, but there may be local skin reactions.

✪ Related entry: Nerisone

diflunisal

is a (NSAID) NON-NARCOTIC ANALGESIC and ANTIRHEUMATIC drug that is derived from aspirin, but is quite powerful and with a longer duration of action. It can be used in the treatment of pain and inflammation (especially in rheumatic disease and other musculoskeletal disorders) and for period pain. Administration is oral in the form of tablets.

+▲ side-effects/warning: see under NSAID. Administer with care to patients who are breast-feeding.

✪ Related entry: Dolobid

Diftavax

(Merieux) is a proprietary, prescription-only VACCINE preparation of adsorbed diphtheria and tetanus vaccine for adults (DT/Vac/Ads for Adults), which combines (toxoid) vaccines for diphtheria and tetanus vaccine adsorbed onto a mineral carrier. It is available in a form for injection.

+▲ side-effects/warning: see DIPHTHERIA VACCINES; TETANUS VACCINE

Digibind

(Wellcome) is a proprietary, prescription-only drug that can be used as an ANTIDOTE

to overdosage by the CARDIAC GLYCOSIDE drugs digoxin and digitoxin. It comprises antibody fragments that react with the glycosides and is administered for emergency use by injection.

digitoxin

is a CARDIAC GLYCOSIDE drug derived from the leaves of *Digitalis* foxgloves. It can be used as a CARDIAC STIMULANT, because it increases the force of contraction in congestive HEART FAILURE TREATMENT and as an ANTI-ARRHYTHMIC to treat certain heartbeat irregularities. Administration is oral as tablets.

+▲ side-effects/warning: see under DIGOXIN

digoxin

is a CARDIAC GLYCOSIDE drug derived from the leaves of *Digitalis* foxgloves. It can be used as a CARDIAC STIMULANT, because it increases the force of contraction in congestive HEART FAILURE TREATMENT and as an ANTI-ARRHYTHMIC to treat certain heartbeat irregularities. It is administered as tablets, an elixir, or by injection.

+ side-effects: there are serious and common side-effects (the minimization of which depends on finding a suitable dosage schedule in each patient and regular monitoring): loss of appetite, nausea and vomiting, with a consequent weight loss; diarrhoea and abdominal pain; visual disturbances; fatigue, confusion, delirium and hallucinations. Overdosage may lead to arrhythmias or heart block.

▲ warning: it should be administered with caution to patients who have had a recent heart attack, certain arrhythmias and heart conditions, hypothyroidism, who are elderly, have impaired kidney function and where there is raised blood potassium. Regular monitoring of the blood potassium level is also recommended.

✪ Related entries: Lanoxin; Lanoxin-PG

dihydrocodeine tartrate

is an (OPIOID) NARCOTIC ANALGESIC drug that is similar to CODEINE PHOSPHATE but

D

more powerful. It is also available in some COMPOUND ANALGESIC preparations (eg.in co-dydramol, where it is combined with paracetamol). Administration can be oral as tablets or a dilute elixir, or in a form for injection.

✚▲ side-effects/warning: see under OPIOID

✪ Related entries: DF118; DF118 Forte; DHC Continus; Galake; Paramol Tablets; Remedeine

dihydrotachysterol

is a synthetic form of vitamin D (related to D_2 and D_3) that is used to make up body deficiencies of this vitamin. Administration is oral.

✚▲ side-effects/warning: see under VITAMIN D

✪ Related entry: AT 10

Dijex

(Seton Healthcare) is a proprietary, non-prescription COMPOUND PREPARATION of the ANTACIDS aluminium hydroxide and magnesium hydroxide. It can be used to relieve acid indigestion and dyspepsia and is available as a liquid suspension. It is not normally given to children under six years, except on medical advice.

✚▲ side-effects/warning: see ALUMINIUM HYDROXIDE; MAGNESIUM HYDROXIDE

Dijex Tablets

(Seton Healthcare) is a proprietary, non-prescription COMPOUND PREPARATION of the ANTACIDS aluminium hydroxide and magnesium carbonate. It can be used to relieve acid indigestion and dyspepsia and is available as tablets. It is not normally given to children under five years, except on medical advice.

✚▲ side-effects/warning: see ALUMINIUM HYDROXIDE; MAGNESIUM CARBONATE

diloxanide furoate

is an ANTIPROTOZOAL and AMOEBICIDAL drug. It can be used to treat chronic

infection of the intestine by amoebae (*Entamoeba histolytica*) that cause amoebic dysentery. Administration is oral as tablets.

✚ side-effects: flatulence; vomiting, pruritus (skin itching) and/or urticaria.

✪ Related entries: Entamizole; Furamide

diltiazem hydrochloride

is a CALCIUM-CHANNEL BLOCKER drug. It is used as an ANTIHYPERTENSIVE treatment and as an ANTI-ANGINA drug in the prevention of attacks. Administration is oral in the form of tablets and capsules (several in long-acting formulations).

✚ side-effects: slowing of the heat and altered heart function, hypotension, flushing; fatigue and malaise, headache; depression, swelling of the ankles; gastrointestinal disturbances; rashes; and altered liver function.

▲ warning: administer with caution and reduce dose, to patients with certain liver, kidney, or heart disorders; and with abnormal blood states. It should not be given to patients who are pregnant.

✪ Related entries: Adizem-60; Adizem-SR; Adizem-XL; Angiozem; Britiazim; Dilzem SR; Dilzem XL; Slozem; Tildiem; Tildiem LA; Tildiem Retard;

Dilzem SR

(Elan) is a proprietary, prescription-only preparation of the CALCIUM-CHANNEL BLOCKER diltiazem hydrochloride. It can be used as an ANTIHYPERTENSIVE treatment and as an ANTI-ANGINA drug in the prevention of attacks. It is available as modified-release capsules.

✚▲ side-effects/warning: see DILTIAZEM HYDROCHLORIDE

Dilzem XL

(Elan) is a proprietary, prescription-only preparation of the CALCIUM-CHANNEL BLOCKER diltiazem hydrochloride. It can be used as an ANTIHYPERTENSIVE treatment and as an ANTI-ANGINA drug in the prevention of attacks. It is available as

modified-release capsules.
✚▲ side-effects/warning: see DILTIAZEM
HYDROCHLORIDE

dimenhydrinate
is an ANTIHISTAMINE drug. It is principally
used as an ANTINAUSEANT, particularly for
treating nausea and vomiting associated
with motion sickness, disorders of the
balance function of the inner ear and
vertigo. Administration is oral in the form
of tablets.
✚▲ side-effects/warning: see under
CYCLIZINE; ANTIHISTAMINE. It should not be
given to patients with porphyria.
✪ Related entry: Dramamine

dimercaprol
(BAL) is a CHELATING AGENT. It is used as
an ANTIDOTE to poisoning with antimony,
arsenic, bismuth, gold, mercury, thallium
and (with sodium calcium edate) lead.
Administration is by injection.
✚ side-effects: hypertension, increase in heart
rate, sweating, malaise, nausea and vomiting,
excessive tears, constriction of the throat and
chest, burning sensation (eyes and mouth),
headache, muscle spasms, pain in the
abdomen, tingling in extremities, raised
temperature in children pain and abscess at
injection site.
▲ warning: it should not be given to patients
with severe liver impairment; administer with
care to those with hypertension.
✪ Related entry: Dimercaprol Injection

Dimercaprol Injection
(Boots) is a proprietary, prescription-only
preparation of the CHELATING AGENT
dimercaprol. It can be used as an
ANTIDOTE to poisoning by a number of
toxic metals and is available in a form for
injection.
✚▲ side-effects/warning: see DIMERCAPROL

dimethicone
is a water-repellent silicone that is used as
an ANTIFOAMING AGENT and, when taken
orally, is thought to reduce flatulence

while protecting mucous membranes. It is
also a constituent in many BARRIER CREAMS
that can be used to protect against
irritation or chapping (eg.nappy rash).
Dimethicone activated is also known as
simethicone.
▲ warning: do not use on acutely inflamed
or weeping skin.
✪ Related articles: Altacite Plus;
**Asilone Liquid; Asilone Suspension;
Asilone Tablets; Bisodol Extra Tablets;
Cobadex; Diovol; Infacol;
Kolanticon Gel; Maalox Plus
Suspension; Maalox Plus Tablets;
Piptalin; Siopel; Sprilon;
Vaseline Dermacare; Vasogen Cream.**

Dimotane Expectorant
(Whitehall Laboratories) is a proprietary,
non-prescription COMPOUND PREPARATION
of the EXPECTORANT drug guaiphenesin,
the ANTIHISTAMINE brompheniramine
maleate and the SYMPATHOMIMETIC and
DECONGESTANT drug pseudoephedrine
hydrochloride. It can be used for the
symptomatic relief of upper respiratory
tract disorders. It is available as a liquid
and is not normally given to children
under two years, except on medical
advice.
✚▲ side-effects/warning: see
BROMPHENIRAMINE MALEATE; GUAIPHENESIN;
PSEUDOEPHEDRINE HYDROCHLORIDE

Dimotane with Codeine
(Whitehall Laboratories) is a
proprietary, non-prescription COMPOUND
PREPARATION of the ANTITUSSIVE drug
codeine phosphate, the ANTIHISTAMINE
brompheniramine maleate and the
SYMPATHOMIMETIC and VASOCONSTRICTOR
drug pseudoephedrine hydrochloride. It
can be used for the symptomatic relief of
coughs associated with colds. It is
available as a liquid and is not normally
given to children under two years, except
on medical advice.
✚▲ side-effects/warning: see
BROMPHENIRAMINE MALEATE;

D

CODEINE PHOSPHATE; PSEUDOEPHEDRINE HYDROCHLORIDE

Dimotane with Codeine Paediatric

(Whitehall Laboratories) is a proprietary, non-prescription COMPOUND PREPARATION of the ANTITUSSIVE drug codeine phosphate, the ANTIHISTAMINE brompheniramine maleate and the SYMPATHOMIMETIC and VASOCONSTRICTOR drug pseudoephedrine hydrochloride. It can be used for the symptomatic relief of coughs associated with colds and other respiratory disorders in children. It is available as a liquid and is not normally given to children under two years, except on medical advice.

✚▲ side-effects/warning: see BROMPHENIRAMINE MALEATE; CODEINE PHOSPHATE; PSEUDOEPHEDRINE HYDROCHLORIDE

Dimotapp Elixir

(Whitehall Laboratories) is a proprietary, non-prescription COMPOUND PREPARATION of the SYMPATHOMIMETIC and DECONGESTANT drugs phenylpropanolamine hydrochloride and phenylephrine hydrochloride and the ANTIHISTAMINE brompheniramine maleate. It can be used for the relief of upper respiratory tract disorders, including congestion, hypersecretion sinusitis and rhinitis. It is available as an elixir and is not normally given to children under two years, except on medical advice.

✚▲ side-effects/warning: see BROMPHENIRAMINE MALEATE; PHENYLEPHRINE HYDROCHLORIDE; PHENYLPROPANOLAMINE HYDROCHLORIDE

Dimotapp Elixir Paediatric

(Whitehall Laboratories) is a proprietary, non-prescription COMPOUND PREPARATION of the SYMPATHOMIMETIC

and DECONGESTANT drugs phenylpropanolamine hydrochloride and phenylephrine hydrochloride and the ANTIHISTAMINE brompheniramine maleate. It can be used for the relief of upper respiratory tract disorders, including congestion, hypersecretion sinusitis and rhinitis. It is available as an elixir and is not normally given to children under two years, except on medical advice.

✚▲ side-effects/warning: see BROMPHENIRAMINE MALEATE; PHENYLEPHRINE HYDROCHLORIDE; PHENYLPROPANOLAMINE HYDROCHLORIDE

Dimotapp LA Tablets

(Whitehall Laboratories) is a proprietary, non-prescription COMPOUND PREPARATION of the SYMPATHOMIMETIC and DECONGESTANT drugs phenylpropanolamine hydrochloride and phenylephrine hydrochloride and the ANTIHISTAMINE brompheniramine maleate. It can be used for the relief of upper respiratory tract disorders, including congestion, hypersecretion sinusitis and rhinitis. It is available as modified-release tablets and is not normally given to children, except on medical advice.

✚▲ side-effects/warning: see BROMPHENIRAMINE MALEATE; PHENYLEPHRINE HYDROCHLORIDE; PHENYLPROPANOLAMINE HYDROCHLORIDE

Dindevan

(Goldshield) is a proprietary, prescription-only preparation of the ANTICOAGULANT drug phenindione. It can be used to treat and prevent thrombosis and is available as tablets.

✚▲ side-effects/warning: see PHENINDIONE

dinoprost

is the PROSTAGLANDIN $F_2\alpha$, which has the effect of causing contractions in the muscular walls of the uterus. It is used almost solely to induce termination of pregnancy (abortion). Administration is by injection, usually into the amniotic sac that surrounds the foetus.

✚▲ side-effects/warning: see under DINOPROSTONE

○ Related entry: Prostin F2 alpha

dinoprostone

is the PROSTAGLANDIN E$_2$, which has the effect of causing contractions in the muscular walls of the uterus. It can be used to induce labour or to assist in termination of pregnancy (abortion). Administration can be oral in the form of tablets, topical in the form of a gel, as vaginal tablets (pessaries), or by injection.

✚ side-effects: there may be nausea, vomiting, flushing and shivering, headache and dizziness, a raised temperature and diarrhoea, severe contractions of the uterus and increased white blood cell count. There will be uterine pain.

▲ warning: when administered by infusion, there may be redness at the injection site. It should be used with caution to those with certain gynaecological or obstetric disorders.

○ Related entries: Prepidil; Prostin E2

Diocalm

(SmithKline Beecham) is a proprietary, non-prescription preparation of the (OPIOID) ANTIDIARRHOEAL drug morphine hydrochloride, along with attapulgite (magnesium aluminium silicate) and activated attapulgite. It can be used for the relief of occasional diarrhoea and its associated pain and discomfort and is available as tablets.

✚▲ side-effects/warning: see under OPIOID

Diocalm Replenisher

(SmithKline Beecham) is a proprietary, non-prescription preparation of sodium chloride, sodium citrate, potassium chloride and glucose. It can be used as an electrolyte replacement in ANTIDIARRHOEAL treatment (usually in conjunction with another preparation that reduces diarrhoea, eg.DIOCALM or

DIOCALM ULTRA). It is available as a powder for the relief of occasional diarrhoea and its associated pain and discomfort.

✚▲ side-effects/warning: see SODIUM CHLORIDE

Diocalm Ultra

(SmithKline Beecham) is a proprietary, non-prescription preparation of the (OPIOID) ANTIDIARRHOEAL drug loperamide hydrochloride. It can be used for the symptomatic relief of acute diarrhoea and its associated pain and discomfort. It is available as capsules and is not normally given to children, except on medical advice.

✚▲ side-effects/warning: see LOPERAMIDE HYDROCHLORIDE

Diocaps

(Berk) is a proprietary, non-prescription preparation of the (OPIOID) ANTIDIARRHOEAL drug loperamide hydrochloride. It can be used for the symptomatic relief of acute diarrhoea and its associated pain and discomfort. It is available as capsules.

✚▲ side-effects/warning: see LOPERAMIDE HYDROCHLORIDE

Dioctyl

(Schwarz) is a proprietary, non-prescription preparation of the (*stimulant*) LAXATIVE docusate sodium. It can be used to relieve constipation and also to evacuate the rectum prior to abdominal procedures. It is available as capsules and a syrup (in two strengths, the weaker one is a *Paediatric Oral Solution*).

✚▲ side-effects/warning: see DOCUSATE SODIUM

Dioctyl Ear Drops

(Schwarz) is a proprietary, non-prescription preparation of docusate sodium (dioctyl sodium sulphosuccinate) and several other ingredients. It can be

D

used for the dissolution and removal of earwax.

✚▲ side-effects/warning: see DOCUSATE SODIUM

dioctyl sodium sulphosuccinate

See DOCUSATE SODIUM

Dioderm

(Dermal) is a proprietary, prescription-only preparation of the CORTICOSTEROID and ANTI-INFLAMMATORY drug hydrocortisone. It can be used to treat mild, inflammatory skin conditions, such as eczema and is available as a cream for topical application.

✚▲ side-effects/warning: see HYDROCORTISONE

Dioralyte

(Rhône-Poulenc Rorer) is a proprietary, non-prescription, preparation of sodium chloride, sodium bicarbonate, potassium chloride, citric acid and glucose. It can be used as an electrolyte and water replacement in dehydration or kidney disease. It is available as soluble tablets and an oral powder.

✚▲ side-effects/warning: see SODIUM CHLORIDE

Diovol

(Pharmax) is a proprietary, non-prescription COMPOUND PREPARATION of the ANTACIDS aluminium hydroxide and magnesium hydroxide and the ANTIFOAMING AGENT dimethicone. It can be used for the symptomatic relief of hyperacidity, hiatus hernia, flatulence and peptic ulcers. It is available as a liquid and is not normally given to children, except on medical advice.

✚▲ side-effects/warning: see ALUMINIUM HYDROXIDE; DIMETHICONE; MAGNESIUM HYDROXIDE

Dip/Ser

is an abbreviation for DIPHTHERIA ANTITOXIN.

Dipentum

(Pharmacia) is a proprietary, prescription-only preparation of the AMINOSALICYLATE drug olsalazine sodium. It can be used to treat patients who suffer from ulcerative colitis and is available as capsules.

✚▲ side-effects/warning: see OLSALAZINE SODIUM

diphenhydramine hydrochloride

is an ANTIHISTAMINE drug. It can be used for the symptomatic relief of allergic symptoms such as hay fever and urticaria (itchy skin rash) and is incorporated into a number of proprietary cough and cold preparations. It has marked SEDATIVE properties and can be used for the relief of occasional insomnia. It is administered in several ways, including orally as tablets, capsules, or syrups.

✚▲ side-effects/warning: see under ANTIHISTAMINE. Because of its sedative side-effects, the performance of skilled tasks such as driving may be impaired.

✪ Related entries: Benylin Chesty Coughs Original; Benylin Children's Coughs Original; Benylin Children's Coughs Sugar Free/Colour Free; Benylin Day and Night; Benylin Dry Coughs Original; Benylin with Codeine; Caladryl Cream; Caladryl Lotion; Medinex Night Time Syrup; Night Cold Comfort Capsules; Nytol; Propain Tablets

diphenoxylate hydrochloride

is an (OPIOID) ANTIDIARRHOEAL drug that is used to treat chronic diarrhoea. It is commonly used in combination with atropine sulphate to form a preparation known as co-phenotrope.

✚ side-effects: see under CODEINE PHOSPHATE; overdosage causes sedation.

Prolonged use may lead to impaired gastrointestinal function and eventual dependence.

▲ warning: overdosage is uncommon but does occur, particularly in young children. However, the symptoms of overdose (chiefly sedation) do not appear until some 48 hours after treatment, so monitoring of patients for at least this period is necessary. Fluid intake must be maintained during treatment. In elderly patients, monitoring is essential to detect possible faecal impaction. The drug should not be used in patients with gastrointestinal obstruction or jaundice. Care should be taken in patients with severe ulcerative colitis.

✪ Related entry: Lomotil

diphenylpyraline hydrochloride

is an ANTIHISTAMINE drug. It is used for the symptomatic relief of allergy such as hay fever and urticaria (itchy skin rash). It is also incorporated into some proprietary cold treatment preparations. Administration is oral in the form of capsules or syrup.

+▲ side-effects/warning: see under ANTIHISTAMINE. Because of its sedative side-effects, the performance of skilled tasks such as driving may be impaired.

✪ Related entries: Eskornade Capsules; Eskornade Syrup

Diphtheria Antitoxin

(Merieux) is a proprietary, prescription-only preparation of diphtheria antitoxin. It can be used to treat suspected cases of diphtheria and is available in a form for injection.

+▲ side-effects/warning: see under IMMUNIZATION

diphtheria antitoxin

(Dip/Ser) is a preparation that neutralizes the toxins produced by diphtheria bacteria (*Corynebacerium diphtheriae*), because IMMUNIZATION

it is not used for prevention, but only to provide *passive immunity* to people who have been exposed to suspected cases of diphtheria. Since the antitoxin is produced in horses, hypersensitivity reactions are common. Administration is by intramuscular injection.

+▲ side-effects/warning: see IMMUNIZATION

✪ Related entry: Diphtheria Antitoxin

diphtheria vaccines

for IMMUNIZATION are VACCINE preparations of inactivated, but still antigenic, toxins (toxoid) of the diphtheria bacteria *Corynebacterium diphtheriae* that provide active immunity to diphtheria. In most instances, they are not administered alone, but as a constituent in the *triple vaccine* ADSORBED DIPHTHERIA, TETANUS, AND PERTUSSIS VACCINE (DTPer/Vac/Ads), or as a *double vaccine* ADSORBED DIPHTHERIA AND TETANUS VACCINE (DT/Vac/Ads). They are used for the primary immunization of children and are administered by intramuscular or subcutaneous injection.

+▲ side effects/warning: see VACCINES

✪ Related entries: Adsorbed Diphtheria Vaccine; Adsorbed Diphtheria Vaccine for Adults; Diftavax; Adsorbed Diphtheria and Tetanus Vaccine for Adults and Adolescents; Trivac-AD

dipipanone

is a rapidly acting and powerful (OPIOID) NARCOTIC ANALGESIC drug. It is used in combination with an ANTI-EMETIC drug (the antihistamine cyclizine) for the relief of acute, moderate and severe pain. Its proprietary form is on the Controlled Drugs List. Administration (in the form of dipipanone hydrochloride) is oral as tablets.

+▲ side-effects/warning: see under OPIOID. It is less sedating than morphine, but in combination with an anti-emetic it is unsuitable for use in chronic pain therapy.

✪ Related entry: Diconal

D

dipivefrine hydrochloride
is a derivative of the SYMPATHOMIMETIC drug adrenaline and is converted in the body to adrenaline. It is often used in GLAUCOMA TREATMENT to reduce intraocular pressure (pressure in the eyeball) and is administered instead of adrenaline because it is thought to pass more rapidly through the cornea. Administration is topical in the form of eye-drops.
+▲ side-effects/warning: see under ADRENALINE
❍ Related entry: Propine

dipotassium clorazepate
See CLORAZEPATE DIPOTASSIUM

Diprivan
(Zeneca) is a proprietary, prescription-only preparation of the GENERAL ANAESTHETIC drug propofol. It can be used for the induction and maintenance of anaesthesia and is available in a form for injection or infusion.
+▲ side-effects/warning: see PROPOFOL

Diprobase
(Schering-Plough) is a proprietary, non-prescription preparation of liquid paraffin (and other paraffins). It can be used as an EMOLLIENT and is available as an ointment and a cream.
+▲ side-effects/warning: see LIQUID PARAFFIN

Diprobath
(Schering-Plough) is a proprietary, non-prescription preparation of liquid paraffin (and isopropyl myristate). It can be used as an EMOLLIENT for dry skin and is available as a bath oil.
+▲ side-effects/warning: see LIQUID PARAFFIN

Diprosalic
(Schering-Plough) is a proprietary, prescription-only COMPOUND PREPARATION of the CORTICOSTEROID and ANTI-INFLAMMATORY drug betamethasone (as dipropionate) and the KERATOLYTIC agent salicylic acid. It can be used to treat severe inflammatory skin disorders such as eczema and psoriasis. It is available as an ointment and a scalp lotion for topical application.
+▲ side-effects/warning: see BETAMETHASONE; SALICYLIC ACID

Diprosone
(Schering-Plough) is a proprietary, prescription-only preparation of the CORTICOSTEROID and ANTI-INFLAMMATORY drug betamethasone (as dipropionate). It can be used to treat severe inflammatory skin disorders such as eczema and psoriasis. It is available as a cream, an ointment and a lotion for topical application.
+▲ side-effects/warning: see BETAMETHASONE

dipyridamole
is an ANTIPLATELET (antithrombotic) drug. It is used to prevent thrombosis (blood-clot formation), but does not have the usual action of an ANTICOAGULANT. It seems to work by stopping platelets sticking to one another or to surgically inserted tubes and valves (particularly artificial heart valves). Administration can be oral as tablets or by injection.
+ side-effects: there may be nausea and diarrhoea, headache and low blood pressure.
▲ warning: it may cause hypotension or worsen migraine. There may be dangerous interactions with adenosine (which is used in heart conditions as an anti-arrhythmic). Administer with caution to patients with certain heart disorders.
❍ Related entry: Persantin

Dirythmin SA
(Astra) is a proprietary, prescription-only preparation of the ANTI-ARRHYTHMIC drug disopyramide (as disopyramide

phosphate). It is available as
modified-release tablets (*Durules*).
✚▲ side-effects/warning: see DISOPYRAMIDE

*disinfectant

is a term that is used to describe agents
which destroy micro-organisms, or inhibit
their activity to such extent that they are
less or no longer harmful to health. It can
be applied to agents used on inanimate
objects (including surgical equipment,
catheters, etc.) as well as to preparations
that are used to treat the skin and living
tissue (although in the latter case the
name ANTISEPTIC is often used instead).

Disipal

(Yamanouchi) is a proprietary,
prescription-only preparation of the
ANTICHOLINERGIC drug orphenadrine
hydrochloride. It can be used to relieve
some of the symptoms of parkinsonism,
especially muscle rigidity and the tendency
to produce an excess of saliva (see
ANTIPARKINSONISM). It also has the
capacity to treat these conditions, in some
cases, where they are produced by drugs.
It is available as tablets.
✚▲ side-effects/warning: see
ORPHENADRINE HYDROCHLORIDE

disodium etidronate

is a drug (a biphosphonate) used to treat
disorders of bone metabolism due to
HORMONE disorders, tumour-induced high
blood calcium levels (hypercalaemia) and
specifically to treat Paget's disease of the
bone. It is also available in a COMPOUND
PREPARATION with calcium carbonate to
treat established osteoporosis of the
vertebrae. It is administered by tablets or
by intravenous infusion.
✚ side-effects: there may be nausea and
diarrhoea. With high dosage, increased bone
pain and the risk of fractures. Rarely, a short-
lived loss of the sense of taste, skin reactions,
abdominal pain and constipation.
▲ warning: administer with caution to
patients with certain kidney disorders. It is not

for use in pregnancy or breast-feeding.
◎ Related entries: Didronel; Didronel
IV; Didronel PMO

disodium pamidronate

is a drug (a biphosphonate) used to treat
disorders of bone metabolism due to
HORMONE disorders and malignant
tumour-induced high blood calcium levels
(hypercalaemia). It is administered by
intravenous infusion.
✚ side-effects: there may be nausea and
diarrhoea, low blood calcium, blood upsets
and transient fever.
▲ warning: administer with caution to
patients with certain kidney disorders. It is not
for use in pregnancy or breast-feeding.
◎ Related entry: Aredia

disopyramide

is an ANTI-ARRHYTHMIC drug. It is used to
regularize the heartbeat, especially
following a heart attack (myocardial
infarction). Administration, as
disopyramide or disopyramide phosphate,
can be oral as capsules, modified-release
capsules, modified-release tablets, or by
slow intravenous injection.
✚ side-effects: there may be hypotension,
gastrointestinal disturbances, dry mouth,
blurred vision, urinary retention and effects
on the heart.
▲ warning: it should be administered with
caution to patients with depressed heart
function (eg.heart failure), certain kidney or
liver disorders, glaucoma, or who are
pregnant or breast-feeding. It should not be
given to patients with certain heart disorders.
◎ Related entries: Dirythmin SA;
Isomide CR; Rythmodan;
Rythmodan Retard

Disprin

(Reckitt & Colman) is a proprietary,
non-prescription preparation of the
(NSAID) NON-NARCOTIC ANALGESIC and
ANTIRHEUMATIC drug aspirin. It can be
used to treat mild to moderate pain and to
relieve flu and cold symptoms,

D

rheumatism and lumbago. It is available as soluble tablets and is not normally given to children under 12 years, except on medical advice.

✚▲ side-effects/warning: see ASPIRIN

Disprin CV

(Reckitt & Colman) is a proprietary, non-prescription preparation of the ANTIPLATELET aggregation drug aspirin. It can be used to help prevent certain cardiovascular diseases, including heart attack.

✚▲ side-effects/warning: see ASPIRIN

Disprin Direct

(Reckitt & Colman) is a proprietary, non-prescription preparation of the (NSAID) NON-NARCOTIC ANALGESIC and ANTIRHEUMATIC drug aspirin. It can be used to treat mild to moderate pain, to relieve flu and cold symptoms and feverishness. It is available as chewable tablets and is not normally given to children under 12 years, except on medical advice.

✚▲ side-effects/warning: see ASPIRIN

Disprin Extra

(Reckitt & Colman) is a proprietary, non-prescription COMPOUND ANALGESIC preparation of the (NSAID) NON-NARCOTIC ANALGESIC and ANTIRHEUMATIC drug aspirin and the non-narcotic analgesic drug paracetamol. It can be used to treat mild to moderate pain, relieve rheumatic aches and pains and flu and cold symptoms. It is available as tablets and is not normally given to children under 12 years, except on medical advice.

✚▲ side-effects/warning: see ASPIRIN; PARACETAMOL

Disprol

(Reckitt & Colman) is a proprietary, non-prescription preparation of the NON-NARCOTIC ANALGESIC drug paracetamol. It can be used to treat mild to moderate pain, relieve flu and cold symptoms,

feverishness and rheumatic aches and pains. It is available as tablets and is not normally given to children under six years, except on medical advice.

✚▲ side-effects/warning: see PARACETAMOL

Disprol Infant

(Reckitt & Colman) is a proprietary, non-prescription preparation of the NON-NARCOTIC ANALGESIC and ANTIPYRETIC drug paracetamol (for children). It can be used to treat mild to moderate pain, including teething and to reduce high body temperature. It is available as a sugar-free suspension and is not normally given to infants under three months, except on medical advice.

✚▲ side-effects/warning: see PARACETAMOL

Disprol Junior

(Reckitt & Colman) is a proprietary, non-prescription preparation of the NON-NARCOTIC ANALGESIC and ANTIPYRETIC drug paracetamol (for children). It can be used to treat mild to moderate pain (including teething), relieve flu and cold symptoms, feverishness and to reduce high body temperature. It is available as effervescent tablets. Even as a paediatric preparation, however, it is not given to children under one year, except on medical advice.

✚▲ side-effects/warning: see PARACETAMOL

Distaclor

(Dista) is a proprietary, prescription-only preparation of the ANTIBACTERIAL and (CEPHALOSPORIN) ANTIBIOTIC drug cefaclor (as monohydrate). It can be used to treat a wide range of bacterial infections, particularly of the urinary tract. It is available as capsules and an oral suspension.

✚▲ side-effects/warning: see CEFACLOR

Distaclor MR

(Lilly) is a proprietary, prescription-only preparation of the ANTIBACTERIAL and (CEPHALOSPORIN) ANTIBIOTIC drug cefaclor (as monohydrate). It can be used to treat a wide range of bacterial infections, particularly of the urinary tract. It is available as tablets.

+▲ side-effects/warning: see CEFACLOR

Distalgesic

(Dista) is a proprietary, prescription-only COMPOUND ANALGESIC preparation of the (OPIOID) NARCOTIC ANALGESIC drug dextropropoxyphene hydrochloride and the NON-NARCOTIC ANALGESIC drug paracetamol (a combination known as CO-PROXAMOL). It can be used to relieve pain anywhere in the body and is available as tablets. It is not not normally given to children, except on medical advice.

+▲ side-effects/warning: see DEXTROPROPOXYPHENE HYDROCHLORIDE; PARACETAMOL

Distamine

(Dista) is a proprietary, prescription-only preparation of the CHELATING AGENT penicillamine. It can be used as an ANTIDOTE to copper or lead poisoning, to reduce copper levels in Wilson's disease and in the long-term treatment of rheumatoid arthritis. It is available as tablets.

+▲ side-effects/warning: see PENICILLAMINE

distigmine bromide

is an ANTICHOLINESTERASE drug, which enhances the effects of the NEUROTRANSMITTER acetylcholine (and certain cholinergic drugs). Because of this it has PARASYMPATHOMIMETIC actions and can be used to stimulate the bladder to treat urinary retention and the intestine to treat paralytic ileus. It can also be used to treat the neuromuscular transmission disorder myasthenia gravis. Administration is either oral as tablets or by injection.

+ side-effects: there may be nausea and vomiting, sweating and blurred vision, slow heart rate and colic.

▲ warning: it should not be administered to patients who suffer from urinary or intestinal blockage, or where increased activity of the intestine or bladder could be harmful. It should be administered with caution to patients with asthma, hyperthyroidism, parkinsonism, epilepsy, peptic ulcer, who have recently had a heart attack, or who are pregnant.

✪ Related entry: Ubretid

disulfiram

Is an ENZYME INHIBITOR, which blocks a stage in the break down of alcohol (ethanol) in the body with a resultant accumulation in a metabolite (acetaldehyde). If even only a very small amount of alcohol is taken, disulfiram causes very unpleasant, potentially dangerous, reactions – such as flushing, headache, palpitations, nausea and vomiting. Therefore, if an alcoholic takes disulfiram on a regular basis there is a powerful disincentive to drink alcoholic beverages. Administration is oral in the form of tablets.

+ side-effects: initial drowsiness and fatigue; nausea and vomiting; halitosis, reduced libido; rarely, there may be psychotic reactions, skin reactions, peripheral nerve and liver damage.

▲ warning: it should not be administered to patients with certain heart disorders, or who are pregnant. Simultaneous use of medications or toiletries containing forms of alcohol should also be avoided.

✪ Related entry: Antabuse 200

dithranol

is the most powerful drug presently used to treat chronic or milder forms of psoriasis in topical application and is incorporated in a number of preparations. Lesions are covered for a period with a dressing on which there is a preparation of dithranol in weak solution; the concentration is adjusted to suit individual response and tolerance of the associated skin irritation. It is thought to work by inhibiting cell division (antimitotic) and may be used in combination with KERATOLYTICS or with agents that have a

D

moisturizing effect (such as UREA). It may also be used in some preparations as dithranol triacetate.

✚ side-effects: irritation and a local sensation of burning.

▲ warning: it is not suitable for the treatment of acute forms of psoriasis. It stains skin, hair and fabrics. Avoid contact with healthy skin and the eyes.

○ Related entries: Anthranol; dithranol ointment, BP; Dithrocream; Dithrolan; Psoradrate; Psorin

dithranol ointment, BP

is a non-proprietary, prescription-only preparation of dithranol. It can be used for subacute and chronic psoriasis and is available as an ointment.

✚▲ side-effects/warning: see DITHRANOL

dithranol triacetate

See DITHRANOL

Dithrocream

(Dermal) is a proprietary, non-prescription preparation of dithranol. It can be used to treat subacute and chronic psoriasis and is available as an ointment in four strengths: 0.1% , 0.25%, 0.5% and 1%. A stronger version, 2%, is available only on prescription.

✚▲ side-effects/warning: see DITHRANOL

Dithrolan

(Dermal) is a proprietary, non-prescription COMPOUND PREPARATION of dithranol and salicylic acid. It can be used for subacute and chronic psoriasis and is available as an ointment.

✚▲ side-effects/warning: see DITHRANOL; SALICYLIC ACID

Ditropan

(Smith & Nephew) is a proprietary, prescription-only preparation of the ANTICHOLINERGIC drug oxybutynin hydrochloride. It can be used as an ANTISPASMODIC in the treatment of urinary frequency and incontinence and is

available as tablets and an elixir.

✚▲ side-effects/warning: see OXYBUTYNIN HYDROCHLORIDE

Diumide-K Continus

(ASTA Medica) is a proprietary, prescription-only COMPOUND PREPARATION of the (*loop*) DIURETIC drug frusemide and the potassium supplement potassium chloride. It can be used to treat oedema and is available as tablets, which should be swallowed whole with plenty of fluid at mealtimes or when in an upright posture.

✚▲ side-effects/warning: see FRUSEMIDE; POTASSIUM CHLORIDE

*diuretics

are drugs used to reduce fluid in the body by increasing the excretion of water and mineral salts by the kidney, so increasing urine production (hence 'water tablets'). They have a wide range of uses, because oedema (accumulation of fluid in the tissues) in sites such as the lungs, ankles and eyeball is symptomatic of a number of disorders. Reducing oedema is, in itself, of benefit in some of these disorders; and diuretic drugs may be used in acute pulmonary (lung) oedema, congestive heart failure, some liver and kidney disorders, glaucoma and in certain electrolyte disturbances such as hypercalaemia (raised calcium levels) and hyperkalaemia (raised potassium levels). Their most common use is in ANTIHYPERTENSIVE treatment, where their action of reducing oedema is of value in relieving the load on the heart, which then (over some days or weeks) gives way to a beneficial reduction in blood pressure (which seems to be associated with VASODILATOR action).

In relation to their specific actions and uses, the diuretics are divided into a number of distinct classes. *Osmotic diuretics* (eg.MANNITOL) are inert compounds secreted into the kidney proximal tubules and are not resorbed and therefore carry water and salts with

them into the urine. *Loop diuretics*
(eg.ETHACRYNIC ACID, FRUSEMIDE and
BUMETANIDE) have a very vigorous action
on the ascending tubules of the loop of
Henlé (inhibiting resorption of sodium
and water and also some potassium) and
are used for short periods, especially in
heart failure. *Thiazide* and *thiazide-like*
diuretics (eg.CHLOROTHIAZIDE,
HYDROCHLOROTHIAZIDE and XIPAMIDE) are
the most commonly used and have a
moderate action in inhibiting sodium
reabsorption at the distal tubule of the
kidney, allowing their prolonged use as
antihypertensives. But they may cause
potassium loss from the blood to the
urine, which needs correction (sometimes
through using preparations that combine
the diuretic and a potassium salt in
tablets). *Potassium-sparing* diuretics
(eg.AMILORIDE HYDROCHLORIDE,
TRIAMTERENE and SPIRONOLACTONE) have a
weak action on the distal tubule of the
kidney and – as the name suggests –
cause retention of potassium, making
them suitable for combination with some
of the other diuretic classes and for some
specific conditions. *Aldosterone
antagonists* (eg.POTASSIUM CANRENOATE
and spironolactone) work by blocking the
action of the normal mineralocorticoid
hormone aldosterone and this makes them
suitable for treating oedema associated
with aldosteronism, liver failure and
certain heart conditions.
Carbonic anhydrase inhibitors
(eg.ACETAZOLAMIDE) are weak diuretics
and are now rarely used to treat systemic
oedema, though they are useful in
reducing fluid in the anterior chamber of
the eye which causes glaucoma. In the
treatment of hypertension, diuretics are
commonly used in combination with other
classes of drugs, particularly BETA-
BLOCKERS.

Diurexan

(ASTA Medica) is a proprietary,
prescription-only preparation of the
(THIAZIDE-like) DIURETIC drug xipamide.
It can be used, either alone of in
conjunction with other drugs, in the
treatment of oedema and as an
ANTIHYPERTENSIVE. It is available as tablets.
✚▲ side-effects/warning: see XIPAMIDE

Dixarit

(Boehringer Ingelheim) is a proprietary,
prescription-only preparation of the
ANTISYMPATHETIC drug clonidine
hydrochloride. It can be used in
ANTIMIGRAINE treatment for reducing the
frequency of attacks and is available as
tablets.
✚▲ side-effects/warning: see
CLONIDINE HYDROCHLORIDE

Doan's Backache Pills

(Zyma Healthcare) is a proprietary, non-
prescription COMPOUND ANALGESIC
preparation of the (NSAID) NON-NARCOTIC
ANALGESIC and ANTIRHEUMATIC drug
paracetamol and the non-narcotic
analgesic drug sodium salicylate. It can be
used for the symptomatic relief of
rheumatic aches and pains, including
lumbago, backache, sprains and other
muscle pains. It is available as tablets.
✚▲ side-effects/warning: see PARACETAMOL;
SODIUM SALICYLATE

dobutamine hydrochloride

is a CARDIAC STIMULANT drug with
SYMPATHOMIMETIC and BETA-RECEPTOR
STIMULANT properties. It is used to treat
serious heart disorders, including
cardiogenic shock, septic shock, during
heart surgery and in cardiac infarction. It
works by increasing the heart's force of
contraction. Administration is by
intravenous infusion.
✚ side-effects: the heart rate following
treatment may increase too much and result
in hypertension.
▲ warning: administer with caution to
patients with severe hypotension (low blood
pressure).
◎ Related entries: Dobutrex; Posiject

217

D

Dobutrex

(Lilly) is a proprietary, prescription-only preparation of the CARDIAC STIMULANT drug dobutamine hydrochloride, which has SYMPATHOMIMETIC and BETA-RECEPTOR STIMULANT properties. It can be used to treat serious heart disorders, including cardiogenic shock, septic shock, during heart surgery and in cardiac infarction. It works by increasing the heart's force of contraction. It is available in a form for intravenous infusion.

✚▲ side-effects/warning: see DOBUTAMINE HYDROCHLORIDE

docusate sodium

(dioctyl sodium sulphosuccinate) is a LAXATIVE with both *stimulant* and *faecal softener* properties. It is used to relieve constipation and also to evacuate the rectum prior to abdominal X-rays. It is a constituent of many proprietary compound laxatives because it seems to have few adverse side-effects. It works like a surfactant, by applying a very thin film of low surface tension (similar to a detergent) over the surface of the intestinal wall. It can also be used to dissolve and remove earwax and is a constituent of proprietary ear-drop preparations. Administration can be as capsules, an oral solution, ear-drops, or an enema.

✚ side-effects: it may cause abdominal cramps.

▲ warning: rectal preparations should not be used in patients with haemorrhoids or an anal fissure.

✪ Related entries: co-danthrusate 50/60; Correctol; Dioctyl; Dioctyl Ear Drops; Fletchers' Enemette; Molcer; Norgalex Micro-enema; Normax; Waxsol

Do-Do Expectorant Linctus

(Zyma Healthcare) is a proprietary, non-prescription preparation of the EXPECTORANT guaiphenesin. It can be used for the relief of productive and non-productive cough associated with irritation due to infection of the upper airways. It is not normally given to children under six years, except on medical advice.

✚▲ side-effects/warning: see GUAIPHENESIN

Do-Do Tablets

(Zyma Healthcare) is a proprietary, non-prescription COMPOUND PREPARATION of the SYMPATHOMIMETIC and DECONGESTANT drug ephedrine hydrochloride, the BRONCHODILATOR drug theophylline anhydrous and the STIMULANT caffeine. It can be used for the relief of bronchial cough, wheezing and breathlessness and to help clear the chest after infections. It is available as tablets and is not normally given to children under 12 years, except on medical advice.

✚▲ side-effects/warning: see CAFFEINE; EPHEDRINE HYDROCHLORIDE; THEOPHYLLINE

Dolmatil

(Delandale) is a proprietary, prescription-only preparation of the ANTIPSYCHOTIC drug sulpiride. It can be used to treat schizophrenia and also other conditions that may cause tremor, tics, involuntary movements, or utterances (such as in Gilles de la Tourette syndrome). It is available as tablets.

✚▲ side-effects/warning: see SULPIRIDE

Dolobid

(Morson) is a proprietary, prescription-only preparation of the (NSAID) NON-NARCOTIC ANALGESIC and ANTIRHEUMATIC drug diflunisal. It can be used to treat moderate to mild pain, the pain of rheumatic disease and other musculoskeletal disorders and period pain. It is available as tablets and is not normally given to children, except on medical advice.

✚▲ side-effects/warning: see DIFLUNISAL

Doloxene

(Lilly) is a proprietary, prescription-only

preparation of the (OPIOID) NARCOTIC ANALGESIC drug dextropropoxyphene hydrochloride. It can be used to treat mild to moderate pain anywhere in the body. It is available as capsules and is not normally given to children, except on medical advice.

✚▲ side-effects/warning: see DEXTROPROPOXYPHENE HYDROCHLORIDE

Doloxene Compound

(Lilly) is a proprietary, prescription-only COMPOUND ANALGESIC preparation of the (NSAID) NON-NARCOTIC ANALGESIC and ANTIRHEUMATIC drug aspirin, the (OPIOID) NARCOTIC ANALGESIC drug dextropropoxyphene (as napsylate) and the STIMULANT caffeine. It can be used to treat mild to moderate pain and is available as capsules.

✚▲ side-effects/warning: see ASPIRIN; CAFFEINE; DEXTROPROPOXYPHENE HYDROCHLORIDE

Domical

(Berk) is a proprietary, prescription-only preparation of the (TRICYCLIC) ANTIDEPRESSANT drug amitriptyline hydrochloride. It can be used to treat depressive illness, especially in cases where some degree of sedation is required and also to treat bed-wetting by children at night. It is available as tablets.

✚▲ side-effects/warning: see AMITRIPTYLINE HYDROCHLORIDE

domiphen bromide

is an ANTISEPTIC agent that is used in throat lozenges.

◒ Related entry: Bradosol Plus

domperidone

is an ANTI-EMETIC and ANTINAUSEANT drug. It is thought to work, in part, as a DOPAMINE antagonist and is used particularly for the relief of nausea and vomiting in patients undergoing treatment with CYTOTOXIC DRUGS. It is also used to prevent vomiting in patients treated for parkinsonism with the drugs levodopa or bromocriptine. Administration is oral in the form of tablets or a suspension, or topical as suppositories.

✚ side-effects: occasionally, spontaneous lactation in women or the development of feminine breasts in men may occur; rashes and changes in libido.

▲ warning: it should be administered with caution to those who suffer from impaired kidney function, or who are pregnant or breast-feeding.

◒ Related entry: Motilium

Dopacard

(Porton) is a proprietary, prescription-only preparation of the CARDIAC STIMULANT and SYMPATHOMIMETIC drug dopexamine hydrochloride. It can be used for the treatment of heart conditions where moderate stimulation of the force of heartbeat with vasodilatation is required in heart failure associated with heart surgery. It is available in a form for intravenous infusion.

✚▲ side-effects/warning: see DOPEXAMINE HYDROCHLORIDE

Dopamet

(Berk) is a proprietary, prescription-only preparation of the ANTISYMPATHETIC drug methyldopa. It can be used in ANTIHYPERTENSIVE treatment and is available as tablets.

✚▲ side-effects/warning: see METHYLDOPA

dopamine

is a NEUROTRANSMITTER and is chemically a catecholamine (like ADRENALINE and NORADRENALINE). It is both an intermediate product in the biosynthetic pathway in the brain and sympathetic nervous system that manufactures and stores noradrenaline and adrenaline and a neurotransmitter in its own right in relaying nerve messages. It is particularly concentrated in the brain and in the adrenal glands. It is possible that some psychoses may in part be caused by

D

abnormalities in the metabolism of dopamine, because drugs that prevent some of its actions (dopamine-receptor antagonists; eg.CHLORPROMAZINE HYDROCHLORIDE, HALOPERIDOL, or PIMOZIDE) can be used as ANTIPSYCHOTICS to relieve some schizophrenic symptoms. Conversely, drugs that lead to increased dopamine production or concentrations in the brain (eg.LEVODOPA) play an important part in the therapy of parkinsonism and drugs that mimic some aspects of the action of dopamine in the brain (eg.BROMOCRIPTINE) can be used both for ANTIPARKINSONISM treatment and to relieve a number of hormone disorders. In the periphery (that is, in the body rather than the brain), dopamine hydrochloride may be administered therapeutically in the treatment of the cardiogenic shock associated with a heart attack or heart surgery, when its beneficial actions are thought to result partly through actions at beta-receptors in the heart and partly at dopamine receptors in blood vessels. Administration of dopamine is by injection or infusion.

✚ side-effects: there may be nausea and vomiting, changes in heart rate and blood pressure, the fingertips and toes may become cold due to constriction of blood vessels.

▲ warning: dopamine hydrochloride should not be administered to patients who suffer from phaeochromocytoma or heartbeat irregularities.

⊘ Related entries: Dopamine Hydrochloride in Dextrose (Glucose) Injection; Intropin; Select-A-Jet Dopamine

dopamine hydrochloride

is the chemical form of the naturally occurring DOPAMINE that is used in medicine.

Dopamine Hydrochloride in Dextrose (Glucose) Injection

(Abbott) is a proprietary, prescription-

only preparation of the SYMPATHOMIMETIC and CARDIAC STIMULANT drug dopamine (as dopamine hydrochloride). It is used to treat cardiogenic shock following a heart attack or during heart surgery. It is available in a form for infusion.

✚▲ side-effects/warning: see DOPAMINE

dopexamine hydrochloride

is a SYMPATHOMIMETIC and CARDIAC STIMULANT drug that is used for the treatment of heart conditions where moderate stimulation of the force of heartbeat with vasodilatation is required in heart failure associated with heart surgery. Its beneficial actions are thought partly to result from stimulation of beta-receptors in the heart and partly of dopamine receptors in the kidney. It is available in a form for intravenous infusion.

✚ side-effects: there may be stimulation of the rate of heartbeat, irregular heartbeats; also, angina pain, nausea, vomiting and muscle tremor.

▲ warning: it should not be used in patients with certain heart outlet obstructions (eg.aortic stenosis), with low blood platelets and with certain endocrine disorders (phaeochromocytoma). Administer with care to those with myocardial infarction (damage to heart muscle, usually after a heart attack) and recent angina, who have low blood potassium, or are hyperglycaemic. Various blood parameters should be monitored (eg.blood pressure, potassium and glucose levels and pulse). Withdrawal of treatment should be gradual.

⊘ Related entry: Dopacard

Dopram

(Wyeth) is a proprietary, prescription-only preparation of the respiratory stimulant drug doxapram hydrochloride. It can be used to relieve severe respiratory difficulties in patients with chronic obstructive airways disease or who undergo respiratory depression following major surgery, particularly where ventilatory support is not possible. It is

available in a form for intranvenous infusion or injection.
+▲ side-effects/warning: see DOXAPRAM HYDROCHLORIDE

Doralese

(Bencard) is a proprietary, prescription-only preparation of the ALPHA-ADRENOCEPTOR BLOCKER drug indoramin. It can be used to treat urinary retention because of its SMOOTH MUSCLE RELAXANT properties (for example, in benign prostatic hyperplasia). It is available as tablets.
+▲ side-effects/warning: see INDORAMIN

Dormonoct

(Roussel) is a proprietary, prescription-only preparation of the BENZODIAZEPINE drug flurazepam. It can be used as a relatively long-acting HYPNOTIC for the short-term treatment of insomnia, where a degree of sedation during the daytime is acceptable. It is available as capsules.
+▲ side-effects/warning: see under BENZODIAZEPINE

Dostinex

(Farmitalia Carlo Erba) is a proprietary, prescription-only preparation of the drug cabergoline. It is used primarily to treat parkinsonism, but not the parkinsonian symptoms caused by certain drug therapies (see ANTIPARKINSONISM) and may also be used to treat a number of other hormonal disorders. It is available as tablets and capsules.
+▲ side-effects/warning: see CABERGOLINE

Dothapax

(Ashbourne) is a proprietary, prescription-only preparation of the (TRICYCLIC) ANTIDEPRESSANT drug dothiepin hydrochloride. It can be used to treat depressive illness, especially in cases where some degree of sedation is required. It is available as tablets and capsules.

+▲ side-effects/warning: see DOTHIEPIN HYDROCHLORIDE

dothiepin hydrochloride

is an ANTIDEPRESSANT drug of the TRICYCLIC group. It can be used to treat depressive illness, especially in cases where some degree of sedation is required. Administration is oral in the form of capsules or tablets.
+▲ side-effects/warning: see under AMITRIPTYLINE HYDROCHLORIDE
○ Related entries: Dothapax; Prepadine; Prothiaden

Double Check

(FP) is a proprietary, non-prescription SPERMICIDAL CONTRACEPTIVE, which is used in combination with barrier methods of contraception (such as a condom). It is available as pessaries containing nonoxinol.
+▲ side-effects/warning: see NONOXINOL

Dovonex

(Leo) is a proprietary, prescription-only preparation of calcipotriol. It can be used for psoriasis and is available as an ointment, a cream and a scalp solution.
+▲ side-effects/warning: see CALCIPOTRIOL

doxapram hydrochloride

is a respiratory stimulant drug. It is used to relieve severe respiratory difficulties in patients who suffer from chronic obstructive airways disease, or who undergo respiratory depression following major surgery, particularly in cases where ventilatory support is not possible. Administration is by injection or intravenous infusion.
+ side-effects: increase in blood pressure and heart rate; dizziness.
▲ warning: it should not be administered to patients with severe hypertension, coronary artery disease, or thyrotoxicosis. Administer with care to those with epilepsy or liver impairment.
○ Related entry: Dopram

D

doxazosin

is an ALPHA-ADRENOCEPTOR BLOCKER drug,
which is used as an ANTIHYPERTENSIVE
treatment, often in conjunction with
other antihypertensives (eg. BETA-
BLOCKERS or (THIAZIDE) DIURETICS).
Administration is oral in the form of
tablets.

✚ side-effects: postural hypotension (fall in
blood pressure on standing); dizziness;
vertigo, headache, tiredness and oedema.

▲ warning: initially, it may cause marked
postural hypotension, so the patient should lie
down, or doses should be given on retiring to
bed. It may cause drowsiness and so a
patient's ability to drive or operate machinery
may be impaired.

● Related entry: Cardura

doxepin

is an ANTIDEPRESSANT drug of the
TRICYCLIC group. It can be used, as
doxepin hydrochloride, to treat depressive
illness, especially in cases where some
degree of sedation is required.
Administration is oral in the form of
capsules.

✚▲ side-effects/warning: see under
AMITRIPTYLINE HYDROCHLORIDE. It should
not be used when breast-feeding.

● Related entry: Sinequan

doxorubicin hydrochloride

is a CYTOTOXIC DRUG (an ANTIBIOTIC
in origin), which is used as an
ANTICANCER treatment particularly
for acute leukaemia, lymphomas and
solid tumours (eg.some bladder
tumours). Administration is by
intravenous infusion or bladder
instillation.

✚▲ side-effects/warning: see CYTOTOXIC
DRUGS. Administer with care to patients with
cardiovascular disease because it has effects
on the heart.

● Related entries:
Doxorubicin Rapid Dissolution;
Doxorubicin Solution for Injection

Doxorubicin Rapid Dissolution

(Pharmacia) is a proprietary,
prescription-only preparation of the
(CYTOTOXIC) ANTICANCER drug doxorubicin
hydrochloride. It is used particularly to
treat acute leukaemias, lymphomas and
some solid tumours and is available in a
form for infusion.

✚▲ side-effects/warning: see
DOXORUBICIN HYDROCHLORIDE

Doxorubicin Solution for Injection

(Pharmacia) is a proprietary,
prescription-only preparation of the
(CYTOTOXIC) ANTICANCER drug doxorubicin
hydrochloride. It is used particularly to
treat acute leukaemias, lymphomas and
some solid tumours and is available in a
form for intravenous infusion.

✚▲ side-effects/warning: see
DOXORUBICIN HYDROCHLORIDE

doxycycline

is a broad-spectrum ANTIBACTERIAL and
ANTIBIOTIC drug, which is one of the
TETRACYCLINES. It can be used to treat
many kinds of infection, for example, of
the respiratory and genital tracts, acne,
chronic sinusitis and prostatitis. It can
also be used, in combination with other
drugs, to treat brucellosis and pelvic
inflammatory disease. Administration is
oral as tablets, capsules, or soluble
tablets.

✚▲ side-effects/warning: see under
TETRACYCLINE; it can be used in patients with
kidney impairment, but not with porphyria.

● Related entries: Cyclodox; Demix;
Doxylar; Nordox; Ramysis; Vibramycin;
Vibramycin D

doxylamine succinate

is an ANTIHISTAMINE drug incorporated
into a proprietary ANALGESIC preparation.

✚▲ side-effects/warning: see under
ANTIHISTAMINE

● Related entry: Syndol

Doxylar

(Lagap) is a proprietary, prescription-only preparation of the ANTIBACTERIAL and (TETRACYCLINE) ANTIBIOTIC drug doxycycline. It can be used to treat infections of many kinds and is available as capsules.

+▲ side-effects/warning: see DOXYCYCLINE

Dozic

(RP Drugs) is a proprietary, prescription-only preparation of the ANTIPSYCHOTIC drug haloperidol. It can be used to treat psychoses, especially schizophrenia and the hyperactive, euphoric condition, mania and to tranquillize patients undergoing behavioural disturbance. It can also be used in the short-term treatment of severe anxiety and to treat some involuntary motor disturbances (and also intractable hiccup). It is available as an oral liquid.

+▲ side-effects/warning: see HALOPERIDOL

Dramamine

(Searle) is a proprietary, non-prescription preparation of the ANTIHISTAMINE and ANTINAUSEANT drug dimenhydrinate. It can be used to treat nausea and vomiting, particularly when it is associated with motion sickness, disorders of the balance function of the inner ear and vertigo. It is available as tablets and is not normally given to children under one year, except on medical advice.

+▲ side-effects/warning: see DIMENHYDRINATE

Drapolene Cream

(Wellcome) is a proprietary, non-prescription COMPOUND PREPARATION of the ANTISEPTIC agents benzalkonium chloride and cetrimide. It can be used for the relief of nappy rash and to dress minor burns and wounds. It is available as a cream.

+▲ side-effects/warning: see BENZALKONIUM CHLORIDE; CETRIMIDE

Driclor

(Stiefel) is a proprietary, non-prescription preparation of aluminium chloride (as hexahydrate). It can be used as an antiperspirant to treat hyperhidrosis (excessive sweating) and is available in a roll-on applicator.

+▲ side-effects/warning: see ALUMINIUM CHLORIDE

DriedTub/Vac/BCG

See BACILLUS CALMETTE-GUÉRIN VACCINE, DRIED

Dristan Decongestant Tablets

(Whitehall Laboratories) is a proprietary, non-prescription COMPOUND PREPARATION of the (NSAID) NON-NARCOTIC ANALGESIC and ANTIRHEUMATIC drug aspirin, the SYMPATHOMIMETIC and DECONGESTANT drug phenylephrine hydrochloride, the ANTIHISTAMINE chlorpheniramine maleate and the STIMULANT caffeine. It can be used to relieve cold and flu symptoms and is available as tablets. It is not normally given to children under six years, except on medical advice.

+▲ side-effects/warning: see ASPIRIN; CAFFEINE; CHLORPHENIRAMINE MALEATE; PHENYLEPHRINE HYDROCHLORIDE

Dristan Nasal Spray

(Whitehall Laboratories) is a proprietary, non-prescription preparation of the SYMPATHOMIMETIC drug oxymetazoline hydrochloride. It can be used as a NASAL DECONGESTANT for the relief of rhinitis in a head cold and is available as a nasal spray. It is not normally given to children under six years, except on medical advice.

+▲ side-effects/warning: see OXYMETAZOLINE HYDROCHLORIDE

Drogenil

(Schering-Plough) is a proprietary, prescription-only preparation of the anti-androgen, HORMONE ANTAGONIST drug flutamide. It can be used as an ANTICANCER

D

drug to treat cancer of the prostate and is available as tablets.
✚▲ side-effects/warning: see
FLUTAMIDE

Droleptan

(Janssen) is a proprietary, prescription-only preparation of the ANTIPSYCHOTIC drug droperidol. It can be used primarily in emergencies to subdue or soothe psychotic (particularly manic) patients during behavioural disturbances. It can also be used in patients about to undergo certain diagnostic procedures that may be difficult or painful, because it promotes a sensation of detachment and to treat nausea and vomiting caused by chemotherapy. It is available as tablets, a liquid and in a form for injection.
✚▲ side-effects/warning: see DROPERIDOL

droperidol

is an ANTIPSYCHOTIC drug. It is used primarily in emergencies to subdue or soothe psychotic (particularly manic) patients during behavioural disturbances. It is also used in patients about to undergo certain diagnostic procedures that may be difficult or painful, because it promotes a sensation of detachment and to treat nausea and vomiting caused by chemotherapy. Administration is either oral as tablets or a liquid, or by injection.
✚▲ side-effects/warning: see under
HALOPERIDOL
✪ Related entry: Droleptan

Dryptal

(Berk) is a proprietary, prescription-only preparation of the (*loop*) DIURETIC drug frusemide. It can be used to treat oedema, particularly pulmonary (lung) oedema in patients with chronic heart failure and low urine production due to kidney failure (oliguria). It is available as tablets.
✚▲ side-effects/warning: see FRUSEMIDE

DTIC-Dome

(Bayer) is a proprietary, prescription-only

preparation of the (CYTOTOXIC) ANTICANCER drug dacarbazine. It can be used in the treatment of melanoma, some soft-tissue sarcomas and the lymphatic cancer Hodgkin's disease. It is available in a form for injection.
✚▲ side-effects/warning: see
DACARBAZINE

DTPer/Vac/Ads

See ADSORBED DIPHTHERIA, TETANUS AND PERTUSSIS VACCINE

DT/Vac/Ads

See ADSORBED DIPHTHERIA AND TETANUS VACCINE

Dubam

(Norma) is a proprietary, non-prescription COMPOUND PREPARATION of methyl salicylate, ethyl salicylate, glycol salicylate and methyl nicotinate, which all have COUNTER-IRRITANT, or RUBEFACIENT, actions. It can be used for the symptomatic relief of underlying muscle or joint pain and is available as an aerosol spray for application to the skin.
✚▲ side-effects/warning: see
ETHYL SALICYLATE; GLYCOL SALICYLATE;
METHYL NICOTINATE; METHYL SALICYLATE

Dulco-lax Suppositories

(Windsor Healthcare) is a proprietary, non-prescription preparation of the (*stimulant*) LAXATIVE bisacodyl. It can be used for the treatment of constipation and is available as suppositories. It is not normally given to children under ten years, except on medical advice.
✚▲ side-effects/warning: see BISACODYL

Dulco-lax Suppositories for Children

(Windsor Healthcare) is a proprietary, non-prescription preparation of the (*stimulant*) LAXATIVE bisacodyl. It can be used for the treatment of constipation and is available as suppositories.
✚▲ side-effects/warning: see BISACODYL

Dulco-lax Tablets

(Windsor Healthcare) is a proprietary, non-prescription preparation of the (*stimulant*) LAXATIVE bisacodyl. It can be used for the treatment of constipation and is available as tablets. It is not normally given to children under ten years, except on medical advice.

✚▲ side-effects/warning: see BISACODYL

Duofilm

(Stiefel) is a proprietary, non-prescription preparation of the KERATOLYTIC agent salicylic acid (with lactic acid). It can be used to remove warts and hard skin and is available as a liquid paint.

✚▲ side-effects/warning: see SALICYLIC ACID

Duovent

(Boehringer Ingelheim) is a proprietary, prescription-only COMPOUND PREPARATION of the SYMPATHOMIMETIC and BETA-RECEPTOR STIMULANT drug fenoterol hydrobromide and the ANTICHOLINERGIC drug ipratropium bromide, which both have BRONCHODILATOR properties. It can be used as an ANTI-ASTHMATIC and chronic bronchitis treatment and is available in a metered-dose *Autoinhaler*, as an aerosol and a nebulizer solution.

✚▲ side-effects/warning: see FENOTEROL HYDROBROMIDE; IPRATROPIUM BROMIDE

Duphalac

(Duphar) is a proprietary, non-prescription preparation of the (*osmotic*) LAXATIVE lactulose. It can be used to relieve constipation and is available as an oral solution.

✚▲ side-effects/warning: see LACTULOSE

Duphaston

(Duphar) is a proprietary, prescription-only preparation of the PROGESTOGEN dydrogesterone. It can be used to treat many conditions of hormonal deficiency in women, including menstrual problems, premenstrual syndrome, endometriosis, recurrent miscarriage and infertility and as part of HRT. It is available in the form of tablets.

✚▲ side-effects/warning: see DYDROGESTERONE

Duracreme

(LRC Products) is a proprietary, non-prescription SPERMICIDAL CONTRACEPTIVE that is used in combination with barrier methods of contraception (such as a condom). It is available as a cream containing nonoxinol.

✚▲ side-effects/warning: see NONOXINOL

Duragel

(LRC Products) is a proprietary, non-prescription SPERMICIDAL CONTRACEPTIVE that is used in combination with barrier methods of contraception (such as a condom). It is available as a gel containing nonoxinol.

✚▲ side-effects/warning: see NONOXINOL

Durogesic

(Janssen) is a proprietary, prescription-only preparation of the (OPIOID) NARCOTIC ANALGESIC drug fentanyl and is on the Controlled Drugs List. It can be used to treat moderate to severe pain and is available as skin patches.

✚▲ side-effects/warning: see FENTANYL

Duromine

(3M Health Care) is a proprietary, prescription-only preparation of the APPETITE SUPPRESSANT phentermine, which is a strong STIMULANT drug and on the Controlled Drugs List. It can be used in the treatment of obesity and is available as modified-release tablets.

✚▲ side-effects/warning: see PHENTERMINE

Dyazide

(SK&F) is a proprietary, prescription-only COMPOUND PREPARATION of the (THIAZIDE) DIURETIC drug hydrochlorothiazide and the (*potassium-sparing*) diuretic triamterene (a combination called co-triamterzide 50/25). It can be used in the

D

D

treatment of oedema and as an ANTIHYPERTENSIVE. It is available as tablets.
+▲ side-effects/warning: see HYDROCHLOROTHIAZIDE; TRIAMTERENE. Also, the urine may be coloured blue.

dydrogesterone

is a PROGESTOGEN, an analogue of the sex hormone PROGESTERONE, that is used to treat many conditions of hormonal deficiency in women, including menstrual problems, premenstrual syndrome, displacement of uterus-lining tissue (endometriosis), recurrent miscarriage and infertility and as part of HRT (hormone replacement therapy). Administration is oral in the form of tablets.
+▲ warning/side-effects: see under PROGESTOGEN. May cause breakthrough bleeding.
۞ Related entry: Duphaston

Dynese

(Galen) is a proprietary, non-prescription preparation of the ANTACID magaldrate. It can be used for the symptomatic relief of dyspepsia and is available as a sugar-free oral suspension.
+▲ side-effects/warning: see MAGALDRATE

Dysman 250

(Ashbourne) is a proprietary, prescription-only preparation of the (NSAID) NON-NARCOTIC ANALGESIC and ANTIRHEUMATIC drug mefenamic acid. It can be used to treat pain and inflammation in rheumatoid arthritis, osteoarthritis and other musculoskeletal disorders and period pain. It is available as capsules.
+▲ side-effects/warning: see MEFENAMIC ACID

Dysman 500

(Ashbourne) is a proprietary, prescription-only preparation of the (NSAID) NON-NARCOTIC ANALGESIC and ANTIRHEUMATIC drug mefenamic acid. It

can be used to treat pain and inflammation in rheumatoid arthritis, osteoarthritis and other musculoskeletal disorders and period pain. It is available as capsules.
+▲ side-effects/warning: see MEFENAMIC ACID

Dyspamet

(SK&F) is a proprietary preparation of the H$_2$-ANTAGONIST cimetidine. It is available on prescription or without a prescription in a limited amount and for short-term uses only. It can be used as an ULCER-HEALING DRUG for benign peptic ulcers (in the stomach or duodenum), gastro-oesophageal reflux, dyspepsia and associated conditions. It is available as chewable tablets (*Chewtab*) and an oral suspension.
+▲ side-effects/warning: see CIMETIDINE

Dysport

(Porton) is a proprietary, prescription-only preparation of botulinum A toxin-haemagglutin complex. It can be used for treating blepharospasm (a tight contraction of the eyelids) and one-sided facial spasm. It is available in a form for injection.

Dytac

(Pharmark) is a proprietary, prescription-only preparation of the (*potassium-sparing*) DIURETIC drug triamterene. It can be used to treat oedema and is available as capsules.
+▲ side-effects/warning: see TRIAMTERENE

Dytide

(Pharmark) is a proprietary, prescription-only COMPOUND PREPARATION of the (THIAZIDE) DIURETIC drug benzthiazide and the (*potassium-sparing*) diuretic triamterene. It can be used to treat oedema and as an ANTIHYPERTENSIVE. It is available as capsules.
+▲ side-effects/warning: see BENZTHIAZIDE; TRIAMTERENE

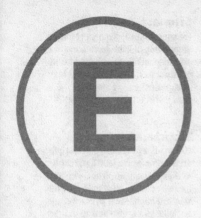

E45 Cream

(Crookes Healthcare) is a proprietary, non-prescription COMPOUND PREPARATION of liquid paraffin, white soft paraffin and wool fat. It can be used as an EMOLLIENT for dry skin and minor abrasions and burns. It is available as a cream, a wash and a bath oil.

✚▲ side-effects/warning: LIQUID PARAFFIN; WHITE SOFT PARAFFIN; WOOL FAT

Ebufac

(DDSA Pharmaceuticals) is a proprietary, prescription-only preparation of the (NSAID) NON-NARCOTIC ANALGESIC and ANTIRHEUMATIC drug ibuprofen. It can be used to relieve pain, particularly the pain of rheumatic disease and other musculoskeletal disorders and is available as tablets.

✚▲ side-effects/warning: see IBUPROFEN

Econacort

(Squibb) is a proprietary, prescription-only COMPOUND PREPARATION of the CORTICOSTEROID drug hydrocortisone and the ANTIFUNGAL drug econazole nitrate. It can be used to treat inflammation in which there is fungal infection and is available as a cream for topical application.

✚▲ side-effects/warning: see ECONAZOLE NITRATE; HYDROCORTISONE

econazole nitrate

is a broad-spectrum (IMIDAZOLE) ANTIFUNGAL drug. It can be used to treat fungal infections of the skin, nails, or mucous membranes, such as vaginal candidiasis. Administration is by creams, ointments, vaginal inserts (pessaries), lotions, sprays, or dusting powders.

✚▲ side-effects/warning: see under CLOTRIMAZOLE

✪ Related entries: Econacort; Ecostatin; Gyno-Pevaryl; Pevaryl; Pevaryl TC

Ecostatin

(Squibb) is a proprietary, prescription-

E

only preparation of the ANTIFUNGAL drug econazole nitrate. It can be used primarily to treat fungal infections of the skin and mucous membranes, especially of the vagina and vulva. It is available as a cream, vaginal pessaries (the stronger form is called *Ecostatin 1*) and a *Twinpack* with pessaries and cream (the cream is available without prescription).

+▲ side-effects/warning: see ECONAZOLE NITRATE

Edecrin

(Merck, Sharp & Dohme) is a proprietary, prescription-only preparation of the (*loop*) DIURETIC drug ethacrynic acid. It can be used to treat oedema, particularly pulmonary (lung) oedema in patients with left ventricular and chronic heart failure and low urine production due to kidney failure (oliguria). It is available as tablets and in a form for injection or infusion.

+▲ side-effects/warning: see ETHACRYNIC ACID

edrophonium chloride

is an ANTICHOLINESTERASE drug that enhances the effects of the NEUROTRANSMITTER acetylcholine (and of certain cholinergic drugs). It has a short duration of action and can be used in the diagnosis of myasthenia gravis and at the termination of operations to reverse the actions of neuromuscular blocking agents (when it is often administered with atropine sulphate). Administration is by injection.

+▲ side-effects/warning: see under NEOSTIGMINE

❂ Related entry: Camsilon

Efalith

(Searle) is a proprietary, prescription-only COMPOUND PREPARATION of lithium succinate and zinc sulphate. It can be used for seborrhoeic dermatitis and is available as an ointment.

+▲ side-effects/warning: see LITHIUM SUCCINATE; ZINC SULPHATE

Efamast

(Searle) is a proprietary, prescripti(
preparation of gamolenic acid (in e
primrose oil). It can be used for th(
of breast pain (mastalgia) and is av
as capsules.

+▲ side-effects/warning: see GAMOLE
ACID

Efcortelan

(Glaxo) is a proprietary, prescripti(
preparation of the CORTICOSTEROID
ANTI-INFLAMMATORY drug hydrocorti
It can be used to treat mild inflamm
skin conditions such as eczema and
available as a cream and an ointme(
+▲ side-effects/warning: see
HYDROCORTISONE

Efcortesol

(Glaxo) is a proprietary, prescripti(
preparation of the CORTICOSTEROID
ANTI-INFLAMMATORY drug hydrocort(
(as sodium phosphate). It can be u
treat inflammation, especially
inflammation caused by allergy, to t
shock, or to make up a deficiency c
steroid hormones. It is available in
for injection.

+▲ side-effects/warning: see
HYDROCORTISONE

Efexor

(Wyeth) is a proprietary, prescripti(
preparation of the (SSRI) ANTIDEPR
drug venlafaxine. It can be used to
depressive illness and is available a
tablets.

+▲ side-effects/warning: see
VENLAFAXINE

Effercitrate

(Typharm) is a proprietary, non-
prescription preparation of potassi
citrate. It can be used as an alkalizi
agent for the relief of discomfort of
urinary tract infection and to make
urine alkaline. It is available as
effervescent tablets for solution.

+▲ side-effects/warning: see POTASSIUM
CITRATE

Efudix
(Roche) is a proprietary, prescription-only
preparation of the (CYTOTOXIC)
ANTICANCER drug fluorouracil. It can be
used to treat malignant skin lesions and is
available as a cream for topical
application.
+▲ side-effects/warning: see
FLUOROURACIL

Elantan
(Schwarz) is a proprietary preparation of
the VASODILATOR and ANTI-ANGINA drug
isosorbide mononitrate. It can be used to
treat and prevent angina pectoris and for
heart failure. It is available as tablets in a
non-prescription preparation, *Elantan 10*
and two prescription-only preparations,
Elantan 20 and *Elantan 40*.
+▲ side-effects/warning: see
ISOSORBIDE MONONITRATE

Elantan LA
(Schwarz) is a proprietary, non-
prescription preparation of the
VASODILATOR and ANTI-ANGINA drug
isosorbide mononitrate. It can be used to
treat and prevent angina pectoris. It is
available as modified-release capsules in
two forms, *Elantan LA 25* and *Elantan LA
50*.
+▲ side-effects/warning: see
ISOSORBIDE MONONITRATE

Elavil
(DDSA Pharmaceuticals) is a proprietary,
prescription-only preparation of the
(TRICYCLIC) ANTIDEPRESSANT drug
amitriptyline hydrochloride. It can be used
to treat depressive illness, especially in
cases where some degree of sedation is
required and has also been used to treat
bed-wetting by children at night. It is
available as tablets.
+▲ side-effects/warning: see AMITRIPTYLINE
HYDROCHLORIDE

Eldepryl
(Britannia) is a proprietary, prescription-
only preparation of the ANTIPARKINSONISM
drug selegiline. It can be used to assist in
the treatment of the symptoms of
parkinsonism and is available as tablets
and a liquid.
+▲ side-effects/warning: see
SELEGILINE

Eldisine
(Lilly) is a proprietary, prescription-only
preparation of the (CYTOTOXIC)
ANTICANCER drug vindesine sulphate. It can
be used to treat acute leukaemia,
lymphomas and some solid tumours. It is
available in a form for injection.
+▲ side-effects/warning: see
VINDESINE SULPHATE

*elixir
is a medicated liquid preparation for
taking by mouth, which is intended to
disguise a potentially unpleasant taste by
including a sweetening substance like
glycerol or alcohol and often with
aromatic agents.

Ellimans Universal Embrocation
(SmithKline Beecham) is a proprietary,
non-prescription preparation of
turpentine oil (with acetic acid). It has a
COUNTER-IRRITANT, or RUBEFACIENT, action
and can be applied to the skin for
symptomatic relief of underlying muscle
or joint pain. It is available as an
embrocation for topical application and is
not normally used for children under 12
years, except on medical advice.
+▲ side-effects/warning: see
TURPENTINE OIL

Eltroxin
(Goldshield) is a proprietary,
prescription-only preparation of thyroxine
sodium, which is a form of thyroid
hormone. It can be used to make up a
hormonal deficiency and to treat

E

associated symptoms. It is available as tablets.

✚▲ side-effects/warning: see THYROXINE SODIUM

Eludril Mouthwash

(Chefaro) is a proprietary, non-prescription COMPOUND PREPARATION of the ANTISEPTIC agents chlorhexidine (as gluconate) and chlorbutol. It can be used in the treatment and prevention of gingivitis, for oral hygiene and minor throat infections. It is not normally given to children, except on medical advice.

✚▲ side-effects/warning: see CHLORBUTOL; CHLORHEXIDINE

Eludril Spray

(Chefaro) is a proprietary, non-prescription COMPOUND PREPARATION of the ANTISEPTIC agent chlorhexidine (as gluconate) and the LOCAL ANAESTHETIC drug amethocaine hydrochloride. It can be used in the local treatment of mouth and throat conditions such as gingivitis and ulcers, minor infections of the throat and mouth and for oral hygiene. It is available as a pressurized spray and is not normally given to children, except on medical advice.

✚▲ side-effects/warning: see AMETHOCAINE HYDROCHLORIDE; CHLORHEXIDINE

Elyzol

(Dumex) is a proprietary, prescription-only preparation of the ANTIMICROBIAL drug metronidazole, which has ANTIBACTERIAL and ANTIPROTOZOAL actions. It can be used for the treatment of local infections in dental surgery and is available as a gel.

✚▲ side-effects/warning: see METRONIDAZOLE

Emblon

(Berk) is a proprietary, prescription-only preparation of the sex HORMONE ANTAGONIST drug tamoxifen, which, because it inhibits the effect of

OESTROGENS, is used primarily as an ANTICANCER treatment for cancers that depend on the presence of oestrogen in women, particularly breast cancer. It can also be used to treat certain conditions of infertility and is available as tablets.

✚▲ side-effects/warning: see TAMOXIFEN

Emcor

(Merck) is a proprietary, prescription-only preparation of the BETA-BLOCKER drug bisoprolol fumarate. It can be used as an ANTIHYPERTENSIVE treatment for raised blood pressure and as an ANTI-ANGINA treatment to relieve symptoms and improve exercise tolerance. It is available as tablets.

✚▲ side-effects/warning: see BISOPROLOL FUMARATE

Emeside

(LAB) is a proprietary, prescription-only preparation of the ANTICONVULSANT and ANTI-EPILEPTIC drug ethosuximide. It can be used to treat absence (petit mal), myoclonic and some other types of seizure. It is available as capsules and a syrup.

✚▲ side-effects/warning: see ETHOSUXIMIDE

*emetic

is a term used to describe any drug that causes vomiting (emesis). Emetics are used primarily to treat poisoning by non-corrosive substances when the patient is conscious, especially drugs taken in overdose. Some affect the vomiting centre in the brain and/or irritate the gastrointestinal tract. Among the best-known and most-used emetics is IPECACUANHA, but several drugs used as EXPECTORANTS can, in higher concentrations, also cause emesis.

Emflex

(Merck) is a proprietary, prescription-only preparation of the (NSAID) NON-NARCOTIC ANALGESIC and ANTIRHEUMATIC drug acemetacin. It can be used to treat the pain of rheumatic and other musculoskeletal disorders and for postoperative pain. It is available as capsules.

✚▲ side-effects/warning: see ACEMETACIN

Eminase

(Beecham) is a proprietary, prescription-only preparation of the FIBRINOLYTIC drug anistreplase. It can be used to treat myocardial infarction and is available in a form for injection.

✚▲ side-effects/warning: see ANISTREPLASE

Emla

(Astra) is a proprietary, prescription-only COMPOUND PREPARATION of the LOCAL ANAESTHETIC drugs lignocaine hydrochloride and prilocaine hydrochloride. It can be used for surface anaesthesia, including preparation for injections and is available as a cream.

l/s side-effects/warning: see lignocaine hydrochloride; prilocaine hydrochloride.

Emmolate

(Bio-Medical) is a proprietary, non-prescription preparation of liquid paraffin, along with acetylated wool alcohol. It has an EMOLLIENT action and can be used for dry skin. It is available as a bath oil.

✚▲ side-effects/warning: see LIQUID PARAFFIN

*emollients

are agents that soothe, soften and moisturize the skin, particularly when it is dry and scaling. They are usually emulsions of water, fats, waxes and oils (eg. LANOLIN and LIQUID PARAFFIN). Emollients can be used alone to help hydrate the skin, or combined with HYDRATING AGENTS such as UREA. A notable example of a skin condition that may be treated with emollients is atopic eczema, when the skin is very dry. They can be applied as creams, ointments, lotions, or added to bath water. Such preparations contain preservatives (eg. parabens) that

in some patients may worsen the condition by causing contact allergic dermatitis and similarly some patients are allergic to some of the major constituents (particularly lanolin or WOOL FAT). There are a number of additives that may help itchiness (eg. MENTHOL, camphor and PHENOL) and some preparations have a beneficial ASTRINGENT action (eg. ZINC OXIDE, CALAMINE). In conditions that also involve a skin infection, emollients may have an ANTIMICROBIAL or ANTIFUNGAL drug added to them, or, in cases of severe inflammation, ANTI-INFLAMMATORY and CORTICOSTEROID drugs may be incorporated.

Emulsiderm

(Dermal) is a proprietary, non-prescription preparation of the ANTISEPTIC agent benzalkonium chloride and the skin EMOLLIENT liquid paraffin (with isopropyl myristate). It is available as a liquid emulsion that can be added to a bath.

✚▲ side-effects/warning:
BENZALKONIUM CHLORIDE;
LIQUID PARAFFIN

emulsifying ointment

is a non-proprietary formulation comprising a combination of wax, white soft paraffin and liquid paraffin. It can be used as a base for medications that require topical application.

enalapril maleate

is an ACE INHIBITOR. It is a powerful VASODILATOR that can be used in ANTIHYPERTENSIVE treatment, HEART FAILURE TREATMENT and to prevent ischaemia (lack of blood supply) in patients with left ventricular failure. It is often used in conjunction with other classes of drug, particularly (THIAZIDE) DIURETICS. Administration is oral in the form of tablets.

✚▲ side-effects/warning: see under CAPTOPRIL

✪ Related entries: Innovace; Innozide

E

Endoxana

(ASTA Medica) is a proprietary, prescription-only preparation of the (CYTOTOXIC) ANTICANCER drug cyclophosphamide. It can be used to treat chronic lymphatic leukaemia, lymphomas and some solid tumours. It is available as tablets and a form for injection.

✚▲ side-effects/warning: see CYCLOPHOSPHAMIDE

Enflurane

(Abbott) is a proprietary preparation of the inhalant GENERAL ANAESTHETIC drug enflurane. It can be used for the induction and maintenance of anaesthesia during major surgery and is available in a form for inhalation.

✚▲ side-effects/warning: see ENFLURANE

enflurane

is an inhalant GENERAL ANAESTHETIC drug, which is similar to HALOTHANE. It is often used along with nitrous oxide-oxygen mixtures for the induction and maintenance of anaesthesia during major surgery. Administration is by inhalation.

✚ side-effects: it depresses heart function (lowers blood pressure) and respiration.

▲ warning: it is not to be used in patients with porphyria.

◎ Related entry: Enflurane

Engerix B

(SmithKline Beecham) is a proprietary, prescription-only VACCINE preparation of hepatitis B vaccine. It can be used to protect people at risk from infection with hepatitis B and is available in a form for injection.

✚▲ side-effects/warning: see HEPATITIS B VACCINE

Eno

(SmithKline Beecham) is a proprietary, non-prescription COMPOUND PREPARATION of the ANTACIDS calcium carbonate and sodium bicarbonate together with citric acid. It can be used for the symptomatic relief of indigestion, flatulence and nausea. It is available as a powder for making up as a sparkling drink and as a flavoured version called *Lemon Eno*. It is not normally given to children, except on medical advice.

✚▲ side-effects/warning: see CALCIUM CARBONATE; SODIUM BICARBONATE

enoxaparin

is a low molecular weight version of heparin. It has some advantages as an ANTICOAGULANT when used for long-duration prevention of venous thrombo-embolism, particularly in orthopaedic use. It is available in a form for injection.

✚▲ side-effects/warning: see under HEPARIN

◎ Related entry: Clexane

enoximone

is a PHOSPHODIESTERASE INHIBITOR. It is used in congestive HEART FAILURE TREATMENT, especially where other drugs have been unsuccessful. Administration is by intravenous injection or infusion.

✚ side-effects: there may be irregular heartbeats, hypotension, headache, nausea and vomiting, insomnia, chills and fever, diarrhoea, retention of urine and pain in the limbs.

▲ warning: it should be given with caution to patients with certain forms of heart failure and vascular disease. The blood pressure and electrocardiogram should be monitored.

◎ Related entry: Perfan

Entamizole

(Boots) is a proprietary, prescription-only preparation of the ANTIPROTOZOAL and AMOEBICIDAL drug diloxanide furoate. It can be used to treat chronic intestinal infection by *Entamoeba histolytica* and is available as tablets.

✚▲ side-effects/warning: see DILOXANIDE FUROATE

*enzyme inhibitor

drugs work by inhibiting enzymes, which are proteins that play an essential part in the metabolism by acting as catalysts in specific, necessary biochemical reactions. Certain drugs have been developed that act only on certain enzymes and so can be used to manipulate the biochemistry of the body.

For example, ANTICHOLINESTERASE drugs (eg. NEOSTIGMINE, PYRIDOSTIGMINE and PHYSOSTIGMINE) inhibit enzymes called cholinesterases, which are normally involved in the rapid break down of ACETYLCHOLINE (an important NEUROTRANSMITTER). Acetylcholine is released from *cholinergic* nerves and has many actions throughout the body. Consequently, since anticholinesterase drugs enhance the effects of acetylcholine on its release from these nerves, they can have a wide range of actions. Their actions at the junction of nerves with skeletal (voluntary) muscles are used in the diagnosis and treatment of the muscle weakness disease myasthenia gravis; also, at the end of surgical operations in which SKELETAL MUSCLE RELAXANTS have been used, the anaesthetist is able to reverse the muscle paralysis by injecting an anticholinesterase. In organs innervated by parasympathetic division of the autonomic nervous system, anticholinesterases cause an exaggeration of the nerves' actions, known as PARASYMPATHOMIMETIC actions and can be used for a number of purposes, such as stimulation of the bladder (in cases of urinary retention), the intestine (in paralytic ileus) and the pupil of the eye (on local application in glaucoma treatment). However, anticholinesterases have a number of undesirable side-effects, including slowing of the heart, constriction of the airways with excessive production of secretions and actions in the brain. In anticholinesterase poisoning, their diverse actions can be life-threatening. Chemicals with anticholinesterase properties are used as insecticides and in chemical warfare. ANTIDOTES are available to treat cases of poisoning, for example due to a farming accident.

MONOAMINE-OXIDASE INHIBITORS, or MAOIs, (eg. ISOCARBOXAZID, PHENELZINE and TRANYLCYPROMINE) are one of the three major classes of ANTIDEPRESSANT drugs. They work by inhibiting an enzyme in the brain that metabolizes monoamines (including NORADRENALINE and SEROTONIN), which results in a change of mood. However, this same enzyme detoxifies other amines, so if certain foods are eaten or medicines taken that contain amines (eg. sympathomimetic amines in cough and cold treatments), then dangerous side-effects could occur. MOCLOBEMIDE is a newly introduced MAOI drug that is an inhibitor of only one type of monoamine oxidase (type A) and is claimed to show less potentiation of the amine in foodstuffs.

ACE INHIBITORS (angiotensin-converting enzyme inhibitors), such as CAPTOPRIL, ENALAPRIL and RAMIPRIL, are drugs that are used as ANTIHYPERTENSIVES and in HEART FAILURE TREATMENT. They work by inhibiting the conversion of the natural circulating HORMONE angiotensin I to angiotensin II and because the latter form is a potent VASOCONSTRICTOR, the overall effect is VASODILATION with a HYPOTENSIVE action.

Further examples of enzyme inhibitor drugs include the CARBONIC ANHYDRASE INHIBITOR drugs (which are used for their DIURETIC actions and in GLAUCOMA TREATMENT), the PHOSPHODIESTERASE INHIBITORS (for congestive heart failure treatment), CARBIDOPA (in ANTIPARKINSONISM treatment), CLAVULANIC ACID (to prolong and enhance the effects of certain ANTIBIOTICS) and DISULFIRAM (which is used in the treatment of alcoholism).

Epanutin

(Parke-Davis) is a proprietary, prescription-only preparation of the ANTICONVULSANT and ANTI-EPILEPTIC drug

E phenytoin. It can be used to treat and prevent most forms of seizure and also the pain of trigeminal (facial) neuralgia. It is available as capsules, chewable tablets (*Epanutin Infatabs*) and as a liquid suspension.

✚▲ side-effects/warning: see PHENYTOIN

Epanutin Ready Mixed Parenteral

(Parke-Davis) is a proprietary, prescription-only preparation of the ANTICONVULSANT and ANTI-EPILEPTIC drug phenytoin. It can be used in the emergency treatment of status epilepticus and convulsive seizures during neurosurgical operations. It is available in a form for injection.

✚▲ side-effects/warning: see PHENYTOIN

ephedrine hydrochloride

is an ALKALOID that is a SYMPATHOMIMETIC drug (also called an *indirect sympathetic*, because it works indirectly through the release of NORADRENALINE from sympathetic nerve endings). It is occasionally used as a BRONCHODILATOR and VASOCONSTRICTOR, but is primarily used as an ANTI-ASTHMATIC and for chronic bronchitis and similar conditions, especially allergy-based ones (this is also the major use of the closely related drug PSEUDOEPHEDRINE). Overall, its effects are similar to those of ADRENALINE, except that in adults it is a quite powerful central nervous STIMULANT, though it has SEDATIVE properties in children. It is also used to treat bed-wetting in children and as a NASAL DECONGESTANT. Administration can be oral as tablets or as an elixir, or topical in the form of nose-drops.

✚ side-effects: there may be changes in heart rate and blood pressure, anxiety, restlessness, tremor, insomnia, dry mouth, cold fingertips and toes and changes in the prostate gland. When used as a nasal decongestant, it may cause irritation in the nose.

▲ warning: administer with caution to patients with certain heart, kidney and thyroid disorders, diabetes and hypertension; care should be taken to avoid interaction with other drugs.

✪ Related entries: Anestan Bronchial Tablets; CAM; Do-Do Tablets; Expulin Decongestant for Babies and Children (Linctus); Franol; Franol Plus; Franolyn for Chesty Coughs; Haymine; Nirolex

Epifoam

(Stafford-Miller) is a proprietary COMPOUND PREPARATION of the CORTICOSTEROID drug hydrocortisone (as acetate) and the LOCAL ANAESTHETIC drug pramoxine hydrochloride. It can be used in the treatment of inflammation and pain in the perineal region, especially in women who have undergone an episiotomy. It is available as a foam.

✚▲ side-effects/warning: see HYDROCORTISONE; PRAMOXINE HYDROCHLORIDE

Epilim

(Sanofi Winthrop) is a proprietary, prescription-only preparation of the ANTICONVULSANT and ANTI-EPILEPTIC drug sodium valproate. It can be used to treat all forms of epilepsy and is available as tablets, a liquid and a syrup.

✚▲ side-effects/warning: see SODIUM VALPROATE

Epilim Chrono

(Sanofi Winthrop) is a proprietary, prescription-only preparation of the ANTICONVULSANT and ANTI-EPILEPTIC drug sodium valproate. It can be used to treat all forms of epilepsy and is available as modified-release tablets.

✚▲ side-effects/warning: see SODIUM VALPROATE

Epilim Intravenous

(Sanofi Winthrop) is a proprietary, prescription-only preparation of the ANTICONVULSANT and ANTI-EPILEPTIC drug sodium valproate. It can be used to treat

all forms of epilepsy and is available in a form for injection.
+▲ side-effects/warning: see SODIUM VALPROATE

Epimaz
(Norton) is a proprietary, prescription-only preparation of the ANTICONVULSANT and ANTI-EPILEPTIC drug carbamazepine. It can be used to treat most forms of epilepsy (except absence seizures), diabetes insipidus, trigeminal neuralgia and in the management of manic-depressive illness. It is available as tablets.
+▲ side-effects/warning: see CARBAMAZEPINE

epinephrine
See ADRENALINE

Epipen
(Allerayde) is a proprietary preparation of the natural HORMONE adrenaline and is available only on special prescription on a 'named-patient' basis (as it is imported from USA). It is used as a SYMPATHOMIMETIC and BRONCHODILATOR drug in emergency treatment of acute and severe bronchoconstriction and other symptoms of acute allergic reaction (eg. an insect sting). It is available as a fully assembled and preloaded disposable syringe and needle for subcutaneous injection (if necessary by a bystander).
+▲ side-effects/warning: see ADRENALINE

epirubicin hydrochloride
is a CYTOTOXIC DRUG (an ANTIBIOTIC in origin), which is used as an ANTICANCER treatment of severe breast and kidney tumours. Administration is by injection or bladder instillation.
+▲ side-effects/warning: see under CYCTOTOXIC DRUGS; but it also has cardiac toxicity.
✪ Related entries: Pharmorubicin Rapid Dissolution; Pharmorubicin Solution for Injection

epoetin
is a synthesized form of human erythropoitetin. It is used as an ANAEMIA TREATMENT for the type of anaemia known to be associated with erythropoetic deficiency in chronic renal failure in dialysis patients. It is available as epoetin alpha and beta and is administered by intravenous administration.
+ side-effects: cardiovascular symptoms including high blood pressure (hypertension) and cardiac complications; anaphylactic reactions, flu-like symptoms, skin reactions; oedema (accumulation of fluid in the tissues) and effects on the blood.
▲ warning: it should be not be administered to patients with uncontrolled hypertension. Administer with care to patients with poorly controlled blood pressure, a history of convulsions, vascular disease, liver failure, or a malignant disease; or who are pregnant or breast-feeding.
✪ Related entries: Eprex; Recormon

Epogam
(Searle) is a proprietary, prescription-only preparation of gamolenic acid (in evening primrose oil). It can be used for the symptomatic relief of atopic eczema and is available as capsules and paediatric capsules.
+▲ side-effects/warning: see GAMOLENIC ACID

epoprostenol
(prostacyclin) is a prostaglandin present naturally in the walls of blood vessels. When administered therapeutically by intravenous infusion it has ANTIPLATELET or antithrombotic activity and so inhibits blood coagulation by preventing the aggregation of platelets. It is also a potent VASODILATOR. Its main use is to act as an ANTICOAGULANT during procedures such as kidney dialysis (though it has a very short lifetime in the body).
+ side-effects: flushing, hypotension and headache.
▲ warning: it must be administered in

E

continuous intravenous infusion since it is rapidly removed from the blood. Blood monitoring is essential, especially when there is simultaneous administration of heparin.
❍ **Related entry: Flolan**

Eppy

(Smith & Nephew) is a proprietary, prescription-only preparation of the SYMPATHOMIMETIC adrenaline. It is used to treat glaucoma and is available as eye-drops.
✚▲ side-effects/warning: see ADRENALINE

Eprex

(Cilag) is a proprietary, prescription-only preparation of epoetin alpha (synthesized human erythropoitetin alpha). It can be used as an ANAEMIA TREATMENT in conditions known to be associated with chronic renal failure in dialysis patients. It is available in a form for injection.
✚▲ side-effects/warning: see EPOETIN

Epsom salt(s)

See MAGNESIUM SULPHATE

Equagesic

(Wyeth) is a proprietary COMPOUND PREPARATION of the potentially habituating (addictive) ANXIOLYTIC and SEDATIVE drug meprobamate, the (NSAID) NON-NARCOTIC ANALGESIC and ANTIRHEUMATIC drug aspirin and ethoheptazine citrate. It is on the Controlled Drugs List. It can be used primarily for the short-term treatment of rheumatic pain and the symptoms of other musculoskeletal disorders and is available as tablets.
✚▲ side-effects/warning: see ASPIRIN; MEPROBAMATE. There are interactions with a wide variety of drugs including alcohol and depressants of the nervous system.

Equanil

(Wyeth) is a proprietary, prescription-only preparation of the ANXIOLYTIC drug meprobamate and is on the Controlled Drugs List. It can be used in the short-term treatment of anxiety and is available as tablets.
✚▲ side-effects/warning: see MEPROBAMATE

Eradacin

(Sanofi Winthrop) is a proprietary, prescription-only preparation of the ANTIBACTERIAL and (QUINOLONE) ANTIBIOTIC drug acrosoxacin. It can be used to treat a range of infections, particularly gonorrhoea in patients who are allergic to penicillin or whose strain of gonorrhoea is resistant to penicillin-type antibiotics. It is available as capsules.
✚▲ side-effects/warning: see ACROSOXACIN

ergocalciferol

is one of the natural forms of calciferol (vitamin D) which are formed in plants by the action of sunlight. It is vitamin D_2 but in medicine it is usually referred to as ergocalciferol or simply calciferol. It is used to make up deficiencies and is available as tablets and in a form for injection.
✚▲ side-effects/warning: see VITAMIN D
❍ **Related entry: calcium and ergocalciferol tablets**

ergometrine maleate

is an alkaloid VASOCONSTRICTOR and uterine stimulant, which is used routinely in obstetric practice. It is administered to women in childbirth to speed up the third stage of labour (the delivery of the placenta), as a measure to prevent excessive postnatal bleeding and also bleeding due to incomplete abortion (when it may be combined with OXYTOCIN). It is available, only on prescription, as tablets and in a form for injection.
✚ side-effects: there may be nausea and vomiting; palpitations, breathlessness, slowing of the heart, temporary high blood pressure; headache, dizziness; abdominal and chest pain; rarely, cardiovascular complications.
▲ warning: it is not administered to patients

for induction or in the first and second stages of labour; it should not be administered to those with vascular disease, certain kidney, liver, or lung disorders, sepsis, severe hypertension, or eclampsia. Administer with caution to those with heart disease, hypertension, blood disorders, multiple pregnancy, or porphyria.

❂ Related entry: Syntometrine

ergot alkaloids

are ALKALOIDS derived, directly or indirectly, from a mould or fungus called *Claviceps purpurea*, which grows on infected damp rye. These alkaloids are powerful VASOCONSTRICTOR substances that narrow the blood vessels in the extremities in particular and cause a tingling sensation that progressively develops into pain then gangrene. Ergot poisoning was known as St. Anthony's Fire and was caused by eating bread made from rye contaminated with ergot. In medicine, the dose of individual alkaloids is adjusted carefully to avoid the development of the more serious side-effects. ERGOTAMINE TARTRATE is the principle vasoconstrictor used in medicine and is mainly given as an ANTIMIGRAINE drug. ERGOMETRINE MALEATE is used to contract the uterus in the last stages of labour and to minimize post-partum haemorrhage (it is the drug of choice because its effects on blood vessels are less pronounced). Some notable examples of semi-synthetic ergot derivatives, which are used for a variety of purposes, include BROMOCRIPTINE, CO-DERGOCRINE MESYLATE, LYSURIDE MALEATE, METHYSERGIDE and PERGOLIDE. All the ergot alkaloids are chemically derivatives of lysergide acid and lysuride (lysergic acid diethylamide) is the medical name for LSD.

ergotamine tartrate

is a vegetable ALKALOID drug. It is given to patients who suffer from migraine that is not relieved by the ordinary forms of painkilling drug. It is most effective if

administered during the aura – the initial symptoms – of an attack and probably works by constricting the cranial arteries. However, although the pain may be relieved other symptoms, such as the visual disturbances and nausea, may not (but other drugs may be used to treat these symptoms separately).

Repeated treatment can, in some patients, eventually lead to addiction and in others it may cause ergot poisoning, which can cause gangrene of the fingers and toes and confusion.

Administration is oral in the form of tablets that are either swallowed or held under the tongue until they dissolve, or as an aerosol inhalant. One proprietary compound preparation is available as suppositories.

✚ side-effects: vomiting, nausea, abdominal pain, repeated high dose causes confusion or gangrene. Sometimes the headache may get worse.

▲ warning: it is not to be used to *prevent* migraine attacks. If there is numbness or tingling in the extremities, stop treatment and seek medical advice. It is not to be used in patients who are pregnant or breast-feeding, who have vascular disease (eg. Raynaud's disease), certain kidney or liver disorders, severe hypertension, sepsis, or hyperthyroidism.

❂ Related entries: Cafergot; Lingraine; Medihaler-Ergotamine; Migril

Ervevax

(SmithKline Beecham) is a proprietary, prescription-only VACCINE preparation of rubella vaccine. It can be used to prevent rubella (German measles) infection and is available in a form for injection.

✚▲ side-effects/warning: see RUBELLA VACCINE

Erwinase

(Porton) is a proprietary, prescription-only preparation of the enzyme cristantaspase. It can be used as an ANTICANCER treatment of acute lymphoblastic leukaemia and is available in a form for injection.

+▲ warning/side-effects: see CRISTANTASPASE

Erycen

(Berk) is a proprietary, prescription-only preparation of the ANTIBACTERIAL and (MACROLIDE) ANTIBIOTIC drug erythromycin. It can be used to treat and prevent many forms of infection and is available as tablets.

+▲ side-effects/warning: see ERYTHROMYCIN

Erymax

(Elan) is a proprietary, prescription-only preparation of the ANTIBACTERIAL and (MACROLIDE) ANTIBIOTIC drug erythromycin. It can be used to treat and prevent many forms of infection and is available as capsules.

+▲ side-effects/warning: see ERYTHROMYCIN

Erythrocin

(Abbott) is a proprietary, prescription-only preparation of the ANTIBACTERIAL and (MACROLIDE) ANTIBIOTIC drug erythromycin. It can be used to treat and prevent many forms of infection and is available as tablets.

+▲ side-effects/warning: see ERYTHROMYCIN

Erythromid

(Abbott) is a proprietary, prescription-only preparation of the ANTIBACTERIAL and (MACROLIDE) ANTIBIOTIC drug erythromycin. It can be used to treat and prevent many forms of infection and is available as tablets (there is also a stronger preparation, *Erythromid DS*).

+▲ side-effects/warning: see ERYTHROMYCIN

erythromycin

is an ANTIBACTERIAL and ANTIBIOTIC drug, which is an original member of the MACROLIDE group. It has a similar spectrum of action to penicillin, but a different mechanism of action (macrolides work by inhibiting microbial protein synthesis). It is effective against many Gram-positive bacteria including streptococci (which causes infections of the soft tissue and respiratory tract), mycoplasma (which causes pneumonia), legionella (which causes legionnaires' disease) and chlamydia (which causes urethritis). It can also be used in the treatment of acne and chronic prostatitis and to prevent diphtheria and whooping cough. Its principal use is as an alternative to penicillin in individuals who are allergic that drug. However, bacterial resistance to erythromycin is quite common. Administration is either oral as tablets, capsules or a dilute suspension, or by injection. Tablets are coated to prevent the drug being inactivated in the stomach.

+ side-effects: depending on the route of administration, there may be nausea and vomiting, abdominal discomfort and diarrhoea after large doses; allergic sensitivity reactions including rashes; reversible hearing loss after large doses; jaundice on prolonged use.

▲ warning: it should not be given to those with porphyria; certain forms that contain the estolate salt should not be given in liver disease. It must be used with caution in patients who have certain heart, liver, or kidney disorders; or who are pregnant or breast-feeding.

۞ Related entries: Arpimycin; Benzamycin; Erycen; Erymax; Erythrocin; Erythromid; Erythroped; Erythroped A; Ilosone; Rommix; Stiemycin; Zineryt

Erythroped

(Abbott) is a proprietary, prescription-only preparation of the ANTIBACTERIAL and (MACROLIDE) ANTIBIOTIC drug erythromycin. It can be used to treat and prevent many forms of infection. It is available as a suspension in several forms: (*Erythroped SF, Forte* or *PI SF*) and as granules (*Erythroped PI* or *Forte*).

+▲ side-effects/warning: see ERYTHROMYCIN

Erythroped A

(Abbott) is a proprietary, prescription-only preparation of the ANTIBACTERIAL and (MACROLIDE) ANTIBIOTIC drug erythromycin. It can be used to treat and prevent many forms of infection and is available as tablets and granules.
+▲ side-effects/warning: see ERYTHROMYCIN

eserine

See PHYSOSTIGMINE

Eskamel

(Goldshield) is a proprietary, non-prescription COMPOUND PREPARATION of the KERATOLYTIC agent resorcinol and sulphur. It can be used to treat acne and is available as a cream.
+▲ side-effects/warning: see RESORCINOL; SULPHUR

Eskazole

(SK&F) is a proprietary, prescription-only preparation of the ANTHELMINTIC drug albendazole. It can be used to provide cover during surgery for the removal of cysts caused by the tapeworm *Echinococcus*, as a treatment when surgery is not possible and also to treat strongyloidiasis. It is available as tablets.
+▲ side-effects/warning: see ALBENDAZOLE

Eskornade Capsules

(Goldshield) is a proprietary, non-prescription COMPOUND PREPARATION of the SYMPATHOMIMETIC, VASOCONSTRICTOR and NASAL DECONGESTANT drug phenylpropanolamine hydrochloride and the ANTIHISTAMINE diphenylpyraline hydrochloride. It can be used for the symptomatic relief of the congestive symptoms of colds, allergy and flu. It is available as capsules and is not normally given to children under 12 years, except on medical advice.
+▲ side-effects/warning: see DIPHENYLPYRALINE HYDROCHLORIDE; PHENYLPROPANOLAMINE HYDROCHLORIDE

Eskornade Syrup

(Goldshield) is a proprietary, non-prescription COMPOUND PREPARATION of the SYMPATHOMIMETIC, VASOCONSTRICTOR and NASAL DECONGESTANT drug phenylpropanolamine hydrochloride and the ANTIHISTAMINE diphenylpyraline hydrochloride. It can be used for the symptomatic relief of the congestive symptoms of colds, allergy and flu. It is available as a syrup and is not normally given to children under two years, except on medical advice.
+▲ side-effects/warning: see DIPHENYLPYRALINE HYDROCHLORIDE; PHENYLPROPANOLAMINE HYDROCHLORIDE

Esmeron

(Organon-Teknika) is a proprietary, prescription-only preparation of the (*non-depolarizing*) SKELETAL MUSCLE RELAXANT drug rocuronium bromide. It can be used to induce muscle paralysis during surgery and is available in a form for injection.
+▲ side-effects/warning: see ROCURONIUM BROMIDE

esmolol hydrochloride

is a BETA-BLOCKER that can be used as an ANTIHYPERTENSIVE treatment for raised blood pressure during operations and as an ANTI-ARRHYTHMIC, in the short term, to regularize heartbeat. Administration is by injection.
+▲ side-effects/warning: see under PROPRANOLOL HYDROCHLORIDE
✪ Related entry: Brevibloc

Estracombi

(Ciba) is a proprietary, prescription-only COMPOUND PREPARATION of the female SEX HORMONES oestradiol (an OESTROGEN) and norethisterone (as acetate; a PROGESTOGEN). It can be used to treat menopausal problems, including in HRT and is available as skin patches.
+▲ side-effects/warning: see NORETHISTERONE; OESTRADIOL

E

Estracyt

(Pharmacia) is a proprietary, prescription-only preparation of the (CYTOTOXIC) ANTICANCER drug estramustine phosphate. It can be used to treat cancer of the prostate gland and is available as capsules.

✚▲ side-effects/warning: see ESTRAMUSTINE PHOSPHATE

Estraderm TTS

(Ciba) is a proprietary, prescription-only preparation of the OESTROGEN oestradiol. It can be used in HRT and is available as skin patches.

✚▲ side-effects/warning: see OESTRADIOL

Estradurin

(Pharmacia) is a proprietary, prescription-only COMPOUND PREPARATION of the SEX HORMONE analogue polyestradiol phosphate (an OESTROGEN), the LOCAL ANAESTHETIC drug mepivacaine and the B vitamin nicotinamide. It can be used to treat cancer of the prostate gland and is available in a form for injection.

✚▲ side-effects/warning: see MEPIVACAINE; NICOTINAMIDE; POLYESTRADIOL PHOSPHATE

estramustine phosphate

is a CYTOTOXIC DRUG and an OESTROGEN. It can be used to treat cancer of the prostate gland and is administered orally in the form of capsules.

✚▲ side-effects/warning: see under CYTOTOXIC DRUGS. It causes some feminization in men (eg. growth of breasts), altered liver function and cardiovascular disorders. It should not be used in patients with peptic ulcer or severe heart or liver disorders.

✪ Related entry: Estracyt

Estrapak 50

(Ciba) is a proprietary, prescription-only COMPOUND PREPARATION of the female SEX HORMONES oestradiol (an OESTROGEN) and norethisterone (a PROGESTOGEN). It can be used in HRT and is available as tablets

in a calendar pack and as skin patches.

✚▲ side-effects/warning: see NORETHISTERONE; OESTRADIOL

Estring

(Pharmacia) is a proprietary, prescription-only preparation of the female SEX HORMONE (an OESTROGEN) oestradiol. It can be used to treat urogenital complaints in postmenopausal women and is available as a vaginal ring.

✚▲ side-effects/warning: see OESTRADIOL

etacrynic acid

See ETHACRYNIC ACID

etamsylate

See ETHAMSYLATE

ethacrynic acid

(etacrynic acid) is a powerful *loop* DIURETIC drug. It can be used to treat oedema, particularly pulmonary (lung) oedema in patients with chronic heart failure or left ventricular heart failure and low urine production due to kidney failure (oliguria). Administration can be oral as tablets or by injection or infusion.

✚▲ side-effects/warning: see under FRUSEMIDE; but more gastrointestinal disturbances; also pain at injection site. Do not use when breast-feeding. Deafness may occur in renal failure.

✪ Related entry: Edecrin

ethambutol hydrochloride

is an ANTIBACTERIAL drug. It is used as an ANTITUBERCULAR treatment for tuberculosis that is resistant to other types of drug. It is used mainly in combination (to cover resistance and for maximum effect) with other antitubercular drugs such as isoniazid or rifampicin. Administration is oral in the form of tablets.

✚ side-effects: side-effects are rare and mostly in the form of visual disturbances (such as loss of acuity or colour-blindness).

▲ warning: it should not be administered to children under six years or to patients who suffer from nervous disorders of the eyes. Administer with caution to patients with poor kidney function, the elderly, or who are pregnant. Eye tests are advised during treatment.

○ Related entry: Myambutol

ethamsylate

(etamsylate) is a drug that can be used in some situations where antifibrinolytic drugs might be used, though it appears not to work in the way such drugs normally do (i.e. preventing clot formation). It seems to improve platelet adhesion (stickiness) and reduce capillary bleeding and can be used for bleeding in premature infants and menorrhagia (excessive periods bleeding).
Administration can be oral as tablets or by injection.

✚ side-effects: headache, nausea and rashes.
▲ warning: it should not be administered to patients with porphyria.

○ Related entry: Dicynene

ethanol

See ETHYL ALCOHOL

Ethanolamine Oleate Injection

(Evans) is a proprietary, prescription-only preparation of ethanolamine oleate. It can be used in sclerotherapy, which is a technique to treat varicose veins by the injection of an irritant solution.

✚▲ side-effects/warning: see ETHANOLAMINE OLEATE

ethanolamine oleate

(monoethanolamine oleate) is a drug that is used in sclerotherapy, which is a technique to treat varicose veins by the injection of an irritant solution.
Administration is by slow injection.

✚ side-effects: some patients experience allergic sensitivity reactions.
▲ warning: leakage of the drug into the tissues at the site of injection may cause tissue damage. It should not be injected into patients whose varicose veins are already inflamed or so painful as to prevent walking, who are obese, or are taking oral contraceptives.

ethinyloestradiol

is a female SEX HORMONE, a synthetic OESTROGEN, that has been used to make up hormonal deficiencies – sometimes in combination with a PROGESTOGEN – to treat menstrual, menopausal or other gynaecological problems. It is also a constituent of many ORAL CONTRACEPTIVES. It can also be used as an ANTICANCER drug in men with cancer of the prostate; and rarely (under specialist care) for hereditary haemorrhagic telangiectasia (hereditary condition of distended blood capillaries and bleeding). One form is available as a COMPOUND PREPARATION with CYPROTERONE ACETATE for the treatment of acne and abnormal bodily hair growth. Administration is oral in the form of tablets.

✚▲ side-effects/warning: these depend on use; also, see under oestrogen. There may be nausea and vomiting. A common effect is weight gain, generally through fluid or sodium retention in the tissues. The breasts may become tender and enlarge slightly. There may also be headache and/or depression; sometimes a rash; thrombosis; in men, impotence and breast enlargement.

○ Related entries: BiNovum; Brevinor; Cilest; Conova 30; Dianette; Eugynon 30; Femodene; Femodene ED; Loestrin 20; Loestrin 30; Logynon; Logynon ED; Marvelon; Mercilon; Microgynon 30; Minulet; Neocon-1/35; Normin; Ovran; Ovran 30; Ovranette; Ovysmen; Schering PC4; Synphase; Triadene; Tri-Minulet; Trinordiol; TriNovum; TriNovum ED

Ethmozine

(Monmouth) is a proprietary, prescription-only preparation of the ANTI-ARRHYTHMIC drug moracizine hydrochloride. It can be used to treat

E

irregularities of the heartbeat and is available as tablets.
✚▲ side-effects/warning: see MORACIZINE HYDROCHLORIDE

ethosuximide

is an ANTICONVULSANT and ANTI-EPILEPTIC drug. It is used to treat absence (petit mal), myoclonic and some other types of seizure. Administration is oral as capsules or a syrup.
✚ side-effects: there may be gastrointestinal disturbances, drowsiness, dizziness, unsteady gait, movement disturbances, headache, hiccup, depression or mild euphoria, rashes, liver changes, effects on blood and psychotic states.
▲ warning: it should be administered with caution to patients with porphyria, kidney or liver impairment, or who are pregnant or breast-feeding. The withdrawal of treatment should be gradual.
✪ Related entries: Emeside; Zarontin

ethyl alcohol

or ethanol, is the form of alcohol that is produced by the fermentation of sugar by yeast and which is found in alcoholic drinks. Therapeutically, it is used as a solvent in some medicines and as an antiseptic.
✚▲ side-effects/warning: see under ALCOHOL

ethyl salicylate

like a number of other SALICYLATES, can exert a COUNTER-IRRITANT, or RUBEFACIENT, action on topical application to relieve inflammatory pain in joints and muscles.
✚▲ side-effects/warning: see under METHYL SALICYLATE
✪ Related entries: Aspellin; Dubam; Ralgex Stick; Transvasin Heat Rub

ethynodiol diacetate

is a PROGESTOGEN that is used as a constituent of the *combined* ORAL CONTRACEPTIVES. Administration is oral as tablets.

✚▲ side-effects/warning: see under PROGESTOGEN
✪ Related entries: Conova 30; Femulen

etodolac

is a (NSAID) NON-NARCOTIC ANALGESIC and ANTIRHEUMATIC drug. It is used primarily to treat the pain and inflammation of rheumatoid arthritis and osteoarthritis. Administration is oral in the form of tablets and capsules.
✚▲ side-effects/warning: see under NSAID
Related entry: Lodine

etomidate

is a GENERAL ANAESTHETIC drug, which is used for the initial induction of anaesthesia. The recovery after treatment is rapid and without any hangover effect. It causes less of a fall in blood pressure than many other anaesthetics. Administration is by intravenous infusion.
✚ side-effects: pain on injection, extraneous muscle movements; repeated doses may suppress the secretion of corticosteroid hormones by the adrenal glands.
▲ warning: it is not to be used in patients with porphyria.
✪ Related entry: Hypnomidate

etoposide

is an ANTICANCER drug, which is used primarily to treat small cell lung cancer, lymphomas and cancer of the testes. It works in much the same way as the VINCA ALKALOIDS by disrupting the replication of cancer cells and so preventing further growth. Administration is either oral in the form of capsules or by injection.
✚▲ side-effects/warning: see under CYTOTOXIC DRUGS
✪ Related entry: Vepesid

Eucardic

(Boehringer Mannheim) is a proprietary, prescription-only preparation of the BETA-BLOCKER drug carvedilol. It can be used as an ANTIHYPERTENSIVE treatment and is available as tablets.

+▲ side-effects/warning: see CARVEDILOL

Eudemine (injection)

(Link) is a proprietary, prescription-only preparation of the drug diazoxide. It can be used, when administered by injection, as an ANTIHYPERTENSIVE to treat hypertensive crisis. It is available in a form for rapid intravenous injection.

+▲ side-effects/warning: see DIAZOXIDE

Eudemine (tablets)

(Evans) is a proprietary, prescription-only preparation of the drug diazoxide, which can be used, when taken orally, as a HYPOGLYCAEMIC to treat chronic hypoglycaemia. It is available as tablets.

+▲ side-effects/warning: see DIAZOXIDE

Euglucon

(Roussel) is a proprietary, prescription-only preparation of the SULPHONYLUREA drug glibenclamide. It is used in DIABETIC TREATMENT of Type II diabetes (non-insulin-dependent diabetes mellitus; NIDDM; maturity-onset diabetes) and is available as tablets.

+▲ side-effects/warning: see GLIBENCLAMIDE

Eugynon 30

(Schering Health) is a proprietary, prescription-only COMPOUND PREPARATION that can be used as a (*monophasic*) ORAL CONTRACEPTIVE (and also for certain menstrual problems) of the type that combines an OESTROGEN and a PROGESTOGEN, in this case ethinyloestradiol and levonorgestrel. It is available in the form of tablets in a calendar pack.

+▲ side-effects/warning: see ETHINYLOESTRADIOL; LEVONORGESTREL

Eumovate

(Glaxo) is a proprietary, prescription-only preparation of the CORTICOSTEROID and ANTI-INFLAMMATORY drug clobetasone butyrate. It can be used to treat non-infective and severe inflammation of the skin caused by conditions such as eczema and various forms of dermatitis. It is used particularly as a maintenance treatment between courses of more potent corticosteroids. It is available as a cream and an ointment for topical application.

+▲ side-effects/warning: see CLOBETASONE BUTYRATE

Eumovate-N

(Cusi) is a proprietary, prescription-only COMPOUND PREPARATION of the ANTI-INFLAMMATORY and CORTICOSTEROID drug clobetasone butyrate and the ANTIBACTERIAL and (AMINOGLYCOSIDE) ANTIBIOTIC drug neomycin sulphate. It can be used to treat inflammation of the eye when infection is also present. It is available as eye-drops.

+▲ side-effects/warning: see CLOBETASONE BUTYRATE; NEOMYCIN SULPHATE

Eurax

(Zyma Healthcare) is a proprietary, non-prescription preparation of the drug crotamiton. It can be used to treat itching, especially in scabies. It is available as a lotion and a cream; the cream is not normally given to children under ten years, except on medical advice.

+▲ side-effects/warning: see CROTAMITON

Eurax-Hydrocortisone

(Zyma Healthcare) is a proprietary, prescription-only COMPOUND PREPARATION of the CORTICOSTEROID and ANTI-INFLAMMATORY drug hydrocortisone and the drug crotamiton. It is used to treat itching (eg. in scabies) and inflammation of the skin and is available as a cream for topical application.

+▲ side-effects/warning: see CROTAMITON; HYDROCORTISONE

Evorel

(Cilag) is a proprietary, prescription-only preparation of the OESTROGEN oestradiol. It can be used in HRT and is available in

E

243

the form of skin patches.
+▲ side-effects/warning: see OESTRADIOL

Evorel Pak
(Cilag) is a proprietary, prescription-only COMPOUND PREPARATION of the OESTROGEN oestradiol and the PROGESTOGEN norethisterone. It can be used in HRT and is available as skin patches.
+▲ side-effects/warning: see NORETHISTERONE; OESTRADIOL

Exelderm
(Zeneca) is a proprietary, prescription-only preparation of the ANTIFUNGAL drug sulconazole nitrate. It can be used to treat fungal skin infections, particularly tinea and is available as a cream for topical application.
+▲ side-effects/warning: see SULCONAZOLE NITRATE

Exirel
(3M Health Care) is a proprietary, prescription-only preparation of the BETA-RECEPTOR STIMULANT pirbuterol. It can be used as a BRONCHODILATOR in reversible obstructive airways disease, as an ANTI-ASTHMATIC treatment in severe acute asthma and for the alleviation of the symptoms of chronic bronchitis and emphysema. It is available in as a metered aerosol inhalant and as capsules.
+▲ side-effects/warning: see PIRBUTEROL

Ex-Lax Chocolate
(Intercare Products) is a proprietary, non-prescription preparation of the (*stimulant*) LAXATIVE phenolphthalein. It can be used to relieve constipation and is available as a chocolate bar. It is not normally given to children under six years, except on medical advice.
+▲ side-effects/warning: see PHENOLPHTHALEIN

Ex-Lax Pills
(Intercare Products) is a proprietary, non-prescription preparation of the

(*stimulant*) LAXATIVE phenolphthalein. It can be used to relieve constipation and is available as pills. It is not normally given to children under six years, except on medical advice.
+▲ side-effects/warning: see PHENOLPHTHALEIN

Exocin
(Allergan) is a proprietary, prescription-only preparation of the ANTIBACTERIAL and (QUINOLONE) ANTIBIOTIC drug ofloxacin. It can be used to treat bacterial infections of the eye and is available as eye-drops.
+▲ side-effects/warning: see OFLOXACIN

*expectorant
is a medicated liquid intended to change the viscosity of sputum (phlegm), so making it more watery and easier to cough up (an action of MUCOLYTICS). In high dosage, most expectorants can be used as EMETICS (to provoke vomiting), which leads to the traditional suggestion that they act as expectorants by stimulating nerves in the stomach to cause reflex secretion of fluid by the bronchioles in the lungs. However, it is not known for sure how they act and, further, there is considerable doubt about their clinical efficacy. Examples include IPECACUANHA, GUAIPHENESIN and AMMONIUM CHLORIDE. See also ELIXIR and LINCTUSES

Expelix
(Cupal) is a proprietary, non-prescription preparation of the ANTHELMINTIC drug piperazine (as citrate). It can be used to treat infestation by threadworms or roundworms and is available as an elixir.
+▲ side-effects/warning: see PIPERAZINE

Expulin Children's Cough Linctus – Sugar Free
(Monmouth) is a proprietary, non-prescription COMPOUND PREPARATION of the ANTIHISTAMINE chlorpheniramine maleate and the (OPIOID) ANTITUSSIVE drug pholcodine. It can be used for the

symptomatic relief of cough in children and is available as an oral liquid. It is not normally given to children under one year, except on medical advice.

+▲ side-effects/warning: see
CHLORPHENIRAMINE MALEATE; PHOLCODINE

Expulin Cough Linctus – Sugar Free

(Monmouth) is a proprietary, non-prescription COMPOUND PREPARATION of the SYMPATHOMIMETIC and DECONGESTANT drug pseudoephedrine hydrochloride, the ANTIHISTAMINE chlorpheniramine maleate and the (OPIOID) ANTITUSSIVE drug pholcodine. It can be used for the symptomatic relief of congestion and cough associated with colds and flu. It is available as an oral liquid and is not normally given to children, except on medical advice.

+▲ side-effects/warning: see
CHLORPHENIRAMINE MALEATE;
PSEUDOEPHEDRINE HYDROCHLORIDE;
PHOLCODINE

Expulin Decongestant for Babies and Children (Linctus)

(Monmouth) is a proprietary, non-prescription COMPOUND PREPARATION of the SYMPATHOMIMETIC and DECONGESTANT drug ephedrine hydrochloride and the ANTIHISTAMINE chlorpheniramine maleate. It can be used for the symptomatic relief of congestion and runny nose associated with colds and flu. It is available as an oral liquid and is not normally given to children under three months, except on medical advice.

+▲ side-effects/warning: see
CHLORPHENIRAMINE MALEATE; EPHEDRINE
HYDROCHLORIDE

Expulin Dry Cough Linctus

(Monmouth) is a proprietary, non-prescription preparation of the (OPIOID) ANTITUSSIVE drug pholcodine. It can be used for the symptomatic relief of dry

persistent cough and is available as an oral liquid. It is not not normally given to children, except on medical advice.

+▲ side-effects/warning: see PHOLCODINE

Exterol

(Dermal) is a proprietary, non-prescription preparation of the ANTISEPTIC agent hydrogen peroxide in a complex with urea in glycerol. It can be used to dissolve and wash out earwax and is available as ear-drops.

+▲ side-effects/warning: see GLYCEROL;
HYDROGEN PEROXIDE; UREA

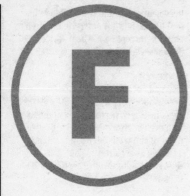

Fabrol

(Zyma Healthcare) is a proprietary,
prescription-only preparation of the
MUCOLYTIC drug acetylcysteine. It can be
used to reduce the viscosity of sputum
and so facilitate expectoration (coughing
up phlegm) in patients with chronic
asthma or bronchitis. It is available in the
form of sachets of granules for
solution in water.

+▲ side-effects/warning: see
ACETYLCYSTEINE

factor IX faction, dried

is prepared from human blood plasma. It
may also contain clotting factor II, VII and
X. It is used in treating patients with a
deficiency in factor IX (haemophilia B)
and hereditary deficiency of factor IX
(Christmas Factor). It is available, only on
prescription, in a form for infusion.

+ side-effects: there may be allergic reactions
with fever or chills.

▲ warning: risk of thrombosis (blood clots);
it should not be used in conditions of
uncontrolled generalized clotting
(disseminated intravascular coagulation).

**✪ Related entries: Alphanine;
Mononine; Replenine**

factor VIII faction, dried

(human antihaemophilic faction, dried) is
a dried principle prepared from blood
plasma obtained from healthy human
donors. It acts as a HAEMOSTATIC drug to
reduce or stop bleeding and is
administered by intravenous infusion or
injection to treat disorders in which
bleeding is prolonged and potentially
dangerous (mainly haemophilia A).

+ side-effects: there may be allergic reactions
with fever or chills; raised fibrin levels in the
blood are rarely seen after extensive use.

▲ warning: clotting within blood vessels is
possible after large or frequent doses (in blood
groups A, B and AB).

**✪ Related entries: Alpha VIII; High
Potency Factor VIII Concentrate;
Kogenate; Monoclate-P; 8SM; 8Y**

factor VIII inhibitor bypassing fraction

is prepared from blood plasma obtained from healthy human donors and used in patients with factor VIII inhibitors. It is available, only on prescription, in a form for infusion.

○ Related entry: Hyate C

famciclovir

is an ANTIVIRAL drug that is similar to ACYCLOVIR, but can be given less often. It is used to treat infection caused by herpes zoster. Administration is oral as tablets.

✚ side-effects: headache and nausea.
▲ warning: it should be administered with caution to patients who are pregnant or breast-feeding, or who have impaired kidney function.

○ Related entry: Famvir

Famel Expectorant

(Seton Healthcare) is a proprietary, non-prescription preparation of the EXPECTORANT guaiphenesin. It can be used for the symptomatic relief of chesty coughs, bronchial congestion and catarrh. It is available as a linctus and is not normally given to children under one year, except on medical advice.

✚▲ side-effects/warning: see GUAIPHENESIN

Famel Honey and Lemon Pastilles

(Seton Healthcare) is a proprietary, non-prescription preparation of the EXPECTORANT guaiphenesin. It can be used for the relief of coughs, sore throats, catarrh and bronchial congestion. It is available as pastilles and is not normally given to children under five years, except on medical advice.

✚▲ side-effects/warning: see GUAIPHENESIN

Famel Linctus

(Seton Healthcare) is a proprietary, non-prescription preparation of the ANTITUSSIVE drug pholcodine. It can be used for the relief of dry and irritating coughs and is available sa a linctus. It is not normally given to children under five years, except on medical advice.

✚▲ side-effects/warning: see PHOLCODINE

Famel Original

(Seton Healthcare) is a proprietary non-prescription preparation of the OPIOID drug codeine phosphate. It can be used as an ANTITUSSIVE to relieve a dry, troublesome cough and is available as a linctus, together with creosote. It is not normally given to children under 12 years, except on medical advice.

✚▲ side-effects/warning: see CODEINE PHOSPHATE

famotidine

is an effective, H_2-ANTAGONIST and ULCER-HEALING DRUG. It can be used to assist in the treatment of benign peptic (gastric and duodenal) ulcers, to relieve heartburn in cases of reflux oesophagitis (caused by regurgitation of stomach contents), Zollinger-Ellison syndrome and a variety of conditions where reduction of acidity is beneficial. It is now also available without prescription – in a limited amount and for short-term uses only – for the relief of heartburn, dyspepsia and hyperacidity. It works by reducing the secretion of gastric acid (by acting as a histamine receptor H_2-receptor antagonist), so reducing erosion and bleeding from peptic ulcers and allowing them a chance to heal. However, treatment with famotidine should not begin before a full diagnosis of gastric bleeding or serious pain has been completed, because its action in restricting gastric secretions may possibly mask the presence of stomach cancer. Administration is oral in the form of tablets.

✚▲ side-effects/warning: see under CIMETIDINE; but it does not significantly inhibit microsomal drug-metabolizing enzymes.

○ Related entries: Pepcid; Pepcid AC

F

Famvir

(SmithKline Beecham) is a proprietary, prescription-only preparation of the ANTIVIRAL drug famciclovir. It can be used to treat infections caused by herpes zoster and is available as tablets.
+▲ side-effects/warning: see FAMCICLOVIR

Fansidar

(Roche) is a proprietary, prescription-only COMPOUND PREPARATION of the ANTIMALARIAL drug pyrimethamine and the SULPHONAMIDE drug sulfadoxine. It can be used to treat patients who are seriously ill with malaria and is available as tablets.
+▲ side-effects/warning: see PYRIMETHAMINE; SULFADOXINE

Farlutal

(Pharmacia) is a proprietary, prescription-only preparation of the SEX HORMONE medroxyprogesterone acetate (a synthetic PROGESTOGEN). It can be used as an ANTICANCER treatment in women for cancer of the breast or uterine endometrium. It is available as tablets and in a form for injection.
+▲ side-effects/warning: see MEDROXYPROGESTERONE ACETATE

Fasigyn

(Pfizer) is a proprietary, prescription-only preparation of the ANTIBACTERIAL and ANTIPROTOZOAL drug tinidazole. It can be used to treat anaerobic infections such as bacterial vaginitis and protozoal infections such as giardiasis, trichomoniasis and amoebiasis. It can also be used to treat acute ulcerative gingivitis and to prevent infection following abdominal surgery. It is available as tablets.
+▲ side-effects/warning: see TINIDAZOLE

Faverin

(Duphar) is a proprietary, prescription-only preparation of the (SSRI) ANTIDEPRESSANT drug fluvoxamine maleate, which has less sedative effects than some other antidepressants. It is available as tablets.
+▲ side-effects/warning: see FLUVOXAMINE MALEATE

Fectrim

(DDSA Pharmaceuticals) is a proprietary, prescription-only COMPOUND PREPARATION of the (SULPHONAMIDE) ANTIBACTERIAL drug sulphamethoxazole and the antibacterial drug trimethoprim, which is a combination called co-trimoxazole. It can be used to treat bacterial infections, especially prostatitis, bronchitis and infections of the urinary tract. It is available as soluble tablets (there is also a stronger preparation, *Fectrim Forte*).
+▲ side-effects/warning: see CO-TRIMOXAZOLE

Fefol

(Evans) is a proprietary, non-prescription COMPOUND PREPARATION of ferrous sulphate and folic acid. It can be used as an IRON and folic acid supplement during pregnancy and is available as capsules.
+▲ side-effects/warning: see FERROUS SULPHATE; FOLIC ACID.

Feldene

(Pfizer) is a proprietary, prescription-only preparation of the (NSAID) NON-NARCOTIC ANALGESIC and ANTIRHEUMATIC drug piroxicam. It can be used to treat acute gout, arthritic and rheumatic pain and other musculoskeletal disorders. It is available as capsules, soluble tablets, as suppositories and in a form for injection. It is also available as a preparation called *Feldene Melt*, which can be taken by placing on the tongue.
+▲ side-effects/warning: see PIROXICAM

Feldene Gel

(Pfizer) is a proprietary, prescription-only preparation of the (NSAID) NON-NARCOTIC ANALGESIC and ANTIRHEUMATIC drug piroxicam, which also has COUNTER-IRRITANT, or RUBEFACIENT, actions. It can be applied to the skin for symptomatic

F

relief of underlying muscle or joint pain and is available as a gel.

+▲ side-effects/warning: see PIROXICAM; but adverse effects on topical application are limited.

felodipine

is a CALCIUM-CHANNEL BLOCKER drug, which is used as an ANTIHYPERTENSIVE treatment. Administration is oral in the form of tablets.

+ side-effects: these include flushing, headache and fatigue; dizziness, palpitations; rashes; oedema (accumulation of fluid in the tissues). There may be an excessive growth of the gums.

▲ warning: it should be administered with care to patients with certain liver disorders, or who are breast-feeding; withdraw treatment if there is ischaemic pain (pain due to lack of blood supply). Do not use in pregnancy.
○ Related entry: Plendil

felypressin

is an analogue of vasopressin, which is used as a VASOCONSTRICTOR and incorporated into LOCAL ANAESTHETIC preparations to prolong their duration of action.

+▲ side-effects/warning: see under VASOPRESSIN
○ Related entry: Citanest with Octapressin

Femeron

(Janssen) is a proprietary, non-prescription preparation of the ANTIFUNGAL drug miconazole (as nitrate). It can be used to soothe and treat external vaginal itching due to *Candida* fungal infections (thrush). It is available as a cream.

+▲ side-effects/warning: see MICONAZOLE

Femeron Soft Pessary

(Janssen) is a of proprietary, non-prescription preparation of the ANTIFUNGAL drug miconazole (as nitrate). It can be used to treat vaginal *Candida*

fungal infections (thrush) and is available as soft, gelatin vaginal pessaries.
+▲ side-effects/warning: see MICONAZOLE

Femigraine

(Roche) is a proprietary, non-prescription COMPOUND PREPARATION of the ANTIHISTAMINE cyclizine hydrochloride and the (NSAID) NON-NARCOTIC ANALGESIC and ANTIRHEUMATIC drug aspirin. It can be used as an ANTIMIGRAINE treatment for acute migraine attacks and associated nausea, but not prophylactically to prevent attacks. It is available as soluble (effervescent) tablets. The preparations are not normally given to children under 12 years, except on medical advice.
+▲ side-effects/warning: see ASPIRIN; CYCLIZINE

Feminax

(Roche) is a proprietary, non-prescription COMPOUND ANALGESIC preparation of the NON-NARCOTIC ANALGESIC drug paracetamol, the NARCOTIC ANALGESIC drug codeine phosphate, the STIMULANT caffeine and the ANTICHOLINERGIC and ANTISPASMODIC drug hyoscine hydrobromide. It can be used specifically for the relief of period pain and is available as capsules.
+▲ side-effects/warning: see CAFFEINE; CODEINE PHOSPHATE; HYOSCINE HYDROBROMIDE; PARACETAMOL

Femodene

(Schering Health) is a proprietary, prescription-only COMPOUND PREPARATION that can be used as a (*monophasic*) ORAL CONTRACEPTIVE (and also for certain menstrual problems) of the type that combines an OESTROGEN and a PROGESTOGEN, in this case ethinyloestradiol and gestodene. It is available in the form of tablets in a calendar pack.
+▲ warning/side-effects: see ETHINYLOESTRADIOL; GESTODENE

F

Femodene ED

(Schering Health) is a proprietary, prescription-only COMPOUND PREPARATION that can be used as a (*monophasic*) ORAL CONTRACEPTIVE (and also for certain menstrual problems) of the type that combines an OESTROGEN and a PROGESTOGEN, in this case ethinyloestradiol and gestodene. It is available in the form of tablets in a calendar pack.

+▲ warning/side-effects: see ETHINYLOESTRADIOL; GESTODENE

Femulen

(Searle) is a proprietary, prescription-only preparation that can be used as an ORAL CONTRACEPTIVE of the PROGESTOGEN-only pill (POP) type and contains ethynodiol acetate. It is available in the form of tablets in a calendar pack.

Fenbid

(Goldshield) is a proprietary, prescription-only preparation of the (NSAID) NON-NARCOTIC ANALGESIC and ANTIRHEUMATIC drug ibuprofen.
It can be used to treat all kinds of pain and inflammation, especially pain from arthritis and rheumatism and other musculoskeletal disorders.
It is available as modified-release capsules (*Spansules*).

+▲ side-effects/warning: see IBUPROFEN

fenbufen

is a (NSAID) NON-NARCOTIC ANALGESIC and ANTIRHEUMATIC drug. It has effects similar to those of aspirin and is used particularly in the treatment of pain associated with rheumatoid arthritis and osteoarthritis.

+▲ side-effect/warning: see under NSAID. It is thought to cause less gastrointestinal bleeding than other NSAIDs. However, it has a greater risk of causing rashes and may cause nasopharyngitis.

✪ Related entries: Fenbuzip; Lederfen; Traxam

Fenbuzip

(Ashbourne) is a proprietary, prescription-only preparation of the (NSAID) NON-NARCOTIC ANALGESIC and ANTIRHEUMATIC drug fenbufen. It can be used to relieve pain and inflammation, particularly rheumatic and arthritic pain and to treat other musculoskeletal disorders. It is available as tablets and capsules.

+▲ side-effects/warning: see FENBUFEN

fenfluramine hydrochloride

is an APPETITE SUPPRESSANT drug. It is used in the short term to aid the slimming regimes of obese patients. It is not a stimulant (unlike most other appetite suppressants of this type) but has sedative properties that may affect a patient's intricacy of thought and movement.

+ side-effects: there may be depression; sedation with headache, disturbed sleep, drowsiness, irritability, impotence and loss of libido, effects on blood pressure, vertigo and gastric upsets. Sometimes there is insomnia, dry mouth, fluid retention, increased frequency of urination; and there may be blood disorders, rashes and schizophrenia-like behaviour. Treatment is only in the short term as tolerance and/or dependence may occur; dosage should be tapered off gradually to avoid withdrawal depression.

▲ warning: it may affect mental concentration and enhances the effect of alcohol. It should not be used in patients with a history of drug abuse, psychiatric illness, epilepsy, glaucoma, or alcoholism; or who are pregnant or breast-feeding.

✪ Related entry: Ponderax

Fennings Children's Cooling Powders

(Fenning) is a proprietary, non-prescription preparation of the NON-NARCOTIC ANALGESIC drug paracetamol. It can be used for the relief of cold symptoms, teething pain, headache, feverishness and pain. It is available as a powder and is not normally given to babies under three months, except on medical advice.

+▲ side-effects/warning: see PARACETAMOL

fenofibrate

can be used as a LIPID-LOWERING DRUG in hyperlipidaemia to reduce the levels, or change the proportions, of various lipids in the bloodstream. It is usually administered only to patients in whom a strict and regular dietary regime, alone, is not having the desired effect. Administration is oral in the form of capsules.

+▲ side-effects/warning: see under BEZAFIBRATE. It is not to be used in patients with gall bladder, severe kidney, or liver disorders; or who are pregnant or breast-feeding.

○ Related entry: Lipantil

fenoprofen

is a (NSAID) NON-NARCOTIC ANALGESIC and ANTIRHEUMATIC drug. It can be used to treat and relieve pain and inflammation, particularly the pain of arthritis and rheumatism and other musculoskeletal disorders. It is available as tablets.

+▲ side-effect/warning: see under NSAID

○ Related entries: Fenopron 300; Fenopron 600; Progesic

Fenopron 300

(Dista) is a proprietary, prescription-only preparation of the (NSAID) NON-NARCOTIC ANALGESIC and ANTIRHEUMATIC drug fenoprofen. It can be used to treat and relieve pain and inflammation, particularly the pain of arthritis and rheumatism and other musculoskeletal disorders. It is available as tablets.

+▲ side-effects/warning: see FENOPROFEN

Fenopron 600

(Dista) is a proprietary, prescription-only preparation of the (NSAID) NON-NARCOTIC ANALGESIC and ANTIRHEUMATIC drug

fenoprofen. It can be used to treat and relieve pain and inflammation, particularly the pain of arthritis and rheumatism and other musculoskeletal disorders. It is available as tablets.

+▲ side-effects/warning: see FENOPROFEN

fenoterol hydrobromide

is a SYMPATHOMIMETIC and BETA-RECEPTOR STIMULANT drug. It is mainly used as a BRONCHODILATOR in reversible obstructive airways disease and as an ANTI-ASTHMATIC treatment in severe acute asthma. It can also be used for the alleviation of symptoms of chronic bronchitis and emphysema. Administration is by aerosol. (Patients should be cautioned not to exceed the stated dose and if a previously effective dose fails to relieve symptoms they must consult their doctor.)

+▲ side-effects/warning: see under SALBUTAMOL

○ Related entry: Berotec

Fenox Nasal Drops

(Seton Healthcare) is a proprietary, non-prescription preparation of the SYMPATHOMIMETIC and DECONGESTANT drug phenylephrine hydrochloride. It can be used for the symptomatic relief of nasal congestion associated with colds, catarrh, sinusitis and hay fever. It is available as viscous nose-drops and is not normally given to children under five years, except on medical advice.

+▲ side-effects/warning: see PHENYLEPHRINE HYDROCHLORIDE

Fenox Nasal Spray

(Seton Healthcare) is a proprietary, non-prescription preparation of the SYMPATHOMIMETIC and DECONGESTANT drug phenylephrine hydrochloride. It can be used for the symptomatic relief of nasal congestion associated with colds, catarrh, sinusitis and hay fever. It is available as a nasal spray and is not normally given to

F

children under five years, except on medical advice.
+▲ side-effects/warning: see PHENYLEPHRINE HYDROCHLORIDE

fentanyl

is an (OPIOID) NARCOTIC ANALGESIC drug. It can be used to treat moderate to severe pain (mainly in operative procedures), to enhance general anaesthetics and to depress spontaneous respiration in patients having their breathing assisted. Administration is either by intravenous injection, with a relatively short duration of action, or by skin patches. Its proprietary preparations are on the Controlled Drugs List.
+▲ side-effects/warning: see under OPIOID
✪ Related entries: Durogesic; Sublimaze

Fentazin

(Forley) is a proprietary, prescription-only preparation of the ANTIPSYCHOTIC drug perphenazine. It can be used to treat schizophrenia and other psychoses and also as an ANTINAUSEANT and ANTI-EMETIC to relieve nausea and vomiting. It is available as tablets.
+▲ side-effects/warning: see PERPHENAZINE

Feospan

(Evans) is a proprietary, non-prescription preparation of the drug ferrous sulphate. It can be used as an IRON supplement in iron deficiency ANAEMIA TREATMENT. It is available in the form of modified-release capsules.
+▲ side-effects/warning: see FERROUS SULPHATE

Ferfolic SV

(Sinclair) is a proprietary, prescription-only COMPOUND PREPARATION of ferrous gluconate, folic acid and ascorbic acid. It can be used as an IRON and folic acid supplement during pregnancy and is available as tablets.

+▲ side-effects/warning: see ASCORBIC ACID; FERROUS GLUCONATE; FOLIC ACID

Fergon

(Sanofi Winthrop) is a proprietary, non-prescription preparation of the drug ferrous gluconate. It can be used as an IRON supplement in iron deficiency ANAEMIA TREATMENT and is available as tablets.
+▲ side-effects/warning: see FERROUS GLUCONATE

ferric ammonium citrate

is an IRON-rich drug that is used in iron deficiency ANAEMIA TREATMENT to restore iron to the body, for example to prevent deficiency in pregnancy.
+▲ side-effects/warning: see under FERROUS SULPHATE
✪ Related entries: Lexpec with Iron; Lexpec with Iron-M

Ferrocap-F 350

(Consolidated) is a proprietary, non-prescription COMPOUND PREPARATION of ferrous fumarate and folic acid. It can be used as an IRON and folic acid supplement during pregnancy and is available as capsules.
+▲ side-effects/warning: see FERROUS FUMARATE; FOLIC ACID

Ferrocontin Continus

(ASTA Medica) is a proprietary, non-prescription preparation of the drug ferrous glycine sulphate. It can be used as an IRON supplement in iron deficiency ANAEMIA TREATMENT and to prevent iron deficiency. It is available as modified-release tablets.
+▲ side-effects/warning: see FERROUS GLYCINE SULPHATE

Ferrocontin Folic Continus

(ASTA Medica) is a proprietary, non-prescription COMPOUND PREPARATION of ferrous glycine sulphate and folic acid. It can be used as an IRON and folic acid

supplement during pregnancy and is available as capsules.
✚▲ side-effects/warning: see FERROUS GLYCINE SULPHATE; FOLIC ACID

Ferrograd

(Abbott) is a proprietary, non-prescription proprietary preparation of ferrous sulphate. It can be used as an IRON supplement in iron deficiency ANAEMIA TREATMENT and is available as modified-release tablets.
✚▲ side-effects/warning: see FERROUS SULPHATE

Ferrograd Folic

(Abbott) is a proprietary, non-prescription COMPOUND PREPARATION of ferrous sulphate and FOLIC ACID. It can be used as an IRON and folic acid supplement during pregnancy and is available as modified-release capsules.
✚▲ side-effects/warning: see FERROUS SULPHATE; FOLIC ACID

ferrous fumarate

is an IRON-rich drug that is used in iron deficiency ANAEMIA TREATMENT to restore iron to the body, for example, to prevent deficiency in pregnancy. Administration is oral as capsules or tablets.
✚▲ side-effects/warning: see under FERROUS SULPHATE
✪ Related entries: Ferrocap-F 350; Folex-350; Galfer; Galfer FA; Meterfolic; Slow-Fe Folic

ferrous gluconate

is an IRON-rich drug that is used in iron deficiency ANAEMIA TREATMENT to restore iron to the body, for example, to prevent deficiency in pregnancy. Administration is oral as tablets.
✚▲ side-effects/warning: see under FERROUS SULPHATE
✪ Related entries: Ferfolic SV; Fergon

ferrous glycine sulphate

is an IRON-rich drug that is used in iron deficiency ANAEMIA TREATMENT to restore iron to the body, for example, to prevent deficiency in pregnancy.
✚▲ side-effects/warning: see under FERROUS SULPHATE
✪ Related entries: Ferrocontin Continus; Ferrocontin Folic Continus; Plesmet

ferrous sulphate

is an IRON-rich drug used in iron deficiency ANAEMIA TREATMENT to restore iron to the body, for example, to prevent deficiency in pregnancy. Administration is oral as tablets, capsules and an oral mixture.
✚ side-effects: large doses may cause gastrointestinal upset and diarrhoea; there may be vomiting. Prolonged treatment may result in constipation.
▲ warning: iron preparations are best absorbed on an empty stomach, but may cause less gastrointestinal upsets if taken with food. Iron salts prevent the absorption of tetracycline antibiotics.
✪ Related entries: Fefol; Feospan; Ferrograd; Ferrograd Folic; ferrous sulphate oral solution, paediatric, BP; Slow-Fe, Slow-Fe Folic

ferrous sulphate oral solution, paediatric, BP

(paediatric ferrous sulphate mixture) is a non-proprietary, non-prescription preparation of ferrous sulphate. It can be used as an IRON supplement in iron deficiency ANAEMIA TREATMENT and is available as modified-release tablets.
✚▲ side-effects/warning: see FERROUS SULPHATE

Fertiral

(Hoechst) is a proprietary preparation of gonadorelin (a synthetic analogue of the HORMONE gonadotrophin-releasing hormone; GnRH) and is available only on prescription at clinics and hospitals. It can be used to treat women for infertility and amenorrhoea (lack of menstruation) due

F

to hormonal insufficiency. In such cases, it is sometimes used in an attempt to determine the cause of infertility. Administration is by pulsatile infusion.
+▲ side-effects/warning: see GONADORELIN

*fibrinolytic drugs

act as thrombolytics, that is, they break up or disperse thrombi (blood clots). They are able to do this by breaking down the protein fibrin, which is the main constituent of many blood clots. They can be used rapidly in serious conditions such as life-threatening venous thrombi, pulmonary embolism and clots in the eye. See: ALTEPLASE; ANISTREPLASE; STREPTOKINASE; UROKINASE

Filair Forte

(3M Health Care) is a proprietary, prescription-only preparation of the CORTICOSTEROID and ANTI-ASTHMATIC drug beclomethasone dipropionate. It can be used to prevent asthmatic attacks and is available in an aerosol for inhalation.
+▲ side-effects/warning: see BECLOMETHASONE DIPROPIONATE

finasteride

is an (*indirect*) ANTI-ANDROGEN, a SEX HORMONE ANTAGONIST, which can be used to treat benign prostatic hyperplasia in men. Administration is oral as tablets.
+ side-effects: impotence, decreased libido and ejaculate volume.
▲ warning: use with caution in patients with urinary obstruction, or cancer of the prostate. It is recommended that a condom is used during sexual intercourse because the drug may enter the woman in semen and have adverse effects.
○ Related entry: Proscar

Fisherman's Friend

(Lofthouse of Fleetwood) is a proprietary, non-prescription lozenge for the relief of cold symptoms and contains liquorice, menthol and aniseed oil.

Flagyl

(Rhône-Poulenc Rorer) is a proprietary, prescription-only preparation of the ANTIMICROBIAL drug metronidazole, which has ANTIBACTERIAL and ANTIPROTOZOAL actions. It can be used to treat many types of anaerobic infection, including bacterial vaginitis, dental infections and following surgery. The antiprotozoal activity is effective against the organisms that cause amoebic dysentery, giardiasis and trichomoniasis. It is available as tablets, suppositories and in a form for injection.
+▲ side-effects/warning: see METRONIDAZOLE

Flagyl Compak

(Rhône-Poulenc Rorer) is a proprietary, prescription-only COMPOUND PREPARATION of the ANTIMICROBIAL drug metronidazole, which has ANTIBACTERIAL properties and the ANTIFUNGAL and ANTIBIOTIC drug nystatin. It can be used to treat mixed infections of the vagina, including trichomoniasis and candidiasis and is available as vaginal pessaries.
+▲ side-effects/warning: see METRONIDAZOLE; NYSTATIN

Flagyl S

(Rhône-Poulenc Rorer) is a proprietary, prescription-only preparation of the ANTIMICROBIAL drug metronidazole, which has ANTIBACTERIAL and ANTIPROTOZOAL properties. It can be used to treat anaerobic infections, including bacterial vaginitis, dental infections and following surgery. The antiprotozoal activity is effective against the organisms that cause amoebic dysentery, giardiasis and trichomoniasis. It is available as a suspension.
+▲ side-effects/warning: see METRONIDAZOLE

Flamatrol

(Berk) is a proprietary, prescription-only preparation of the (NSAID) NON-NARCOTIC ANALGESIC and ANTIRHEUMATIC drug piroxicam. It can be used to relieve pain and inflammation, particularly rheumatic and arthritic pain and to treat other musculoskeletal disorders (including juvenile arthritis) and acute gout. It is available as capsules.

+▲ side-effects/warning: see PIROXICAM

Flamazine

(Smith & Nephew) is a proprietary, prescription-only preparation of the ANTIBACTERIAL drug silver sulphadiazine. It can be used to treat wounds, burns and ulcers, bedsores and skin-graft donor sites. It is available as a cream.

+▲ side-effects/warning: see SILVER SULPHADIAZINE

Flamrase SR

(Berk) is a proprietary, prescription-only preparation of the (NSAID) NON-NARCOTIC ANALGESIC and ANTIRHEUMATIC drug diclofenac sodium. It can be used to treat pain and inflammation, particularly arthritic and rheumatic pain and other musculoskeletal disorders. It is available as modified-release capsules.

+▲ side-effects/warning: see DICLOFENAC SODIUM

flavoxate hydrochloride

is an ANTICHOLINERGIC drug that can be used as an ANTISPASMODIC to treat urinary frequency and incontinence. It is available as tablets.

+▲ side-effects/warning: see under OXYBUTYNIN HYDROCHLORIDE; but it usually has fewer side-effects.

✪ Related entry: Urispas

Flaxedil

(Rhône-Poulenc Rorer) is a proprietary, prescription-only preparation of the (*non-depolarizing*) SKELETAL MUSCLE RELAXANT drug gallamine triethiodide. It can be used to induce muscle paralysis during surgery and is available in a form for injection.

+▲ side-effects/warning: see GALLAMINE TRIETHIODIDE

flecainide acetate

is an ANTI-ARRHYTHMIC drug. It is used to regularize the heartbeat in certain specific conditions. Administration is normally in hospital and is either oral or by slow intravenous injection.

+ side-effects: dizziness; photosensitivity and cornea disturbances; nausea and vomiting; jaundice; changed liver enzymes.

▲ warning: administer with caution to patients with certain heart, kidney, or liver disorders; jaundice; who are pregnant or breast-feeding.

✪ Related entry: Tambocor

Fleet Ready-to-use Enema

(De Witt) is a proprietary, non-prescription COMPOUND PREPARATION of the (*osmotic*) LAXATIVE agents sodium phosphate and sodium acid phosphate. It can be used to relieve constipation and to evacuate the rectum prior to abdominal procedures.

+▲ side-effects/warning: see SODIUM ACID PHOSPHATE

Flemoxin Solutab

(Yamanouchi) is a proprietary, prescription-only preparation of the broad-spectrum ANTIBACTERIAL and (PENICILLIN) ANTIBIOTIC drug amoxycillin. It can be used to treat systemic bacterial infections, infections of the upper respiratory tract, of the ear, nose and throat and of the urinogenital tracts. It is available as dispersible tablets.

+▲ side-effects/warning: see AMOXYCILLIN

Fletchers' Arachis Oil Retention Enema

(Pharmax) is a proprietary, non-prescription preparation of arachis oil. It can be used as a (*faecal softener*) LAXATIVE.

+▲ side-effects/warning: see ARACHIS OIL

F

F

Fletchers' Enemette
(Pharmax) is a proprietary, non-prescription preparation of the (*stimulant*) LAXATIVE docusate sodium and glycerol (along with macrogol and sorbic acid). It can be used to relieve constipation and to evacuate the rectum prior to abdominal procedures. It is available as an enema.

+▲ side-effects/warning: see DOCUSATE SODIUM; GLYCEROL.

Fletchers' Phosphate Enema
(Pharmax) is a proprietary, non-prescription COMPOUND PREPARATION of the (*osmotic*) LAXATIVE agents sodium phosphate and sodium acid phosphate. It can be used to relieve constipation and to evacuate the rectum prior to abdominal procedures.

+▲ side-effects/warning: see SODIUM ACID PHOSPHATE

Flexin Continus
(Napp) is a proprietary, prescription-only preparation of the (NSAID) NON-NARCOTIC ANALGESIC and ANTIRHEUMATIC drug indomethacin. It can be used to treat the pain and inflammation of rheumatic and other acute, severe musculoskeletal disorders. It is available as modified-release tablets.

+▲ side-effects/warning: see INDOMETHACIN

Flexin-25 Continus
(Napp) is a proprietary, prescription-only preparation of the (NSAID) NON-NARCOTIC ANALGESIC and ANTIRHEUMATIC drug indomethacin. It can be used to treat the pain and inflammation of rheumatic and other acute, severe musculoskeletal disorders and also period pain. It is available as modified-release tablets.

+▲ side-effects/warning: see INDOMETHACIN

Flexin-LS Continus
(Napp) is a proprietary, prescription-only preparation of the (NSAID) NON-NARCOTIC

ANALGESIC and ANTIRHEUMATIC drug indomethacin. It can be used to treat the pain and inflammation of rheumatic and other acute, severe musculoskeletal disorders. It is available as modified-release tablets.

+▲ side-effects/warning: see INDOMETHACIN

Flixonase
(Allen & Hanburys) is a proprietary, prescription-only preparation of the CORTICOSTEROID drug fluticasone propionate. It can be used to treat nasal allergy such as hay fever and is available as a nasal spray.

+▲ side-effects/warning: see FLUTICASONE PROPIONATE

Flolan
(Wellcome) is a proprietary, prescription-only preparation of the ANTIPLATELET aggregation drug epoprostenol. It can be used to prevent formation of clots; for example, in conjunction with HEPARIN in kidney dialysis. It is available in a form for infusion.

+▲ side-effects/warning: see EPOPROSTENOL

Florinef
(Squibb) is a proprietary, prescription-only preparation of the CORTICOSTEROID and ANTI-INFLAMMATORY drug fludrocortisone acetate, which can be used for its *mineralocorticoid* activity to treat adrenal gland insufficiency. It is available as tablets.

+▲ side-effects/warning: see FLUDROCORTISONE ACETATE

Floxapen
(Beecham) is a proprietary, prescription-only preparation of the ANTIBACTERIAL and (PENICILLIN) ANTIBIOTIC drug flucloxacillin. It can be used to treat bacterial infections, particularly staphylococcal infections that prove to be resistant to penicillin. It is available as capsules, a syrup and in a form for injection.

+▲ side-effects/warning: see
FLUCLOXACILLIN

Flu-Amp

(Generics) is a proprietary prescription-only COMPOUND PREPARATION of the broad-spectrum ANTIBACTERIAL and (PENICILLIN) ANTIBIOTIC drug ampicillin and the *penicillinase-resistant*, antibacterial and (penicillin) antibiotic drug flucloxacillin (a combination called co-fluampicil). It can be used to treat severe infection where the causative organism has not been identified, but Gram-positive staphylococcal infection is suspected, or where penicillin-resistant bacterial infection is probable. It is available as capsules, a syrup and in a form for injection.

+▲ side-effects/warning: see AMPICILLIN;
FLUCLOXACILLIN

Fluanxol

(Lundbeck) is a proprietary, prescription-only preparation of the drug flupenthixol, which has ANTIPSYCHOTIC properties and also ANTIDEPRESSANT actions. It can be used in the short-term treatment of depressive illness and is available as tablets.

+▲ side-effects/warning: see FLUPENTHIXOL

Fluarix

(SmithKline Beecham) is a proprietary, prescription-only preparation of influenza VACCINE (split viron vaccine). It can be used for the prevention of influenza and is available in a form for injection.

+▲ side-effects/warning: see INFLUENZA
VACCINE

Fluclomix

(Ashbourne) is a proprietary, prescription-only preparation of the ANTIBACTERIAL and (PENICILLIN) ANTIBIOTIC drug flucloxacillin. It can be used to treat bacterial infections, particularly staphylococcal infections that prove to be resistant to penicillin. It is

available as capsules.

+▲ side-effects/warning: see
FLUCLOXACILLIN

fluclorolone acetonide

is a CORTICOSTEROID with ANTI-INFLAMMATORY properties. It is used in the treatment of severe, acute inflammatory skin disorders, such as eczema and psoriasis, that are unresponsive to less potent corticosteroids. Administration is by topical application in the form of a cream or ointment.

+▲ side-effects/warning: see under
CORTICOSTEROIDS; though systemic effects are unlikely with topical application, but there may be local skin reactions.

○ Related entry: Topilar

flucloxacillin

is an ANTIBACTERIAL and ANTIBIOTIC drug, which is one of the PENICILLIN family. It can be used to treat bacterial infections, particularly those resistant to penicillin (eg. penicillinase-producing staphylococcal infections) and in the treatment of ear infections, pneumonia, impetigo, cellulitis and staphylococcal endocarditis. Administration can be by capsules, a syrup, an oral suspension, or by injection.

+▲ side-effects/warning: see under
BENZYLPENICILLIN. Adminsiter with caution to patients with porphyria. There have been reports of hepatic (liver) and cholestatic jaundice.

○ Related entries: co-fluampicil;
Floxapen; Flu-Amp; Fluclomix;
Galfloxin; Ladropen; Magnapen;
Stafoxil

fluconazole

is an (AZOLE) ANTIFUNGAL drug. It can be used in the treatment of many fungal infections, especially candidiasis, of the mucous membranes, of the vagina (candidiasis) or mouth, oesophagitis, athlete's foot and cytococcal meningitis. It can also be used to prevent fungal

F infections in immunocompromised patients following chemotherapy or radiotherapy. Administration can be by capsules, an oral liquid suspension, or by intravenous infusion.

✚ side-effects: nausea, abdominal discomfort and flatulence, diarrhoea, headaches, rash, angio-oedema, anaphylaxis and alteration in liver enzymes.

▲ warning: it should be administered with care to patients with certain kidney disorders, or who are pregnant or breast-feeding.

❂ Related entry: Diflucan

flucytosine

is an (AZOLE) ANTIFUNGAL drug. It can be used to treat systemic infections by yeasts such as systemic candidiasis. Administration is either oral by tablets or by intravenous infusion.

✚ side-effects: there may be diarrhoea with nausea and vomiting; rashes may occur, confusion, hallucinations and headaches.

▲ warning: it should be administered with caution to patients who suffer from certain kidney or liver disorders, blood disorders; or who are pregnant or breast-feeding. During treatment, there should be regular blood counts and liver-function tests.

❂ Related entry: Alcobon

Fludara

(Schering Health) is a proprietary, prescription-only preparation of the (CYTOTOXIC) ANTICANCER drug fludarabine phosphate. It can be used in the treatment of acute leukaemia and is available in a form for injection.

✚▲ side-effects/warning: see FLUDARABINE PHOSPHATE

fludarabine phosphate

is a CYTOTOXIC DRUG, which can be used as an ANTICANCER drug primarily in the treatment of certain leukaemias. Administration is by injection.

✚▲ side-effects/warning: see under CYTOTOXIC DRUGS

❂ Related entry: Fludara

fludrocortisone acetate

is a CORTICOSTEROID, which is used for its *mineralocorticoid* activity to correct a deficiency of HORMONE from the adrenal gland and is used to treat the resulting salt-and-water imbalance in the body. Administration is oral as tablets.

✚▲ side-effects/warning: see under CORTICOSTEROIDS

❂ Related entry: Florinef

fludroxycortide

See FLURANDRENOLONE

flumazenil

is a BENZODIAZEPINE antagonist. It can be used to reverse the sedative effects of benzodiazepine drugs on the central nervous system induced during anaesthesia, in intensive care, or for diagnostic procedures. Administration is by intravenous infusion or injection.

✚ side-effects: nausea, vomiting, flushing; on waking rapidly, agitation, anxiety and fear; rarely, convulsions (particularly epileptics).

▲ warning: it should be given with caution to those with impaired liver function; or who are pregnant or breast-feeding.

❂ Related entry: Anexate

flunisolide

is an ANTI-ALLERGIC and CORTICOSTEROID drug, which is used to treat nasal allergy such as hay fever. Administration is by nasal spray.

✚▲ side-effects/warning: see under BECLOMETHASONE DIPROPIONATE

❂ Related entry: Syntaris

flunitrazepam

is a BENZODIAZEPINE drug, which is used as a HYPNOTIC in the short-term treatment of insomnia. Administration is oral in the form of tablets.

✚▲ side-effects/warning: see under BENZODIAZEPINE.

❂ Related entry: Rohypnol

fluocinolone acetonide

is a CORTICOSTEROID with ANTI-INFLAMMATORY properties. It is used in the treatment of inflammatory skin disorders such as eczema and psoriasis. Administration is by topical application in the form of a cream, gel, or ointment. It is also a constituent in several COMPOUND PREPARATIONS containing ANTIBACTERIAL or ANTIMICROBIAL drugs.

+▲ side-effects/warning: see under CORTICOSTEROIDS; though systemic effects are unlikely with topical application, but there may be local skin reactions.

○ Related entries: Synalar; Synalar C; Synalar N

fluocinonide

is a CORTICOSTEROID with ANTI-INFLAMMATORY properties. It is used in the treatment of severe, acute inflammatory skin disorders, such as eczema and psoriasis, that are unresponsive to less powerful corticosteroids. Administration is by topical application in the form of a cream, ointment, or scalp lotion.

+▲ side-effects/warning: see under CORTICOSTEROIDS; though systemic effects are unlikely with topical application, but there may be local skin reactions.

○ Related entry: Metosyn

fluocortolone

is a CORTICOSTEROID with ANTI-INFLAMMATORY properties. It is used in the treatment of severe, acute inflammatory skin disorders, such as eczema and psoriasis, that are unresponsive to less powerful corticosteroids. Administration is by topical application in the form of a cream or ointment.

+▲ side-effects/warning: see under CORTICOSTEROIDS; though systemic effects are unlikely with topical application, but there may be local skin reactions.

○ Related entries: Ultradil Plain; Ultralanum Plain

fluorescein sodium

is a dye that is used on the surface of an eye in ophthalmic diagnostic procedures. Administration is topical as eye-drops.

○ Related entry: Minims Fluorescein Sodium

fluorometholone

is a CORTICOSTEROID with ANTI-INFLAMMATORY properties. It is used as a short-term treatment of inflammatory eye conditions and is administered as eye-drops.

+▲ side-effects/warning: see under CORTICOSTEROIDS; though systemic effects are unlikely with topical application, but there may be local skin reactions.

○ Related entries: FML; FML-Neo

fluorouracil

is a CYTOTOXIC DRUG, which is used as an ANTICANCER treatment primarily of solid tumours (eg. of the colon and breast) and malignant skin lesions. It works by preventing the cancer cells from replicating and so prevents the growth of the cancer. Administration can be oral as capsules, topical as a cream, or by injection.

+▲ side-effects/warning: see under CYTOTOXIC DRUGS

○ Related entries: Efudix; Fluoro-uracil

Fluoro-uracil

(Roche) is a proprietary, prescription-only preparation of the (CYTOTOXIC) ANTICANCER drug fluorouracil. It can be used to treat solid tumours (eg. of the colon or breast) and is available in a form for injection.

+▲ side-effects/warning: see FLUOROURACIL

Fluothane

(Zeneca) is a proprietary preparation of the inhalant GENERAL ANAESTHETIC drug halothane. It can be used for the induction and maintenance of anaesthesia during surgery and is

F

available in a form for inhalation.
✚▲ side-effects/warning: see HALOTHANE

fluoxetine

is an ANTIDEPRESSANT drug of the SSRI
group. It is used to treat depressive illness
and has the advantage over some other
antidepressants because it has relatively
less SEDATIVE and ANTICHOLINERGIC side-
effects. It has recently been used for
bulimia nervosa and obsessive-compulsive
disorders. The onset of action may take
some weeks to reach full effect and offset
on discontinuation is also slow. It is
available as tablets.
✚ side-effects: gastrointestinal symptoms,
including nausea, vomiting and diarrhoea
(which may be severe); abdominal pain, acid
stomach, constipation, anorexia with weight
loss, dry mouth, anxiety or drowsiness, tremor,
palpitations, may cause a rash (if so,
discontinue treatment), convulsions, fever,
headache, tremor, insomnia, confusion,
sweating, weakness, hypothermia, sexual
dysfunction; occasionally, blood disorders,
including lowered sodium and liver
dysfunction. A hypersensitivity syndrome has
been described involving symptoms in the
skin and inflammation of inner organs. A
number of other disorders have been reported,
including vaginal bleeding on withdrawal,
several different blood disorders, violent
behaviour and hair loss.
▲ warning: it should be given with caution
to patients with liver, kidney or heart disorders
and those who have a history of mania,
epilepsy, diabetes, or who are pregnant or
breast-feeding.
❂ Related entry: Prozac

flupenthixol

(flupentixol) is chemically one of the
thioxanthenes, which have properties
similar to the PHENOTHIAZINE DERIVATIVES.
It is used as an ANTIPSYCHOTIC drug in the
treatment of schizophrenia and other
psychoses, particularly where there is
apathy and withdrawal, but not for mania
or psychomotor hyperactivity. It is also

used (at a lower dose) in the short-term
treatment of depressive illness.
Administration is oral as tablets.
See also FLUPENTHIXOL DECANOATE.
✚▲ side-effects/warning: see under
CHLORPROMAZINE HYDROCHLORIDE; but it is
less sedating and extrapyramidal symptoms
(muscle tremor and rigidity) are more
common; avoid its use in senile, overactive, or
excitable patients and in those with porphyria.
There may be pain, redness and swelling at
the injection site.

flupenthixol decanoate

is a salt of FLUPENTHIXOL and has a longer
duration of action. It is used as an
ANTIPSYCHOTIC drug for long-term
maintenance in schizophrenia and other
psychoses, particularly where there is
apathy and withdrawal, but not for mania
or psychomotor hyperactivity.
Administration is by depot deep
intramuscular injection.
✚▲ side-effects/warning: see under
CHLORPROMAZINE HYDROCHLORIDE; but it
may have mood-elevating effects and
extrapyramidal symptoms (muscle tremor
and rigidity) are more common; avoid its use
in senile, overactive, or excitable patients and
in those with porphyria.
❂ Related entries: Depixol; Depixol
Conc; Depixol Low Volume

flupentixol

See FLUPENTHIXOL

flupentixol deconate

See FLUPENTHIXOL DECONATE

fluphenazine decanoate

is a powerful ANTIPSYCHOTIC drug, which
is chemically a PHENOTHIAZINE DERIVATIVE.
It is used for the long-term treatment of
psychoses, such as schizophrenia. The
decanoate salt is administered by depot
deep intramuscular injection.
✚▲ side-effects/warning: see under
CHLORPROMAZINE HYDROCHLORIDE; but with
less sedation, fewer anticholinergic and

hypotensive side-effects; but there are extrapyramidal symptoms (muscle tremor and rigidity and also dystonic and akinesic motor movements). Avoid its use in patients with depression.
○ **Related entries: Decazate; Modecate**

fluphenazine hydrochloride

is a powerful ANTIPSYCHOTIC drug, which is chemically a PHENOTHIAZINE DERIVATIVE. It is used in the treatment of psychoses, such as schizophrenia and for the short-term control of severe manic, violent, or agitated states. It can also be used for the short-term treatment of severe anxiety. Administration of the hydrochloride salt is oral as tablets and the decanoate salt by depot deep intramuscular injection.
+▲ side-effects/warning: see under CHLORPROMAZINE HYDROCHLORIDE; but with less sedation, fewer anticholinergic and hypotensive side-effects, but there are extrapyramidal symptoms (muscle tremor and rigidity and also dystonic and akinesic motor movements). Avoid using it in patients with depression.
○ **Related entries: Moditen; Motipress; Motival**

flurandrenolone

(fludroxycortide) is a CORTICOSTEROID with ANTI-INFLAMMATORY properties. It is used in the treatment of inflammatory skin disorders such as eczema and is also a constituent in a COMPOUND PREPARATION with the ANTIBACTERIAL drug clioquinol. Administration is by topical application in the form of a cream or ointment.
+▲ side-effects/warning: see under CORTICOSTEROIDS; though systemic effects are unlikely with topical application, but there may be local skin reactions.
○ **Related entries: Haelan; Haelan-C**

flurazepam

is a BENZODIAZEPINE drug, which is used as a HYPNOTIC to treat insomnia in cases where some degree of sedation during the daytime is acceptable. Administration is oral in the form of capsules.
+▲ side-effects/warning: see under BENZODIAZEPINE
○ **Related entry: Dalmane**

flurbiprofen

is a (NSAID) NON-NARCOTIC ANALGESIC and ANTIRHEUMATIC drug with effects similar to those of aspirin. It is used particularly in the treatment of pain and inflammation in musculoskeletal disorders, period pain and postoperative pain. Administration can be oral as capsules or tablets, or topical as eye-drops or suppositories.
+▲ side-effects/warning: see under NSAID. Suppositories may cause irritation.
○ **Related entries: Froben; Ocufen**

Flurex Cold/Flu Capsules with Cough Suppressant

(Seton Healthcare) is a proprietary, non-prescription preparation of the SYMPATHOMIMETIC and VASOCONSTRICTOR drug phenylephrine hydrochloride, the NON-NARCOTIC ANALGESIC and ANTIPYRETIC drug paracetamol and the (OPIOID) NARCOTIC ANALGESIC and ANTITUSSIVE drug dextromethorphan hydrobromide. It can be used for the relief of nasal congestion during colds and flu, aches, cough and fever. It is available as a liquid and is not normally given to children under six years, except on medical advice.
+▲ side-effects/warning: see DEXTROMETHORPHAN HYDROBROMIDE; PARACETAMOL; PHENYLEPHRINE HYDROCHLORIDE

Flurex Tablets

(Seton Healthcare) is a proprietary, non-prescription COMPOUND PREPARATION of the NON-NARCOTIC ANALGESIC and ANTIPYRETIC drug paracetamol, the SYMPATHOMIMETIC and DECONGESTANT drug phenylephrine hydrochloride and the STIMULANT caffeine. It can be used for the symptomatic relief of colds, flu, congested and blocked nose and catarrh. It is

F available in the form of a liquid and is not normally given to children under six years, except on medical advice.

✚▲ side-effects/warning: see CAFFEINE; PARACETAMOL; PHENYLEPHRINE HYDROCHLORIDE

fluspirilene

is an ANTIPSYCHOTIC drug, which is used in the treatment of schizophrenia. Administration is by injection.

✚▲ side-effects/warning: see under CHLORPROMAZINE HYDROCHLORIDE; but is less sedating, however, there is a a greater frequency of extrapyramidal symptoms (muscle tremor and rigidity), restlessness, headache and sweating.

✪ Related entry: Redeptin

flutamide

is a HORMONE ANTAGONIST (an anti-androgen) that is used as an ANTICANCER drug for the treatment of prostate cancer. It is available as tablets.

✚ side-effects: there may be gynaecomastia (growth of breasts) and milk secretion, diarrhoea, nausea and vomiting, increased appetite, tiredness and sleep disturbances, decreased libido, gastrointestinal and chest pain, blurred vision, oedema, rashes, blood disturbances, headache, dizziness, thirst, rash, blood and liver disorders.

▲ warning: administer with caution to patients suffering certain heart disorders. Liver function should be monitored.

✪ Related entry: Drogenil

fluticasone propionate

is a CORTICOSTEROID drug. It is used as an ANTI-INFLAMMATORY treatment for inflammatory skin disorders, such as dermatitis and eczema, that are unresponsive to less potent corticosteroids and also for psoriasis. Administration is by topical application as a cream. It can also be used as an ANTI-ALLERGIC treatment for nasal allergy such as hay fever and is administered by a nasal spray.

✚▲ side-effects/warning: see under HYDROCORTISONE

✪ Related entries: Cultivate; Flixonase

fluvastatin

can be used as a LIPID-LOWERING DRUG in hyperlipidaemia to reduce the levels, or change the proportions, of various lipids in the bloodstream. It is usually administered only to patients in whom a strict and regular dietary regime, alone, is not having the desired effect. Administration is oral in the form of capsules.

✚▲ side-effects/warning: see under SIMVASTATIN

✪ Related entry: Lescol

Fluvirin

(Evans) is a proprietary, prescription-only preparation of influenza VACCINE. It can be used for the prevention of influenza and is available in a form for injection.

✚▲ side-effects/warning: see INFLUENZA VACCINE

fluvoxamine maleate

is an ANTIDEPRESSANT drug of the SSRI group. It is used to treat depressive illness and has the advantage over some other antidepressant drugs because it has less SEDATIVE and ANTICHOLINERGIC side-effects. Administration is by tablets.

✚▲ side-effects/warning: see under FLUOXETINE; there may also be slowing of the heart.

✪ Related entry: Faverin

Fluzone

(Servier) is a proprietary, prescription-only preparation of influenza VACCINE. It can be used for prevention of influenza and is available in a form for injection.

✚▲ side-effects/warning: see INFLUENZA VACCINE

FML

(Allergan) is a proprietary, prescription-only preparation of the CORTICOSTEROID

and ANTI-INFLAMMATORY drug
fluorometholone. It can be used for the
short-term treatment of inflammatory eye
conditions and is available as eye-drops.
+▲ side-effects/warning: see
FLUOROMETHOLONE

FML-Neo

(Allergan) is a proprietary, prescription-
only COMPOUND PREPARATION of the ANTI-
INFLAMMATORY and CORTICOSTEROID drug
fluorometholone and the ANTIBACTERIAL
and (AMINOGLYCOSIDE) ANTIBIOTIC drug
neomycin sulphate. It can be used in cases
where inflammation is not primarily
caused by infection and is available as eye-
drops.
+▲ side-effects/warning: see
FLUOROMETHOLONE; NEOMYCIN SULPHATE

Folex-350

(Rybar) is a proprietary, non-prescription
COMPOUND PREPARATION of ferrous
fumarate and folic acid. It can be used as
an IRON and folic acid supplement during
pregnancy and is available as tablets.
+▲ side-effects/warning: see FERROUS
FUMARATE; FOLIC ACID

folic acid

is a vitamin of the B complex and is also
known as pteroylglutamic acid. It has an
important role in the synthesis of nucleic
acids (DNA and RNA). Good food sources
of folic acid include liver and vegetables
and its consumption is particularly
necessary during pregnancy. The
Department of Health now agree that folic
acid supplements help prevent neural tube
defects when taken before and during
pregnancy. There are also certain forms of
anaemia (eg. megaloblastic anaemia) that
can be treated with folic acid (as well as
supplements of cyanocobalamin).
Administration is oral as tablets, a syrup,
or capsules.
▲ warning: treatment with folic acid
generally also indicates parallel treatment
with cyanocobalamin (vitamin B_{12}).

◑ Related entries: Fefol; Ferfolic SV;
Ferrocap-F 350; Ferrocontin Folic
Continus; Ferrograd Folic; Folex-350;
Galfer FA; Lexpec; Lexpec with Iron;
Lexpec with Iron-M; Meterfolic;
Pregaday; Slow-Fe Folic

folinic acid

is a derivative of FOLIC ACID (a vitamin of
the VITAMIN B complex) and is used to
counteract the folate-antagonist activity
and resulting toxicity of certain
ANTICANCER drugs, especially
METHOTREXATE. Administration is either
oral in the form of tablets or by injection
or intravenous infusion.
+ side-effects: rarely, fever after injections.
◑ Related entries: Calcium Leucovorin;
Refolinon

follicle-stimulating hormone (FSH)

is a HORMONE secreted by the anterior
pituitary gland and is one of the
GONADOTROPHIN hormones (along with
LUTEINIZING HORMONE; LH). In women (in
conjunction with LH), it causes the
monthly ripening in one ovary
of a follicle and stimulates ovulation. In
men, it stimulates the production of sperm
in the testes. It may be injected
therapeutically in infertility treatment to
stimulate ovulation. It is available, in
combination with luteinizing
hormone, as HUMAN MENOPAUSAL
GONADOTROPHIN.
See also CHORIONIC GONADOTROPHIN.
◑ Related entries: Humegon; Metrodin
High Purity; Normegon; Orgafol;
Pergonal

Fomac

(Berk) is a proprietary, prescription-only
preparation of the ANTISPASMODIC drug
mebeverine hydrochloride. It can be used
to treat gastrointestinal spasm and is
available as tablets.
+▲ side-effects/warning: see MEBEVERINE
HYDROCHLORIDE

F

formaldehyde

is a powerful KERATOLYTIC agent, which is used in mild solution to dissolve away layers of toughened or warty skin, especially in the treatment of verrucas (plantar warts) on the soles of the feet.
+▲ side-effects/warning: see under SALICYLIC ACID
○ Related entry: Veracur

formestane

is an ANTICANCER drug used to treat advanced breast cancer in post-menopausal women. It is thought to work by inhibiting the conversion of the male SEX HORMONE androgen to the female sex hormone OESTROGEN. Administration is by deep intramuscular injection.
s side-effects: there may be drowsiness and lethargy; rashes and allergic reactions; vomiting and constipation; hot flushes and headache, vaginal bleeding; joint pain, pelvic and muscle cramps; sore throat; growth of facial hair; emotional instability, clots in the blood vessels of the leg, or irritation at the site of injection.
▲ warning: it should not be used in pre-menopausal women or in those who are pregnant of breast-feeding.
○ Related entry: Lentaron

Fortagesic

(Sanofi Winthrop) is a proprietary, prescription-only COMPOUND ANALGESIC preparation of the (OPIOID) NARCOTIC ANALGESIC drug pentazocine (as hydrochloride) and the NON-NARCOTIC ANALGESIC drug paracetamol. It can be used to relieve pain anywhere in the body and is available as tablets. It is not normally given to children under seven years, except on medical advice.
+▲ side-effects/warning: SEE PARACETAMOL; PENTAZOCINE

Fortral

(Sanofi Winthrop) is a proprietary, prescription-only preparation of the (OPIOID) NARCOTIC ANALGESIC drug

pentazocine. It can be used to relieve pain and is available as capsules, tablets, suppositories and in a form for injection.
+▲ side-effects/warning: see PENTAZOCINE

Fortum

(Glaxo) is a proprietary, prescription-only preparation of the ANTIBACTERIAL and (CEPHALOSPORIN) ANTIBIOTIC drug CEFTAZIDIME. It can be used particularly to treat infections of the respiratory tract, during surgery and in patients whose immune systems are defective. It is available in a form for injection or infusion.
+▲ side-effects/warning: see CEFTAZIDIME

foscarnet sodium

is an ANTIVIRAL drug. It can be used to treat cytomegaloviral retinitis in patients with AIDS when the more commonly used antiviral drug GANCICLOVIR is inappropriate. Administration is by intravenous infusion.
+ side-effects: there may be various blood-cell deficiencies, effects on the functioning of the kidney and liver and gastrointestinal disturbances, nausea, vomiting, rash and fatigue.
▲ warning: it should not be administered to patients who have impaired kidney function, or who are pregnant or breast-feeding.
○ Related entry: Foscavir

Foscavir

(Astra) is a proprietary, non-prescription preparation of the ANTIVIRAL drug foscarnet sodium. It can be used to treat viral infections, especially of the eye (cytomegaloviral retinitis) in patients with AIDS. It is available in a form for intravenous infusion.
+▲ side-effects/warning: see FOSCARNET SODIUM

fosfestrol tetrasodium

is a drug that is converted in the body to STILBOESTROL, which is a drug with OESTROGEN activity. It is used in men as an

ANTICANCER treatment for cancer of the prostate gland.

✚▲ side-effects/warning: see under STILBOESTROL

⊙ **Related entry: Honvan**

fosfomycin

is an ANTIBACTERIAL and ANTIBIOTIC drug. It is used mainly to treat urinary tract infections, including uncomplicated infections of the lower urinary tract and to prevent infection during certain surgical procedures. Administration is oral as granules, which come in adult and paediatric strengths.

✚ side-effects: diarrhoea, heartburn, nausea, or rash.

▲ warning: it should be used with care in patients with severe kidney dysfunction, or who are pregnant or breast-feeding.

⊙ **Related entry: Monuril**

fosinopril

is an ACE INHIBITOR. It is a powerful VASODILATOR that can be used in ANTIHYPERTENSIVE treatment, often when other treatments cannot be used. It is frequently administered in conjunction with other classes of drug, particularly (THIAZIDE) DIURETICS. Administration is oral in the form of tablets.

✚▲ side-effects/warning: see under CAPTOPRIL

⊙ **Related entry: Staril**

Fragmin

(Pharmacia) is a proprietary, prescription-only preparation of the ANTICOAGULANT drug dalteparin, which is a low molecular weight version of heparin. It can be used for long-duration prevention of venous thrombo-embolism, particularly in orthopaedic use. It is available in a form for injection.

✚▲ side-effects/warning: see DALTEPARIN

framycetin sulphate

is a broad-spectrum ANTIBACTERIAL and ANTIBIOTIC drug, which is one of the AMINOGLYCOSIDE family. As with all aminoglycoside antibiotics, framycetin is active against some Gram-positive and many Gram-negative bacteria and is used to treat infections of the eye, ear and open wounds (when it is used in a gauze dressing). It is largely restricted to topical use because of its toxicity. Administration is by eye-drops or an ointment.

✚▲ side-effects/warning: see under GENTAMICIN; but topical application limits its toxic side-effects.

⊙ **Related entries: Sofradex; Soframycin**

Franol

(Sanofi Winthrop) is a proprietary, prescription-only COMPOUND PREPARATION of the BRONCHODILATOR drug theophylline and the SYMPATHOMIMETIC drug ephedrine hydrochloride. It can be used as an ANTI-ASTHMATIC and to treat chronic bronchitis and is available as tablets.

✚▲ side-effects/warning: see EPHEDRINE HYDROCHLORIDE; THEOPHYLLINE

Franol Plus

(Sanofi Winthrop) is a proprietary, prescription-only COMPOUND PREPARATION of the BRONCHODILATOR drug theophylline and the SYMPATHOMIMETIC drug ephedrine hydrochloride. It can be used as an ANTI-ASTHMATIC and to treat chronic bronchitis and is available as tablets.

✚▲ side-effects/warning: see EPHEDRINE HYDROCHLORIDE; THEOPHYLLINE

Franolyn for Chesty Coughs

(Janssen) is a proprietary, non-prescription COMPOUND PREPARATION of the BRONCHODILATOR and ANTI-ASTHMATIC drug theophylline, the SYMPATHOMIMETIC and DECONGESTANT drug ephedrine hydrochloride and the EXPECTORANT guaiphensin. It can be used for the symptomatic relief of coughs, especially when associated with asthma, bronchitis and hay fever. It is available as a liquid and

F

is not normally used in children under seven years, except on medical advice.

+▲ side-effects/warning: see EPHEDRINE HYDROCHLORIDE; GUAIPHENSIN; THEOPHYLLINE

Franolyn for Dry Coughs

(Janssen) is a proprietary, non-prescription preparation of the (OPIOID) ANTITUSSIVE and NARCOTIC ANALGESIC drug dextromethorphan hydrobromide. It can be used for the symptomatic relief of dry, irritating cough and is available as a syrup. It is not normally given to children under seven years, except on medical advice.

+▲ side-effects/warning: see DEXTROMETHORPHAN HYDROBROMIDE

Frisium

(Hoechst) is a proprietary, prescription-only preparation of the (BENZODIAZEPINE) ANXIOLYTIC drug clobazam. It can be used in the short-term treatment of anxiety and, in conjunction with other drugs, in ANTI-EPILEPTIC therapy. It is available as capsules.

+▲ side-effects/warning: see CLOBAZAM

Froben

(Boots) is a proprietary, prescription-only preparation of the (NSAID) NON-NARCOTIC ANALGESIC and ANTIRHEUMATIC drug flurbiprofen. It can be used to treat arthritic and rheumatic pain and inflammation, other musculoskeletal disorders, period pain and pain after surgical operations. It is available as tablets, as modified-release capsules (*Froben SR*) and as suppositories.

+▲ side-effects/warning: see FLURBIPROFEN

Froop

(Ashbourne) is a proprietary, prescription only preparation of the (*loop*) DIURETIC drug frusemide. It can be used to treat oedema, particularly pulmonary (lung) oedema in patients with chronic heart failure and low urine production due to kidney failure (oliguria). It is available as tablets.

+▲ side-effects/warning: see FRUSEMIDE

Fru-Co

(Baker Norton) is a proprietary, prescription-only COMPOUND PREPARATION of the (*potassium-sparing*) DIURETIC drug amiloride hydrochloride and the (*loop*) diuretic frusemide (a combination called co-amilofruse 5/40). It can be used to treat oedema and is available as tablets.

+▲ side-effects/warning: see AMILORIDE HYDROCHLORIDE; FRUSEMIDE

fructose

(laevulose; fruit sugar) is a simple sugar (a monosaccharide). Fructose and GLUCOSE, when chemically combined, make up the disaccharide sucrose, which is found naturally in cane sugar and sugar-beet and is a major source of carbohydrate and energy. In the body, sucrose is metabolized into the simple sugars. The glucose level in the blood is closely regulated by INSULIN and GLUCAGON. Fructose, as part of a normal diet, can therefore be used as a source of energy and is a constituent of honey and in certain fruits (such as figs). It offers no particular advantage in normal individuals, but medically may be recommended for use, without prescription, by patients who suffer from glucose or galactose intolerance.

Frumil

(Rhône-Poulenc Rorer) is a proprietary, prescription-only COMPOUND PREPARATION of the (*potassium-sparing*) DIURETIC drug amiloride hydrochloride and the (*loop*) diuretic frusemide (a combination called co-amilofruse 5/40). It can be used to treat oedema and is available as tablets.

+▲ side-effects/warning: see AMILORIDE HYDROCHLORIDE; FRUSEMIDE

Frumil Forte

(Rhône-Poulenc Rorer) is a proprietary, prescription-only COMPOUND PREPARATION of the (*potassium-sparing*) DIURETIC drug amiloride hydrochloride and the (*loop*) diuretic frusemide (a combination called co-amilofruse 10/80). It can be used to treat oedema and is available as tablets.

✚▲ side-effects/warning: see AMILORIDE HYDROCHLORIDE; FRUSEMIDE

Frumil LS

(Rhône-Poulenc Rorer) is a proprietary, prescription-only COMPOUND PREPARATION of the (*potassium-sparing*) DIURETIC drug amiloride hydrochloride and the (*loop*) diuretic frusemide (a combination called co-amilofruse 2.5/20). It can be used to treat oedema and is available as tablets.

✚▲ side-effects/warning: see AMILORIDE HYDROCHLORIDE; FRUSEMIDE

frusemide

(furosemide) is a powerful DIURETIC drug, one of the class of *loop diuretics*. It can be used to treat oedema (accumulation of fluid in the tissues), particularly pulmonary (lung) oedema in patients with left ventricular or chronic heart failure and low urine production due to kidney failure (oliguria). Administration can be oral as tablets or oral liquid solutions, or in a form for injection or infusion.

✚ side-effects: there may be lowered blood levels of potassium, sodium, magnesium and chloride. There may be an abnormally low blood pressure (hypotension), gastrointestinal disturbances, raised levels of urea in the blood, raised blood glucose, changes in fats in the blood, tinnitus (ringing in the ears) and deafness. There may be skin rashes, photosensitivity, bone marrow depression, pancreatitis. Many of these effects are only seen with high or prolonged dosage.

▲ warning: it should be administered with care to patients with certain kidney disorders, who are pregnant or breast-feeding, who have

gout, diabetes, an enlarged prostate gland, or liver failure or porphyria. It should not be used in patients with kidney failure and anuria (no urine produced).

❍ Related entries: Diumide-K Continus; Dryptal; Froop; Fru-Co; Frumil; Frumil Forte; Frumil LS; Frusene; Lasikal; Lasilactone; Lasix; Lasix+K; Lasix Paediatric Liquid; Lasoride; Min-I-Jet Frusemide; Rusyde

Frusene

(Fisons) is a proprietary, prescription-only COMPOUND PREPARATION of the (*potassium-sparing*) DIURETIC drug triamterene and the (*loop*) diuretic frusemide. It can be used to treat oedema and is available as tablets.

✚▲ side-effects/warning: see FRUSEMIDE; TRIAMTERENE

FSH

See FOLLICLE-STIMULATING HORMONE

Fucibet

(Leo) is a proprietary, prescription-only COMPOUND PREPARATION of the CORTICOSTEROID drug betamethasone and the ANTIBACTERIAL and ANTIBIOTIC drug fusidic acid. It can be used to treat skin disorders, such as psoriasis and eczema, in which bacterial infection is present. It is available as a cream.

✚▲ side-effects/warning: see BETAMETHASONE; FUSIDIC ACID

Fucidin

(Leo) is a proprietary, prescription-only preparation of the narrow-spectrum ANTIBACTERIAL and ANTIBIOTIC drug fusidic acid. It can be used against staphylococcal infections, especially infections of the skin and bone and also abscesses, that prove to be resistant to penicillin. It is available in many forms: for topical application as a gel, as a cream, as an ointment; for oral administration as tablets or suspension; and in a form for intravenous injection (all contain as their active constituent

F

either fusidic acid or one of its salts).

+▲ side-effects/warning: see FUSIDIC ACID

Fucidin H

(Leo) is a proprietary, prescription-only COMPOUND PREPARATION of the narrow-spectrum ANTIBACTERIAL and ANTIBIOTIC drug fusidic acid and the ANTI-INFLAMMATORY and CORTICOSTEROID drug hydrocortisone (as acetate). It can be used to treat skin inflammation where there is bacterial infection, such as eczema and nappy rash. It is available for topical application as a cream, ointment and a gel.

+▲ side-effects/warning: see FUSIDIC ACID; HYDROCORTISONE

Fucidin Intertulle

(Leo) (sodium fusidate gauze dressing, BP) is a proprietary, prescription-only preparation of the narrow-spectrum ANTIBACTERIAL and ANTIBIOTIC drug fusidic acid (as sodium fusidate). It can be used to treat staphylococcal infections that prove to be resistant to penicillin and is available as a gauze dressing.

+▲ side-effects/warning: see FUSIDIC ACID

Fucithalmic

(Leo) is a proprietary, prescription-only preparation of the narrow-spectrum ANTIBACTERIAL and ANTIBIOTIC drug fusidic acid. It can be used against staphylococcal infections of the eye that prove to be resistant to penicillin and is available as eye-drops.

+▲ side-effects/warning: see FUSIDIC ACID

Fulcin

(Zeneca) is a proprietary, prescription-only preparation of the ANTIFUNGAL and ANTIBIOTIC drug griseofulvin. It can be used to treat fungal infections of the scalp, skin and nails and is available as tablets and an oral suspension.

+▲ side-effects/warning: see GRISEOFULVIN

Full Marks Lotion

(Napp) is a proprietary, non-prescription preparation of the PEDICULICIDAL drug phenothrin. It can be used for the treatment of lice and is available as a lotion. It is not normally given to infants under six months, except on medical advice.

+▲ side-effects/warning: see PHENOTHRIN

fungicidal

See ANTIFUNGAL

Fungilin

(Squibb) is a proprietary, prescription-only preparation of the ANTIFUNGAL and ANTIBIOTIC drug amphotericin. It can be used used to treat fungal infections, especially candidiasis (thrush) of the mouth and gastrointestinal tract. It is available as tablets, a liquid oral suspension and as lozenges.

+▲ side-effects/warning: see AMPHOTERICIN

Fungizone

(Squibb) is a proprietary, prescription-only preparation of the ANTIFUNGAL drug amphotericin. It can be used to treat systemic fungal infections and is available in a form for intravenous infusion.

+▲ side-effects/warning: see AMPHOTERICIN

Furadantin

(Procter & Gamble) is a proprietary, prescription-only preparation of the ANTIBACTERIAL drug nitrofurantoin. It can be used to treat infections of the urinary tract and is available as tablets and an oral suspension.

+▲ side-effects/warning: see NITROFURANTOIN

Furamide

(Boots) is a proprietary, prescription-only preparation of the ANTIPROTOZOAL and AMOEBICIDAL drug diloxanide furoate. It can be used to treat chronic intestinal infection by *Entamoeba histolytica* and is available as tablets.

✚▲ side-effects/warning: see DILOXANIDE FUROATE

furosemide
See FRUSEMIDE

fusafungine
is an ANTI-INFLAMMATORY and ANTIBIOTIC drug, which is used in a proprietary preparation to treat infection and inflammation in the nose and throat. Administration is by topical application as an aerosol.
○ Related entry: Locabiotal

fusidic acid
is a narrow-spectrum ANTIBACTERIAL and ANTIBIOTIC drug. It is commonly used in combination with other antibiotics to treat staphylococcal infections, especially skin infections, infections of the lining of the heart, infections of the bone (osteomyelitis) and the eye, that prove to be resistant to penicillin. The drug works by inhibiting protein synthesis at the ribosome level in sensitive organisms (Gram-positive bacteria).

Administration can be oral as tablets and as a suspension, or by infusion, or by topical application as a cream, gel, or ointment. It is also used in the form of its salt sodium fusidate and as diethanolamine fusidate.
✚ side-effects: nausea and vomiting; rash; jaundice.
▲ warning: regular monitoring of liver function during treatment is essential.
○ Related entries: Fucidin; Fucidin H; Fucidin Intertulle, Fucithalmic

Fybogel
(Reckitt & Colman) is a proprietary, non-prescription preparation of the (*bulking agent*) LAXATIVE ispaghula husk. It can be used to treat a number of gastrointestinal disorders and is available as effervescent granules. It is not normally given to children under six years, except on medical advice.

✚▲ side-effects/warning: see ISPAGHULA HUSK

Fybogel Mebeverine
(Reckitt & Colman) is a proprietary, prescription-only COMPOUND PREPARATION of the ANTISPASMODIC drug mebeverine hydrochloride and the (*bulking agent*) LAXATIVE ispaghula husk. It can be used to treat conditions characterized by gastrointestinal spasm, such as irritable bowel syndrome. It is available as effervescent granules.
✚▲ side-effects/warning: see ISPAGHULA HUSK; MEBEVERINE HYDROCHLORIDE

Fynnon Calcium Aspirin
(SmithKline Beecham) is a proprietary, non-prescription COMPOUND ANALGESIC preparation of the (NSAID) NON-NARCOTIC ANALGESIC and ANTIRHEUMATIC drug aspirin and the ANTACID calcium carbonate. It can be used to treat rheumatic pain, stiffness and swelling of the joints and to provide relief from the symptoms of minor upper respiratory tract infections. It is available as tablets and is not normally given to children, except on medical advice.
✚▲ side-effects/warning: see ASPIRIN; PARACETAMOL; CALCIUM CARBONATE

Fynnon Salt
(Seton Healthcare) is a proprietary, non-prescription preparation of the (*osmotic*) LAXATIVE sodium sulphate. It can be used to relieve constipation and is available as a powder. It is not normally given to children under 12 years, except on medical advice.

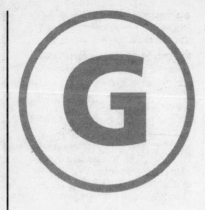

gabapentin

is an ANTICONVULSANT and ANTI-EPILEPTIC drug. It can be used to assist in the control of seizures that have not responded to other anti-epileptics. Administration is oral as capsules.

✚ side-effects: sleepiness, dizziness, unsteady gait, fatigue, eye flicker and double vision, headache, tremor, nausea and vomiting, rhinitis, weight gain, convulsions, dyspepsia, cough, nervousness and amnesia.

▲ warning: administer with care in certain seizures, to patients with certain kidney disorders, or who are pregnant or breast-feeding. Withdrawal of treatment should be gradual.

✺ Related entry: Neurontin

Galake

(Galen) is a proprietary, non-prescription COMPOUND ANALGESIC preparation of the (OPIOID) NARCOTIC ANALGESIC and ANTITUSSIVE drug dihydrocodeine tartrate and the NON-NARCOTIC ANALGESIC and ANTIPYRETIC drug paracetamol; in the ratio 500:10 (mg) (a combination known as co-dydramol). It can be used to treat pain and to reduce high body temperature and is available as tablets.

✚▲ side-effects/warning: see DIHYDROCODEINE TARTRATE; PARACETAMOL

Galcodine

(Galen) is a proprietary, prescription-only preparation of the (OPIOID) ANTITUSSIVE drug codeine phosphate. It can be used to relieve a dry, painful cough and is available as a sugar-free linctus.

✚▲ side-effects/warning: see CODEINE PHOSPHATE

Galcodine Paediatric

(Galen) is a proprietary, prescription-only preparation of the (OPIOID) ANTITUSSIVE drug codeine phosphate. It can be used to relieve a dry, painful cough and is available as a sugar-free linctus. It is not normally given to children under one year, except on medical advice

+▲ side-effects/warning: see CODEINE PHOSPHATE

Galenamet

(Galen) is a proprietary preparation of the H$_2$-ANTAGONIST drug cimetidine and is available on prescription or without a prescription in a limited amount and for short-term uses only. It can be used as an ULCER HEALING DRUG for benign peptic ulcers (in the stomach or duodenum), gastro-oesophageal reflux and for dyspepsia and associated conditions. It is available as tablets.

+▲ side-effects/warning: see CIMETIDINE

Galenamox

(Galen) is a proprietary, prescription-only preparation of the broad-spectrum ANTIBACTERIAL and (PENICILLIN) ANTIBIOTIC drug amoxycillin. It can be used to treat systemic bacterial infections, infections of the upper respiratory tract, of the ear, nose and throat and of the urinogenital tracts. It is available as capsules and an oral suspension.

+▲ side-effects/warning: see AMOXYCILLIN

Galenphol Linctus

(Galen) is a proprietary, non-prescription preparation of the (OPIOID) ANTITUSSIVE drug pholcodine. It can be used for a dry, painful cough and is available as a sugar-free linctus.

+▲ side-effects/warning: see PHOLCODINE

Galenphol Linctus, Strong

(Galen) is a proprietary, non-prescription preparation of the (OPIOID) ANTITUSSIVE drug pholcodine. It can be used for a dry, painful cough and is available as a sugar-free linctus.

+▲ side-effects/warning: see PHOLCODINE

Galenphol Paediatric Linctus

(Galen) is a proprietary, non-prescription preparation of the (OPIOID) ANTITUSSIVE drug pholcodine. It can be used for a dry, painful cough and is available as a sugar-free linctus. It is not normally given to children under one year, except on medical advice.

+▲ side-effects/warning: see PHOLCODINE

Galfer

(Galen) is a proprietary, non-prescription preparation of the drug ferrous fumarate. It can be used as an IRON supplement in iron deficiency ANAEMIA TREATMENT and is available as capsules and a syrup.

+▲ side-effects/warning: see FERROUS FUMARATE

Galfer FA

(Galen) is a proprietary, non-prescription COMPOUND PREPARATION of ferrous fumarate and folic acid. It can be used as an IRON and folic acid supplement during pregnancy and is available as capsules.

+▲ side-effects/warning: see FERROUS FUMARATE; FOLIC ACID

Galfloxin

(Galen) is a proprietary, prescription-only preparation of the ANTIBACTERIAL and (PENICILLIN) ANTIBIOTIC drug flucloxacillin. It can be used to treat bacterial infections, especially staphylococcal infections that prove to be resistant to penicillin. It is available as capsules.

+▲ side-effects/warning: see FLUCLOXACILLIN

gallamine triethiodide

is a *non-depolarizing* SKELETAL MUSCLE RELAXANT drug. It is used to induce muscle paralysis during surgery and is administered by injection.

+▲ side-effects/warning: see under TUBOCURARINE CHLORIDE; but causes greater speeding of the heart. Avoid its use in patients with severe kidney disease.

✪ Related entry: Flaxedil

Galpseud

(Galen) is a proprietary, non-prescription

preparation of the SYMPATHOMIMETIC drug pseudoephedrine hydrochloride. It can be used as a NASAL DECONGESTANT and is available as tablets or an orange-flavoured, sugar-free linctus for dilution.

+▲ side-effects/warning: see PSEUDOEPHEDRINE HYDROCHLORIDE

Galpseud Plus

(Galen) is a proprietary, non-prescription COMPOUND PREPARATION of the SYMPATHOMIMETIC drug pseudoephedrine hydrochloride and the ANTIHISTAMINE chlorpheniramine maleate. It can be used as a NASAL DECONGESTANT and for the relief of cold symptoms. It is available as tablets or a linctus.

+▲ side-effects/warning: see CHLORPHENIRAMINE MALEATE; PSEUDOEPHEDRINE HYDROCHLORIDE

Gamanil

(Merck) is a proprietary, prescription-only preparation of the (TRICYCLIC) ANTIDEPRESSANT drug lofepramine (as hydrochloride). It can be used to treat depressive illness and is available as tablets.

+▲ side-effects/warning: see LOFEPRAMINE

Gammabulin

(Immuno) is a proprietary, prescription-only preparation of human NORMAL IMMUNOGLOBULIN. It can be used to confer immediate *passive immunity* against infection by viruses, including hepatitis A virus, rubeola (measles) and rubella (German measles). It is available in a form for intramuscular injection.

+▲ side-effects/warning: see normal IMMUNOGLOBULIN

gamma globulin

See NORMAL IMMUNOGLOBULIN

gamolenic acid

is used in preparations that are taken by mouth for the relief of atopic eczema and breast pain.

+ side-effects: there may be nausea, headache, or indigestion.

▲ warning: use with caution in patients who are pregnant or epileptics.

✪ Related entries: Efamast; Epogam

ganciclovir

is an ANTIVIRAL drug that is related to acyclovir, but is more toxic. Its use is therefore restricted to the treatment of life-threatening or sight-threatening cytomegalovirus infections in immunocompromised patients and to prevent cytomegalovirus disease during immunosuppressive therapy following organ transplant operations. Administration is by intravenous infusion.

+ side-effects: there are many side-effects; various blood cell deficiencies; sore throat and swelling of the face; fever and rash; effects on liver function, gastrointestinal disturbances; and a number of other reactions.

▲ warning: it should not be given to patients who are pregnant or breast-feeding. Blood monitoring is necessary. Administer with caution to patients with blood-cell deficiency or kidney impairment. An adequate fluid intake must be maintained.

✪ Related entry: Cymevene

Ganda

(Smith & Nephew) is a proprietary, prescription-only COMPOUND PREPARATION of the ADRENERGIC NEURONE BLOCKER drug guanethidine monosulphate and the SYMPATHOMIMETIC drug adrenaline. It can be used as a GLAUCOMA TREATMENT and is available as eye-drops.

+▲ side-effects/warning: see ADRENALINE; GUANETHIDINE MONOSULPHATE

*ganglion-blocker

drugs are a class of drugs that block transmission in the peripheral autonomic nervous system at the nervous junction called ganglia. These drugs work by preventing the actions of ACETYLCHOLINE, which is the NEUROTRANSMITTER at these junctions and so in effect ganglion-blocking drugs are a type of ANTICHOLINERGIC drug. The cholinergic receptors at which ganglion-blockers act are called *nicotinic receptors* (since NICOTINE is a strong stimulant at such receptors) and these are similar, but not identical, to the cholinergic receptors of the same name that are found at the skeletal neuromuscular junction. One result of this, is that some of the SKELETAL MUSCLE RELAXANT drugs (eg. TUBOCURARINE CHLORIDE and GALLAMINE TRIETHIODIDE) have some ganglion-blocking side-effects and vice versa. The ganglion-blockers were introduced as ANTIHYPERTENSIVE drugs (and are very effective as such), but their actions and side-effects are so widespread that they are now rarely used in medicine. However, TRIMETAPHAN CAMSYLATE is still in use because it reduces blood pressure by reducing vascular tone normally induced by the sympathetic nervous system and since it is short-acting it makes a useful HYPOTENSIVE for controlling blood pressure during surgery.

A quite different group of anticholinergic drugs, the ANTIMUSCARINIC drugs, have very extensive uses in medicine. For this reason, the term 'anticholinergic' is commonly used synonymously with antimuscarinic drugs, though not really correct. (Examples of drugs such block the actions of acetylcholine at muscarinic receptors are: ATROPINE SULPHATE; BENZHEXOL HYDROCHLORIDE; HYOSCINE HYDROBROMIDE).

Garamycin

(Schering-Plough) is a proprietary, prescription-only preparation of the ANTIBACTERIAL and (AMINOGLYCOSIDE) ANTIBIOTIC drug gentamicin (as sulphate). It can be used to treat many forms of infection, particularly serious infections caused by Gram-negative bacteria. It is available as eye- and ear-drops.

+▲ side-effects/warning: see GENTAMICIN

Gardenal Sodium

(Rhône-Poulenc Rorer) is a proprietary, prescription-only preparation of the BARBITURATE drug phenobarbitone (as sodium) and is on the Controlled Drugs List. It can be used as an ANTICONVULSANT and ANTI-EPILEPTIC to treat most forms of epilepsy and is available in a form for injection.

+▲ side-effects/warning: see PHENOBARBITONE

Gastrobid Continus

(Napp) is a proprietary, prescription-only preparation of the ANTI-EMETIC and ANTINAUSEANT drug metoclopramide hydrochloride. It can be used to treat nausea and vomiting, particularly in gastrointestinal disorders and after treatment with radiation or cytotoxic drugs. It also has gastric MOTILITY STIMULANT actions and can be used in the treatment of non-ulcer dyspepsia, gastric stasis and for the prevention of reflux oesophagitis. It is available as modified-release tablets.

+▲ side-effects/warning: see METOCLOPRAMIDE HYDROCHLORIDE

Gastrocote

(Boehringer Mannheim) is a proprietary, non-prescription COMPOUND PREPARATION of the ANTACIDS aluminium hydroxide, sodium bicarbonate and magnesium trisilicate and the DEMULCENT alginic acid. It can be used for the symptomatic relief of heartburn, reflux oesophagitis and hiatus hernia. It is available as chewable tablets.

+▲ side-effects/warning: see ALGINIC ACID; ALUMINIUM HYDROXIDE; MAGNESIUM TRISILICATE; SODIUM BICARBONATE

Gastroflux

(Ashbourne) is a proprietary, prescription-only preparation of the ANTI-EMETIC and ANTINAUSEANT drug metoclopramide hydrochloride. It can be used to treat nausea and vomiting,

G

particularly of gastrointestinal disorders and after treatment with radiation or cytotoxic drugs. It also has gastric MOTILITY STIMULANT actions and can be used in the treatment of non-ulcer dyspepsia, gastric stasis and for the prevention of reflux oesophagitis. It is available as tablets.

+▲ side-effects/warning: see METOCLOPRAMIDE HYDROCHLORIDE

Gastromax

(Pharmacia) is a proprietary, prescription-only preparation of the ANTI-EMETIC and ANTINAUSEANT drug metoclopramide hydrochloride. It can be used to treat nausea and vomiting, particularly of gastrointestinal disorders and after treatment with radiation or cytotoxic drugs. It also has gastric MOTILITY STIMULANT actions and can be used in the treatment of non-ulcer dyspepsia, gastric stasis and for the prevention of reflux oesophagitis. It is available as modified-release capsules.

+▲ side-effects/warning: see METOCLOPRAMIDE HYDROCHLORIDE

Gastron

(Sanofi Winthrop) is a proprietary, non-prescription COMPOUND PREPARATION of the ANTACIDS aluminium hydroxide, sodium bicarbonate and magnesium trisilicate and the DEMULCENT alginic acid. It can be used for the relief of dyspepsia due to gastro-oesophageal reflux and is available as chewable tablets.

+▲ side-effects/warning: see ALGINIC ACID; ALUMINIUM HYDROXIDE; MAGNESIUM TRISILICATE; SODIUM BICARBONATE

Gastrozepin

(Boots) is a proprietary, prescription-only preparation of the ANTICHOLINERGIC drug pirenzepine. It can be used as an ULCER-HEALING DRUG for gastric and duodenal ulcers and is available as tablets.

+▲ side-effects/warning: see PIRENZEPINE

Gaviscon 250

(Reckitt & Colman) is a proprietary, non-prescription COMPOUND PREPARATION of the ANTACIDS aluminium hydroxide, sodium bicarbonate and magnesium trisilicate and the DEMULCENT alginic acid. It can be used for the symptomatic relief of indigestion and heartburn and is available as tablets.

+▲ side-effects/warning: see ALGINIC ACID; ALUMINIUM HYDROXIDE; MAGNESIUM TRISILICATE; SODIUM BICARBONATE

Gaviscon Liquid

(Reckitt & Colman) is a proprietary, non-prescription COMPOUND PREPARATION of the ANTACIDS calcium carbonate and sodium bicarbonate and the DEMULCENT alginic acid (as sodium alginate). It can be used for the symptomatic relief of heartburn and indigestion due to gastric reflux and is available as a liquid. It is not normally given to children, except on medical advice.

+▲ side-effects/warning: see ALGINIC ACID; CALCIUM CARBONATE; SODIUM BICARBONATE

Geangin

(Cusi) is a proprietary, prescription-only preparation of the CALCIUM-CHANNEL BLOCKER drug verapamil hydrochloride. It can be used as an ANTIHYPERTENSIVE treatment, as an ANTI-ANGINA drug in the prevention of attacks and as an ANTI-ARRHYTHMIC to correct heart irregularities. It is available as tablets.

+▲ side-effects/warning: see VERAPAMIL HYDROCHLORIDE

Gee's Linctus

is a compound, non-prescription preparation that combines several soothing liquids, including tolu syrup, the (OPIOID) ANTITUSSIVE camphorated tincture of opium and anhydrous morphine, in a cough linctus (also known as *Squill Linctus, Opiate*).

+▲ side-effects/warning: see under OPIOID.

Gelcosal

(Quinoderm) is a proprietary, non-prescription COMPOUND PREPARATION of salicylic acid and coal tar (and pine tar). It can be used to treat psoriasis or dermatitis and is available as a gel and a liquid scalp preparation.

✚▲ side-effects/warning: see COAL TAR; SALICYLIC ACID

Gelcotar

(Quinoderm) is a proprietary, non-prescription preparation of coal tar (and pine tar). It can be used to treat psoriasis and eczema and is available as a gel (with pine tar) and a liquid (with cade oil).

✚▲ side-effects/warning: see COAL TAR

Gemeprost

(Farillon) is a proprietary, prescription-only preparation of the PROSTAGLANDIN analogue gemeprost. It is used during induction of labour and earlier in operative procedures. It is administered to the cervix by pessary to cause softening and dilation.

✚▲ side-effects/warning: see GEMEPROST

gemeprost

is a PROSTAGLANDIN (an analogue of prostaglandin E_1), which is a LOCAL HORMONE naturally involved in the control of uterine motility) that is used in early pregnancy in operative procedures. It is administered to the cervix by pessary to cause softening and dilation. It is also used in pregnancy to cause therapeutic abortion and to remove the foetus following intra-uterine death.

✚ side-effects: vaginal bleeding and uterine pain; nausea, vomiting, flushing and shivering, headache and dizziness, a raised temperature and diarrhoea, muscle weakness, chills, backache, chest pain and breathing difficulties. Uterine rupture has been reported.

▲ warning: it should not be administered to patients who have vaginal or cervical infections, or cardiovascular insufficiency. Administer with caution to those with asthma or glaucoma.

○ Related entry: Gemeprost

gemfibrozil

can be used as a LIPID-LOWERING DRUG in hyperlipidaemia to reduce the levels, or change the proportions, of various lipids in the bloodstream. It is usually administered only to patients in whom a strict and regular dietary regime, alone, is not having the desired effect.
Administration is oral in the form of capsules or tablets.

✚ side-effects: dizziness, blurred vision, gastrointestinal disturbances, skin disorders, pain in the extremities, muscle pain and impotence.

▲ warning: it is not to be given to alcoholics, patients with liver damage, gallstones, or who are pregnant. Blood and liver function should be monitored and eyes tested.

○ Related entry: Lopid

*general anaesthetic

drugs reduce sensation in the whole body with a loss of consciousness and are used for surgical procedures. LOCAL ANAESTHETIC drugs, in contrast, affect sensation in a specific, local area without the loss of consciousness. The general anaesthetic drug that is used to initially induce anaesthesia is often different from the drug, or drugs, administered to maintain the anaesthesia. For induction, short-acting general anaesthetics that can be injected are convenient (eg. THIOPENTONE SODIUM, ETOMIDATE and METHOHEXITONE SODIUM), but for maintenance during long operations, inhalation anaesthetics are commonly used (eg. HALOTHANE and ENFLURANE). In order to minimize the depth of anaesthesia necessary for a surgical procedure, premedication with, or concurrent use of, other drugs is usually necessary. A range of ancillary drugs are also valuable, including TRANQUILLIZER or SEDATIVE drugs (eg. BENZODIAZEPINES), ANALGESICS (eg. MORPHINE), SKELETAL MUSCLE

G RELAXANTS (eg. TUBOCURARINE CHLORIDE) and concurrent use of local anaesthetics (eg. LIGNOCAINE HYDROCHLORIDE). See also: CYCLOPROPANE; DESFLURANE; DIETHYL ETHER; ISOFLURANE; KETAMINE; PROPOFOL

Genisol

(Roche) is a proprietary preparation of coal tar (and sodium sulphosuccinate undecylenic monoalklolamide). It can be used to treat skin conditions such as dandruff and psoriasis of the scalp and is available as a shampoo.

+▲ side-effects/warning: see COAL TAR

Genotropin

(Pharmacia) is a proprietary, prescription-only preparation of somatropin, which is the biosynthetic form of human growth hormone. It is used to treat growth hormone deficiency and associated symptoms (in particular, short stature). It is available in several forms for injection, including a powder for reconstitution, in cartridges (*KabiPen* and *KabiVial*) and in preloaded syringes (*KabiQuick*).

+▲ side-effects/warning: see SOMATROPIN

gentamicin

is a broad-spectrum ANTIBACTERIAL and ANTIBIOTIC drug, which is the most widely used of the AMINOGLYCOSIDE family. Although it does have activity against Gram-positive bacteria, it is used primarily against serious infections caused by Gram-negative bacteria. It is not orally absorbed and is therefore given by injection or infusion for the treatment of, for example, septicaemia, meningitis, infections of the heart (usually in conjunction with penicillin), the kidney, prostate gland, eye and ear and skin infections. Because of its potential toxicity to the ear (ototoxicity), which could result in deafness and its toxicity to the kidney (nephrotoxicity), treatment should be short term. It is also available in the form of drops, creams and ointments for topical application.

+ side-effects: these depend on the route of administration. Prolonged or high dosage may be damaging to the ear (especially in the elderly, children and patients with renal damage) and cause deafness and balance disorders – treatment must be discontinued if this occurs; there may also be reversible kidney damage.

▲ warning: again, these depend on the route of administration. It should not be administered to patients who are pregnant, breast-feeding, or who suffer from myasthenia gravis, or impaired kidney function. Kidney and neuronal function and gentamicin blood concentrations must be monitored.

✪ **Related entries: Cidomycin; Cidomycin Topical; Garamycin; Genticin; Gentisone HC; Isotonic Gentamicin Injection; Minims Gentamicin**

gentian violet

See CRYSTAL VIOLET

Genticin

(Roche) is a proprietary, prescription-only preparation of the ANTIBACTERIAL and (AMINOGLYCOSIDE) ANTIBIOTIC drug gentamicin (as sulphate). It can be used to treat many forms of infection, particularly serious infections caused by Gram-negative bacteria. It is available in a form for injection and as eye- and ear-drops.

+▲ side-effects/warning: see GENTAMICIN

Gentisone HC

(Roche) is a proprietary, prescription-only COMPOUND PREPARATION of the ANTIBACTERIAL and (AMINOGLYCOSIDE) ANTIBIOTIC drug gentamicin (as sulphate) and the ANTI-INFLAMMATORY and CORTICOSTEROID drug hydrocortisone (as acetate). It can be used to treat bacterial infections of the middle ear and is available as ear-drops.

+▲ side-effects/warning: see HYDROCORTISONE; GENTAMICIN

Geref 50

(Serono) is a proprietary, prescription-only preparation of sermorelin. It is used to test the release of GROWTH HORMONE and is administered by injection.

+▲ side-effects/warning: see SERMORELIN

Germoline Cream

(SmithKline Beecham) is a proprietary, non-prescription COMPOUND PREPARATION of the ANTISEPTIC agents chlorhexidine (as gluconate) and phenol. It can be used for cleaning all types of lesions, ranging from minor skin disorders or blisters to minor burns and small wounds and preventing them from becoming infected. It is available as a cream.

+▲ side-effects/warning: see CHLORHEXIDINE; PHENOL

Germoline Ointment

(SmithKline Beecham) is a proprietary, non-prescription COMPOUND PREPARATION of the ASTRINGENT agent zinc oxide, the ANTISEPTIC agents phenol, octaphonium and methyl salicylate and the EMOLLIENTS white petroleum jelly, liquid paraffin and lanolin. It can be used for cleaning minor skin disorders, blisters, sunburn, minor burns and small wounds and preventing them from becoming infected. It is available as an ointment.

+▲ side-effects/warning: see LANOLIN; LIQUID PARAFFIN; METHYL SALICYLATE; PHENOL; ZINC OXIDE

Germoloids

(SmithKline Beecham) is a proprietary, non-prescription COMPOUND PREPARATION of the LOCAL ANAESTHETIC drug lignocaine hydrochloride and the ASTRINGENT agent zinc oxide. It can be used for the symptomatic relief of the pain and itching of haemorrhoids and pruritus ani. It is available as an ointment, a cream and as suppositories. It is not normally given to children, except on medical advice.

+▲ side-effects/warning: see LIGNOCAINE HYDROCHLORIDE; ZINC OXIDE

gestodene

is a PROGESTOGEN. It is used as a constituent of the *combined* ORAL CONTRACEPTIVES that contain OESTROGEN and a progestogen. Administration is oral as tablets.

+▲ warning/side-effects: see PROGESTOGEN
✪ Related entries: Femodene; Femodene ED; Minulet; Tri-Minulet; Triadene

Gestone

(Paines & Byrne) is a proprietary, prescription-only preparation of the PROGESTOGEN progesterone. It can be used to treat many hormonal deficiency disorders in women, abnormal bleeding from the uterus and for maintenance of early pregnancy in recurrent miscarriage. It is available in a form for injection.

+▲ side-effects/warning: see PROGESTERONE

gestronol hexanoate

is a synthetic form of PROGESTOGEN, a SEX HORMONE, that is used primarily in women as an ANTICANCER treatment for cancer of the uterine lining (endometrium), but it can also be used to treat (malignant) enlargement of the kidneys (hypernephroma) and benign enlargement of the prostate gland in men. It is administered by intramuscular injection.

+▲ side-effects/warning: see under MEDROXYPROGESTERONE ACETATE
✪ Related entry: Depostat

Glandosane

(Fresenius) is a proprietary, non-prescription COMPOUND PREPARATION of carmellose sodium, sorbitol, potassium chloride, sodium chloride and other salts. It can be used as a form of ARTIFICIAL SALIVA for application to the mouth and throat in conditions that make the mouth abnormally dry. It is available as an aerosol.

+▲ side-effects/warning: see CARMELLOSE

G

G SODIUM; POTASSIUM CHLORIDE; SODIUM CHLORIDE; SORBITOL

Glaucol

(Baker Norton) is a proprietary, prescription-only preparation of the BETA-BLOCKER drug timolol maleate. It can be used for GLAUCOMA TREATMENT and is available as eye-drops.

✚▲ side-effects/warning: see under TIMOLOL MALEATE

*glaucoma treatment

involves the use of drugs to lower the raised intraocular pressure (pressure in the eyeball) that is characteristic of the group of eye conditions in which the optic nerve and consequently vision, is damaged within the eye. A number of types of drug help reduce this pressure (which has nothing to do with blood pressure) and which one is used depends on what sort of glaucoma is being treated (eg. simple, open-angle, closed-angle, etc.). BETA-BLOCKER drugs are effective in most cases (eg. BETAXOLOL HYDROCHLORIDE, CARTEOLOL HYDROCHLORIDE, LEVOBUNOLOL HYDROCHLORIDE and METIPRANOLOL), some SYMPATHOMIMETIC drugs (eg. APRACLONIDINE and DIPIVEFRINE HYDROCHLORIDE) and certain cholinergic drugs (eg. CARBACHOL, PHYSOSTIGMINE SULPHATE and PILOCARPINE). It is important to note that certain classes of drugs, such as the CORTICOSTEROIDS and ANTICHOLINERGICS (eg. ATROPINE SULPHATE), cause a rise in intraocular pressure and if administered to patients predisposed to glaucoma may precipitate an acute attack.

glibenclamide

is a drug of the SULPHONYLUREA class and is used in DIABETIC TREATMENT of Type II diabetes (non-insulin-dependent diabetes mellitus; NIDDM; maturity-onset diabetes). It works by augmenting what remains of INSULIN production in the pancreas and is available as tablets.

✚ side-effects: these are generally minor and rare, but there may be some sensitivity reaction, such as a rash and also blood disorders. There may be headache and gastrointestinal upsets.

▲ warning: it should not be administered to patients with certain liver, kidney, or endocrine disorders, or who are under stress, pregnant or breast-feeding; and should be avoided in the elderly because of possible hypoglycaemia. There may be weight gain so diet should be controlled.

⊙ Related entries: Calabren; Daonil; Diabetamide; Euglucon; Libanil; Malix; Semi-Daonil

Glibenese

(Pfizer) is a proprietary, prescription-only preparation of the SULPHONYLUREA drug glipizide. It can be used in DIABETIC TREATMENT of Type II diabetes (non-insulin-dependent diabetes mellitus; NIDDM; maturity-onset diabetes) and is available as tablets.

✚▲ side-effects/warning: see GLIPIZIDE

gliclazide

is a drug of the SULPHONYLUREA class and is used in DIABETIC TREATMENT of Type II diabetes (non-insulin-dependent diabetes mellitus; NIDDM; maturity-onset diabetes). It works by augmenting what remains of INSULIN production in the pancreas and is available as tablets.

✚▲ side-effects/warning: see under GLIBENCLAMIDE; except it may be used in patients with renal impairment and in the elderly.

⊙ Related entry: Diamicron

glipizide

is a drug of the SULPHONYLUREA class and is used in DIABETIC TREATMENT of Type II diabetes (non-insulin-dependent diabetes mellitus; NIDDM; maturity-onset diabetes). It works by augmenting what remains of INSULIN production in the pancreas and is available as tablets.

✚▲ side-effects/warning: see under
GLIBENCLAMIDE
○ **Related entries: Glibenese; Minodiab**

gliquidone

is a drug of the SULPHONYLUREA class and
is used in DIABETIC TREATMENT of Type II
diabetes (non-insulin-dependent diabetes
mellitus; NIDDM; maturity-onset
diabetes). It works by augmenting what
remains of INSULIN production in the
pancreas and is available as tablets.
✚▲ side-effects/warning: see under
GLIBENCLAMIDE; but it may be used in
patients with kidney impairment.
○ **Related entry: Glurenorm**

glucagon

is a HORMONE produced and secreted by
the pancreas in order to cause an increase
in blood sugar levels, that is, it is a
hyperglycaemic agent. In most people it is
part of a balancing mechanism with
INSULIN, which has the opposite effect.
Therapeutically, glucagon is therefore
administered to patients with low blood
sugar levels (hypoglycaemia), usually in
an emergency. Administration is by
injection.
✚ side-effects: diarrhoea, nausea; vomiting;
occasionally hypersensitivity.
▲ warning: insulinoma,
phaeochromocytoma and glucagonoma.

Glucobay

(Bayer) is a proprietary, prescription-only
preparation of the drug acarbose, which is
used in DIABETIC TREATMENT. It is available
as tablets.
✚▲ side-effects/warning: see
ACARBOSE

Glucophage

(Lipha) is a proprietary, prescription-only
preparation of the BIGUANIDE drug
metformin hydrochloride. It is used in
DIABETIC TREATMENT of Type II diabetes
(non-insulin-dependent diabetes mellitus;
NIDDM; maturity-onset diabetes) and is

available as tablets.
✚▲ side-effects/warning: see METFORMIN
HYDROCHLORIDE

glucose

or dextrose, is a simple sugar, which is an
important source of energy for the body –
and the sole source of energy for the
brain. Once digested, it is stored in the
liver and muscles in the form of glycogen
and its break down in the muscles back
into glucose produces energy. The level of
glucose in the blood is critical and
harmful symptoms can occur if the level is
too high or too low. Therapeutically, it may
be administered as a dietary supplement
in conditions of low blood sugar level, to
treat abnormally high acidity of body fluids
(acidosis), or to increase glucose levels in
the liver following liver damage.
Administration is either oral or by
intravenous infusion.

Glurenorm

(Sanofi Winthrop) is a proprietary,
prescription-only preparation of the
SULPHONYLUREA drug gliquidone. It is used
in DIABETIC TREATMENT of Type II diabetes
(non-insulin-dependent diabetes mellitus;
NIDDM; maturity-onset diabetes) and is
available as tablets.
✚▲ side-effects/warning: see GLIQUIDONE

glutaraldehyde

is a DISINFECTANT, or ANTISEPTIC, agent that
is similar to formaldehyde, but is stronger
and faster-acting. It is mostly used to
sterilize medical and surgical equipment.
Therapeutically, it can be used in solution
for warts (particularly verrucas) and as a
KERATOLYTIC to remove hard, dead skin.
✚▲ side-effects/warning: see under
SALICYLIC ACID. Its effects as a treatment are
not always predictable; skin treated may
become irritated or sensitized.
○ **Related entries: Glutarol; Verucasep**

Glutarol

(Dermal) is a proprietary, non-

G prescription preparation of the KERATOLYTIC agent glutaraldehyde. It can be used by topical application to treat warts and to remove hard, dead skin. It is available as a solution.
✚▲ side-effects/warning: see GLUTARALDEHYDE

glycerin(e)
See GLYCEROL

glycerol
or glycerin(e), is a colourless viscous liquid that is a mixture of hydrolysed fats and oils. It is used therapeutically as a constituent in many EMOLLIENT skin preparations, as a sweetening agent for medications and as a LAXATIVE in the form of anal suppositories. Taken orally, glycerol can be used for short-term GLAUCOMA TREATMENT.
○ Related entries: compund thymol glycerin, BP; Exterol; Fletchers' Enemette; Massé Breast Cream; Micolette Micro-enema; Neutrogena Dematological Cream; Otex

glyceryl trinitrate
is a short-acting VASODILATOR and ANTI-ANGINA drug. It is used to prevent attacks of angina pectoris (ischaemic heart pain) when taken before exercise, for symptomatic relief during an acute attack and to treat heart failure. It works by dilating the blood vessels returning blood to the heart and so reducing the workload of the heart. It is short-acting, but its effect is extended through use of modified-release tablets kept under the tongue (sublingual tablets). It is also administered by aerosol spray, by intravenous injection, or in ointments and dressings to be placed on the surface of the chest for absorption through the skin.
✚ side-effects: there may be a throbbing headache, flushing, dizziness; some patients experience an increase in heart rate and postural hypotension (fall in blood pressure on standing); when given by injection, there

may be additional side-effects.
▲ warning: it should be administered with caution to patients who suffer from hypotension and certain other cardiovascular disorders and those with severe liver, kidney, or thyroid impairment.
○ Related entries: Coro-Nitro Spray; Deponit; Glytrin Spray; GTN 300 mcg; Minitran; Nitrocine; Nitrocontin Continus; Nitro-Dur; Nitrolingual Spray; Nitronal; Percutol; Suscard; Sustac; Transiderm-Nitro; Tridil

glycol salicylate
like a number of other SALICYLATES, has a COUNTER-IRRITANT, or RUBEFACIENT, action on topical application to relieve inflammatory pain in joints and muscles.
✚▲ side-effects/warning: see under METHYL SALICYLATE
○ Related entries: Cremalgin Balm; Dubam

glycopyrronium bromide
is an ANTICHOLINERGIC drug that is used in preoperative medication for drying up saliva and other secretions. It is administered by injection.
✚▲ side-effects/warning: see under ATROPINE SULPHATE
○ Related entries: Robinul; Robinul-Neostigmine

Glypressin
(Ferring) is a proprietary preparation of the pituitary HORMONE antidiuretic hormone (ADH, or vasopressin). It is used as a VASOCONSTRICTOR to treat bleeding from varices (varicose veins) in the oesophagus. It is available in a form for injection.
✚▲ side-effects/warning: see TERLIPRESSIN

Glytrin Spray
(Sherwin) is a proprietary, non-prescription preparation of the VASODILATOR and ANTI-ANGINA drug glyceryl trinitrate. It can be used to treat and prevent angina pectoris and is available as

an aerosol spray in metered doses.
✚▲ side-effects/warning: see GLYCERYL
TRINITRATE

GnRH
See GONADORELIN

Goddard's Embrocation
(LRC Products) is a proprietary, non-
prescription preparation of turpentine oil
(with ammonia and acetic acid), which
has COUNTER-IRRITANT, or RUBEFACIENT,
action. It can be applied to the skin for
symptomatic relief of underlying muscle
or joint pain. It is available as an
embrocation for topical application.
▲ warning: do not use on inflamed or
broken skin, or on mucous membranes.
✚▲ side-effects/warning:
see: TURPENTINE OIL

gold
in the form of the chemical compounds
sodium aurothiomalate and auranofin, is
used therapeutically as an ANTIRHEUMATIC
treatment for rheumatoid arthritis and
juvenile arthritis. Gold compounds work
very slowly and it may take several months
of treatment before there are any
beneficial effects. Administration is by
injection.
✚▲ side-effects/warning: see AURANOFIN;
SODIUM AUROTHIOMALATE

Golden Eye Drops
(Typharm) is a proprietary, non-
prescription preparation of the
ANTIBACTERIAL drug propamidine
isethionate. It can be used to treat
infections of the eyelids or conjunctiva
(including acanthamoeba keratitis) and is
available as eye-drops.
✚▲ side effects/warnings: see PROPAMIDINE
ISETHIONATE

Golden Eye Ointment
(Typharm) is a proprietary, non-
prescription preparation of the
ANTIBACTERIAL drug dibromopropamidine

isethionate. It can be used to treat
infections of the eyelids or conjunctiva
(specifically acanthamoeba keratitis) and
is available as an eye ointment and as eye-
drops.
✚▲ side effects/warnings: see
DIBROMOPROPAMIDINE ISETHIONATE

gonadorelin
(gonadotrophin-releasing hormone;
GnRH) is the hypothalamic HORMONE that
acts on the pituitary gland to release the
GONADOTROPHINS (luteinizing hormone,
LH and follicle-stimulating hormone,
FSH). It is therefore also known as
luteinizing-hormone releasing hormone,
LH-RH, or more correctly LH-FSH-RH.
Gonadorelin is in fact the synthetic
analogue of the naturally occurring
gonadotrophin-releasing hormone and is
used for diagnostic purposes (to assess
pituitary function) or as an infertility
treatment, when it is given by pulsatile
subcutaneous or intravenous infusion.
Synthetic analogues of gonadorelin
(BUSERELIN, GOSERELIN, LEUPRORELIN
ACETATE and NAFARELIN) are used to treat
endometriosis, infertility, breast and
prostate cancer.
✚ side-effects: rarely, there may be headache,
abdominal pain and nausea; the site of
infusion may become painful.
▲ warning: administration of gonadorelin to
treat infertility or absence of menstruation
has to be by pulsed subcutaneous infusion,
which is a form of treatment generally
available only in specialist units.
**✪ Related entries: Fertiral; HRF;
Relefact LH-RH; Relefact LH-RH/TRH**

Gonadotraphon LH
(Paines & Byrne) is a proprietary,
prescription-only preparation of the
HORMONE human chorionic
gonadotrophin (HCG). It can be used to
treat undescended testicles and delayed
puberty in boys and also women who are
suffering from specific hormonal
deficiency for infertility. It is available in a

G

form for injection.
+▲ side-effects/warning: see CHORIONIC
GONADOTROPHIN

gonadotrophin

is the name of any of several HORMONES
that are produced and secreted by the
anterior pituitary gland and which act on
the ovary in women and on the testes in
men to promote the production in turn of
other SEX HORMONES and of ova (eggs) or
sperm, respectively. The major
gonadotrophins are FOLLICLE STIMULATING
HORMONE (FSH) and LUTEINIZING HORMONE
(LH). In pregnancy, large amounts of a
similar hormone are released by the
placenta, so it is called CHORIONIC
GONADOTROPHIN and this is the basis of
most pregnancy tests. These hormones are
used as an infertility treatment.

gonadotrophin-releasing hormone

See GONADORELIN

Gopten

(Knoll) is a proprietary, prescription-only
preparation of the ACE INHIBITOR
trandolapril. It can be used as an
ANTIHYPERTENSIVE treatment and often in
conjunction with other classes of drug. It
is available as capsules.
+▲ side-effects/warning: see TRANDOLAPRIL

goserelin

is an analogue of the hypothalamic
HORMONE GONADORELIN (gonadotrophin-
releasing hormone; GnRH). Its effect is to
down-regulate secretion by the pituitary
gland of gonadotrophin (after an initial
surge). The end result of this is to, in turn,
inhibit secretion of steroid hormones by
the ovaries, which is of benefit in
endometriosis (a growth of the lining of
the uterus at inappropriate sites).
Goserelin is used therapeutically as an
ANTICANCER drug for cancer of the prostate
gland. Administration is by subcutaneous
injection.

+▲ side-effects/warning: see under
BUSERELIN. Additionally, there may be rashes,
bruises at the sight of injection and rarely
high blood calcium levels in patients with
breast cancer.
✪ Related entry: Zoladex

gramicidin

is an ANTIMICROBIAL and ANTIBIOTIC drug,
which is incorporated into a number of
eye- and ear-drop preparations along with
NEOMYCIN SULPHATE and NYSTATIN.
**✪ Related entries: Adcortyl with
Graneodin; Neosporin; Tri-Adcortyl; Tri-
Adcortyl Otic**

Graneodin

(Squibb) is a proprietary, prescription-
only preparation of the ANTIBACTERIAL and
(AMINOGLYCOSIDE) ANTIBIOTIC drug
neomycin sulphate. It can be used to treat
bacterial infections of the skin and to
prevent infection following minor surgery.
It is available as an ointment for topical
application.
+▲ side-effects/warning: see NEOMYCIN
SULPHATE

granisetron

is a recently introduced ANTI-EMETIC and
ANTINAUSEANT drug. It gives relief from
nausea and vomiting, especially in patients
receiving cytotoxic radiotherapy or
chemotherapy. It acts by blocking the
action of the natural mediator SEROTONIN.
Administration is either oral as tablets or
by intravenous injection or infusion.
+ side-effects: headache, rash, constipation
and change in liver function.
▲ warning: administer with care to patients
who are pregnant or breast-feeding.
✪ Related entry: Kytril

Gregoderm

(Unigreg) is a proprietary, prescription-
only COMPOUND PREPARATION of the ANTI-
INFLAMMATORY and CORTICOSTEROID drug
hydrocortisone, the ANTIBACTERIAL and
(AMINOGLYCOSIDE) ANTIBIOTIC drug

neomycin sulphate, the antibacterial and (POLYMYXIN) antibiotic drug polymyxin B sulphate and the ANTIFUNGAL and antibiotic drug nystatin. It can be used to treat inflammation of the skin in which infection is also present and is available as an ointment for topical application.

✚▲ side-effects/warning: see HYDROCORTISONE; NEOMYCIN SULPHATE; NYSTATIN, POLYMYXIN B SULPHATE

griseofulvin

is a powerful ANTIFUNGAL and ANTIBIOTIC drug. It is most commonly used for large-scale skin infections, especially those that prove resistant to other drugs. During treatment, which may be prolonged, it is deposited selectively in the skin, hair and nails and so prevents further fungal invasion. Administration is oral as tablets or a suspension.

✚ side-effects: there may be headache with nausea and vomiting; some patients experience sensitivity to light, rash, dizziness, fatigue and blood disorders.

▲ warning: it should not be administered to patients who suffer from liver failure, porphyria, or who are pregnant. Administer with caution to patients who are breast-feeding. Avoid alcohol because its effects are enhanced.

✪ Related entries: Fulcin; Grisovin

Grisovin

(Glaxo) is a proprietary, prescription-only preparation of the ANTIFUNGAL and ANTIBIOTIC drug griseofulvin. It can be used to treat fungal infections of the scalp, skin and nails and is available as tablets.

✚▲ side-effects/warning: see GRISEOFULVIN

growth hormone

See SOMATOTROPIN; SOMATROPIN

GTN 300 mcg

(Martindale) is a proprietary, non-prescription preparation of the VASODILATOR and ANTI-ANGINA drug glyceryl trinitrate. It can be used to treat and prevent angina pectoris and in HEART FAILURE TREATMENT. It is available as short-acting sublingual tablets.

✚▲ side-effects/warning: see GLYCERYL TRINITRATE

guaiphenesin

is incorporated into a number of proprietary preparations as an EXPECTORANT, though evidence of its efficacy is lacking. Administration is oral as a linctus.

✪ Related articles: Actifed Expectorant; Benylin Chesty Coughs Non-Drowsy; Covonia Bronchial Balsam; Dimotane Expectorant; Do-Do Expectorant Linctus; Famel Expectorant; Famel Honey and Lemon Pastilles; Jackson's All Fours; Lemsip Chesty Cough; Meltus Junior Expectorant Linctus; Nirolex; Nirolex for Children; Robitussin Chesty Cough with Congestion; Sudafed Expectorant; Veno's Expectorant; Vicks Original Formula Cough Syrup; Vicks Vaposyrup for Chesty Coughs; Vicks Vaposyrup for Chesty Coughs and Nasal Congestion.

guanethidine monosulphate

is an ADRENERGIC NEURONE BLOCKER, which is an ANTISYMPATHETIC class of drug that prevents release of noradrenaline from sympathetic nerves. It can be used in ANTIHYPERTENSIVE treatment of moderate to severe high blood pressure, especially when other treatments have failed and usually in conjunction with other antihypertensive drugs (eg. a DIURETIC or BETA-BLOCKER). Administration can be oral as tablets or in a form for injection.

✚ side-effects: postural hypotension (fall in blood pressure on standing); fluid retention; nasal congestion; diarrhoea, failure to ejaculate; drowsiness.

▲ warning: it should not be administered to patients with certain renal or heart disorders, or who have phaeochromocytoma; it should be administered with caution to those who are

G elderly, pregnant, or have peptic ulcers, asthma, or coronary or cerebral arteriosclerosis.
○ **Related entries: Ganda; Ismelin**

Guarem

(Rybar) is a proprietary, non-prescription preparation of guar gum, which is a form of DIABETIC TREATMENT. It is available as sachets of granules that are dissolved in fluid and drunk before a meal or sprinkled onto food.
+▲ side-effects/warning: see GUAR GUM

guar gum

is a form of DIABETIC TREATMENT in as much that if it is taken in sufficient quantities it reduces the rise in blood glucose which occurs after meals, probably by delaying absorption of food. It may be used to relieve the symptoms of Dumping Syndrome. It is available as sachets of granules that are dissolved in fluid and drunk before a meal or sprinkled onto food.
+ side-effects: flatulence, distension of the intestine with possible obstruction.
▲ warning: do not use when there is pre-existing intestinal obstruction. Fluid intake should be maintained. Gum preparations should usually be taken with plenty of water and not last thing at night.
○ **Related entries: Guarem; Guarina**

Guarina

(Norgine) is a proprietary, non-prescription preparation of guar gum, which is a form of DIABETIC TREATMENT. It is available as sachets of granules that are dissolved in fluid and drunk before a meal or sprinkled onto food.
+▲ side-effects/warning: see GUAR GUM

Gyno-Daktarin

(Janssen) is a proprietary, prescription-only range of preparations of the ANTIFUNGAL drug miconazole (as nitrate). The various preparations can be used to treat fungal infections of the vagina or

vulva (eg. candidiasis; thrush). They are available as an intravaginal cream (with its own applicator), vaginal inserts (pessaries), an *Ovule* (a vaginal capsule) called *Gyno-Daktarin 1* and a *Combipack* that combines the cream and the pessaries. The preparations are also available, under certain conditions, without prescription.
+▲ side-effects/warning: see MICONAZOLE

Gynol II

(Ortho) is a proprietary, non-prescription SPERMICIDAL CONTRACEPTIVE for use in combination with barrier methods of contraception (such as a condom). It is available as a jelly containing nonoxinol.
+▲ side effects/warning: see NONOXINOL

Gyno-Pevaryl

(Cilag) is a proprietary, prescription-only range of preparations of the ANTIFUNGAL drug econazole nitrate. The various preparations can be used to treat fungal infections of the vagina or vulva (eg. candidiasis; thrush) and the penis (applied under the foreskin). They are available as a cream for topical application to the anogenital area, as vaginal inserts (pessaries) in two formulations with one under the name *Gyno-Pevaryl 1* and *Combipacks* that combine the cream and one or other formulation of the pessaries. The cream is also available, under certain conditions, without prescription.
+▲ side-effects/warning: see ECONAZOLE NITRATE

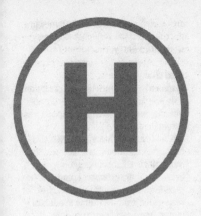

H

*H₂-antagonist

drugs act to block the actions of
histamine at a class of histamine receptor
called H_2, which is found in the gastric
mucosa (stomach lining) and promotes
secretion of peptic (hydrochloric) acid.
The over-production of peptic acid may be
involved in ulceration of the gastric
(stomach) and duodenal (first part of
small intestine) linings, or be the cause of
pain in reflux oesophagitis (regurgitation
of acid and enzymes into the oesophagus).
H_2-antagonists are commonly used as
ULCER-HEALING DRUGS and for a wide
variety of other peptic acid complaints.
Technically, these drugs are
ANTIHISTAMINES, but somewhat confusingly
this term is not applied to them because it
is reserved for the much earlier class of
drugs that act at H_1 receptors and which
have quite different actions (they are used,
among other purposes, to treat allergic
reactions).
See: CIMETIDINE; FAMOTIDINE; NIZATIDINE;
RANITIDINE.

Haelan

(Dista) is a proprietary, prescription-only
preparation of the CORTICOSTEROID and
ANTI-INFLAMMATORY drug flurandrenolone.
It can be used to treat inflammatory skin
disorders such as eczema and is available
as a cream and an ointment for topical
application.
+▲ side-effects/warning: see
FLURANDRENOLONE

Haelan-C

(Dista) is a proprietary, prescription-only
COMPOUND PREPARATION of the
CORTICOSTEROID drug flurandrenolone
and the ANTIMICROBIAL drug clioquinol. It
can be used as a topical application to
treat severe, non-infective inflammation of
the skin, particularly eczema that is
unresponsive to less-powerful drugs. It is
available as a cream and an ointment.
+▲ side-effects/warning: see CLIOQUINOL;
FLURANDRENOLONE

H

Haemophilus Influenzae Type B Vaccine

(District Health Authorities) (Hib) is a non-proprietary prescription-only preparation of the VACCINE used to prevent *Haemophilus influenzae* infection and is available in a form for injection.

+▲ side-effects/warning: see HAEMOPHILUS INFLUENZAE TYPE B VACCINE

Haemophilus influenzae type b vaccine

(Hib) vaccine for IMMUNIZATION prevents *Haemophilus influenzae* infection (bacteria that cause respiratory infection). It is given as a routine childhood preventive vaccination and is administered by injection.

+▲ side-effects/warning: see VACCINE

✪ Related entries: Act-HIB; Haemophilus Influenzae Type B Vaccine; HibTITER

*haemostatic

drugs slow or prevent bleeding (haemorrhage). They are used mostly to treat disorders in which bleeding is prolonged and potentially dangerous (eg. haemophilia).

Halciderm Topical

(Squibb) is a proprietary, prescription-only preparation of the CORTICOSTEROID and ANTI-INFLAMMATORY drug halcinonide. It can be used to treat inflammatory skin disorders such as eczema and is available as a cream for topical application.

+▲ side-effects/warning: see HALCINONIDE

halcinonide

is a CORTICOSTEROID with ANTI-INFLAMMATORY properties. It is used to treat inflammatory skin disorders, such as recalcitrant eczema and psoriasis, that are unresponsive to less potent corticosteroids. Administration is by topical application in the form of a cream.

+▲ side-effects/warning: see under CORTICOSTEROIDS; though systemic effects are unlikely with topical application, but there may be local skin reactions.

✪ Related entry: Halciderm Topical

Haldol

(Janssen) is a proprietary, prescription-only preparation of the ANTIPSYCHOTIC drug haloperidol. It can be used to treat psychotic disorders, especially schizophrenia or the hyperactive, euphoric condition mania and to tranquillize patients undergoing behavioural disturbance. It can also be used for the short-term treatment of severe anxiety and of some involuntary motor (movement) disturbances. Additionally, it can be used for intractable hiccups. It is available as a liquid, tablets and in a form for injection and depot deep intramuscular injection.

+▲ side-effects/warning: see HALOPERIDOL

Haldol Decanoate

(Janssen) is a proprietary, prescription-only preparation of the ANTIPSYCHOTIC drug haloperidol (as undecanoate). It can be used in the maintenance of schizophrenia and other psychoses and is available in a form for depot deep intramuscular injection.

+▲ side-effects/warning: see HALOPERIDOL

Halfan

(SK&F) is a proprietary, prescription-only preparation of the ANTIMALARIAL drug halofantrine hydrochloride. It is available as tablets.

+▲ side-effects/warning: see HALOFANTRINE HYDROCHLORIDE

Half-Betadur CR

(Monmouth) is a proprietary, prescription-only preparation of the BETA-BLOCKER drug propranolol hydrochloride. It can be used as an ANTIHYPERTENSIVE treatment for raised blood pressure, as an ANTI-ANGINA treatment to relieve symptoms and improve exercise tolerance and as an ANTI-ARRHYTHMIC to regularize heartbeat and to treat myocardial infarction. It can also be used as an ANTITHYROID drug for short-term treatment of thyrotoxicosis, as an ANTIMIGRAINE treatment to prevent attacks, as an ANXIOLYTIC treatment, particularly for symptomatic relief of tremor and palpitations and, with an ALPHA-ADRENOCEPTOR BLOCKER, in the acute treatment of phaeochromocytoma. It is available as modified-release capsules.

+▲ side-effects/warning: see PROPRANOLOL HYDROCHLORIDE

Half-Beta-Prograne

(Tillomed) is a proprietary, prescription-only preparation of the BETA-BLOCKER drug propranolol hydrochloride. It can be used as an ANTIHYPERTENSIVE treatment for raised blood pressure, as an ANTI-ANGINA treatment to relieve symptoms and improve exercise tolerance and as an ANTI-ARRHYTHMIC to regularize heartbeat and to treat myocardial infarction. It can also be used as an ANTITHYROID drug for short-term treatment of thyrotoxicosis, as an ANTIMIGRAINE treatment to prevent attacks, as an ANXIOLYTIC treatment, particularly for symptomatic relief of tremor and palpitations and, with an ALPHA-ADRENOCEPTOR BLOCKER, in the acute treatment of phaeochromocytoma. It is available as modified-release capsules.

+▲ side-effects/warning: see PROPRANOLOL HYDROCHLORIDE

Half-Inderal LA

(Zeneca) is a proprietary, prescription-only preparation of the BETA-BLOCKER drug propranolol hydrochloride. It can be used as an ANTIHYPERTENSIVE treatment for raised blood pressure, as an ANTI-ANGINA treatment to relieve symptoms and improve exercise tolerance and as an ANTI-ARRHYTHMIC to regularize heartbeat and to treat myocardial infarction. It can also be used as an ANTITHYROID drug for short-term treatment of thyrotoxicosis, as an ANTIMIGRAINE treatment to prevent attacks, as an ANXIOLYTIC treatment,

particularly for symptomatic relief of tremor and palpitations and, with an ALPHA-ADRENOCEPTOR BLOCKER, in the acute treatment of phaeochromocytoma. It is available as modified-release capsules.

+▲ side-effects/warning: see PROPRANOLOL HYDROCHLORIDE

Half Securon SR

(Knoll) is a proprietary, prescription-only preparation of the CALCIUM-CHANNEL BLOCKER verapamil hydrochloride. It can be used as an ANTIHYPERTENSIVE treatment and as an ANTI-ANGINA drug in the prevention of attacks. It is available as modified-release tablets.

+▲ side-effects/warning: see VERAPAMIL HYDROCHLORIDE

Half Sinemet CR

(Du Pont) is a proprietary, prescription-only COMPOUND PREPARATION of the drugs levodopa and carbidopa, which is a combination called co-careldopa. It can be used to treat parkinsonism, but not the parkinsonian symptoms induced by drugs (see ANTIPARKINSONISM) and is available as modified-release tablets.

+▲ side-effects/warning: see LEVODOPA

halibut-liver oil

is an excellent source of retinol (vitamin A) and also contains VITAMIN D. A non-proprietary preparation is available in the form of tablets, but it should not be taken without initial medical diagnosis. Retinol deficiency is rare and if any treatment should be required it must be under medical supervision in order to avoid the potentially unpleasant side-effects of excess vitamin A in the body. It is available as capsules.

+▲ side-effects/warning: see RETINOL

halofantrine hydrochloride

is an ANTIMALARIAL drug. It is used to treat infection by uncomplicated, chloroquine-resistant *Plasmodium falciparum* species malaria, or chloroquine-resistant

Plasmodium vivax species malaria in areas of the world where this is common. Administration is oral as tablets.

✚ side-effects: diarrhoea, nausea, vomiting, rash and pruritus and abdominal pain.

▲ warning: it may cause serious heart arrhythmias in susceptible patients; it should not be taken with food. It should not be administered to patients with certain heart disorders (such as arrhythmias), or who are pregnant or breast-feeding.

❍ Related entry: Halfan

haloperidol

is a powerful ANTIPSYCHOTIC drug. It is used to treat and tranquillize patients with psychotic disorders (such as schizophrenia) and is particularly suitable for treating manic forms of behavioural disturbance, especially for emergency control. It can also be used in the short-term treatment of severe anxiety. Quite separately from the previous uses, it can be administered to treat other conditions that may cause tremor, tics, involuntary movements, or involuntary utterances (eg. Gilles de la Tourette syndrome). Administration is either oral as capsules, tablets, or a liquid, or by injection or depot deep intramuscular injection (in the form of the undecanoate salt).

✚▲ side-effects/warning: see under CHLORPROMAZINE HYDROCHLORIDE; but with less sedative effects, fewer anticholinergic and hypotensive symptoms and photosensitivity and skin pigmentation are rare. However, extrapyramidal symptoms (muscle tren.or and rigidity) are more frequent and there may be weight loss. Avoid in basal ganglia disease.

❍ Related entries: Dozic; Haldol; Haldol Decanoate; Serenace

Halothane

(Rhône-Poulenc Rorer) is a proprietary preparation of the inhalant GENERAL ANAESTHETIC drug halothane. It can be used for the induction and maintenance of anaesthesia during surgery. It is available in a form for inhalation.

✚▲ side-effects/warning: see HALOTHANE

halothane

is an inhalant GENERAL ANAESTHETIC drug, which is widely used both for induction and maintenance of anaesthesia during surgical operations. It is relatively non-irritant and does not induce coughing and seldom causes postoperative vomiting. Administration is by inhalation as a liquid through a calibrated vaporizer.

✚ side-effects: there may be liver damage, cardiodepression and peripheral vasodilation.

▲ warning: it should not be given to patients with porphyria.

❍ Related entries: Fluothane; Halothane

Hamarin

(Roche) is a proprietary, prescription-only preparation of the (xanthine oxidase) ENZYME INHIBITOR allopurinol. It can be used to treat excess uric acid in the blood and to prevent renal stones and attacks of gout. It is available as tablets.

✚▲ side-effects/warning: see ALLOPURINOL

Harmogen

(Upjohn) is a proprietary, prescription-only preparation of the OESTROGEN piperazine oestrone sulphate. It can be used in HRT and is available as tablets

✚▲ side-effects/warning: see PIPERAZINE OESTRONE SULPHATE

HAV

See HEPATITIS A VACCINE

Havrix

(SmithKline Beecham) is a proprietary, prescription-only VACCINE preparation of hepatitis A vaccine. It can be used to protect people at risk from infection with hepatitis A; there is also a paediatric preparation called *Havrix Junior*. It is available in a form for injection.

✚▲ side-effects/warning: see HEPATITIS A VACCINE

Havrix Monodose

(SmithKline Beecham) is a proprietary, prescription-only VACCINE preparation of the hepatitis A vaccine. It can be used to protect people at risk from infection with hepatitis A and is available in a form for injection.
+▲ side-effects/warning: see HEPATITIS A VACCINE

Hay-Crom

(Baker Norton) is a proprietary, prescription-only preparation of the ANTI-ALLERGIC drug sodium cromoglycate. It can be used to treat allergic conjunctivitis and is available as eye-drops and an eye ointment.
+▲ side-effects/warning: see SODIUM CROMOGLYCATE

Haymine

(Pharmax) is a proprietary, non-prescription COMPOUND PREPARATION of the ANTIHISTAMINE chlorpheniramine maleate and the SYMPATHOMIMETIC drug ephedrine hydrochloride. It can be used as a NASAL DECONGESTANT for the symptomatic relief of the allergic symptoms of hay fever and allergic rhinitis. It is available as tablets.
+▲ side-effects/warning: see CHLORPHENIRAMINE MALEATE; EPHEDRINE HYDROCHLORIDE

HBIG

See HEPATITIS B IMMUNOGLOBULIN (HBIG)

H-B-Vax II

(Merck, Sharp & Dohme) is a proprietary, prescription-only VACCINE preparation of hepatitis B vaccine. It can be used to give protection from hepatitis B in people at risk and is available in a form for injection.
+▲ side-effects/warning: see HEPATITIS B VACCINE

HCG

See CHORIONIC GONADOTROPHIN

Healonid

(Pharmacia) is a proprietary, prescription-only preparation of sodium hyaluronate, which is a visco-elastic polymer normally present in the aqueous and vitreous humour of the eye. It can be used during surgical procedures on the eye and is available in a form for injection.
+▲ side-effects/warning: see SODIUM HYALURONATE

*heart failure treatment

is used to rectify the functioning of a failing heart. It can involve the administration of a number of different drug types. The causes of heart failure include disease within the heart (mainly ischaemia – an inadequate supply of blood to the muscle that can cause angina pain) or an excessive load imposed on the heart by arterial and other forms of hypertension. CARDIAC GLYCOSIDES increase the force of contraction and have been widely used in congestive heart failure treatment, though nowadays they are usually used in conjunction with other drugs. ANTIHYPERTENSIVE treatment is often the first course of treatment to be used and here both the DIURETIC drugs (eg. AMILORIDE HYDROCHLORIDE, BUMETANIDE, CHLOROTHIAZIDE, ETHACRYNIC ACID, FRUSEMIDE, HYDROCHLOROTHIAZIDE and TRIAMTERENE) and the ACE INHIBITORS (eg. CAPTOPRIL and ENALAPRIL MALEATE) may be valuable. Alternatively, VASODILATOR drugs can be used, such as the NITRATES (eg. GLYCERYL TRINITRATE, ISOSORBIDE DINITRATE, ISOSORBIDE MONONITRATE and PENTAERYTHRITOL TETRANITRATE) or HYDRALAZINE HYDROCHLORIDE. Lastly, CARDIAC STIMULANT drugs, such the SYMPATHOMIMETIC drugs DOPEXAMINE HYDROCHLORIDE and DOBUTAMINE HYDROCHLORIDE, are reserved more for emergencies.

Hedex Extra Tablets

(Sterling Health) is a proprietary, non-

H

prescription COMPOUND ANALGESIC preparation of the NON-NARCOTIC ANALGESIC and ANTIPYRETIC drug paracetamol and the STIMULANT caffeine. It can be used for the pain of headache (including migraine), neuralgia, period pain and to relieve cold symptoms. It is available as tablets and is not normally given to children under 12 years, except on medical advice.

✚▲ side-effects/warning: see CAFFEINE; PARACETAMOL

Hedex Tablets

(Sterling Health) is a proprietary, non-prescription preparation of the NON-NARCOTIC ANALGESIC and ANTIPYRETIC drug paracetamol. It can be used for the pain of headache (including migraine), tension headaches, backache, period pain and to relieve cold and flu symptoms. It is available as tablets and is not normally given to children under six years, except on medical advice.

✚▲ side-effects/warning: see PARACETAMOL

Hemabate

(Upjohn) is a proprietary, prescription-only preparation of the PROSTAGLANDIN analogue carboprost. It can be used to treat haemorrhage following childbirth, especially where other drugs have proved to be ineffective. It is available in a form for injection.

✚▲ side-effects/warning: see CARBOPROST

Heminevrin

(Astra) is a proprietary, prescription-only preparation of the drug chlormethiazole (as base or edisylate). It can be used as a HYPNOTIC for treating severe insomnia (especially in the elderly), as an ANTICONVULSANT and ANTI-EPILEPTIC for treating status epilepticus, eclampsia, the symptoms caused by withdrawal from alcohol and for maintaining unconsciousness under regional anaesthesia. It is available as capsules, a syrup and in a form for intravenous infusion.

✚▲ side-effects/warning: see CHLORMETHIAZOLE

Hemocane

(Intercare Products) is a proprietary, non-prescription COMPOUND PREPARATION of the LOCAL ANAESTHETIC drug lignocaine hydrochloride and the ASTRINGENT agents zinc oxide, bismuth oxide and benzoic acid. It can be used for the symptomatic relief of the pain and itching of haemorrhoids and other ano-rectal conditions. It is available as a cream and is not normally given to children, except on medical advice.

✚▲ side-effects/warning: see BENZOIC ACID; BISMUTH OXIDE; LIGNOCAINE HYDROCHLORIDE; ZINC OXIDE

heparin

is a natural ANTICOAGULANT in the body, which is produced mainly by the liver, leucocytes (white blood cells) and at some other sites. It inhibits the action of the enzyme thrombin, which is needed for the final stages of blood coagulation. For therapeutic use, it is purified after extraction from bovine lungs and bovine and porcine intestinal mucosa. It is available in several forms, including DALTEPARIN, ENOXAPARIN, TINZAPARIN and DANAPAROID SODIUM. Administration is generally by injection (eg. during surgery) to prevent or treat thrombosis and similar conditions. Its effect does not last long and treatment may have to be repeated frequently, or it can be given by constant infusion.

✚ side-effects: should haemorrhage occur, it may be difficult to stop the bleeding for a time – although because heparin is so short-acting merely discontinuing treatment is usually effective fairly quickly. There may be sensitivity reactions. Prolonged use may cause a loss of calcium from the bones and of hair from the head. There may be skin damage.

▲ warning: it should not be administered to patients with haemophilia, thrombocytopenia, peptic ulcer, hypertension, severe kidney or liver disorders, or who have recently undergone eye surgery. It should be administered with caution to those who are pregnant.

○ Related entries: Calciparine; Fragmin; Innohep; Minihep; Minihep Calcium; Monoparin; Monoparin Calcium; Multiparin; Orgaran; Pump-Hep; Unihep; Uniparin; Uniparin Calcium

heparinoid

is a version of the drug HEPARIN. It is used to improve circulation in the skin in the treatment of conditions such as bruising, chilblains, thrombophlebitis, varicose veins and haemorrhoids, though it is not entirely clear how it works. There are various versions with different molecular weights (some that are used are called *Bayer HDB-U*). There is also a version called danaparoid (Org 10172), which is thought to have some advantages as an ANTICOAGULANT and is used to prevent deep vein thrombosis, particularly in orthopaedic surgery.

○ Related entries: Anacal Rectal Ointment; Anarcal Suppositories; danaparoid sodium; Lasonil; Movelat Cream

hepatitis A vaccine

consists of a VACCINE, used for IMMUNIZATION, that is prepared from biosynthetic inactivated hepatitis A virus (HAV). It is an alternative to human NORMAL IMMUNOGLOBULIN for frequent travellers to moderate to high risk areas. Administration is by intramuscular injection.

✚▲ side-effects/warning: see VACCINE

Hepatitis B Immunoglobulin

(Public Health Laboratory Service) (Antihepatatis B Immunoglobulin) is a non-proprietary, prescription-only preparation of hepatitis B

immunoglobulin, which is a SPECIFIC IMMUNOGLOBULIN used to give immediate immunity against infection by the hepatitis B virus. It is available in a form for intramuscular injection.

hepatitis B immunoglobulin (HBIG)

(HBIG) is a SPECIFIC IMMUNOGLOBULIN that is used for IMMUNIZATION to give immediate *passive immunity* against infection by the hepatitis B virus. It is used specifically to immunize personnel in medical laboratories and hospitals who may be infected and to treat babies of mothers infected by the virus during pregnancy. Administration is by intramuscular injection. See also HEPATITIS B VACCINE

○ Related entry: Hepatitis B Immunoglobulin

hepatitis B vaccine

consists of a VACCINE, used for IMMUNIZATION, that is prepared from biosynthetic inactivated hepatitis B virus surface antigen (HBsAg). It is given to patients with a high risk of infection from the hepatitis B virus mostly through contact with a carrier. Administration is by intramuscular injection.

✚▲ side-effects/warning: see VACCINE
○ Related entries: Engerix B; H-B-Vax

heroin

is the common term for the (OPIOID) NARCOTIC ANALGESIC drug DIAMORPHINE HYDROCHLORIDE.

Herpid

(Yamanouchi) is a proprietary, prescription-only preparation of the ANTIVIRAL drug idoxuridine (in the organic solvent dimethyl sulphoxide; DMSO). It can be used to treat infections of the skin by herpes simplex or herpes zoster. It is available in a form for topical application with its own applicator.

✚▲ side-effects/warning: see IDOXURIDINE

H

Hewletts Cream

(Bioglan) is a proprietary, non-prescription preparation of zinc oxide in hydrous wool fat. It can be used for minor abrasions and burns and is available as a cream for topical application to the skin.
✚▲ side-effects/warning: see: WOOL FAT; ZINC OXIDE

hexachlorophane

(hexachlorophene) is an ANTISEPTIC agent. It can be used on the skin for many purposes, including to prevent staphylococcal infections of the skin in newborn babies and to treat recurrent boils. It is available as a dusting powder.
✚ side-effects: rarely, there may be sensitivity reactions and increased sensitivity to light.
▲ warning: it should not be used on areas of raw or badly burned skin. It is not for use by pregnant women.
○ Related entry: Dermalex

hexachlorophene

See HEXACHLOROPHANE

hexamine hippurate

(methenamine hippurate) is an ANTIBACTERIAL drug. It is used to treat recurrent infections of the urinary tract and to prevent infections during urinogenital surgery. Administration is oral in the form of tablets.
✚ side-effects: gastrointestinal upsets, rash and bladder irritation.
▲ warning: it should not be used in patients with severe kidney impairment; administer with care to those who are pregnant.
○ Related entry: Hiprex

hexetidine

is an ANTISEPTIC mouthwash or gargle, which is used for routine oral hygiene and to cleanse and freshen the mouth.
○ Related entry: Oraldene

Hexopal

(Sanofi Winthrop) is a proprietary, non-prescription preparation of the VASODILATOR drug inositol nicotinate. It can be used to help improve blood circulation to the hands and feet when this is impaired, for instance in peripheral vascular disease (Raynaud's phenomenon). It is available as tablets and a suspension.
✚▲ side-effects/warning: see INOSITOL NICOTINATE

Hib

is an abbreviation for HAEMOPHILUS INFLUENZAE TYPE B VACCINE.

Hibicet Hospital Concentrate

(Zeneca) is a proprietary, non-prescription COMPOUND PREPARATION of the ANTISEPTIC agents chlorhexidine (as gluconate) and cetrimide. It can be used, after dilution, for cleaning, disinfecting and swabbing wounds. It is available as a cream.
✚▲ side-effects/warning: see CETRIMIDE; CHLORHEXIDINE

Hibisol

(Zeneca) is a proprietary, non-prescription preparation of the ANTISEPTIC agent chlorhexidine (as gluconate). It can be used to treat minor wounds and burns on the skin and hands and is available as a solution.
✚▲ side-effects/warning: see CHLORHEXIDINE

Hibitane

(Zeneca) is the name of a range of proprietary, non-prescription ANTISEPTIC preparations that are based on solutions of chlorhexidine. The standard preparation is a powder, which is used to prepare solutions of chlorhexidine and powdered antiseptic compounds. There are two solutions: *Hibitane 5% Concentrate*, which is diluted in water or alcohol and then used to disinfect the skin; and *Hibitane Gluconate 20%*, which can be used to disinfect cavities and the

bladder and to treat urethral infections. *Hibitane Antiseptic*, which is a cream, can be used to treat minor wounds and burns.
+▲ side-effects/warning: see CHLORHEXIDINE

HibTITER
(Lederle) is a proprietary, prescription-only VACCINE preparation used to provide protection against *Haemophilus influenzae* infection. It is available in a form for injection.
+▲ side-effects/warning: see HAEMOPHILUS INFLUENZAE TYPE B VACCINE

High Potency Factor VIII Concentrate
(SNBTS) is a proprietary, prescription-only preparation of dried human factor VIII fraction. It acts as a HAEMOSTATIC drug to reduce or stop bleeding in the treatment of disorders in which bleeding is prolonged and potentially dangerous (mainly haemophilia A). It is available in a form for infusion or injection.
+▲ side-effects/warning: see FACTOR VIII FRACTION, DRIED

Hioxyl
(Quinoderm) is a proprietary, non-prescription preparation of the ANTISEPTIC agent hydrogen peroxide. It can be used to treat bedsores, leg ulcers, minor wounds and burns and is available as a cream for topical application.
+▲ side-effects/warning: see HYDROGEN PEROXIDE

Hiprex
(3M Health Care) is a proprietary, non-prescription preparation of the ANTIBACTERIAL drug hexamine hippurate. It can be used to treat infections of the urinary and gastrointestinal tracts and to prevent infections during urinogenital surgery. It is available as capsules.
+▲ side-effects/warning: see HEXAMINE HIPPURATE

Hirudoid

H

(Panpharma) is a proprietary, non-prescription preparation of heparinoids. It can be used to improve circulation in conditions such as bruising, haematoma, chilblains, thrombophlebitis and varicose veins. It is available as a cream and a gel.
+▲ side-effects/warning: see HEPARINOID

Hismanal
(Janssen) is a proprietary, prescription-only preparation of the ANTIHISTAMINE drug astemizole. It can be used to treat the symptoms of allergic disorders such as hay fever and urticaria. It is available as tablets and a sugar-free suspension. (It can be sold without a prescription only for the treatment of hay fever and to patients over 12 years old.)
+▲ side-effects/warning: see ASTEMIZOLE

Hivid
(Roche) is a proprietary, prescription-only preparation of zalcitabine (DDC). It can be used as an ANTIVIRAL drug in the treatment of AIDS and is available as tablets.
+▲ side-effects/warning: see ZALCITABINE

HNIG
See NORMAL IMMUNOGLOBULIN

Honvan
(ASTA Medica) is a proprietary, prescription-only preparation of the drug fosfestrol tetrasodium, which is converted in the body to STILBOESTROL (which has OESTROGEN activity as a SEX HORMONE). It can be used in men as an ANTICANCER drug for cancer of the prostate gland. It is available as tablets and in a form for injection.
+▲ side-effects/warning: see FOSFESTROL TETRASODIUM

*hormone antagonists
are a class of drugs that prevent the action of HORMONES at their receptors (special recognition sites on cells). They act either

H

directly by competing for these sites (eg. TAMOXIFEN at oestrogen receptors and CYPROTERONE ACETATE at androgen receptors), or indirectly where the antagonist acts on other receptors to inhibit the production, or the release, of the hormone (eg. OCTREOTIDE inhibits the release of hormones from cancerous cells).

hormone replacement therapy

See HRT

*hormones

are substances produced and secreted by glands. In the case of endocrine hormones there are carried by the bloodstream to the organs on which they have their effect. Hormones can be divided into several families.

The *adrenal hormones* are secreted by the adrenal glands (a small paired-gland just above the kidneys), of which there are two distinct types: adrenal cortical hormones and adrenal medullary hormones. The adrenocortical hormones come from the cortical (outer) region of the adrenal gland (eg. CORTICOSTEROID hormones, which are STEROIDS with glucocorticoid or mineralocorticoid activity). The adrenalomedullary hormones come from the medullary (outer) region of the adrenal gland (eg. ADRENALINE and NORADRENALINE).

The THYROID HORMONES and the *parathyroid hormones* come from the thyroid and parathyroid glands at the base of the neck (eg. CALCITONIN, parathormone, THYROXINE and TRIIODOTHYRONINE). The *glucose-regulatory hormones* are produced by the pancreas (eg. GLUCAGON and INSULIN).

The SEX HORMONES come mainly from the ovaries or the testes (eg. the androgens, such as TESTOSTERONE; the OESTROGENS such as OESTRADIOL and OESTRIOL; and the PROGESTOGENS such as PROGESTERONE).

The *pituitary gland*, situated at the base of the skull, is an important producer of several vital hormones. There are two distinct classes of pituitary hormones: the posterior pituitary hormones OXYTOCIN and VASOPRESSIN (antidiuretic hormone; ADH); and the anterior pituitary hormones, which include CORTICOTROPHIN (adrenocorticotrophic hormone; ACTH), SOMATOTROPIN (growth hormone; GH); PROLACTIN and THYROTROPHIN (thyroid-stimulating hormone; TSH); or the GONADOTROPHINS – FOLLICLE-STIMULATING HORMONE (FSH) and LUTEINIZING HORMONE (LH).

The release of anterior pituitary hormones is controlled, in turn, by factors that travel, in a specialized system of portal blood vessels, the short distance from the hypothalamus (an adjacent brain area). These *hypothalamic hormones* include corticotrophin-releasing hormone (CRH; or corticotrophin-releasing factor, CRF); GONADORELIN (gonadotrophin-releasing hormone, GnRH; or gonadotropin-releasing factor, GRF; LH-RH); growth hormone-releasing hormone (GHRH, or growth hormone-releasing factor, GRF); growth hormone release-inhibiting hormone (GHRIH; somatostatin, or growth hormone-release-inhibiting factor, GHRIF); and PROTIRELIN (thyrotrophin-releasing hormone; TRH). Many of these hormones can be administered therapeutically to people with a hormonal deficiency, sometimes in synthetic form. Synthetic HORMONE ANTAGONISTS have been developed either to reduce the release of hormones (eg. in cancers of endocrine glands) or, with sex hormones, to reduce normal release, or the effects of normal levels, of hormone, for example where this inhibition benefits cancers of certain organs such as the prostate gland, the endometrium of the uterus, or of the breast (eg. TAMOXIFEN).

Hormonin

(Shire) is a proprietary, prescription-only

COMPOUND PREPARATION of the natural, OESTROGEN SEX HORMONES oestradiol and oestriol. It can be used in HRT and is available as tablets.

+▲ side-effects/warning: see OESTRADIOL; OESTRIOL

HRF

(Monmouth) is a proprietary, prescription-only preparation of the HORMONE gonadorelin (gonadotrophin-releasing hormone, GnRH). It can be used as a diagnostic aid in assessing the functioning of the pituitary gland. It is available in a form for injection or infusion.

+▲ side-effects/warning: see GONADORELIN

*HRT

hormone replacement therapy, is a drug treatment for women to supplement the diminished production of the SEX HORMONE OESTROGEN by the body during the menopause. HRT consists of the administration of small amounts of an oestrogen and is used to alleviate menopausal vasomotor symptoms and vaginitis (vaginal atrophy) in women whose lives are inconvenienced by these conditions. Additionally, there is evidence that HRT will reduce post-menopausal osteoporosis, stroke and myocardial infarction (especially if started prior to the menopause). It may also be suggested for women undergoing early natural, or surgical, menopause; since they are at high risk of osteoporosis (brittle bones). In some women, a PROGESTOGEN may also be prescribed (to reduce the risk of endometrial cystic hyperplasia and possible cancer). Administration of HRT drugs can be oral as tablets, by topical application as skin patches, or implants.

HTIG

See TETANUS IMMUNOGLOBULIN, HUMAN

Human Actraphane 30/70

(Novo Nordisk) is a proprietary, non-

prescription preparation of human BIPHASIC ISOPHANE INSULIN. It is used in DIABETIC TREATMENT to treat and maintain diabetic patients. It contains both isophane and neutral insulins in a proportion of 70% to 30% respectively. It is available in vials for injection and has an intermediate duration of action.

+▲ side-effects/warning: see INSULIN

Human Actrapid

(Novo Nordisk) is a proprietary, non-prescription preparation of synthesized neutral SOLUBLE INSULIN. It is used in DIABETIC TREATMENT to treat and maintain diabetic patients. It is available in vials for injection, in cartridges (*Penfil*) for use with *NovoPen* injectors and as prefilled disposable injectors (*Actrapid*). It has a short duration of action.

+▲ side-effects/warning: see INSULIN

human antihaemophilic fraction, dried

See FACTOR VIII FRACTION, DRIED

human chorionic gonadotrophin

See CHORIONIC GONADOTROPHIN

human growth hormone

See SOMATOTROPIN; SOMATROPIN

Human Initard 50/50

(Novo Nordisk, Wellcome) is a proprietary, non-prescription preparation of BIPHASIC ISOPHANE INSULIN. It is used to treat and maintain diabetic patients and contains isophane and neutral insulins in equal proportions. It is available in vials for injection and has an intermediate duration of action.

+▲ side-effects/warning: see INSULIN

Human Insulatard

(Novo Nordisk, Wellcome) is a proprietary, non-prescription preparation of human ISOPHANE INSULIN. It is used to treat and maintain diabetic patients. It is

H

available in vials for injection and has an intermediate duration of action.
✚▲ side-effects/warning: see INSULIN

human menopausal gonadotrophins

is a pituitary HORMONE preparation and is a collective name for combinations of the GONADOTROPHINS follicle-stimulating hormone (FSH) and luteinizing hormone (LH) (one form of which is called MENOTROPHIN). It is extracted from the urine of post-menopausal women and has various uses, including as an infertility treatment for women with proven hypopituitarism, or who do not respond to the drug CLOMIPHENE CITRATE (another drug commonly used to treat infertility) and in superovulation treatment in assisted conception (as with *in vitro* fertilization). It is available in a form for injection.
✚ side-effects: hyperstimulation of the ovaries, multiple pregnancy and local reactions.
▲ warning: it should be given with caution to women with ovarian cysts; thyroid, adrenal, or pituitary gland tumours or certain other disorders.
❍ Related entries: Humegon; Normegon; Pergonal

Human Mixtard 30/70

(Novo Nordisk, Wellcome) is a proprietary, non-prescription preparation of BIPHASIC ISOPHANE INSULIN. It is used to treat and maintain diabetic patients and contains both isophane and neutral insulins in a proportion of 70% to 30% respectively. It is available in vials for injection and has an intermediate duration of action.
✚▲ side-effects/warning: see INSULIN

Human Monotard

(Novo Nordisk) is a proprietary, non-prescription preparation of human INSULIN ZINC SUSPENSION. It is used in DIABETIC TREATMENT to treat and maintain diabetic

patients. It is available in vials for injection and has a long duration of action.
✚▲ side-effects/warning: see INSULIN

human normal immunoglobulin

See NORMAL IMMUNOGLOBULIN

Human Protaphane

(Novo Nordisk) is a proprietary, non-prescription preparation of human ISOPHANE INSULIN. It is used in DIABETIC TREATMENT to maintain diabetic patients. It is available in vials for injection and as cartridges (*Penfill*) for *Human Protaphane Novopen* injection devices. It has an intermediate duration of action.
✚▲ side-effects/warning: see INSULIN

Human Ultratard

(Novo Nordisk) is a proprietary, non-prescription preparation of human INSULIN ZINC SUSPENSION (CRYSTALLINE). It is used in DIABETIC TREATMENT to treat and maintain diabetic patients. It is available in vials for injection and has a long duration of action.
✚▲ side-effects/warning: see INSULIN

Human Velosulin

(Novo Nordisk, Wellcome) is a proprietary, non-prescription preparation of human SOLUBLE INSULIN. It is used in DIABETIC TREATMENT to treat and maintain diabetic patients. It is available in vials for injection and has a short duration of action.
✚▲ side-effects/warning: see INSULIN

Humatrope

(Lilly) is a proprietary, prescription-only preparation of somatropin, which is the biosynthetic form of the pituitary HORMONE human growth hormone. It can be used to treat hormonal deficiency and associated symptoms (in particular, short stature). It is available in a form for injection.
✚▲ side-effects/warning: see SOMATROPIN

Humegon

(Organon) is a proprietary, prescription-only HORMONE preparation of human menopausal gonadotrophins, which contains FOLLICLE-STIMULATING HORMONE (FSH) and LUTEINIZING HORMONE (LH). It can be used to treat infertile women with proven hypopituitarism and who do not respond to CLOMIPHENE CITRATE (another drug commonly used to treat infertility) and in superovulation treatment in assisted conception (as with *in vitro* fertilization). It is available in a form for injection.

+▲ side-effects/warning: see HUMAN MENOPAUSAL GONADOTROPHINS

Humiderm

(BritCair) is a proprietary, non-prescription preparation of pyrrolidone carboxylic acid. It can be used as an EMOLLIENT to treat dry skin and is available as a cream.

Humulin I

(Lilly) is a proprietary, non-prescription preparation of human ISOPHANE INSULIN. It is used in DIABETIC TREATMENT to treat and maintain diabetic patients. It is available in vials for injection and as cartridges for the *B-D Pen* device and has an intermediate duration of action.

+▲ side-effects/warning: see INSULIN

Humulin Lente

(Lilly) is a proprietary, non-prescription preparation of human INSULIN ZINC SUSPENSION. It is used in DIABETIC TREATMENT to treat and maintain diabetic patients. It is available in vials for injection and has a relatively long duration of action.

+▲ side-effects/warning: see INSULIN

Humulin M1

(Lilly) is a proprietary, non-prescription preparation of BIPHASIC ISOPHANE INSULIN, human insulins. It is used in DIABETIC TREATMENT to treat and maintain diabetic patients and contains both isophane and neutral insulins in a proportion of 90% to 10% respectively. It is available in vials for injection or as cartridges for the *B-D Pen* device and has an intermediate duration of action.

+▲ side-effects/warning: see INSULIN

Humulin M2

(Lilly) is a proprietary, non-prescription preparation of BIPHASIC ISOPHANE INSULIN, human insulins. It is used in DIABETIC TREATMENT to treat and maintain diabetic patients and contains both isophane and neutral insulins in a proportion of 80% to 20% respectively. It is available in vials for injection or as cartridges for the *B-D Pen* device and has an intermediate duration of action.

+▲ side-effects/warning: see INSULIN

Humulin M3

(Lilly) is a proprietary, non-prescription preparation of BIPHASIC ISOPHANE INSULIN, human insulins. It is used in DIABETIC TREATMENT to treat and maintain diabetic patients and contains human isophane insulin (30% soluble/70% isophane). It is available in vials for injection or as cartridges for the *B-D pen* device and has an intermediate duration of action.

+▲ side-effects/warning: see INSULIN

Humulin M4

(Lilly) is a proprietary, non-prescription preparation of BIPHASIC ISOPHANE INSULIN, mixed human insulins. It is used in DIABETIC TREATMENT to treat and maintain diabetic patients and contains human isophane insulin (40% soluble/60% isophane). It has a short duration of action.

+▲ side-effects/warning: see INSULIN

Humulin S

(Lilly) is a proprietary, non-prescription preparation of human synthesized neutral SOLUBLE INSULIN. It is used in DIABETIC TREATMENT to treat and maintain diabetic

H

patients and is available in vials for injection or as cartridges for the *B-D Pen* device. It has a short duration of action.
＋▲ side-effects/warning: see INSULIN

Humulin Zn

(Lilly) is a proprietary, non-prescription preparation of human INSULIN ZINC SUSPENSION (CRYSTALLINE). It is used in DIABETIC TREATMENT to treat and maintain diabetic patients and is available in vials for injection. It has an intermediate duration of action.
＋▲ side-effects/warning: see INSULIN

Hyalase

(CP Pharmaceuticals) is a proprietary, prescription-only preparation of the enzymehyaluronidase. It can be used to increase the permeability of soft tissues to injected drugs. It is available in a form for injection.
＋▲ side-effects/warning: see HYALURONIDASE

hyaluronidase

is an enzyme, which can be used to increase the permeability of soft tissues to injected drugs. Administration is by injection.
＋ side-effects: sometimes there are allergic sensitivity reactions.
▲ warning: it should not be administered directly to the cornea of the eye, or where there is malignant infection; it is not to be used to reduce swelling in stings and bites.
✪ Related entries: Hyalase; Lasonil

Hyate C

(Porton) is a porcine, prescription-only preparation of factor VIII inhibitor bypassing fraction and is used in patients with factor VIII inhibitors.
＋▲ side-effects/warning: see FACTOR VIII INHIBITOR BYPASSING FRACTION

Hydergine

(Sandoz) is a proprietary, prescription-only preparation of the mixture of drugs

known as co-dergocrine mesylate, which is a VASODILATOR of blood vessels in the brain. It is used primarily to assist in the management of elderly patients with mild to moderate dementia. It is available as tablets.
＋▲ side-effects/warning: see CO-DERGOCRINE MESYLATE

hydralazine hydrochloride

is a VASODILATOR drug that is used to treat acute and chronic cardiovascular disorders, such as a hypertensive crisis and as an ANTIHYPERTENSIVE for long-term high blood pressure (where it is often administered with a BETA-BLOCKER and a DIURETIC). Administration can be oral as tablets or in a form for injection or infusion.
＋ side-effects: there may be nausea and vomiting. Prolonged high-dosage may cause lupus erythematosus (inflamed connective tissue), blood disorders, headache, fast heartbeat and fluid retention.
▲ warning: there may be a swift and severe fall in blood pressure. Special care must be taken when used with certain cardiovascular disorders, in pregnancy and when breast-feeding.
✪ Related entry: Apresoline

*hydrating agents

are drugs that soothe and soften the skin. They are incorporated into ointments and skin creams that are used to treat conditions where the skin is dry or flaky (eg. eczema). They are usually fats or oils, such as LANOLIN and LIQUID PARAFFIN and can be combined with other hydrating agents such as UREA. In conditions where there is a skin infection, hydrating agents can be combined with ANTIMICROBIAL or ANTIFUNGAL drugs and where there is severe inflammation ANTI-INFLAMMATORY and CORTICOSTEROID drugs can be added.

Hydrea

(Squibb) is a proprietary, prescription-only preparation of the (CYTOTOXIC)

ANTICANCER drug hydroxyurea. It can be used to treat myeloid leukaemia and is available as capsules.

+▲ side-effects/warning: see HYDROXYUREA

Hydrenox

(Boots) is a proprietary, prescription-only preparation of the (THIAZIDE) DIURETIC drug hydroflumethiazide. It can be used in the treatment of oedema, either alone or in conjunction with other drugs and as an ANTIHYPERTENSIVE. It is available as tablets.

+▲ side-effects/warning: see HYDROFLUMETHIAZIDE

Hydrocal

(Bioglan) is a proprietary, prescription-only COMPOUND PREPARATION of the CORTICOSTEROID and ANTI-INFLAMMATORY drug hydrocortisone (as acetate) and the ASTRINGENT agent calamine. It can be used to treat mild inflammatory skin conditions (such as eczema) and is available as a cream for topical application.

+▲ side-effects/warning: see CALAMINE; HYDROCORTISONE

hydrochloric acid

is a strong acid that, within the body, is part of the gastric juice secreted from special cells within the mucosal lining of the stomach. It provides the acid environment that is essential for the working of the enzyme pepsin, which begins the process of digestion that then continues within the small intestine. Over-production of acid (hyperacidity) can cause the symptoms of dyspepsia (indigestion) and this can be exacerbated by alcohol and NSAID drugs. ANTACIDS give symptomatic relief of acute dyspepsia and gastritis. But for chronic problems associated with peptic ulcers (gastric or duodenal ulcers) and oesophagitis, ULCER-HEALING DRUGS are required (see H$_2$-ANTAGONISTS and PROTON-PUMP INHIBITOR). Under-production of acid (hypochlorhydria and achlorhydria) can also be a problem and one treatment is to administer a preparation that releases hydrochloric acid (eg. *Muripsin*).

hydrochlorothiazide

is a DIURETIC of the THIAZIDE class. It can be used as an ANTIHYPERTENSIVE, either alone or in conjunction with other drugs and in the treatment of oedema (accumulation of fluid in the tissues) associated with congestive heart failure. Administration is oral in the form of tablets.

+▲ side-effects/warning: see under BENDROFLUAZIDE

✪ Related entries: Accuretic; Acezide; Amil-Co; Capozide; Carace Plus; Delvas; Dyazide; Hydromet; HydroSaluric; Innozide; Kalten; Moducren; Moduret-25; Moduretic; Monozide 10; Secadrex; Sotazide; Tolerzide; Triam-Co; TrimaxCo; Zestoretic

hydrocortisone

is a CORTICOSTEROID with ANTI-INFLAMMATORY properties, which can be administered therapeutically (sometimes in COMPOUND PREPARATIONS with ANTIBACTERIAL, ANTIBIOTIC, or ANTIFUNGAL drugs) to treat any kind of inflammation, including arthritis, to treat allergic conditions, adrenocortical insufficiency, shock, inflammatory bowel disease, haemorrhoids, eye and skin inflammation and hypersensitivity reactions. It can be administered in a number of forms: hydrocortisone, hydrocortisone acetate, hydrocortisone butyrate, hydrocortisone sodium phosphate, or hydrocortisone sodium succinate; and by several different routes, including by topical application as a lotion, ointment, eye ointment, cream, lozenge, gel, suppositories, spray, foam, ear-drops, scalp lotion or tablets or by injection.

+▲ side-effects/warning: see under CORTICOSTEROIDS. Side-effects depend on the route of administration, but are unlikely with topical application.

✪ Related entries: Actinac; Alphaderm;

H

Alphosyl HC; Anugesic-HC; Anusol-HC; Calmurid HC; Canesten-HC; Carbo-Cort; Chloromycetin Hydrocortisone; Cobadex; Colifoam; Corlan; Daktacort; Dioderm; Econacort; Efcortelan; Efcortesol; Epifoam; Eurax-Hydrocortisone; Fucidin H; Gentisone HC; Gregoderm; Hydrocal; Hydrocortistab; Hydrocortisyl; Hydrocortone; Locoid; Locoid C; Mildison; Neo-Cortef; Nystaform-HC; Otosporin; Perinal; Proctofoam HC; Proctosedyl; Quinocort; Solu-Cortef; Tarcortin; Terra-Cortril; Terra-Cortril Nystatin; Timodine; Uniroid-HC; Vioform-Hydrocortisone; Xyloproct

hydrocortisone acetate
See HYDROCORTISONE

hydrocortisone butyrate
See HYDROCORTISONE

hydrocortisone sodium phosphate
See HYDROCORTISONE

hydrocortisone sodium succinate
See HYDROCORTISONE

Hydrocortistab
(Boots) is a proprietary, prescription-only preparation of the CORTICOSTEROID and ANTI-INFLAMMATORY drug hydrocortisone (as acetate). It can be used to treat mild inflammatory skin conditions (such as eczema) and is available as a cream, an ointment and tablets.
+▲ side-effects/warning: see HYDROCORTISONE

Hydrocortisyl
(Roussel) is a proprietary, prescription-only preparation of the CORTICOSTEROID and ANTI-INFLAMMATORY drug hydrocortisone. It can be used to treat mild inflammatory skin conditions (such as eczema) and is available as a cream

and an ointment.
+▲ side-effects/warning: see HYDROCORTISONE

Hydrocortone
(Merck, Sharp & Dohme) is a proprietary, prescription-only preparation of the CORTICOSTEROID and ANTI-INFLAMMATORY drug hydrocortisone. It can be used to make up hormonal deficiency and to treat inflammation, shock and certain allergic conditions. It is available as tablets.
+▲ side-effects/warning: see HYDROCORTISONE

hydroflumethiazide
is a DIURETIC drug of the THIAZIDE class. It can be used, either alone or in conjunction with other drugs, as an ANTIHYPERTENSIVE and in the treatment of oedema (accumulation of fluid in the tissues) associated with congestive heart failure. Administration is oral in the form of tablets.
+▲ side-effects/warning: see under BENDROFLUAZIDE
✪ Related entries: Aldactide 25; Aldactide 50; Hydrenox; Spiro-Co; Spiro-Co 50

hydrogen peroxide
is a general ANTISEPTIC agent. It can be used for a wide range of purposes and is available in several forms: in solution and as a cream to cleanse and deodorize wounds and ulcers; as drops to clean ears; and as a mouthwash and gargle for oral hygiene.
✪ Related entries: Exterol; Hioxyl; Otex

Hydromet
(Merck, Sharp & Dohme) is a proprietary, prescription-only COMPOUND PREPARATION of the (THIAZIDE) DIURETIC drug hydrochlorothiazide and the ANTISYMPATHETIC drug methyldopa. It can be used as an ANTIHYPERTENSIVE and is available as tablets.
+▲ side-effects/warning: see

HYDROCHLOROTHIAZIDE; METHYLDOPA

Hydromol

(Quinoderm) is a proprietary, non-prescription COMPOUND PREPARATION of liquid paraffin and arachis oil (and several other constituents). It has EMOLLIENT properties and can be used for treating dry skin. It is available as a cream and a bath additive (*Emollient*).

+▲ side-effects/warning: ARACHIS OIL; LIQUID PARAFFIN

HydroSaluric

(Merck, Sharp & Dohme) is a proprietary, prescription-only preparation of the (THIAZIDE) DIURETIC drug hydrochlorothiazide. It can be used, either alone or in conjunction with other drugs, in the treatment of oedema and as an ANTIHYPERTENSIVE. It is available as tablets.

+▲ side-effects/warning: see HYDROCHLOROTHIAZIDE

hydrotalcite

is an ANTACID complex of aluminium magnesium carbonate hydroxide hydrate. It is used for the relief of dyspepsia and also reduces flatulence. Administration is oral in the form of chewable tablets or a suspension.

✪ Related entries: Altacite Plus; Altacite Suspension; Altacite Tablets

hydroxocobalamin

is the form of VITAMIN B_{12} that is now used therapeutically, having replaced CYANOCOBALAMIN. Supplements of hydroxocobalamin are administered only by injection (because vitamin B_{12} deficiency is usually caused by malabsorption, which renders oral administration futile).

✪ Related entries: Cobalin-H; Neo-Cytamen

hydroxychloroquine sulphate

is a drug that has ANTI-INFLAMMATORY and ANTIRHEUMATIC properties. It can be used primarily to treat rheumatoid arthritis (including juvenile arthritis) and is usually used when other, more common treatments (eg. with NSAIDs) are unsuccessful. Its effects may not be seen for four to six months. It is available as tablets.

+▲ side-effects/warning: see under CHLOROQUINE. (Although it is not used for malaria, it is a similar chemical and has similar side-effects and warnings.)

✪ Related entry: Plaquenil

hydroxyethylcellulose

is a constituent of a preparation that is used as artificial tears and which is given to patients with dry eyes due to disease. Administration is by eye-drops.

✪ Related entry: Minims Artificial Tears

hydroxyprogesterone caproate

See HYDROXYPROGESTERONE HEXANOATE

hydroxyprogesterone hexanoate

(hydroxyprogesterone caproate) is a PROGESTOGEN that can be used to treat recurrent abortion (habitual abortion). Administration is by long-lasting, intramuscular depot injection.

+▲ side-effects/warning: see under PROGESTOGEN

✪ Related entry: Proluton Depot

hydroxyurea

is a CYTOTOXIC DRUG, which is used as an ANTICANCER treatment for chronic myeloid leukaemia and sometimes for polycythaemia. Administration is oral in the form of capsules.

+▲ side-effects/warning: see under CYTOTOXIC DRUGS

✪ Related entry: Hydrea

hydroxyzine hydrochloride

is an ANTIHISTAMINE drug with some additional ANXIOLYTIC properties. It can be

H

used for the relief of allergic symptoms such as itching and mild rashes and also for short-term treatment of anxiety. Administration is oral as tablets or a syrup.

✚▲ side-effects/warning: see under ANTIHISTAMINE. Because of its sedative side-effects, the performance of skilled tasks such as driving may be impaired.

○ Related entries: Atarax; Ucerax

Hygroton

(Geigy) is a proprietary, prescription-only preparation of the (THIAZIDE-like) DIURETIC drug chlorthalidone. It can be used, either alone or in conjunction with other drugs, in the treatment of oedema and as an ANTIHYPERTENSIVE. It is available as tablets.

✚▲ side-effects/warning: see CHLORTHALIDONE

hyoscine butylbromide

is an ANTICHOLINERGIC drug, which can be used as an ANTISPASMODIC for the symptomatic relief of smooth muscle spasm in the gastrointestinal tract. Administration is oral as tablets or by injection.

✚▲ side-effects/warning: see under ATROPINE SULPHATE; but with less actions on the central nervous system. Avoid in porphyria.

○ Related entry: Buscopan

hyoscine hydrobromide

(known as scopolamine hydrobromide in the USA) is a BELLADONNA ALKALOID drug derived from plants of the belladonna family and is a powerful ANTICHOLINERGIC. By itself it is an effective SEDATIVE and is commonly used for premedication prior to surgery and in obstetric practice. It also has ANTINAUSEANT properties and can be used to prevent motion sickness. In a solution, it can be used in ophthalmic treatments to paralyse the muscles of the pupil either for surgery or to rest the eye following surgery. Administration is topical

as eye-drops or skin patches, or by injection. See HYOSCINE BUTYLBROMIDE for use as an ANTISPASMODIC.

✚ side-effects: depending on the route of administration, there may be drowsiness, dry mouth, dizziness, blurred vision and difficulty in urination; in doses for premedication and obstetrics it may cause confusion, hallucinations, behavioural disturbances, amnesia, ataxia, occasionally excitement and slowing of the heartbeat (especially in the elderly).

▲ warning; it is not to be given to patients with porphyria or closed-angle glaucoma. Administer with caution to those who are pregnant or breast-feeding, elderly, or have urinary retention, cardiovascular disease, or liver or kidney impairment. Because it has sedative properties, the performance of skilled tasks such as driving may be impaired.

○ Related entries: Boots Travel Calm Tablets; Feminax; Joy-Rides; Kwells Junior; Kwells Tablets; Scopoderm TTS

hyoscyamine

See ATROPINE SULPHATE

Hypnomidate

(Janssen) is a proprietary, prescription-only preparation of the GENERAL ANAESTHETIC drug etomidate. It can be used for the induction of anaesthesia and is available in a form for injection.

✚▲ side-effects/warning: see ETOMIDATE

*hypnotic

drugs induce sleep by an action on the brain. They are used mainly to treat insomnia and to calm patients who are mentally ill, but can also be used for the short-term treatment of insomnia due to jet lag, shiftwork, emotional problems, or serious illness. The best-known and most-used hypnotics are the BENZODIAZEPINES (which can also be used as ANXIOLYTICS) such as DIAZEPAM, NITRAZEPAM, FLUNITRAZEPAM and FLURAZEPAM, which have a relatively long duration of action and may cause drowsiness the next day.

There are some more recently introduced benzodiazepines that have a comparatively short duration of action and cause less drowsiness (eg. LOPRAZOLAM, LORMETAZEPAM and TEMAZEPAM). Other types of drug that are used as hypnotics include CHLORAL HYDRATE, TRICLOFOS SODIUM and CHLORMETHIAZOLE. The BARBITURATES (eg. AMYLOBARBITONE) are now rarely used, because they can readily cause dependence and are extremely dangerous in overdose.

Hypnovel

(Roche) is a proprietary, prescription-only preparation of the BENZODIAZEPINE drug midazolam. It can be used as an ANXIOLYTIC and SEDATIVE, where its ability to cause amnesia is useful in preoperative medication, dental surgery and local anaesthesia, because the patient forgets the unpleasant procedure. It is available in a form for injection.
+▲ side-effects/warning: see MIDAZOLAM

*hypoglycaemic

drugs reduce the levels of glucose (sugar) in the bloodstream. They are used mainly in the treatment of diabetes mellitus. The ORAL HYPOGLYCAEMIC drugs are primarily used to treat Type II diabetes (non-insulin-dependent diabetes mellitus; NIDDM; maturity-onset diabetes), for example, the SULPHONYLUREA drugs (eg. CHLORPROPAMIDE and GLIBENCLAMIDE), the BIGUANIDE drug METFORMIN HYDROCHLORIDE and ACARBOSE and GUAR GUM. Administration of INSULIN, which is mainly used in Type I diabetes (insulin-dependent diabetes mellitus; IDDM; juvenile-onset diabetes), is by injection.

Hypotears

(CIBA Vision) is a proprietary, non-prescription preparation of polyvinyl alcohol. It can be used as artificial tears in conditions where there is dryness of the eye due to disease. It is available as eye-drops.

+▲ side-effects/warning: see POLYVINYL ALCOHOL

*hypotensive

literally means a drug that lowers blood pressure and there are many drugs that have such an action. Some drugs do so on acute (short-term) administration as a deliberate part of their medical use. For instance, NITRATES, which are used to treat angina attacks, have an immediate and powerful VASODILATOR action which redistributes blood flow in the body and beneficially reduces the workload of the heart. In a hypertensive crisis the aim is an immediate fall in blood pressure and this can be achieved by the injection of a vasodilator such as HYDRALAZINE HYDROCHLORIDE. However, other types of drug may cause an unwanted fall in blood pressure to below normal levels as one of their side-effects, which may limit their usefulness in susceptible patients. This undesirable side-effect usually occurs as postural hypotension (a fall in blood pressure on standing quickly, where the brain is starved of blood causing the patient to feel dizzy or faint) and can be minimized, or avoided, by taking the drug in question on retiring to bed. Also, this side-effect often becomes less of a problem if the drug is taken as part of a chronic (long-term) treatment.

The term ANTIHYPERTENSIVE is, by convention, commonly used in medicine to describe the class of drug that is used to lower abnormally high blood pressure (hypertension) and usually administered on a long-term basis. Such drugs are not necessarily hypotensive in normal individuals.

Hypovase

(Invicta) is a proprietary, prescription-only preparation of the ALPHA-ADRENOCEPTOR BLOCKER drug prazosin hydrochloride. It can be used in ANTIHYPERTENSIVE treatment, in peripheral vascular disease and in congestive HEART

H

FAILURE TREATMENT. It is available as tablets.

✚▲ side-effects/warning: see PRAZOSIN HYDROCHLORIDE

Hypovase Benign Prostatic Hypertrophy

(Invicta) is a proprietary, prescription-only preparation of the ALPHA-ADRENOCEPTOR BLOCKER drug prazosin hydrochloride. It can be used to treat urinary retention (eg. in benign prostatic hypertrophy) because of its SMOOTH MUSCLE RELAXANT properties. It is available as tablets.

✚▲ side-effects/warning: see PRAZOSIN HYDROCHLORIDE

hypromellose

is a constituent of artificial tears, which are used to treat extremely dry eyes due to certain disorders. It is available as eye-drops and often in combination with a variety of drugs.

○ Related entries: Isopto Alkaline; Isopto Carpine; Isopto Frin; Isopto Plain; Maxidex

Hypurin Isophane

(CP Pharmaceuticals) is a proprietary, non-prescription preparation of highly purified bovine ISOPHANE INSULIN. It is used in DIABETIC TREATMENT to treat and maintain diabetic patients and is available in vials for injection. It has an intermediate duration of action.

✚▲ side-effects/warning: see INSULIN

Hypurin Lente

(CP Pharmaceuticals) is a proprietary, non-prescription preparation of highly purified bovine INSULIN ZINC SUSPENSION. It is used in DIABETIC TREATMENT to treat and maintain diabetic patients and is available in vials for injection. It has a relatively long duration of action.

✚▲ side-effects/warning: see INSULIN

(CP Pharmaceuticals) is a proprietary, non-prescription preparation of highly purified bovine SOLUBLE INSULIN. It is used in DIABETIC TREATMENT to treat and maintain diabetic patients and is available in vials for injection. It has a relatively short duration of action.

✚▲ side-effects/warning: see INSULIN

Hypurin Protamine Zinc

(CP Pharmaceuticals) is a proprietary, non-prescription preparation of highly purified bovine PROTAMINE ZINC INSULIN. It is used in DIABETIC TREATMENT to treat and maintain diabetic patients and is available in vials for injection. It has a long duration of action.

✚▲ side-effects/warning: see INSULIN

Hytrin

(Abbott) is a proprietary, prescription-only preparation of the ALPHA-ADRENOCEPTOR BLOCKER drug terazosin (as terazosin hydrochloride). It can be used in ANTIHYPERTENSIVE treatment and is available as tablets.

✚▲ side-effects/warning: see TERAZOSIN

Hytrin BPH

(Abbott) is a proprietary, prescription-only preparation of the ALPHA-ADRENOCEPTOR BLOCKER drug terazosin (as terazosin hydrochloride). It can be used to treat urinary retention (eg. in benign prostatic hyperplasia) because of its SMOOTH MUSCLE RELAXANT properties. It is available as tablets.

✚▲ side-effects/warning: see TERAZOSIN

Ibugel

(Dermal) is a proprietary, prescription-only preparation of the (NSAID) NON-NARCOTIC ANALGESIC and ANTIRHEUMATIC drug ibuprofen, which has COUNTER-IRRITANT, or RUBEFACIENT, actions. It can be applied to the skin for symptomatic relief of underlying rheumatic and muscular pain, sprains and neuralgia. It is available as a gel for topical application to the skin and is not normally used for children, except on medical advice.
✚▲ side-effects/warning: see IBUPROFEN; but adverse effects on topical application are limited.

Ibular

(Lagap) is a proprietary, prescription-only preparation of the (NSAID) NON-NARCOTIC ANALGESIC and ANTIRHEUMATIC drug ibuprofen. It can be used to relieve pain, particularly the pain and inflammation of rheumatic disease and other musculoskeletal disorders. It is available as tablets.
✚▲ side-effects/warning: see IBUPROFEN

Ibuleve Gel

(DDD) is a proprietary, non-prescription preparation of the (NSAID) NON-NARCOTIC ANALGESIC and ANTIRHEUMATIC drug ibuprofen, which has COUNTER-IRRITANT, or RUBEFACIENT actions. It can be used for the symptomatic relief of rheumatic and muscular pain, backache, sprains, strains and neuralgia. It is available as a gel for massage into the effected area and is not normally used for children under 14 years, except on medical advice.
✚▲ side-effects/warning: see IBUPROFEN

Ibuleve Sports Gel

(DDD) is a proprietary, non-prescription preparation of the (NSAID) NON-NARCOTIC ANALGESIC and ANTIRHEUMATIC drug ibuprofen, which has COUNTER-IRRITANT, or RUBEFACIENT actions. It can be used for the symptomatic relief of muscular aches, sprains and strains. It is available as a non-greasy gel, in a pump-action tube, for massage into the effected area. It is not normally used for children under 14 years, except on medical advice.

+▲ side-effects/warning: see IBUPROFEN

Ibumed

(Medipharma) is a proprietary, prescription-only preparation of the (NSAID) NON-NARCOTIC ANALGESIC and ANTIRHEUMATIC drug ibuprofen, which also has valuable ANTIPYRETIC properties. It can be used to relieve pain, particularly the pain of rheumatic disease and other musculoskeletal disorders. It is available as tablets.

+▲ side-effects/warning: see IBUPROFEN

ibuprofen

is a (NSAID) NON-NARCOTIC ANALGESIC and ANTIRHEUMATIC drug. It is used primarily to treat the pain of rheumatism and other musculoskeletal disorders, moderate pain of inflammatory origin and postoperative pain. Although its anti-inflammatory property is not as powerful as a number of other NSAIDs, its side-effects tend to be relatively well tolerated, so higher dosage may be used to compensate. Accordingly, it was the first and only, modern NSAID licensed for non-prescription, over-the-counter sale in the UK. It has extensive use both in its own right and as the major active constituent in COMPOUND ANALGESIC preparations for the treatment of minor to moderate pain, including headache, period pain, toothache and muscle ache. Its ANTIPYRETIC action helps symptomatic relief of the fever associated with colds and flu. It is also available for use in babies and children (including juvenile arthritis) and also during breast-feeding. Administration is oral as tablets, capsules, suspensions or syrups, or as a gel for topical application.

+▲ side-effects/warning: see under NSAID; but ibuprofen is better tolerated and causes less gastrointestinal disturbances than the majority of its class.

☉ Related entries: Apsifen; Arthrofen; Brufen; Brufen Retard; Codafen Continus; Cuprofen Ibuprofen Tablets; Ebufac; Fenbid; Ibugel; Ibular; Ibuleve Gel; Ibuleve Sports Gel; Ibumed; Inoven; Isisfen; Junifen; Librofem; Lidifen; Motrin; Nurofen; Nurofen Soluble; Pacifene; Pacifene Maximum Strength; PhorPain; PhorPain Double Strength; Proflex Pain Relief; Proflex Sustained Relief Capsules; Proflex Tablets; Rimafen

Ibuspray

(Dermal) is a proprietary, prescription-only preparation of the (NSAID) NON-NARCOTIC ANALGESIC and ANTIRHEUMATIC drug ibuprofen, which has COUNTER-IRRITANT, or RUBEFACIENT, actions. It can be used for the symptomatic relief of underlying rheumatic and muscular pain, sprains and neuralgia. It is available as a spray for topical application to the skin and is not normally used for children, except on medical advice.

+▲ side-effects/warning: see IBUPROFEN; but adverse effects on topical application are limited.

ichthammol

is a thick, dark brown liquid derived from bituminous oils. It is used in ointments or in glycerol solution for the topical treatment of ulcers and inflammation on the skin. It is milder than coal tar and is useful in treating the less-severe forms of eczema. A popular mode of administration is as an impregnated bandage with ZINC PASTE.

+ side-effects: some patients experience skin irritation; the skin may become sensitized.

▲ warning: it must not be placed in contact with broken skin surfaces.

+▲ side-effects/warning: see under COAL TAR

idarubicin hydrochloride

is a recently introduced CYTOTOXIC DRUG (of ANTIBIOTIC origin) with properties similar to doxorubicin. It is used as an

ANTICANCER drug particularly to treat acute leukaemia and breast cancer. Administration is oral as capsules or by infusion.

+▲ side-effects/warning: see under CYTOTOXIC DRUGS. Administer with care to patients with liver or kidney impairment.
✪ Related entry: Zavedos

Idoxene

(Spodefell) is a proprietary, prescription-only preparation of the ANTIVIRAL drug idoxuridine. It can be used to treat local viral infections, particularly herpes simplex eye infections. It is available as an eye ointment.
+▲ side-effects/warning: see IDOXURIDINE

idoxuridine

is an ANTIVIRAL drug. It can be used in solution to treat infections caused by herpes viruses in and around the mouth or eye, on external genitalia and the skin. It has rather weak and variable results when used topically and is too toxic to be used systemically. It works by stopping the virus multiplying by interfering with DNA synthesis. Administration is as a paint, eye-drops, or an eye ointment.
+ side-effects: it may cause initial irritation and/or stinging on application; changes in taste; overuse may cause softening of the skin.
▲ warning: avoid contact with the eyes and mucous membranes. It should not be used in pregnancy or when breast-feeding. It will damage fabrics.
✪ Related entries: Herpid; Idoxene; Iduridin; Virudox

Iduridin

(Ferring) is a proprietary, prescription-only preparation of the ANTIVIRAL drug idoxuridine (in the organic solvent dimethyl sulphoxide; DMSO). It can be used to treat infections of the skin by herpes simplex (cold sores) or by herpes zoster. It is available as a solution for topical application either with a dropper or its own applicator.

+▲ side-effects/warning: see IDOXURIDINE

ifosfamide

is a CYTOTOXIC DRUG, which is used in ANTICANCER treatment. It works by interfering with cellular DNA and so inhibits cell replication. Administration is by injection or infusion and often simultaneously with the synthetic drug MESNA (which reduces the toxic side-effects).
+▲ side-effects/warning: see under CYTOTOXIC DRUGS
✪ Related entry: Mitoxana

Ikorel

(Rhône-Poulenc Rorer) is a proprietary, prescription-only preparation of the POTASSIUM-CHANNEL ACTIVATOR and VASODILATOR drug nicorandil. It can be used as an ANTI-ANGINA drug to prevent and treat angina pectoris and is available as tablets.
+▲ side-effects/warning: see NICORANDIL

Ilosone

(Dista) is a proprietary, prescription-only preparation of the ANTIBACTERIAL and (MACROLIDE) ANTIBIOTIC drug erythromycin. It can be used to treat and prevent many forms of infection. It is available as capsules, tablets and as a suspension, which is a stronger preparation called *Suspension Forte*.
+▲ side-effects/warning: see ERYTHROMYCIN

Ilube

(Cusi) is a proprietary, prescription-only preparation of the MUCOLYTIC drug acetylcysteine and a small proportion of the synthetic tear fluid hypromellose. It can be used to treat a deficiency of tears in the eyes (eg. in rheumatoid arthritis), which may lead to eye dryness and inflammation. It is available as eye-drops.
+▲ side-effects/warning: see ACETYLCYSTEINE; HYPROMELLOSE

Imbrilon

(Berk) is a proprietary, prescription-only preparation of the (NSAID) NON-NARCOTIC ANALGESIC and ANTIRHEUMATIC drug indomethacin. It can be used to treat the pain and inflammation of rheumatic disease and other musculoskeletal disorders (including gout). It is available as capsules and suppositories.

✚▲ side-effects/warning: see INDOMETHACIN

Imdur

(Astra) is a proprietary, prescription-only preparation of the VASODILATOR and ANTI-ANGINA drug isosorbide mononitrate. It can be used to treat and prevent angina pectoris and is available as modified-release tablets (*Durules*).

✚▲ side-effects/warning: see ISOSORBIDE MONONITRATE

*imidazoles

(or AZOLE) drugs are a chemical group that includes drugs with a variety of ANTIMICROBIAL and ANTIPROTOZOAL actions, but the term is mainly used as a convenient, collective description of a group of broad-spectrum ANTIFUNGAL drugs that are active against most fungi and yeasts. The most common conditions that they are used to treat are vaginal infections (such as candidiasis; thrush), infections of the skin surface, of the mucous membranes, the hair and the nails. The best-known and most-used imidazoles include CLOTRIMAZOLE, MICONAZOLE, KETOCONAZOLE, ISOCONAZOLE and ECONAZOLE NITRATE. Miconazole and ketoconazole can be used systemically, though the latter can cause hepatoxicity (liver damage). They work by interfering with fungal enzymes, causing a lethal accumulation of hydrogen peroxide and by interfering with the fungal cell wall.

Imigran

(Glaxo) is a proprietary, prescription-only preparation of the ANTIMIGRAINE drug sumatriptan. It can be used to treat acute migraine attacks and for cluster headache. It is available as tablets and in a form for self-injection.

✚▲ side-effect/warning: see SUMATRIPTAN

imipenem with cilastin

is an ANTIBACTERIAL and ANTIBIOTIC drug, which is a new sort of BETA-LACTAM with a broad-spectrum of activity against many Gram-positive and Gram-negative bacteria. However, it is partly degraded by an enzyme in the kidney and is therefore combined with CILASTIN, which is an ENZYME INHIBITOR. It can be used to treat infections in the periphery, such as the urethra and cervix and to prevent infection during surgery. Administration is by injection or infusion.

✚ side-effects: vomiting and nausea, diarrhoea and abdominal pain; altered taste and mouth ulcers; skin rashes; hepatitis, jaundice and blood disorders; pain at site of injection; brain and nerve disturbances. The urine may be coloured red.

▲ warning: administer with caution to those who have impaired kidney function, who are pregnant, or have brain disorders such as epilepsy.

○ Related entry: Primaxin

imipramine hydrochloride

is an ANTIDEPRESSANT drug of the TRICYCLIC class, which has fewer SEDATIVE properties than many other tricyclics. It is therefore more suited for the treatment of withdrawn and apathetic patients, rather than those who are agitated and restless. As is the case with many such drugs, it can also be used to treat bed-wetting at night by children. Administration is oral as tablets or a syrup.

✚▲ side-effects/warning: see under AMITRIPTYLINE HYDROCHLORIDE

○ Related entry: Tofranil

Immukin

(Boehringer Ingelheim) is a proprietary, prescription-only preparation of the drug interferon (in the form of gamma-1b). It can be used in conjunction with ANTIMICROBIAL and ANTBIOTIC drugs to reduce the frequency of serious infections in patients with chronic glanulomatous disease. It is available in a form for injection.

✚▲ side-effects/warning: see INTERFERON

*immunization

prevents an individual from contracting specific diseases and is achieved by using one of two methods, *active immunity* or *passive immunity*. Active immunity is conferred by vaccination (that is, administering a VACCINE), which involves the injection of *live* infective agents that are harmless (*attenuated*), dead (*inactivated*), or toxoid (chemically-modified toxin) and so triggering the body's own defence mechanisms to manufacture antibodies. This method gives long-lasting, but not permanent, protection. Passive immunity is conferred by the injection of a quantity of blood serum already containing mixed antibodies (NORMAL IMMUNOGLOBULIN) or of the purified (SPECIFIC IMMUNOGLOBULIN) and prevents the person contracting the disease. This method gives immediate but short-lived protection. See also ANTISERUM and IMMUNOGLOBULIN

✚▲ side-effects/warning: these vary greatly depending on the particular vaccine or immunoglobulin and the individual. However, all involve administering foreign protein so some sort of sensitivity reaction is usual. Commonly, there is malaise, fever and chills.

*immunocompromised

is a term used to describe a patient whose immune defences are abnormally low due to either a congenital or acquired condition. The commonest deficiencies are: of the various white blood cells, the *neutrophils* – which are the first line of defence in actute infections ; the *macrophages* and *T-lymphocytes* – which

are involved in cell-mediated killing of foreign or 'parasitized' host cells; and of blood proteins, the *antibodies* – which neutralize and bind to foreign antigens. Examples of immunocompromised hosts are patients receiving immunosuppressant drugs to prevent rejection of transplanted organs. Individuals suffering from leukaemia, or being treated with high doses of cytotoxic drugs to treat cancer, will also be immunocompromised, as will individuals with AIDS. In any of these circumstances *opportunistic* infections are apt to occur where microbes that normally pose little threat to a healthy person become highly invasive and pose a serious threat. Prophylaxis (prevention) with ANTIBACTERIAL drugs may be required, but once infections are established they are much more difficult to eradicate even with vigorous antibiotic treatment.

*immunoglobulin

is a term used to describe any of five classes of proteins in the immune system that naturally act as *antibodies* in the bloodstream. They are created in response to the presence of a specific *antigen* (any substance the body regards as foreign or dangerous) and circulate within the blood. Immunoglobulin deficiencies are often associated with increased risk of infection. They can be administered therapeutically, by injection or infusion to confer immediate immunity, commonly known as *passive immunity*, against certain diseases. To minimize the risk of allergic reactions, immunoglobulins are normally of human origin rather than from an animal (when they are usually referred to as *antiserum* or *antisera*). Two classes of human immunoglobulins are used to protect either patients suffering from infection or individuals exposed to infection: NORMAL IMMUNOGLOBULIN and SPECIFIC IMMUNOGLOBULIN. Normal immunoglobulin is prepared from the pooled serum of at least 1000 donors who have antibodies to viruses prevalent in a normal population (including for hepatitis A, measles and rubella). Specific immunoglobulin is prepared in a similar way, except that the pooled blood plasma used to obtain the immunoglobulins is from donors with high levels of the particular antibody that is required (eg. for hepatitis B, rabies, rubella, tetanus, or varicella-zoster). See also ANTISERUM; IMMUNIZATION.

✪ Related entries:anti-D (Rh$_0$) immuno-globulin; hepatitis B immunoglobulin (HBIG); rabies immunoglobulin; rubella immunoglobulin; tetanus immuno-globulin; varicella-zoster immunoglobulin (VZIG);

Immunoprin

(Ashbourne) is a proprietary, prescription-only preparation of the IMMUNOSUPPRESSANT drug azathioprine. It can be used to treat a variety of autoimmune diseases and also tissue rejection in transplant patients. It is available as tablets.
✚▲ side-effects/warning: see AZATHIOPRINE

*immunostimulant

is an agent that is used to treat the presence of malignant fluids inside body cavities. A preparation of inactivated bacteria of the species *Corynebacterium parvum*, for example, can be injected into the lung (pleural) cavity of the chest or the abdominal (peritoneal) cavity to treat the presence of such fluids (effusions) there. The effect is to increase the local antibacterial activity by the natural immune system. However, this type of therapy did not prove to be very successful and has largely been discontinued.

*immunosuppressant

drugs are used to inhibit the body's resistance to the presence of infection or foreign bodies. Because of this property, such drugs can be used to prevent tissue rejection following donor grafting or transplant surgery (although there is then the risk of unopposed infection). They are also commonly used to treat autoimmune disease (when the immune system is triggered into acting against part of the body itself). Immunosuppressant drugs can be used to treat conditions such as rheumatoid arthritis, lupus erythematosus and collagen disorders. The best-known and most-used immunosuppressants are the the CORTICOSTEROIDS (eg. PREDNISOLONE) and the non-steroid drugs AZATHIOPRINE, CHLORAMBUCIL, CYCLOPHOSPHAMIDE and CYCLOSPORIN.

Imodium Capsules

(Janssen) is a proprietary, non-prescription preparation of the (OPIOID) ANTIDIARRHOEAL drug loperamide hydrochloride. It can be used for the symptomatic relief of acute diarrhoea and its associated pain and discomfort and is available as capsules.
✚▲ side-effects/warning: see LOPERAMIDE HYDROCHLORIDE

Imtack Spray

(Astra) is a proprietary, non-prescription preparation of the VASODILATOR and ANTI-ANGINA drug isosorbide dinitrate. It can be used to treat and prevent angina pectoris and also in HEART FAILURE TREATMENT. It is available as an aerosol spray.
✚▲ side-effects/warning: see ISOSORBIDE DINITRATE

Imunovir

(Leo) is a proprietary, prescription-only preparation of the ANTIVIRAL drug inosine pranobex. It can be used to treat herpes simplex infections and warts in mucous membranes and adjacent skin (eg. genital warts). It is available as tablets.
✚▲ side-effects/warning: see INOSINE PRANOBEX

Imuran

(Wellcome) is a proprietary, prescription-only preparation of the IMMUNO-SUPPRESSANT drug azathioprine. It can be used to a variety of autoimmune diseases and to treat tissue rejection in transplant patients. It is available as tablets and in a form for injection.

✚▲ side-effects/warning: see AZATHIOPRINE

Inactivated Influenza Vaccine (Split Viron)

(Merieux) is a proprietary, prescription-only VACCINE preparation of influenza vaccine (split viron vaccine). It can be used to prevent an individual from contracting influenza and is available in a form for injection.

✚▲ side-effects/warning: see INFLUENZA VACCINE

indapamide

is a DIURETIC drug of the THIAZIDE-like class. It can be used in ANTIHYPERTENSIVE treatment, either alone or in conjunction with other drugs. Administration is oral in the form of tablets.

✚ side-effects: headache, dizziness, fatigue; nausea and anorexia; muscle cramps; gastrointestinal upsets; skin rashes and other disorders; hypotension; low blood potassium; raised blood urea and glucose; loss of feeling in the extremities; photosensitivity; impotence; kidney impairment, myopia (reversible shortsightedness).

▲ warning: it is not to be used after recent stroke, or where there is severe liver impairment; care must be taken when administering to patients with certain kidney disorders, parathyroid disease (blood electrolytes must be measured), or who are pregnant or breast-feeding.

⊙ **Related entries: Indaxa 25; Natrilix**

Indaxa 25

(Ashbourne) is a proprietary, prescription-only preparation of the (THIAZIDE-like) DIURETIC drug indapamide. It can be used, either alone or in conjunction with other drugs, in ANTIHYPERTENSIVE treatment. It is available as tablets .

✚▲ side-effects/warning: see INDAPAMIDE

Inderal

(Zeneca) is a proprietary, prescription-only preparation of the BETA-BLOCKER drug propranolol hydrochloride. It can be used as an ANTIHYPERTENSIVE treatment for raised blood pressure, as an ANTI-ANGINA treatment to relieve symptoms and improve exercise tolerance and as an ANTI-ARRHYTHMIC to regularize heartbeat and to treat myocardial infarction. It can also be used as an ANTITHYROID drug for short-term treatment of thyrotoxicosis, as an ANTIMIGRAINE treatment to prevent attacks, as an ANXIOLYTIC treatment, particularly for symptomatic relief of tremor and palpitations and, with an ALPHA-ADRENOCEPTOR BLOCKER, in the acute treatment of phaeochromocytoma. It is available as tablets and in a form for injection.

✚▲ side-effects/warning: see PROPRANOLOL HYDROCHLORIDE

Inderal-LA

(Zeneca) is a proprietary, prescription-only preparation of the BETA-BLOCKER drug propranolol hydrochloride. It can be used as an ANTIHYPERTENSIVE treatment for raised blood pressure, as an ANTI-ANGINA treatment to relieve symptoms and improve exercise tolerance and as an ANTI-ARRHYTHMIC to regularize heartbeat and to treat myocardial infarction. It can also be used as an ANTITHYROID drug for short-term treatment of thyrotoxicosis, as an ANTIMIGRAINE treatment to prevent attacks, as an ANXIOLYTIC treatment, particularly for symptomatic relief of tremor and palpitations and, with an ALPHA-ADRENOCEPTOR BLOCKER, in the acute treatment of phaeochromocytoma. It is available as modified-release capsules.

✚▲ side-effects/warning: see PROPRANOLOL HYDROCHLORIDE

Inderetic

(Zeneca) is a proprietary, prescription-only COMPOUND PREPARATION of the BETA-BLOCKER drug propranolol hydrochloride and the (THIAZIDE) DIURETIC drug bendrofluazide. It can be used as an ANTIHYPERTENSIVE treatment for raised blood pressure and is available as capsules.

✚▲ side-effects/warning: see BENDROFLUAZIDE; PROPRANOLOL HYDROCHLORIDE

Inderex

(Zeneca) is a proprietary, prescription-only COMPOUND PREPARATION of the BETA-BLOCKER drug propranolol hydrochloride and the (THIAZIDE) DIURETIC drug bendrofluazide. It can be used as an ANTIHYPERTENSIVE treatment for raised blood pressure and is available as capsules.

✚▲ side-effects/warning: see BENDROFLUAZIDE; PROPRANOLOL HYDROCHLORIDE

Indocid

(Morson) is a proprietary, prescription-only preparation of the (NSAID) NON-NARCOTIC ANALGESIC and ANTIRHEUMATIC drug indomethacin. It can be used to treat the pain of rheumatic disease and other musculoskeletal disorders. It is available as capsules, as modified-release capsules (under the name *Indocid-R*), as suppositories and as a sugar-free suspension.

✚▲ side-effects/warning: see INDOMETHACIN

Indocid PDA

(Morson) is a proprietary, prescription-only preparation of the (NSAID) NON-NARCOTIC ANALGESIC and ANTIRHEUMATIC drug indomethacin. It can be used (in this preparation only) for specialist, emergency, short-term treatment of premature infants with a heart defect (patent ductus arteriosus), while preparations are being made for surgery. It is administered by intravenous infusion.

✚▲ side-effects/warning: see INDOMETHACIN

Indolar SR

(Lagap) is a proprietary, prescription-only preparation of the (NSAID) NON-NARCOTIC ANALGESIC and ANTIRHEUMATIC drug indomethacin. It can be used to relieve the pain of rheumatic disease, gout and other inflammatory musculoskeletal disorders. It is available as modified-release capsules.

✚▲ side-effects/warning: see INDOMETHACIN

Indomax

(Ashbourne) is a proprietary, prescription-only preparation of the (NSAID) NON-NARCOTIC ANALGESIC and ANTIRHEUMATIC drug indomethacin. It can be used to relieve the pain of rheumatic disease and other musculoskeletal disorders. It is available as capsules.

✚▲ side-effects/warning: see INDOMETHACIN

indometacin

See INDOMETHACIN

indomethacin

(indometacin) is a (NSAID) NON-NARCOTIC ANALGESIC and ANTIRHEUMATIC drug. It can be used to treat rheumatic and muscular pain caused by inflammation and/or bone degeneration, particularly at the joints. It can also be used to treat period pain and acute gout. Administration is mainly oral as tablets, capsules, modified-release capsules, or a liquid; but its use in suppositories is especially effective for the relief of overnight pain and stiffness in the morning. Most of its proprietary preparations are not normally given to children, but one form is used (under specialist supervision with extensive monitoring) in premature babies who have patent ductus arteriosus (failure of this connecting vessel between the pulmonary artery and aorta to close after birth).

+▲ side-effects/warning: see under NSAID; there may also be pronounced intestinal disturbances; headaches, dizziness and, though rarely, drowsiness, confusion, insomnia, depression, convulsions, blood disorders, blurred vision, blood pressure changes. It is not to be used in patients who are breast-feeding, who have blood coagulation defects, or kidney and certain other disorders.

۞ Related entries: Artracin; Flexin Continus; Flexin-25 Continus; Flexin-LS Continus; Imbrilon; Indocid; Indocid PDA; Indolar SR; Indomax; Indomod; Mobilan; Rheumacin LA; Rimacid; Slo-Indo

Indomod

(Pharmacia) is a proprietary, prescription-only preparation of the (NSAID) NON-NARCOTIC ANALGESIC and ANTIRHEUMATIC drug indomethacin. It can be used to treat the pain of rheumatic disease and other musculoskeletal disorders. It is available as modified-release capsules.

+▲ side-effects/warning: see INDOMETHACIN

indoramin

is an ALPHA-ADRENOCEPTOR BLOCKER drug. It is used as an ANTIHYPERTENSIVE treatment, often in conjunction with other classes of drug (eg. BETA-BLOCKERS or DIURETICS). It is also used, because of its SMOOTH MUSCLE RELAXANT properties, in the treatment of urinary retention (in prostatic hyperplasia). Administration is oral in the form of tablets.

+ side-effects: dizziness; dry mouth and nasal congestion; failure to ejaculate; there may be depression, drowsiness and weight gain.

▲ warning: it may cause drowsiness, so ability to drive or operate machinery may be impaired. Avoid alcohol. Administer with care in the elderly, or where there are certain kidney or liver disorders, in Parkinson's disease, epilepsy, or depression. It should not

be used by patients who have heart failure.

۞ Related entries: Baratol; Doralese

Infacol

(Pharmax Healthcare) is a proprietary, non-prescription preparation of the ANTIFOAMING AGENT dimethicone (as simethicone). It can be used for the relief of infant colic and griping pain and is available as an oral liquid.

+▲ side-effects/warning: see DIMETHICONE

Infant Gaviscon Liquid

(Reckitt & Colman) is a proprietary, non-prescription preparation of the DEMULCENT agent alginic acid (as sodium alginate and magnesium alginate) and colloidal silica and mannitol. It can be used for gastric reflux and regurgitation and is available as an oral powder.

+▲ side-effects/warning: see ALGINIC ACID

influenza vaccine

for IMMUNIZATION prevents people from catching influenza. It is recommended only for persons at high risk of catching known strains of influenza such as the elderly. This is because, unlike some viruses, the influenza viruses A and B are constantly changing in physical form and antibodies manufactured in the body to deal with one strain at one time will have no effect at all on the same strain at another time. Administration is by injection.

+▲ side-effects/warning: see under VACCINE. Because these vaccines are prepared from virus strains grown in chicken embryos, they should be used with caution in individuals known to be sensitive to eggs.

۞ Related entries: Fluarix; Fluvirin; Fluzone; Inactivated Influenza Vaccine (Split Viron); Influvac Sub-unit

Influvac Sub-unit

(Duphar) is a proprietary, prescription-only VACCINE preparation of influenza vaccine (surface antigen). It can be used to prevent an individual from contracting influenza and is available in a form for injection.

+▲ side-effects/warning: see INFLUENZA VACCINE

Initard 50/50

(Novo Nordisk; Wellcome) is a proprietary, non-prescription preparation of (mixed) BIPHASIC ISOPHANE INSULIN. It is used in DIABETIC TREATMENT to treat and maintain diabetic patients and contains both neutral and isophane porcine insulins in equal proportions. It is available in vials for injection and has an intermediate duration of action.

+▲ side-effects/warning: see INSULIN

Innohep

(Leo) is a proprietary, prescription-only preparation of the ANTICOAGULANT drug tinzaparin, which is a low molecular weight version of heparin. It can be used for long-duration prevention of venous thrombo-embolism, particularly in orthopaedic use. It is available in a form for injection.

+▲ side-effects/warning: see TINZAPARIN

Innovace

(Merck, Sharp & Dohme) a proprietary, prescription-only preparation of the ACE INHIBITOR enalapril maleate. It can be used as an ANTIHYPERTENSIVE and in HEART FAILURE TREATMENT. It is available as tablets.

+▲ side-effects/warning: see ENALAPRIL MALEATE

Innozide

(Merck, Sharp & Dohme) is a proprietary, prescription-only COMPOUND PREPARATION of the ACE INHIBITOR enalapril maleate and the DIURETIC drug hydrochlorothiazide. It can be used as an ANTIHYPERTENSIVE treatment and is available as tablets.

+▲ side-effects/warning: see ENALAPRIL MALEATE; HYDROCHLOROTHIAZIDE

inosine pranobex

is an ANTIVIRAL drug. It is used to treat herpes simplex infections in mucous membranes and adjacent skin (eg. genital warts). Administration is oral as tablets.

+ side-effects: increased uric acid levels in the blood and urine.

▲ warning: it should not be administered to patients with impaired kidney function or high blood levels of uric acid (for instance in gout).

O Related entry: Imunovir

inositol nicotinate

is a VASODILATOR that can be used to help improve blood circulation to the hands and feet when this is impaired, for example in peripheral vascular disease (Raynaud's phenomenon). It is available as tablets and an oral suspension.

+▲ side-effects/warning: see under NICOTINIC ACID

O Related entry: Hexopal

Inoven

(Janssen) is a proprietary, non-prescription preparation of the (NSAID) NON-NARCOTIC ANALGESIC and ANTIRHEUMATIC drug ibuprofen. It can be used for the relief of headache, period pain, muscular pain, dental pain and feverishness. It is available as tablets and is not normally given to children under 12 years, except on medical advice.

+▲ side-effects/warning: see IBUPROFEN

Instillagel

(CliniFlex) is a proprietary, non-prescription COMPOUND PREPARATION of the ANTISEPTIC agent chlorhexidine (as gluconate) and the LOCAL ANAESTHETIC drug lignocaine hydrochloride. It can be used to treat painful inflammations of the urethra and is available as a gel in disposable syringes.

+▲ side-effects/warning: see CHLORHEXIDINE; LIGNOCAINE HYDROCHLORIDE

Insulatard

(Novo Nordisk, Wellcome) is a proprietary, non-prescription preparation of porcine ISOPHANE INSULIN. It is used in DIABETIC TREATMENT to treat and maintain diabetic patients. It is available in vials for injection and has an intermediate duration of action.

✚▲ side-effects/warning: see INSULIN

insulin

is a protein HORMONE produced and secreted by the Islets of Langerhans within the pancreas. It has the effect of reducing the level of glucose (blood sugar) in the bloodstream and is part of a balancing mechanism with the opposing hormone glycogen (which increases blood sugars). Its deficiency (in the disorder called diabetes mellitus) results in high levels of blood sugar, which can rapidly lead to severe symptoms and potentially coma and death. Patients suffering from diabetes can be divided into two groups, which largely determines the nature of their treatment. Those who have Type I diabetes (insulin-dependent diabetes mellitus; IDDM; juvenile-onset diabetes) are generally maintained for life on one or other of the insulin preparations. Those who develop Type II diabetes (non-insulin-dependent diabetes mellitus; NIDDM; maturity-onset diabetes) can usually be managed by treatment with ORAL HYPOGLYCAEMIC drugs or by diet alone and less commonly require insulin injections. Most diabetics take some form of insulin on a regular (daily) basis, generally by subcutaneous injection. Modern genetic engineering has enabled the production of quantities of the human form of insulin, which is now replacing the former insulins extracted from cows (bovine insulin) or pigs (porcine insulin). There are marked differences in absorption time – which dictates both the rate of onset and duration of action – between insulin preparations. This depends on their pH and whether preparations are solutions,

suspensions, or complexes with zinc or protamine. Consequently, forms are available that are short-acting (eg. soluble insulin), or intermediate-acting (eg. insulin zinc suspension (amorphous)), or long-acting (eg. insulin zinc suspension (crystalline)). Many diabetic patients use more than one type of insulin in proportions relative to their own specific needs. Insulin is usually administered by patients themselves, by subcutaneous injection into the thigh, buttock, upper arm, or abdomen.

✚ side-effects: hypoglycaemia in overdose. Local reactions at injection site.

▲ warning: expert counselling, initial training and blood-glucose monitoring is required because patients must maintain a stable blood-glucose level over long periods. Choice of suitable preparations, or combination of preparations, for injection may take some time to establish. Patients should be warned of possible hazards in driving over long periods and should only drive if *hypoglycaemic aware*.

❍ Related entries: biphasic insulin; **biphasic isophane insulin; Human Actraphane 30/70; Human Actrapid; Human Initard 50/50; Human Insulatard; Human Mixtard 30/70; Human Monotard; Human Protaphane; Human Ultratard; Human Velosulin; Humulin I; Humulin Lente; Humulin M1; Humulin M2; Humulin M3; Humulin M4; Humulin S; Humulin Zn; Hypurin Isophane; Hypurin Lente; Hypurin Neutral; Hypurin Protamine Zinc; Initard 50/50; Insulatard; insulin zinc suspension; insulin zinc suspension (amorphous); insulin zinc suspension (crystalline); Lentard MC; Mixtard 30/70; PenMix 10/90; PenMix 20/80; PenMix 30/70; PenMix 40/60; PenMix 50/50; protamine zinc insulin; Pur-In Isophane; Pur-In Mix 15/85; Pur-In Mix 25/75; Pur-In Mix 50/50; Pur-In Neutral; Rapitard MC; Semitard MC; soluble insulin; Velosulin**

insulin injection
See SOLUBLE INSULIN

insulin zinc suspension
(Insulin Zinc Suspension (Mixed; *I.Z.S.*) is a form of highly purified purified bovine and/or porcine insulin, prepared as a sterile neutral complex with zinc salts, that is used in DIABETIC TREATMENT to maintain diabetic patients. It is available in vials for injection and has a long duration of action.
+▲ side-effects/warning: see INSULIN
☉ Related entries: Human Monotard; Humulin M1; Hypurin Lente; Lentard MC

insulin zinc suspension (amorphous)
(*Amorph.I.Z.S.*) is a form of highly purified purified animal (porcine or bovine) insulin, prepared as a sterile neutral complex with zinc salts, that is used in DIABETIC TREATMENT to maintain diabetic patients. It is available in vials for injection and has an intermediate duration of action.
+▲ side-effects/warning: see INSULIN
☉ Related entry: Semitard MC

insulin zinc suspension (crystalline)
(*Cryst.I.Z.S.*) is a form of highly purified bovine or human insulin, prepared as a sterile complex with zinc salts, that is used in DIABETIC TREATMENT to maintain diabetic patients. It is available in vials for injection and is medium- to long-acting.
+▲ side-effects/warning: see INSULIN
☉ Related entries: Human Ultratard; Humulin Zn

Intal
(Fisons) is a proprietary, prescription-only preparation of sodium cromoglycate (sodium cromoglicate). It can be used as a prophylactic (preventive) ANTI-ASTHMATIC treatment. It is available as a liquid in aerosol units (available with a spacer device, *Syncroner* and large volume inhaler, *Fisonair*), as a nebulizer solution, or as a powder for inhalation in *Spincaps* (which can be used with the *Spinhaler Insufflator*).
+▲ side-effects/warning: see ISOPRENALINE; SODIUM CROMOGLYCATE

*interferon
is a protein produced in tiny quantities by cells infected by a virus and which has the ability to inhibit further growth of the virus. Genetic engineering, including the use of bacteria as host cells has enabled interferons to be mass-produced, but they have been less effective against viruses than was hoped. They also have complex effects on cells, cell function and immunity, which has limited their use. *Interferon alpha* is used as an ANTICANCER treatment for particular cancers, particularly lymphomas (eg. AIDS-related Kaposi's sarcoma), certain cancers of the kidney, some solid tumours and other conditions including chronic active hepatitis B. *Interferon gamma* is used in conjunction with ANTIMICROBIAL and ANTIBIOTIC drugs to reduce the frequency of serious infection in patients with chronic granulatomatous disease.
+ side-effects: severe flu-like symptoms; there may also be lethargy and depression. The blood-producing capacity of the bone marrow may be reduced. Some patients experience high or low blood pressure and heartbeat irregularities. Liver toxicity has been reported. There may be thyroid abnormalities, rashes and confusion.
▲ warning: regular blood counts are essential during treatment, particularly to check the levels of white blood cells.
☉ Related entries: Immukin; Intron A; Roferon-A; Viraferon; Wellferon

Intralgin
(3M Health Care) is a proprietary, non-prescription COMPOUND PREPARATION of the LOCAL ANAESTHETIC drug benzocaine and salicylamide, which has a COUNTER-

IRRITANT, or RUBEFACIENT, action. It can be applied to the skin for symptomatic relief of underlying muscle or joint pain and is available as a gel.

+▲ side-effects/warning: see BENZOCAINE

Intraval Sodium

(Rhône-Poulenc Rorer) is a proprietary, prescription-only preparation of the BARBITURATE drug thiopentone sodium. It can be used as a GENERAL ANAESTHETIC for the induction of anaesthesia and is available in a form for injection.

+▲ side-effects/warning: see THIOPENTONE SODIUM

Intron A

(Schering-Plough) is a proprietary, prescription-only preparation of interferon (in the form alpha-2b, rbe). It can be used as an ANTICANCER treatment mainly for leukaemia, AIDS-related Kaposi's sarcoma and chronic active hepatitis B. It is available in a form for injection.

+▲ side-effects/warning: see INTERFERON

Intropin

(Du Pont) is a proprietary, prescription-only preparation of the SYMPATHOMIMETIC and CARDIAC STIMULANT drug dopamine hydrochloride. It can be used to treat cardiogenic shock following a heart attack, or during heart surgery. It is available as a liquid in vials for dilution and infusion.

+▲ side-effects/warning: see DOPAMINE

iodine

is a non-metallic element, which is accumulated by the body in the thyroid gland (situated at the base of the neck) and is used by the cells of this gland to synthesize the thyroid HORMONES THYROXINE and TRIIODOTHYRONINE, which control a number of normal metabolic processes and growth. Nutritional sources of iodine include seafood, vegetables grown in soil containing iodine and iodinated table salt. A deficiency is one of the possible causes of *goitre*, where the thyroid gland becomes enlarged. Therapeutically, iodine (as AQUEOUS IODINE ORAL SOLUTION) can be used in thyrotoxicosis prior to surgery and in solution as an ANTISEPTIC.

Ionamin

(Lipha) is a proprietary preparation of the APPETITE SUPPRESSANT drug phentermine. It can be used, in the short term only, to assist in the medical treatment of obesity and is on the Controlled Drugs List. It is available as modified-release capsules.

+▲ side-effects/warning: see PHENTERMINE

Ionax Scrub

(Novex) is a proprietary, non-prescription preparation of the ANTISEPTIC agent benzalkonium chloride with abrasive polyethylene granules within a foaming aqueous-alcohol base. It can be used in the treatment of acne.

+▲ side-effects/warning: see BENZALKONIUM CHLORIDE

Ionil T

(Novex) is a proprietary, non-prescription COMPOUND PREPARATION of the ANTISEPTIC agent benzalkonium chloride, the KERATOLYTIC agent salicylic acid and coal tar. It can be used as a treatment for dandruff and other scalp conditions and is available as a shampoo.

+▲ side-effects/warning: see BENZALKONIUM CHLORIDE; COAL TAR; SALICYLIC ACID

ipecac

See IPECACUANHA

ipecacuanha

is an extract from the ipecac plant. It contains two ALKALOIDS (emetine and cephaeline) that have an irritant action on the gastrointestinal tract and is therefore a powerful EMETIC. It can be used to clear the stomach in certain cases of non-corrosive poisoning when the patient is conscious (particularly in children). In smaller doses it can also be used as an EXPECTORANT in non-proprietary mixtures and proprietary tinctures and syrups. Emetine (and certain derivatives) has been used as an AMOEBICIDAL drug.

✚ side-effects: excessive vomiting, effects on the heart (if absorbed), damage to epithelium (surface tissues) of the gastrointestinal tract.

▲ warning: in high dosage it can cause severe gastric upset.

❂ Related entry: ammonia and ipecacuanha mixture, BP; ipecacuanha and morphine mixture, BP

ipecacuanha and morphine mixture, BP

is a COMPOUND PREPARATION that combines the (OPIOID) NARCOTIC ANALGESIC drug morphine (anhydrous) as tincture with chloroform and used here as an ANTITUSSIVE in combination with a tincture of the EMETIC drug ipecacuanha and liquorice liquid extract. Administration is oral as a liquid.

✚▲ side-effects/warning: see IPECACUANHA; MORPHINE SULPHATE

Ipral

(Squibb) is a proprietary, prescription-only preparation of the ANTIBACTERIAL drug trimethoprim. It can be used to treat infections of the upper respiratory tract (particularly bronchitis) and the urinary tract. It is available as tablets.

✚▲ side-effects/warning: see TRIMETHOPRIM

ipratropium bromide

is an ANTICHOLINERGIC drug with BRONCHODILATOR properties. It can be used to treat obstructive airways disease, where it is more often used for chronic bronchitis than as an ANTI-ASTHMATIC treatment. For this treatment it is administered by inhalation from an aerosol or a nebulizer. It is also used, in the form of a nasal spray, as a NASAL DECONGESTANT to treat watery rhinitis.

✚ side-effects: there may be dryness of mouth; rarely, there is urinary retention and/or constipation.

▲ warning: administer with caution to patients with glaucoma or enlargement of the prostate gland, or who are pregnant.

❂ Related entries: Atrovent; Rinatec; Steri-Neb Ipratropium

iron

is a metallic element essential to the body in several ways, particularly its role, as the red blood cell constituent haemoglobin, as the transporter of oxygen around the body and in a similar form in muscle to accept the oxygen. Iron deficiency due to disease states that prevent its proper absorption or because of its deficiency in the diet, lead to forms of anaemia (*iron-deficiency anaemia*). It is used therapeutically usually to treat anaemia caused by dietary deficiency. Supplements can be administered orally (in the form of FERROUS FUMARATE, FERROUS GLUCONATE, FERROUS GLYCINE SULPHATE, FERROUS SULPHATE and other salts) or by injection or intravenous infusion (in the form of iron dextran and other preparations). There are numerous iron-and-vitamin supplements available and can be particularly useful during pregnancy. Excellent foods sources of iron include meat and liver.

Isclofen

(Isis) is a proprietary, prescription-only preparation of the (NSAID) NON-NARCOTIC ANALGESIC and ANTIRHEUMATIC drug diclofenac sodium. It can be used to treat the pain and inflammation of arthritis and rheumatism and other musculoskeletal disorders. It is available as tablets.

✚▲ side-effects/warning: see DICLOFENAC SODIUM

Isisfen

(Isis) is a proprietary, prescription-only preparation of the (NSAID) NON-NARCOTIC ANALGESIC and ANTIRHEUMATIC drug ibuprofen. It can be used to relieve the pain of rheumatism and other musculoskeletal disorders and is available as tablets.

+▲ side-effects/warning: see
IBUPROFEN

Ismelin

(Ciba) is a proprietary, prescription-only preparation of the ADRENERGIC NEURONE BLOCKER drug guanethidine monosulphate. It can be used in ANTIHYPERTENSIVE treatment of moderate to severe high blood pressure. It is available as tablets and in a form for injection.

+▲ side-effects/warning: see GUANETHIDINE
MONOSULPHATE

Ismo

(Boehringer Mannheim) is a proprietary, non-prescription preparation of the VASODILATOR and ANTI-ANGINA drug isosorbide mononitrate. It can be used to treat and prevent angina pectoris and in HEART FAILURE TREATMENT. It is available as tablets.

+▲ side-effects/warning: see ISOSORBIDE
MONONITRATE

Ismo Retard

(Boehringer Mannheim) is a proprietary, non-prescription preparation of the VASODILATOR and ANTI-ANGINA drug isosorbide mononitrate. It can be used to treat and prevent angina pectoris and is available as modified-release tablets.

+▲ side-effects/warning: see ISOSORBIDE
MONONITRATE

isocarboxazid

is an ANTIDEPRESSANT drug of the MONOAMINE-OXIDASE INHIBITOR (MAOI) class. It can be used to treat depressive illness. Administration is oral in the form of tablets.

+▲ side-effects/warning: see under
PHENELZINE; but it has a more stimulant action.

✪ Related entry: Marplan

isoconazole

is an (IMIDAZOLE) ANTIFUNGAL drug, which is used particularly to treat fungal infections (candidiasis) of the vagina. Administration is in the form of vaginal tablets (pessaries).

+ side-effects: there may be local irritation.

✪ Related entry: Travogyn

Isoflurane

(Abbott) is a proprietary, prescription-only preparation of the inhalant GENERAL ANAESTHETIC drug isoflurane. It can be used for the induction and maintenance of anaesthesia and is available in a form for inhalation.

+▲ side-effects/warning: see ISOFLURANE

isoflurane

is an inhalant GENERAL ANAESTHETIC drug, which is similar to ENFLURANE. It can be used with nitrous oxide-oxygen for the induction and maintenance of anaesthesia during surgical operations. Administration is by inhalation.

+ side-effects: there may be an increase in heart rate accompanied by a fall in blood pressure; it may depress respiration.

✪ Related entry: Isoflurane

Isogel

(Charwell) is a proprietary, non-prescription preparation of the (*bulking agent*) LAXATIVE ispaghula husk. It can be used to treat a number of gastrointestinal disorders, including irritable bowel syndrome and is available as granules.

+▲ side-effects/warning: see ISPAGHULA
HUSK

Isoket

(Schwarz) is a proprietary, prescription-only preparation of the VASODILATOR and ANTI-ANGINA drug isosorbide dinitrate. It can be used in HEART FAILURE TREATMENT and to treat and, in particular, prevent angina pectoris. It is available in a form for injection.

+▲ side-effects/warning: see ISOSORBIDE DINITRATE

Isoket Retard

(Schwarz) is a proprietary, non-prescription preparation of the VASODILATOR and ANTI-ANGINA drug isosorbide dinitrate. It can be used to prevent angina pectoris and is available as modified-release tablets in two strengths, *Isoket Retard-20* and *Isoket Retard-20*.
+▲ side-effects/warning: see ISOSORBIDE DINITRATE

isometheptene mucate

is a SYMPATHOMIMETIC drug, which is used in the treatment of acute ANTIMIGRAINE. Administration is oral in the form of capsules.
+ side-effects: dizziness, peripheral circulation disturbances and rashes; blood disturbances have been reported.
▲ warning: administer with caution to patients with cardiovascular disease, diabetes, or hyperthyroidism; do not administer to those with glaucoma, severe heart, liver, or kidney disorders, porphyria; or who are pregnant or breast-feeding.
❍ Related entry: Midrid

Isomide CR

(Monmouth) is a proprietary, prescription-only preparation of the ANTI-ARRHYTHMIC drug disopyramide (as disopyramide phosphate). It is available as modified-release tablets.
+▲ side-effects/warning: see DISOPYRAMIDE

isoniazid

is an ANTIBACTERIAL drug that is used, in combination with other drugs, in ANTITUBERCULAR treatment. It can also be administered to prevent the contraction of tuberculosis by close associates of an infected patient. Administration is in the form of tablets, an elixir, or by injection.
+ side-effects: these include nausea and vomiting; sensitivity reactions including rash and fever and peripheral neuritis (which may

be prevented by taking the drug pyridoxine), convulsions and/or psychotic episodes, blood disorders and other complications.
▲ warning: it is not to be administered to patients with liver disease induced by drug treatment; administer with caution to patients with impaired kidney or liver function, epilepsy, alcoholism, who are pregnant or breast-feeding, or who have porphyria. (Patients with abnormal metabolism (slow acetylators) are known to need the dose to be adjusted to avoid unacceptable side-effects.)
❍ Related entry: Rifater; Rifinah; Rimactazid; Rimifon

isophane insulin

is a form of purified bovine, porcine, or human, insulin, prepared as a sterile complex with protamine, that is used in DIABETIC TREATMENT to maintain diabetic patients. It is available in vials for injection and has an intermediate duration of action.
+▲ side-effects/warning: see under INSULIN
❍ Related entries: Human Insulatard; Human Protaphane; Humulin I; Hypurin Isophane; Insulatard; Pur-In Isophane

isoprenaline

is a synthetic SYMPATHOMIMETIC substance similar to ADRENALINE. As isoprenaline sulphate, it is used as a BETA-RECEPTOR STIMULANT and SMOOTH MUSCLE RELAXANT. These properties have allowed its administration, in a form suitable for use in an aerosol inhalant, as a BRONCHODILATOR in ANTI-ASTHMATIC treatment. However, isoprenaline's use for this purpose has largely been superseded by drugs that are more selective of the $beta_2$-receptors of the airways and therefore are far less likely to produce cardiac arrhythmias by stimulating the $beta_1$-receptors of the heart. Since isoprenaline does stimulate the heart, it may be used to produce an increased rate and force of contraction (eg. in heart block or severe bradycardia), when it is administered (as isoprenaline

hydrochloride) as tablets or by injection.
+▲ side-effects/warning: see under
SALBUTAMOL. There may be headache, tremor,
sweating, increased heart rate and heartbeat
irregularities and a decrease in blood
pressure. Administer with caution to patients
with certain heart diseases, or excessive
secretion of thyroid hormones
(hyperthyroidism), or who are diabetic.
**✪ Related entries; Medihaler-iso; Min-I-
Jet Isoprenaline; Saventrine**

Isopto Alkaline

(Alcon) is a proprietary, non-prescription
preparation of hypromellose. It can be
used as artificial tears to treat dryness of
the eyes due to disease and is available as
eye-drops.
+▲ side-effects/warning: see HYPROMELLOSE

Isopto Atropine

(Alcon) is a proprietary, prescription-only
preparation of the ANTICHOLINERGIC drug
atropine sulphate. It can be used to dilate
the pupil and so facilitate inspection of the
eye and for refraction procedures in
young children. It is available as eye-
drops.
+▲ side-effects/warning: see
ATROPINE SULPHATE

Isopto Carbachol

(Alcon) is a proprietary, prescription-only
preparation of the PARASYMPATHOMIMETIC
drug carbachol. It can be used as in
GLAUCOMA TREATMENT because it lowers
intraocular pressure (pressure in the
eyeball) and constricts the pupil. It is
available as eye-drops.
+▲ side-effects/warning: see CARBACHOL

Isopto Carpine

(Alcon) is a proprietary, prescription-only
COMPOUND PREPARATION of the
PARASYMPATHOMIMETIC drug pilocarpine
and hypromellose ('artificial tears'). It can
be used as in GLAUCOMA TREATMENT
because it lowers intraocular pressure
(pressure in the eyeball) and constricts

the pupil. It is available as eye-drops.
+▲ side-effects/warning: see
HYPROMELLOSE; PILOCARPINE

Isopto Frin

(Alcon) is a proprietary, non-prescription
preparation of the SYMPATHOMIMETIC drug
phenylephrine hydrochloride and
hypromellose ('artificial tears'). It can be
used to treat tear deficiency and is
available as eye-drops.
+▲ side-effects/warning: see
HYPROMELLOSE; PHENYLEPHRINE
HYDROCHLORIDE

Isopto Plain

(Alcon) is a proprietary, non-prescription
preparation of hypromellose. It can be
used as artificial tears to treat dryness of
the eyes due to disease and is available as
eye-drops.
+▲ side-effects/warning: see
HYPROMELLOSE

Isordil

(Monmouth) is a proprietary, non-
prescription preparation of the
VASODILATOR and ANTI-ANGINA drug
isosorbide dinitrate. It can be used in
HEART FAILURE TREATMENT and to treat and
prevent angina pectoris. It is available as
short-acting oral and sublingual tablets.
+▲ side-effects/warning: see ISOSORBIDE
DINITRATE

Isordil Tembids

(Monmouth) is a proprietary, non-
prescription preparation of the
VASODILATOR and ANTI-ANGINA drug
isosorbide dinitrate. It can be used to
prevent angina pectoris and is available as
modified-release capsules.
+▲ side-effects/warning: see ISOSORBIDE
DINITRATE

isosorbide dinitrate

is a short-acting VASODILATOR and ANTI-
ANGINA drug. It is used to prevent attacks
of angina pectoris (ischaemic heart pain)

when taken before exercise, for symptomatic relief during an acute attack and to treat left ventricular heart failure. It works by dilating the veins returning blood to the heart and so reducing the heart's workload. It is short-acting, but its effect can be extended through the use of modified-release tablets kept under the tongue (sublingual tablets).

Administration can be oral as tablets (for swallowing, chewing, or holding under the tongue), as modified-release capsules, as a spray or aerosol (applied under the tongue), or in a form for injection or infusion.

✚▲ side-effects/warning: see under GLYCERYL TRINITRATE

✪ Related entries; Cedocard; Cedocard Retard; Imtack Spray; Isoket; Isoket Retard; Isordil; Isordil Tembids; Soni-Slo; Sorbichew; Sorbid SA; Sorbitrate

isosorbide mononitrate

is a short-acting VASODILATOR and ANTI-ANGINA drug. It is used to prevent attacks of angina pectoris (ischaemic heart pain) when taken before exercise, for symptomatic relief during an acute attack and in HEART FAILURE TREATMENT. It works by dilating the blood vessels returning blood to the heart and so reducing the heart's workload. It is short-acting, but its effect is extended through the use of modified-release tablets kept under the tongue (sublingual tablets).

Administration is oral in the form of tablets or capsules.

✚▲ side-effects/warning: see under GLYCERYL TRINITRATE

✪ Related entries: Elantan; Elantan LA; Imdur; Ismo; Ismo Retard; Isotrate; MCR-50; Monit; Monit SR; Mono-Cedocard

Isotonic Gentamicin Injection

(Baxter) is a proprietary, prescription-only preparation of the ANTIBACTERIAL and (AMINOGLYCOSIDE) ANTIBIOTIC drug

gentamicin (as sulphate). It can be used to treat many forms of infection, particularly serious infections by Gram-negative bacteria. It is available in a form for intravenous infusion.

✚▲ side-effects/warning: see GENTAMICIN

Isotrate

(Bioglan) is a proprietary, non-prescription preparation of the VASODILATOR and ANTI-ANGINA drug isosorbide mononitrate. It can be used to treat and prevent angina pectoris and in HEART FAILURE TREATMENT. It is available as tablets.

✚▲ side-effects/warning: see ISOSORBIDE MONONITRATE

isotretinoin

is chemically a retinoid (a derivative of RETINOL, or vitamin A) and has a marked effect on the cells that make up the skin epithelium (surface tissues). It can be used for the long-term, systemic treatment of severe acne. Administration is either oral as capsules or by topical application as a gel.

✚▲ side-effects/warning: see under TRETINOIN for the side-effects of topical application. There are many side-effects with oral administration, including effects on the skin, mucous membranes (eg. nasal mucosa), visual disturbances and other effects on the eyes, hair thinning, headache, nausea, drowsiness, sweating, muscle and joint pain, effects on the liver and blood function.

▲ warning: see under tretinoin for topical application. For oral administraion, do not use when pregnant (or one month before or after treatment), breast-feeding, or in certain liver or kidney disorders.

✪ Related entries: Isotrex; Roaccutane

Isotrex

(Stiefel) is a proprietary, prescription-only preparation of isotretinoin (a retinoid). It can be used for the long-term treatment of severe acne and is available as tablets and a gel.

+▲ side-effects/warning: see ISOTRETINOIN

ispaghula husk

is a *bulking agent* LAXATIVE. It works by increasing the overall mass of faeces (and retaining a lot of water) so stimulating bowel movement (the full effect may not be achieved for many hours). It can be used in patients who cannot tolerate bran for treating a range of bowel conditions, including diverticular disease and irritable bowel syndrome. Administration is oral as granules or a powder for dissolving in water.

+ side-effects: there may be flatulence, abdominal distention, faecal impaction and lack of tone in the colon. Hypersensitivity has been reported.

▲ warning: preparations of ispaghula husk should not be administered to patients with obstruction of the intestines, lack of tone in the colon, or faecal impaction. Fluid intake during treatment should be higher than usual. Preparations containing ispaghula husk swell on contact with liquids and should be carefully swallowed with water and should not be taken last thing at night.

○ Related entries:
Fybogel; Fybogel Mebeverine; Isogel; Manevac; Metamucil; Regulan

isradipine

is a CALCIUM-CHANNEL BLOCKER drug, which is used as an ANTIHYPERTENSIVE treatment. Administration is oral in the form of tablets.

+ side-effects: these include flushing, headache; dizziness, hypotension and palpitations; rashes and itching; rarely, increased body weight, oedema and gastrointestinal upsets.

▲ warning: the dose should be reduced when treating patients with certain liver or kidney disorders and avoided if possible in pregnancy. It should be given with caution to patients with some types of heart defect.

○ Related entry: Prescal

Istin

(Pfizer) is a proprietary, prescription-only preparation of the CALCIUM-CHANNEL BLOCKER drug amlodipine besylate. It can be used as an ANTIHYPERTENSIVE treatment and as an ANTI-ANGINA drug in the prevention of attacks. It is available as tablets.

+▲ side-effects/warning: see AMLODIPINE BESYLATE

itraconazole

is a broad-spectrum (AZOLE) ANTIFUNGAL drug. It can be used to treat resistant forms of candidiasis (thrush) of the vagina, vulva or oropharyngeal region, infections of the skin and mucous membranes and infections of the fingernails by tinea organisms, including ringworm and athlete's foot. It is available as capsules.

+ side-effects: nausea and gastrointestinal disturbances, abdominal pains, dyspepsia, skin disorders, headaches and liver disorders.

▲ warning: it should not be administered to patients with certain liver or kidney disorders; or who are pregnant or breast-feeding.

○ Related entry: Sporanox

ivermectin

is an ANTHELMINTIC drug that, although it is not available in the UK, is very effective in the treatment of the tropical disease onchocerciasis (infestation by the filarial worm-parasite *Onchocerca volvulus*). The destruction of the worms, however, may cause an allergic response. It is now the drug of choice because a single treatment produces a large reduction in the level of parasites, though more than one course of treatment with ivermectin may be necessary to eradicate the infestation. It is available in a form for oral administration.

+ side-effects: headache with nausea and vomiting; the dermatitis associated with onchocerciasis may temporarily be aggravated, causing itching and rash, as may any associated conjunctivitis or other eye

inflammation.
▲ warning: medical supervision is essential
during treatment.
✪ Related entry: Mectizan

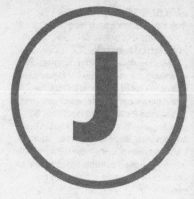

Jackson's All Fours

(Rosmarine) is a proprietary, non-prescription preparation of the EXPECTORANT guaiphenesin. It can be used for the symptomatic relief of coughs, and is available as a syrup. It is not normally given to children under 12 years, except on medical advice.

+▲ side-effects/warning: see GUAIPHENESIN

Jackson's Febrifuge

(Rosmarine) is a proprietary, non-prescription preparation of the (NSAID) NON-NARCOTIC ANALGESIC and ANTIRHEUMATIC drug sodium salicylate. It can be used for the symptomatic relief of flu, sore throat, feverish colds and muscle pains. It is available as a liquid preparation and is not normally given to children under 12 years, except on medical advice.

+▲ side-effects/warning: see SODIUM SALICYLATE

J Collis Browne's Mixture

(Napp) is a proprietary, non-prescription preparation of the (OPIOID) ANTIDIARRHOEAL drug morphine anhydrous and peppermint oil. It can be used for the symptomatic relief of occasional diarrhoea and its associated pain and discomfort and is also an effective ANTITUSSIVE. It is available as a liquid.

+▲ side-effects/warning: see OPIOID

J Collis Browne's Tablets

(Napp) is a proprietary, non-prescription preparation of the (OPIOID) ANTIDIARRHOEAL drug morphine hydrochloride, kaolin and calcium carbonate. It can be used for the symptomatic relief of occasional diarrhoea and its associated pain and discomfort and is available as tablets. It is not normally given to children under six years, except on medical advice.

+▲ side-effects/warning: see CALCIUM CARBONATE; KAOLIN; OPIOID

Japps Health Salts

(Roche) is a proprietary, non-prescription COMPOUND PREPARATION of the ANTACID and (*osmotic*) LAXATIVE salts sodium bicarbonate and sodium potassium tartrate (with tartaric acid). It can be used for the symptomatic relief of indigestion and heartburn and for the mild relief of constipation. It is available as an effervescent powder.

+▲ side-effects/warning: see SODIUM BICARBONATE; SODIUM POTASSIUM TARTRATE

Jexin

(Evans) is a proprietary, prescription-only preparation of the (*non-depolarizing*) SKELETAL MUSCLE RELAXANT drug tubocurarine chloride. It can be used to induce muscle paralysis during surgery and is available in a form for injection.

+▲ side-effects/warning: see TUBOCURARINE CHLORIDE

Joy-Rides

(Stafford Miller) is a proprietary, non-prescription preparation of the ANTICHOLINERGIC drug hyoscine hydrobromide. It can be used as an ANTINAUSEANT in the treatment of motion sickness and is available as chewable tablets. It is not normally given to children under three years, except on medical advice.

+▲ side-effects/warning: see HYOSCINE HYDROBROMIDE

Junifen

(Crookes Healthcare) is a proprietary, non-prescription preparation of the (NSAID) NON-NARCOTIC ANALGESIC, ANTIRHEUMATIC and ANTIPYRETIC drug ibuprofen. It can be used to relieve pain such as earache, sore throats, minor aches and sprains and flu and cold symptoms in children. It is available as a sugar-free, oral suspension and is not normally given to children under one year, except on medical advice.

+▲ side-effects/warning: see IBUPROFEN

K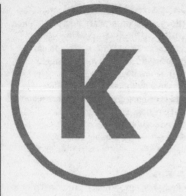

Kabiglobulin

(Pharmacia) is a proprietary, prescription-only preparation of human NORMAL IMMUNOGLOBULIN. It can be used in IMMUNIZATION to confer immediate *passive immunity* to infection by viruses such as hepatitis A virus, rubeola (measles) and rubella (German measles). It is available in a form for intramuscular injection.

+▲ side-effects/warning: see NORMAL IMMUNOGLOBULIN

Kabikinase

(Pharmacia) is a proprietary, prescription-only preparation of the FIBRINOLYTIC drug streptokinase. It can be used to treat thrombosis and embolism and is available in a form for injection.

+▲ side-effects/warning: see STREPTOKINASE

Kalspare

(Cusi) is a proprietary, prescription-only COMPOUND PREPARATION of the (THIAZIDE-related) DIURETIC drug chlorthalidone and the (*potassium-sparing*) diuretic triamterene. It can be used as an ANTIHYPERTENSIVE treatment and is available as tablets.

+▲ side-effects/warning: see CHLORTHALIDONE; TRIAMTERENE

Kalten

(Stuart) is a proprietary, prescription-only COMPOUND PREPARATION of the BETA-BLOCKER drug atenolol and the DIURETIC drugs hydrochlorothiazide and amiloride hydrochloride. It can be used as an ANTIHYPERTENSIVE treatment for raised blood pressure and is available as capsules.

+▲ side-effects/warning: see AMILORIDE HYDROCHLORIDE; ATENOLOL; HYDROCHLOROTHIAZIDE

Kamillosan

(Norgine) is a proprietary, non-prescription COMPOUND PREPARATION of

arachis oil and liquid paraffin (and some other constituents). It can be used as an EMOLLIENT to treat and soothe nappy rash, sore nipples, chapped hands and dry skin. It is available as an ointment.
+▲ side-effects/warning: see ARACHIS OIL; LIQUID PARAFFIN

kanamycin
is a broad-spectrum ANTIBACTERIAL and (AMINOGLYCOSIDE) ANTIBIOTIC drug. Although it does have activity against Gram-positive bacteria, it is primarily used against serious infections caused by Gram-negative bacteria. It has largely been replaced by other aminoglycosides. Administration is by injection.
+▲ side-effects/warning: see under GENTAMICIN
✪ Related entry: Kannasyn

Kannasyn
(Sanofi Winthrop) is a proprietary, prescription-only preparation of the ANTIBACTERIAL and (AMINOGLYCOSIDE) ANTIBIOTIC drug kanamycin. It can be used to treat many forms of infection, particularly serious Gram-negative ones. It is available in a form for injection.
+▲ side-effects/warning: see KANAMYCIN

Kaodene
(Knoll/Boots) is a proprietary, non-prescription COMPOUND PREPARATION of the absorbent substance KAOLIN and the OPIOID drug codeine phosphate. It can be used as an ANTIDIARRHOEAL treatment and is available as an oral mixture.
+▲ side-effects/warning: see CODEINE PHOSPHATE

kaolin
is a purified and sometimes powdered white clay (china clay) that is used as an adsorbent, particularly in ANTIDIARRHOEAL preparations (with or without OPIOIDS such as codeine phosphate or morphine sulphate)

and also to treat food poisoning and some digestive disorders. Additionally, it can be used in some poultices and dusting powders.
✪ Related entries: J Collis Browne's Tablets; Kaodene; Kaopectate; KLN

kaolin and morphine mixture, BP
is a COMPOUND PREPARATION of kaolin and the (OPIOID) ANTIDIARRHOEAL and ANTIMOTILITY drug tincture of morphine (anhydrous). It is available as an oral suspension.
✪ Related entry: OPIOID

Kaopectate
(Upjohn) is a proprietary, non-prescription preparation of KAOLIN. It can be used as an absorbent in ANTIDIARRHOEAL treatment and is available as a suspension.

Kapake
(Galen) is a proprietary, prescription-only COMPOUND PREPARATION of the (OPIOID) NARCOTIC ANALGESIC drug codeine phosphate and the NON-NARCOTIC ANALGESIC drug paracetamol (a combination known as co-codamol 30/500). It can be used as a painkiller and is available in as tablets.
+▲ side-effects/warning: see CODEINE PHOSPHATE; PARACETAMOL

Karvol Decongestant Capsules
(Crookes Healthcare) is a proprietary, non-prescription preparation of menthol, chlorbutol and thymol (with aromatic oils). It can be used as a NASAL DECONGESTANT for the symptomatic relief of colds. It is available as capsules which are sprinkled over bedding or added to hot water for the essences to be inhaled. It is not normally given to children under three months, except on medical advice.
+▲ side-effects/warning: see CHLORBUTOL; MENTHOL; THYMOL

K

Kefadim

(Lilly) is a proprietary, prescription-only preparation of the ANTIBACTERIAL and (CEPHALOSPORIN) ANTIBIOTIC drug ceftazidime. It can be used to treat many infections, particularly of the respiratory tract and to prevent infection during surgery and in patients whose immune systems are defective. It is available in a form for injection or infusion.
✚▲ side-effects/warning: see CEFTAZIDIME

Kefadol

(Dista) is a proprietary, prescription-only preparation of the ANTIBACTERIAL and (CEPHALOSPORIN) ANTIBIOTIC drug cephamandole. It can be used to treat infections caused by both Gram-positive and Gram-negative bacteria and also to prevent infections following abdominal surgery. It is available in a form for injection or infusion.
✚▲ side-effects/warning: see CEPHAMANDOLE

Keflex

(Lilly) is a proprietary, prescription-only preparation of the ANTIBACTERIAL and (CEPHALOSPORIN) ANTIBIOTIC drug cephalexin. It can be used to treat many forms of infection, including of the urinogenital tract. It is available as capsules, tablets and an oral suspension.
✚▲ side-effects/warning: see CEPHALEXIN

Kefzol

(Lilly) is a proprietary, prescription-only preparation of the ANTIBACTERIAL and (CEPHALOSPORIN) ANTIBIOTIC drug cephazolin. It can be used used to treat bacterial infections and to prevent infection during surgery. It is available in a form for injection or infusion.
✚▲ side-effects/warning: see CEPHAZOLIN

Kelfizine W

(Pharmacia) is a proprietary, prescription-only preparation of the (SULPHONAMIDE) ANTIBACTERIAL drug sulfametopyrazine. It can be used primarily to treat chronic bronchitis and infections of the urinary tract. It is available as tablets.
✚▲ side-effects/warning: see SULFAMETOPYRAZINE

Kelocyanor

(Lipha) is a proprietary, prescription-only preparation of the CHELATING AGENT dicobalt edetate. It can be used as an ANTIDOTE to acute cyanide poisoning and is available in a form for injection.
✚▲ side-effects/warning: see DICOBALT EDETATE

Kemadrin

(Wellcome) is a proprietary, prescription-only preparation of the ANTICHOLINERGIC drug procyclidine hydrochloride. It can be used in the treatment of parkinsonism and is available as tablets and in a form for injection.
✚▲ side-effects/warning: see PROCYCLIDINE HYDROCHLORIDE

Kemicetine

(Pharmacia) is a proprietary, prescription-only preparation of the broad-spectrum ANTIBACTERIAL and ANTIBIOTIC drug chloramphenicol. It can be used to treat life-threatening infections and is available in a form for injection.
✚▲ side-effects/warning: see CHLORAMPHENICOL

Kenalog ·

(Squibb) is a proprietary, prescription-only preparation of the CORTICOSTEROID and ANTI-INFLAMMATORY drug triamcinolone acetonide. It can be used to treat inflammation and allergic conditions and is available in a form for injection.
✚▲ side-effects/warning: see TRIAMCINOLONE ACETONIDE

Kenalog Intra-articular/Intramuscular

(Squibb) is a proprietary, prescription-only preparation of the CORTICOSTEROID and ANTI-INFLAMMATORY drug triamcinolone acetonide. It can be used to treat inflammation of the joints and the soft tissues and is available in a form for injection.

✚▲ side-effects/warning: see TRIAMCINOLONE ACETONIDE

*keratolytic

(desquamating agents) agents are used to clear the skin of hyperkeratoses (thickened and horny patches) and scaly areas that occur in some forms of eczema, ichthyosis and psoriasis and also in the treatment of acne. The standard keratolytic is SALICYLIC ACID, but there are others such as BENZOIC ACID, COAL TAR, DITHRANOL, ICHTHAMMOL and ZINC PASTE (several of which can usefully be applied in the form of a paste inside an impregnated bandage).

Keri

(Bristol-Myers) is a proprietary, non-prescription COMPOUND PREPARATION of liquid paraffin and lanolin oil. It can be used as an EMOLLIENT to soften dry skin, relieve itching and to treat nappy rash. It is available as a lotion.

✚▲ side-effects/warning: LIQUID PARAFFIN; LANOLIN

Kerlone

(Lorex) is a proprietary, prescription-only preparation of the BETA-BLOCKER drug betaxolol hydrochloride. It can be used as an ANTIHYPERTENSIVE treatment for raised blood pressure, as an ANTI-ANGINA treatment to relieve symptoms and improve exercise tolerance and as an ANTI-ARRHYTHMIC to regularize heartbeat and to treat myocardial infarction. It is available as tablets.

✚▲ side-effects/warning: see BETAXOLOL HYDROCHLORIDE

Keromask

(Network Management) is a proprietary, non-prescription preparation that is used

to mask scars and other skin disfigurements. It is available as a cream and a powder and may be obtained on prescription under certain circumstances.

Ketalar

(Parke-Davis) is a proprietary, prescription-only preparation of the GENERAL ANAESTHETIC drug ketamine (as hydrochloride). It is available in a form for injection.

✚▲ side-effects/warning: see KETAMINE

ketamine

is a GENERAL ANAESTHETIC drug, which can be used for the induction or maintenance of anaesthesia. Administration is by intramuscular or intravenous injection or infusion.

✚ side-effects: transient psychotic episodes such as hallucinations may occur. There is cardiovascular stimulation and blood pressure may rise.

▲ warning: it should not be administered to patients with hypertension or prone to hallucinations. Recovery is slow.

⊘ Related entry: Ketalar

ketoconazole

is an (IMIDAZOLE) ANTIFUNGAL drug. It can be used to treat deep-seated, serious fungal infections (mycoses) and to prevent infection in immunosuppressed patients. In particular, it is used to treat resistant candidiasis (thrush), gastrointestinal infections and serious infections of the skin (including the scalp) and fingernails. Administration can be oral in the form of tablets or a liquid suspension, or as a topical cream or shampoo.

✚ side-effects: these depend on the route of administration; serious liver damage may occur; there may be an itching skin rash, nausea, abdominal pain, blood disorders and breast enlargement in men.

▲ warning: it should not be administered to patients who have impaired liver function, or who are pregnant. Because it may cause serious liver toxicity, it should not be used for

K

minor fungal infections. Liver function
should be monitored.
❍ Related entry: Nizoral

ketoprofen

is a (NSAID) NON-NARCOTIC ANALGESIC and
ANTIRHEUMATIC drug. It can be used to
treat rheumatic and muscular pain caused
by inflammation, pain after orthopaedic
surgery, acute gout and period pain. It is
available as capsules and in a form for
injection.
✚▲ side-effects/warning: see under NSAID.
There is also an intermediate risk of
gastrointestinal disturbances; there may be
pain at the site of injection, or irritation with
suppositories.
❍ Related entries: Alrheumat;
Ketoprofen CR; Ketovail; Larafen CR;
Orudis; Oruvail 25%

Ketoprofen CR

(Du Pont) is a proprietary, prescription-
only preparation of the (NSAID) NON-
NARCOTIC ANALGESIC and ANTIRHEUMATIC
drug ketoprofen. It can be used to relieve
the pain of arthritis and rheumatism and
other musculoskeletal disorders. It is
available as modified-release capsules.
✚▲ side-effects/warning: see KETOPROFEN

ketorolac trometamol

is a (NSAID) NON-NARCOTIC ANALGESIC
drug. It is used in the short-term
management of moderate to severe, acute
postoperative pain. Administration is
either oral as tablets or by injection.
✚▲ side-effect/warning: see under NSAID;
but use with care, because it is a recently
introduced drug and it✚ side-effects have not
been thoroughly established.
❍ Related entry: Toradol

ketotifen

is an ANTIHISTAMINE drug, which has
additional ANTI-ALLERGIC properties
somewhat like those of SODIUM
CROMOGLYCATE. It can be used as an ANTI-
ASTHMATIC drug to prevent asthmatic

attacks. Administration is oral as capsules,
tablets, or an elixir.
✚ side-effects: it may cause drowsiness with
dryness in the mouth; dizziness and weight
gain.
▲ warning: it may impair the performance
of skilled tasks such as driving; effects of
alcohol are enhanced.
❍ Related entry: Zaditen

Ketovail

(APS) is a proprietary, prescription-only
preparation of the (NSAID) NON-NARCOTIC
ANALGESIC and ANTIRHEUMATIC drug
ketoprofen. It can be used to relieve the
pain of arthritis and rheumatism and other
musculoskeletal disorders. It is available
as modified-release capsules.
✚▲ side-effects/warning: see KETOPROFEN

Kinidin Durules

(Astra) is a proprietary, prescription-only
preparation of the ANTI-ARRHYTHMIC drug
quinidine (as quinidine bisulphate). It can
be used to treat heartbeat irregularities
and is available as modified-release
tablets.
✚▲ side-effects/warning: see QUINIDINE

Klaricid

(Abbott) is a proprietary, prescription-
only preparation of the ANTIBACTERIAL and
(MACROLIDE) ANTIBIOTIC drug
clarithromycin. It can be used to treat and
prevent many forms of infection, including
of the respiratory tract, skin and soft
tissues. It is available as tablets, a
paediatric suspension and in a form for
intravenous infusion.
✚▲ side-effects/warning: see
CLARITHROMYCIN

Klean-Prep

(Norgine) is proprietary, non-prescription
preparation of macrogol (polyethylene
glycol) with sodium and potassium salts. It
can be used as a bowel-cleansing solution
prior to colonic surgery, colonoscopy, or a
barium enema to ensure that the bowel is

free of solid contents. It is available in a form to make up in water.

✚▲ side-effects/warning: see BOWEL-CLEANSING SOLUTIONS

KLN Suspension

(Roche) is a proprietary, non-prescription COMPOUND PREPARATION of KAOLIN, peppermint oil and sodium citrate (with pectin). It can be used as an absorbent in ANTIDIARRHOEAL treatment for children and for minor stomach upsets caused by diet. It is available as an oral suspension.

✚▲ side-effects/warning: PEPPERMINT OIL; SODIUM CITRATE

Kogenate

(Bayer) is a proprietary, prescription-only preparation of dried human factor VIII fraction, which acts as a HAEMOSTATIC drug to reduce or stop bleeding in the treatment of disorders in which bleeding is prolonged and potentially dangerous (mainly haemophilia A). It is available in a form for infusion or injection.

✚▲ side-effects/warning: see FACTOR VIII FRACTION, DRIED

Kolanticon Gel

(Merrell) is a proprietary, non-prescription COMPOUND PREPARATION of the ANTACIDS aluminium hydroxide and magnesium oxide, the ANTICHOLINERGIC drug dicyclomine hydrochloride and the ANTIFOAMING AGENT dimethicone. It can be used to treat gastrointestinal spasm, hyperacidity, flatulence and the symptoms of peptic ulceration. It is available as a gel and is not normally given to children, except on medical advice.

✚▲ side-effects/warning: see ALUMINIUM HYDROXIDE; DICYCLOMINE HYDROCHLORIDE; DIMETHICONE

Konakion

(Roche) is a proprietary, non-prescription preparation of VITAMIN K₁ (phytomenadione). It can be used to treat deficiency of vitamin K and is available as

tablets and in a form for injection (only with a prescription).

✚▲ warning/side-effects: see PHYTOMENADIONE

Kwells Junior

(Roche) is a proprietary, non-prescription preparation of the ANTICHOLINERGIC drug hyoscine hydrobromide. It can be used as an ANTINAUSEANT in the treatment of motion sickness and is available as chewable tablets. It is not normally given to children under four years, except on medical advice.

✚▲ side-effects/warning: see HYOSCINE HYDROBROMIDE

Kwells Tablets

(Roche) is a proprietary, non-prescription preparation of the ANTICHOLINERGIC drug hyoscine hydrobromide. It can be used as an ANTINAUSEANT in the treatment of motion sickness and is available as chewable tablets. It is not normally given to children under ten years, except on medical advice.

✚▲ side-effects/warning: see HYOSCINE HYDROBROMIDE

Kytril

(SmithKline Beecham) is a proprietary, prescription-only preparation of the ANTI-EMETIC and ANTINAUSEANT drug granisetron. It can be used to give relief from nausea and vomiting, especially in patients receiving radiotherapy or chemotherapy. It is available as tablets and in a form for intravenous injection or infusion.

✚▲ side-effects/warning: see GRANISETRON

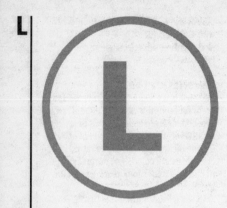

labetalol hydrochloride

is an unusual drug that combines BETA-BLOCKER properties with ALPHA-ADRENOCEPTOR BLOCKER properties. It can be used as an ANTIHYPERTENSIVE to reduce high blood pressure, including in pregnancy, after myocardial infarction, in angina and during surgery. Administration can be oral as tablets or by injection.

✚ side-effects: there may be lethargy, weakness, headache, and/or tingling of the scalp, nausea and vomiting; rashes may occur; there may be liver damage; pain in the upper body; difficulty in urinating. Higher dosages may lead to postural hypotension (low blood pressure and dizziness on standing).

▲ warning: see under PROPRANOLOL HYDROCHLORIDE. Also, it should be administered with caution to patients who are in late pregnancy, or who are breast-feeding. It should not be given to patients with certain liver disorders. Withdrawal of treatment must be gradual.

✪ Related entry: Trandate

Labophylline

(LAB) is a proprietary, prescription-only preparation of the BRONCHODILATOR drug theophylline. It can be used as an ANTI-ASTHMATIC and to treat chronic bronchitis. It is available in a form for injection or intravenous infusion.

✚▲ side-effects/warning: see THEOPHYLLINE

Labosept Pastilles

(LAB) is a proprietary, non-prescription preparation of the ANTISEPTIC agent dequalinium chloride. It can be used to treat sore throats.

✚▲ side-effects/warning: see: DEQUALINIUM CHLORIDE

lacidipine

is a CALCIUM-CHANNEL BLOCKER drug, which is used as an ANTIHYPERTENSIVE treatment. Administration is oral in the form of tablets.

✚ side-effects: include flushing, headache;

dizziness, palpitations; rashes and itching; gastrointestinal upsets and increased production of urine; chest pains. There may be an excessive growth of the gums.
▲ warning: administer with caution to patients with certain heart and liver disorders, or who are breast-feeding. Do not use in pregnancy.
○ Related entry: Motens

Lacri-Lube
(Allergan) is a proprietary, non-prescription COMPOUND PREPARATION of liquid paraffin and white soft paraffin. It can be used as an eye lubricant in patients with tear deficiency and is available as an eye ointment.
✚▲ side-effects/warning: see LIQUID PARAFFIN; WHITE SOFT PARAFFIN

Lacticare
(Stiefel) is a proprietary, non-prescription COMPOUND PREPARATION of sodium pyrrolidone carboxylate and lactic acid. It can be used as an EMOLLIENT for dry skin conditions and is available as a lotion for topical application.

lactilol
is an *osmotic* LAXATIVE and is a sugar-like compound. It can be used to relieve constipation and works by retaining fluid in the intestine and may take up to 48 hours to have full effect. Administration is oral in the form of a powder for solution.
✚▲ side-effects/warning: see under LACTULOSE

Lactugal
(Galen) is a proprietary, non-prescription preparation of the (*osmotic*) LAXATIVE lactulose. It can be used to relieve constipation and is available as a solution.
✚▲ side-effects/warning: see LACTULOSE

lactulose
is an *osmotic* LAXATIVE and is a sugar-like compound. It can be used to relieve constipation and works by retaining fluid

in the intestine and may take up to 48 hours to have full effect. It can also be used to treat hepatic encephalopathy. Administration is oral as a solution.
✚ side-effects: there may be flatulence, intestinal cramps and abdominal discomfort.
▲ warning: it should not be administered to patients with any form of intestinal obstruction. Because lactulose is itself a form of sugar, patients who have blood sugar abnormalities should be checked before using it.
○ Related entries: Duphalac; Lactugal; Laxose; Osmolax; Regulose

Ladropen
(Berk) is a proprietary, prescription-only preparation of the ANTIBACTERIAL and (PENICILLIN) ANTIBIOTIC drug flucloxacillin. It can be used to treat bacterial infections, especially staphylococcal infections that prove to be resistant to penicillin. It is available as capsules, an oral solution and in a form for injection.
✚▲ side-effects/warning: see FLUCLOXACILLIN

Lamictal
(Wellcome) is a proprietary, prescription-only preparation of the ANTICONVULSANT and ANTI-EPILEPTIC drug lamotrigine. It can be used to treat partial and tonic-clonic seizures that have not responded to other drugs. It is available as tablets and dispersible tablets.
✚▲ side-effects/warning: see LAMOTRIGINE

Lamisil
(Sandoz) is a proprietary, prescription-only preparation of the ANTIFUNGAL drug terbinafine. It can be used to treat fungal infections of the nails and ringworm and is available as tablets and a cream.
✚▲ side-effects/warning: see TERBINAFINE

lamotrigine
is a recently introduced ANTICONVULSANT and ANTI-EPILEPTIC drug. It is used, in

L

L

conjunction with other drugs, to treat partial and tonic-clonic seizures that have not responded to other drugs. Administration is oral in the form of tablets.

✚ side-effects: rashes, fever, malaise, flu-like symptoms, drowsiness; rarely, liver dysfunction, blood changes, blurred vision, headache, drowsiness, gastrointestinal upsets and nausea

▲ warning: it should not be administered to patients with kidney or liver impairment. Administer with caution to those who are pregnant or breast-feeding. All the body functions known to be influenced by the drug should be monitored.

○ Related entry: Lamictal

Lamprene

(Geigy) is a proprietary, prescription-only preparation of the ANTIBACTERIAL drug clofazimine. It can be used, in combination with other drugs, in the treatment of the major form of leprosy. It is available as capsules.

✚▲ side-effects/warning: see CLOFAZIMINE

lanolin

is a non-proprietary constituent of WOOL FAT and is incorporated into several EMOLLIENT preparations. It can be is used on cracked, dry, or scaling skin, where it encourages hydration and is commonly combined with LIQUID PARAFFIN.

✚▲ side-effects/warning: some people are sensitive to wool fat preparations; there may be an eczematous rash.

○ Related entries: Alpha Keri Bath; Bengués Balsam; Germoline Ointment; Keri; Panda Baby Cream & Caster Oil Cream with Lanolin; Sudocrem Antiseptic Cream

Lanoxin

(Wellcome) is a proprietary, prescription-only preparation of the CARDIAC GLYCOSIDE drug digoxin. It can be used in congestive HEART FAILURE TREATMENT and as an ANTI-ARRHYTHMIC to treat heartbeat

irregularities. It is available as tablets and in a form for injection.

✚▲ side-effects/warning: see DIGOXIN

Lanoxin-PG

(Wellcome) is a proprietary, prescription-only preparation of the CARDIAC GLYCOSIDE drug digoxin. It can be used in congestive HEART FAILURE TREATMENT and as an ANTI-ARRHYTHMIC to treat heartbeat irregularities. It is available as tablets and an elixir.

✚▲ side-effects/warning: see DIGOXIN

lansoprazole

is an ULCER-HEALING DRUG. It works as an inhibitor of gastric acid secretion in the parietal (acid-producing) cells of the stomach lining by acting as a PROTON-PUMP INHIBITOR. It is used for the treatment of benign gastric and duodenal ulcers (including those complicating NSAID therapy), Zollinger-Ellison syndrome and reflux oesophagitis (inflammed oesophagus due to regurgitation of acid and enzymes). Administration is oral as capsules.

✚▲ side-effects/warning: see under OMEPRAZOLE

○ Related entry: Zoton

Lanvis

(Wellcome) is a proprietary, prescription-only preparation of the (CYTOTOXIC) ANTICANCER drug thioguanine. It can be used in the treatment of leukaemia and is available as tablets.

✚▲ side-effects/warning: see THIOGUANINE

Laractone

(Lagap) is a proprietary, prescription-only preparation of the (*aldosterone-antagonist* and *potassium-sparing*) DIURETIC drug spironolactone. It can be used, in conjunction with other types of diuretic (such as the THIAZIDES, which cause loss of potassium) to treat oedema associated with aldosteronism, heart disease, or kidney disease; and fluid

retention and ascites caused by cirrhosis of the liver. It is available as tablets.
✛▲ side-effects/warning: see
SPIRONOLACTONE

Larafen CR

(Lagap) is a proprietary, prescription-only preparation of the (NSAID) NON-NARCOTIC ANALGESIC and ANTIRHEUMATIC drug ketoprofen. It can be used to relieve arthritic and rheumatic pain and to treat other musculoskeletal disorders. It is available as modified-release capsules.
✛▲ side-effects/warning: see KETOPROFEN

Laraflex

(Lagap) is a proprietary, prescription-only preparation of the (NSAID) NON-NARCOTIC ANALGESIC and ANTIRHEUMATIC drug naproxen. It can be used to relieve pain, particularly rheumatic and arthritic pain and to treat other musculoskeletal disorders. It is available as tablets.
✛▲ side-effects/warning: see NAPROXEN

Larapam

(Lagap) is a proprietary, prescription-only preparation of the (NSAID) NON-NARCOTIC ANALGESIC and ANTIRHEUMATIC drug piroxicam. It can be used to relieve pain, particularly rheumatic and arthritic pain and inflammation and to treat other musculoskeletal disorders (including juvenile arthritis) and acute gout. It is available as tablets.
✛▲ side-effects/warning: see PIROXICAM

Laratrim

(Lagap) is a proprietary, prescription-only COMPOUND PREPARATION of the (SULPHONAMIDE) ANTIBACTERIAL drug sulphamethoxazole and the antibacterial drug trimethoprim, which is a combination called co-trimoxazole. It can be used to treat bacterial infections, especially infections of the urinary tract, prostatitis and bronchitis. It is available as soluble tablets, a suspension and a paediatric suspension.

✛▲ side-effects/warning: see
CO-TRIMOXAZOLE

Largactil

(Rhône-Poulenc Rorer) is a proprietary, prescription-only preparation of the (PHENOTHIAZINE) ANTIPSYCHOTIC drug chlorpromazine hydrochloride. It can be used to treat patients undergoing behavioural disturbances, who are psychotic (especially schizophrenics), or with severe anxiety where a degree of sedation is useful. It can also be used as an ANTINAUSEANT and ANTI-EMETIC to relieve nausea and vomiting, particularly in terminal illness, as a preoperative medication and for intractable hiccup. It is available as tablets, a syrup, a suspension, as suppositories and in a form for injection.
✛▲ side-effects/warning: see
CHLORPROMAZINE HYDROCHLORIDE

Lariam

(Roche) is a proprietary, prescription-only preparation the ANTIMALARIAL drug mefloquine. It can be used to prevent or treat malaria and is available as tablets.
✛▲ side-effects/warning: see MEFLOQUINE

Larodopa

(Cambridge) is a proprietary, prescription-only preparation of the ANTIPARKINSONISM drug levodopa. It can be used to treat parkinsonism and is available as tablets.
✛▲ side-effects/warning: see LEVODOPA

Lasikal

(Hoechst) is a proprietary, prescription-only COMPOUND PREPARATION of the (*loop*) DIURETIC drug frusemide and the potassium supplement potassium chloride. It can be used to treat oedema. It is available as tablets, which should be swallowed whole with plenty of fluid at mealtimes, or when in an upright posture.
✛▲ side-effects/warning see FRUSEMIDE;
POTASSIUM CHLORIDE

L

Lasilactone

(Hoechst) is a proprietary, prescription-only COMPOUND PREPARATION of the (*aldosterone-antagonist* and *potassium-sparing*) DIURETIC drug spironolactone and the (*loop*) diuretic frusemide. It can be used to treat resistant oedema and is available as capsules.

+▲ side-effects/warning: see FRUSEMIDE; SPIRONOLACTONE

Lasix

(Hoechst) is a proprietary, prescription only preparation of the (*loop*) DIURETIC drug frusemide. It can be used to treat oedema, particularly pulmonary (lung) oedema in patients with chronic heart failure and low urine production due to kidney failure (oliguria). It is available as tablets and in a form for injection or infusion.

+▲ side-effects/warning: see FRUSEMIDE

Lasix+K

(Hoechst) is a proprietary, prescription-only COMPOUND PREPARATION of the (*loop*) DIURETIC drug frusemide and the potassium supplement potassium chloride. It can be used to treat oedema. It is available as tablets, which should be swallowed whole with plenty of fluid at mealtimes, or when in an upright posture.

+▲ side-effects/warning see FRUSEMIDE; POTASSIUM CHLORIDE

Lasix Paediatric Liquid

(Hoechst) is a proprietary, prescription-only preparation of the (*loop*) DIURETIC drug frusemide. It can be used to treat oedema and is available as an oral solution.

+▲ side-effects/warning: see FRUSEMIDE

Lasma

(Pharmax) is a proprietary, non-prescription preparation of the BRONCHODILATOR drug theophylline. It can be used as an ANTI-ASTHMATIC and to treat chronic bronchitis. It is available as

modified-release tablets.

+▲ side-effects/warning: see THEOPHYLLINE

Lasonil

(Bayer) is a proprietary, non-prescription COMPOUND PREPARATION of heparinoids (*Bayer HDB-U*) and hyaluronidase. It can be used to improve circulation to the skin in conditions such as bruising, chilblains, thrombophlebitis and varicose veins. It is available as an ointment.

+▲ side-effects/warning: see HEPARINOID; HYALURONIDASE

Lasoride

(Hoechst) is a proprietary, prescription-only COMPOUND PREPARATION of the (*potassium-sparing*) DIURETIC drug amiloride hydrochloride and the (*loop*) diuretic frusemide (a combination called co-amilofruse 5/40). It can be used to treat oedema and is available in as tablets.

+▲ side-effects/warning: see AMILORIDE HYDROCHLORIDE; FRUSEMIDE

Lassar's paste

See ZINC AND SALICYLIC ACID PASTE, BP

*laxatives

(or purgatives) are preparations that promote defecation and so relieve constipation. They can be divided into several different types. The *faecal softener laxatives*, eg. LIQUID PARAFFIN, soften the faeces for easier evacuation. The *bulking agent laxatives* increase the overall volume of the faeces, which then stimulates bowel movement. Bulking agents are usually some form of fibre, eg. BRAN, ISPAGHULA HUSK, METHYLCELLULOSE and STERCULIA. The *stimulant laxatives* act on the intestinal muscles to increase motility.

Many traditional remedies for constipation are stimulants, such as cascara, CASTOR OIL, FIGS ELIXIR and SENNA. However, there are modern variants with less of a stimulant action and which also have other properties, eg. BISACODYL,

DANTHRON, DOCUSATE SODIUM (dioctyl sodium sulphosuccinate) and SODIUM PICOSULPHATE. Finally, the *osmotic laxatives*, which are chemical salts that work by retaining water in the intestine so increasing overall liquidity, eg. LACTULOSE, MAGNESIUM HYDROXIDE and MAGNESIUM SULPHATE (note that magnesium salts are also used as ANTACIDS). Suppositories and enemas also aid in promoting defecation.

Laxoberal
(Windsor Healthcare) is a proprietary, non-prescription preparation of the (*stimulant*) LAXATIVE sodium picosulphate. It can be used for the relief of constipation and is available as an elixir.
+▲ side-effects/warning: see SODIUM PICOSULPHATE

Laxose
(Berk) is a proprietary, non-prescription preparation of the (*osmotic*) LAXATIVE lactulose. It can be used to relieve constipation and is available as an oral solution.
+▲ side-effects/warning: see LACTULOSE

Ledclair
(Sinclair) is a proprietary, prescription-only preparation of the CHELATING AGENT sodium calciumedetate. It can be used as an ANTIDOTE to poisoning by heavy metals, especially by lead and is available in a form for injection.
+▲ side-effects/warning: see SODIUM CALCIUMEDETATE

Ledercort
(Lederle) is a proprietary, prescription-only preparation of the CORTICOSTEROID and ANTI-INFLAMMATORY drug triamcinolone. It can be used to treat severe inflammatory and allergic disorders of the skin, such as severe eczema and is available as tablets.
+▲ side-effects/warning: see TRIAMCINOLONE

Lederfen
(Lederle) is a proprietary, prescription-only preparation of the (NSAID) NON-NARCOTIC ANALGESIC and ANTIRHEUMATIC drug fenbufen. It can be used to relieve pain, particularly rheumatic and arthritic pain and inflammation and to treat other musculoskeletal disorders. It is available as tablets and capsules.
+▲ side-effects/warning: see FENBUFEN

Ledermycin
(Lederle) is a proprietary, prescription-only preparation of the ANTIBACTERIAL and (TETRACYCLINE) ANTIBIOTIC drug demeclocycline hydrochloride. It can be used to treat a wide range of infections and is available as capsules.
+▲ side-effects/warning: see DEMECLOCYCLINE HYDROCHLORIDE

Lederspan
(Lederle) is a proprietary, prescription-only preparation of the CORTICOSTEROID and ANTI-INFLAMMATORY drug triamcinolone hexacetonide. It can be used to treat inflammation of the joints and the soft tissues and is available in a form for injection.
+▲ side-effects/warning: see TRIAMCINOLONE HEXACETONIDE

Lemsip
(Reckitt & Colman) is a proprietary, non-prescription preparation of the NON-NARCOTIC ANALGESIC and ANTIPYRETIC drug paracetamol, the SYMPATHOMIMETIC and DECONGESTANT drug phenylephrine hydrochloride, sodium citrate and vitamin C. It can be used for the relief of cold and flu symptoms. It is available as sachets of powder for making up in hot water and is not normally given to children under 12 years, except on medical advice.
+▲ side-effects/warning: see PARACETAMOL; PHENYLEPHRINE HYDROCHLORIDE

Lemsip Chesty Cough
(Reckitt & Colman) is a proprietary, non-

L prescription preparation of the EXPECTORANT guaiphenesin. It can be used for the relief of sore throats and deep chesty coughs. It is available as a linctus and is not normally given to children under two years, except on medical advice.

+▲ side-effects/warning: see GUAIPHENESIN

Lemsip Cold Relief Capsules

(Reckitt & Colman) is a proprietary, non-prescription preparation of the NON-NARCOTIC ANALGESIC and ANTIPYRETIC drug paracetamol, the SYMPATHOMIMETIC and DECONGESTANT drug phenylephrine hydrochloride and the STIMULANT caffeine. It can be used for the relief of cold and flu symptoms and is available as capsules. It is not normally given to children under 12 years, except on medical advice.

+▲ side-effects/warning: see CAFFEINE; PARACETAMOL; PHENYLEPHRINE HYDROCHLORIDE

Lemsip Flu Strength

(Reckitt & Colman) is a proprietary, non-prescription preparation of the NON-NARCOTIC ANALGESIC and ANTIPYRETIC drug paracetamol, the SYMPATHOMIMETIC and DECONGESTANT drug phenylephrine hydrochloride and vitamin C. It can be used for the relief of flu and cold symptoms, including aches and pains, nasal congestion and fever. It is available as sachets for making up in hot water and is not normally given to children under 12 years, except on medical advice.

+▲ side-effects/warning: see PARACETAMOL; PHENYLEPHRINE HYDROCHLORIDE

Lemsip, Junior

(Reckitt & Colman) is a proprietary, non-prescription preparation of the NON-NARCOTIC ANALGESIC and ANTIPYRETIC drug paracetamol, the SYMPATHOMIMETIC and DECONGESTANT drug phenylephrine hydrochloride, sodium citrate and vitamin C. It can be used for the relief of cold symptoms in children, but not children under three years, except on medical advice. It is available as a powder.

+▲ side-effects/warning: see PARACETAMOL; PHENYLEPHRINE HYDROCHLORIDE

Lemsip Menthol Extra

(Reckitt & Colman) is a proprietary, non-prescription preparation of the NON-NARCOTIC ANALGESIC and ANTIPYRETIC drug paracetamol, the SYMPATHOMIMETIC and DECONGESTANT drug phenylephrine hydrochloride, the STIMULANT caffeine and vitamin C. It can be used for the relief of flu and cold symptoms, including aches and pains, nasal congestion and fever. It is available as sachets for making up in hot water and is not to be given to children under 12 years, except on medical advice.

+▲ side-effects/warning: see CAFFEINE; PARACETAMOL; PHENYLEPHRINE HYDROCHLORIDE

Lemsip Night-Time

(Reckitt & Colman) is a proprietary, non-prescription preparation of the ANTIHISTAMINE chlorpheniramine maleate, the SYMPATHOMIMETIC and VASOCONSTRICTOR drug phenylpropanolamine, the NON-NARCOTIC ANALGESIC and ANTIPYRETIC drug paracetamol, the narcotic analgesic and ANTITUSSIVE drug dextromethorphan hydrobromide and alcohol. It can be used as a NASAL DECONGESTANT during colds and flu, with relief of aches, cough and fever. It is available as a liquid and is not normally given to children under 13 years, except on medical advice.

+▲ side-effects/warning: see ALCOHOL; CHLORPHENIRAMINE MALEATE; DEXTROMETHORPHAN HYDROBROMIDE; PARACETAMOL; PHENYLPROPANOLAMINE

Lenium

(Cilag) is a proprietary, non-prescription preparation of selenium sulphide. It can be used as an antidandruff agent and is available as a cream.

✚▲ side-effects/warning: see SELENIUM
SULPHIDE

Lentard MC
(Novo Nordisk) is a proprietary, non-
prescription preparation of INSULIN ZINC
SUSPENSION. It is used in DIABETIC
TREATMENT to treat and maintain diabetic
patients and contains highly purified
bovine and porcine insulin. It is available
in vials for injection and has a relatively
long duration of action.
✚▲ side-effects/warning: see INSULIN

Lentaron
(Ciba) is a proprietary, prescription-only
preparation of the sex HORMONE
ANTAGONIST drug formestane. It can be
used as an ANTICANCER drug in the
advanced stages of breast cancer and is
available in a form for injection.
✚▲ side-effects/warning: see FORMESTANE

Lentizol
(Parke-Davis) is a proprietary,
prescription-only preparation of the
(TRICYCLIC) ANTIDEPRESSANT drug
amitriptyline hydrochloride. It can be used
to treat depressive illness, particularly in
cases where some degree of sedation is
required and is available as capsules.
✚▲ side-effects/warning: see AMITRIPTYLINE
HYDROCHLORIDE

Lescol
(Sandoz) is a proprietary, prescription-
only preparation of fluvastatin. It can be
used as a LIPID-LOWERING DRUG in
hyperlipidaemia to reduce the levels, or
change the proportions, of various lipids
in the bloodstream. It is available as
capsules.
✚▲ side-effects/warning: see FLUVASTATIN

Leukeran
(Wellcome) is a proprietary, prescription-
only preparation of the
IMMUNOSUPPRESSANT and CYTOTOXIC
(ANTICANCER) drug chlorambucil. It can

be used to treat various forms of cancer
and rheumatoid arthritis and is available
as tablets.
✚▲ side-effects/warning: see CHLORAMBUCIL

leuprorelin acetate
is an analogue of GONADORELIN
(gonadothrophin-releasing hormone;
GnRH), which is a hypothalamic
HORMONE. It reduces the pituitary gland's
secretion of gonadotrophin, which results
in reduced secretion of SEX HORMONES by
the ovaries or testes. It can be used to
treat endometriosis (a growth of the lining
of the uterus at inappropriate sites) and is
also used as an ANTICANCER drug for
cancer of the prostate gland. It is
administered by injection.
✚▲ side-effects/warning: see under
BUSERELIN. There may also be fatigue,
peripheral oedema, nausea and irritation at
the injection site.
✪ Related entry: Prostap SR

levamisole
is an ANTHELMINTIC drug, which, although
not available in the UK, is very effective in
treating infestation by roundworms
(*Ascaris lumbricoides*) and is well
tolerated with rarely any side-effects. It is
administered orally.
✚▲ side-effects/warning: rarely, mild nausea
and vomiting.

levobunolol hydrochloride
is a BETA-BLOCKER that can be used as a
GLAUCOMA TREATMENT for chronic simple
glaucoma. It is thought to work by slowing
the rate of production of the aqueous
humour in the eye and is available as eye-
drops.
✚ side-effects: there may be some systemic
absorption after using eye-drops, so some of
the side-effects listed under propranolol
hydrochloride may be seen. Also, dry eyes and
some local allergic reactions, including
conjunctivitis, may occur.
▲ warning: in view of possible absorption,
dangerous side-effects should be borne in

L

mind, particularly bronchospasm in asthmatics and interactions with calcium-channel blockers.

○ Related entry: Betagen

levodopa

is a powerful ANTIPARKINSONISM drug. It is used to treat parkinsonism, but not the symptoms of parkinsonism induced by drugs. Levodopa is converted into the NEUROTRANSMITTER DOPAMINE within the brain and works by replenishing dopamine levels in the part of the brain (striatum) where there is depletion in Parkinson's disease. It is effective in reducing the slowness of movement and rigidity associated with parkinsonism, but is not as successful in controlling the tremor. Administration is oral in the form of capsules or tablets. It is often combined with other types of drug (eg. CARBIDOPA) that inhibit the conversion of levodopa to dopamine outside the brain, therefore enabling as much levodopa as possible to reach the brain before it is converted, so maximizing its effect. It is the presence of such an inhibitor that may produce involuntary movements.

✚ side-effects: anorexia, nausea, vomiting, insomnia, agitation, postural hypotension (or sometimes short-lived hypertension), dizziness, heart rate changes, red discolouration of the urine and other fluids, rarely sensitivity reactions, abnormal involuntary muscle movements, psychiatric changes, depression, drowsiness, headache, flushing, sweating, gastrointestinal bleeding, changes in liver enzymes and peripheral nerve disturbances.

▲ warning: it is not to be administered to patients with closed-angle glaucoma; administer with caution to those with lung disease, peptic ulcers, cardiovascular disease, diabetes, certain bone disorders, open-angle glaucoma, skin melanoma, or psychiatric disorders; or who are pregnant or breast-feeding. Monitoring of heart, blood, liver and kidney functions is advisable during prolonged treatment.

○ Related entries: Brocadopa; co-beneldopa; co-careldopa; Half Sinemet CR; Larodopa; Madopar; Sinemet; Sinemet CR; Sinemet LS; Sinemet-Plus

levomepromazine

See METHOTRIMEPRAZINE

levonorgestrel

is a PROGESTOGEN. It is used as a constituent of the *combined* ORAL CONTRACEPTIVES that contain OESTROGEN with a progesterone and also in progesterone-only pills. It is also used (in combination with oestrogens) in HRT (hormone replacement therapy) and as an emergency 'morning-after' pill. Administration is either oral as tablets or as capsules for implanting.

✚▲ warning/side-effects: see PROGESTOGEN

○ Related entries: Eugynon 30; Logynon; Logynon ED; Microgynon 30; Microval; Norgeston; Noriday; Norplant; Nuvelle; Ovran; Ovran 30; Ovranette; Schering PC4; Trinordiol

Levophed

(Sanofi Winthrop) is a proprietary, prescription-only preparation of the VASOCONSTRICTOR and SYMPATHOMIMETIC drug noradrenaline (as noradrenaline acid tartrate). It can be used in emergencies to raise the blood pressure in cases of dangerous hypotension and cardiac arrest. It is available in a form for injection.

✚▲ side-effects/warning: see NORADRENALINE

Lexotan

(Roche) is a proprietary, prescription-only preparation of the (BENZODIAZEPINE) ANXIOLYTIC drug bromazepam. It can be used in the short-term treatment of anxiety and is available as tablets.

✚▲ side-effects/warning: see BROMAZEPAM

Lexpec

(RP Drugs) is a proprietary, prescription-

only preparation of folic acid.
It can be used as a VITAMIN supplement,
for example, during pregnancy or to treat
a deficiency. It is available
as a syrup.
+▲ side-effects/warning: see FOLIC ACID

Lexpec with Iron
(RP Drugs) is a proprietary,
prescription-only COMPOUND PREPARATION
of ferric ammonium citrate and folic acid.
It can be used as an IRON and folic acid
supplement during pregnancy and is
available as a syrup.
+▲ side-effects/warning: see FERRIC
AMMONIUM CITRATE; FOLIC ACID

Lexpec with Iron-M
(RP Drugs) is a proprietary,
prescription-only COMPOUND PREPARATION
of ferric ammonium citrate and folic acid.
It can be used as an IRON and folic acid
supplement during pregnancy and is
available as a syrup.
+▲ side-effects/warning: see FERRIC
AMMONIUM CITRATE; FOLIC ACID

LH
See LUTEINIZING HORMONE

Libanil
(APS) is a proprietary, prescription-only
preparation of the SULPHONYLUREA drug
glibenclamide. It is used in DIABETIC
TREATMENT of Type II diabetes (non-
insulin-dependent diabetes mellitus;
NIDDM; maturity-onset diabetes) and is
available as tablets.
+▲ side-effects/warning: see
GLIBENCLAMIDE

Librium
(Roche) is a proprietary, prescription-only
preparation of the (BENZODIAZEPINE)
ANXIOLYTIC drug chlordiazepoxide. It can
be used in the short-term treatment of
anxiety and acute alcohol withdrawal
symptoms. It is available as capsules and
tablets.

+▲ side-effects/warning: see
CHLORDIAZEPOXIDE

Librofem (200 mg)
(Zyma Healthcare) is a proprietary, non-
prescription preparation of the (NSAID)
NON-NARCOTIC ANALGESIC, ANTIRHEUMATIC
and ANTIPYRETIC drug ibuprofen. It can be
used for the relief of period pain and also
for headache, muscular pain and
feverishness. It is available as tablets and
is not to be given to children under 12
years, except on medical advice.
+▲ side-effects/warning: see IBUPROFEN

Lidifen
(Berk) is a proprietary, prescription-only
preparation of the (NSAID) NON-NARCOTIC
ANALGESIC and ANTIRHEUMATIC drug
ibuprofen. It can be used to relieve pain
and inflammation, particularly the pain of
rheumatic disease and other
musculoskeletal disorders. It is available
as tablets.
+▲ side-effects/warning: see IBUPROFEN

Lignocaine in Glucose Injection
(Baxter) is a prescription-only
preparation of the LOCAL ANAESTHETIC drug
lignocaine hydrochloride, which can be
used as an ANTI-ARRHYTHMIC drug to treat
irregularities in the heartbeat, especially
after a heart attack. It is available in a
form for infusion.
+▲ side-effects/warning: see LIGNOCAINE
HYDROCHLORIDE

lignocaine hydrochloride
is the most commonly used of all the
LOCAL ANAESTHETIC drugs. It can be
administered by a number of routes and
always close to its site of action. When
administered by injection or infiltration, it
can be used for dental and minor surgery
(such as sutures). By epidural injection
(into a space surrounding the nerves of
the spinal cord), it is used in childbirth or
major surgery (sometimes in combination

L

with a GENERAL ANAESTHETIC). When
injected into a vascular region, it is co-
injected with ADRENALINE which acts as a
VASOCONSTRICTOR and so limits the rate at
which the lignocaine is washed away.
When applied topically, it is well absorbed
from mucous membranes and abraded
skin and can be used to treat discomfort at
many sites. It is also used in eye-drops as
an anaesthetic for minor surgery on the
eye. Additionally, lignocaine is also used as
an ANTI-ARRHYTHMIC drug (particularly in
the emergency treatment of arrhythmias
and fibrillation following heart attack),
when it is administered by intravenous
injection. It is available in forms suitable
for infiltration, injection or infusion, or
topically as a gel, an ointment, a spray, a
lotion, lozenges, or as eye-drops.
✚ side-effects: these depend on what it is
being used for and the route of
administration. There may be a slowing of the
heartbeat, a fall in blood pressure and
depression of respiration. There may be
allergic hypersensitivity reactions, tingling in
the extremities, dizziness and confusion.
▲ warning: depending on the route of
administration; it should not be administered
to patients with certain heart disorders, or
porphyria. It should be used with caution in
those with liver or respiratory impairment, or
epilepsy.
❂ Related entries: Anbesol Liquid;
Anbesol Teething Gel; Anodesyn;
Betnovate; Bonjela Antiseptic Pain-
Relieving Pastilles; Bradosol Plus;
Depo-Medrone with Lidocaine; Emla;
Instillagel; Lignocaine in Glucose
Injection; Min-I-Jet Lignocaine; Min-I-
Jet Lignocaine Hydrochloride with
Adrenaline; Minims Lignocaine and
Fluorescein; Xylocaine; Xylocard

Li-Liquid

(RP Drugs) is a proprietary, prescription-
only preparation of the ANTIMANIA drug
lithium (as lithium citrate). It can be used
to prevent and treat mania, manic-
depressive bouts and recurrent

depression. It is available as an oral
solution.
✚▲ side-effects/warning: see LITHIUM

Limclair

(Sinclair) is a proprietary, prescription-
only preparation of the drug trisodium
edetate. It can be used to treat the
symptoms of hypercalcaemia (excess
calcium in the blood) and calcification of
the cornea, or lime burns, of the eyeball.
It is available in a form for injection.
✚▲ side-effects/warning: see TRISODIUM
EDETATE

*linctuses

are medicated syrups that are thick and
soothing enough to relieve sore throats or
loosen a cough. However, a linctus is not
the same thing as an EXPECTORANT, which
is a drug that changes the viscosity of
sputum, making it easier to cough up and
so clear the lungs. Also, a linctus is not
necessarily an ELIXIR, which is a
formulation that disguises a potentially
unpleasant taste and is often a sweetening
substance such as glycerol, a sweetener,
or alcohol.

lindane

is a SCABICIDAL and PEDICULICIDAL drug. It
is used to treat parasitic infestation by
itch-mites (scabies) on the skin surface,
particularly under the hair and crab lice
(pubic lice). Administration is topical in
the form of a lotion.
✚ side-effects: skin irritation
▲ warning: avoid contact with the eyes and
do not use on broken or infected skin. It
should not be used on patients who are
pregnant or breast-feeding, or who are
epileptics.
❂ Related entry: Quellada

Lingraine

(Sanofi Winthrop) is a proprietary,
prescription-only preparation of the
VASOCONSTRICTOR drug ergotamine
tartrate. It can be used as an ANTIMIGRAINE

treatment for acute attacks and is available as tablets.

+▲ side-effects/warning: see ERGOTAMINE TARTRATE

liniments

are medicated lotions for rubbing into the skin. Many of them contain alcohol and/or camphor and are intended to relieve minor muscle aches and pains.

Lioresal

(Geigy) is a proprietary, prescription-only preparation of the SKELETAL MUSCLE RELAXANT drug baclofen. It can be used to treat muscle spasm caused by an injury to or a disease of the central nervous system. It is available as tablets and an oral liquid.

+▲ side-effects/warning: see BACLOFEN

liothyronine sodium

is a form of the natural THYROID HORMONE L-tri-iodothyronine sodium that can be used to make up a hormonal deficiency (hypothyroidism). It is rapidly absorbed by the body and is administered by intravenous injection in emergency treatment of hypothyroid coma. It is available as tablets and in a form for intravenous injection.

+▲ side-effects/warning: see under THYROXINE SODIUM

○ Related entries: Tertroxin; Triiodothyronine

Lipantil

(Fournier) is a proprietary, prescription-only preparation of fenofibrate. It can be used as a LIPID-LOWERING DRUG in hyperlipidaemia to reduce the levels, or change the proportions, of various lipids in the bloodstream. It is available as capsules.

+▲ side-effects/warning: see FENOFIBRATE

*lipid-lowering drugs

are used in clinical conditions of hyperlipidaemia; where the blood plasma contains very high levels of the lipids cholesterol and/or triglycerides (natural fats of the body). Current medical opinion suggests that if diet, or drugs, can be used to lower levels of LDL-cholesterol (low-density lipoprotein) while raising HDL-cholesterol (high-density lipoprotein), then there may be a regression of the progress of coronary atherosclerosis (a diseased state of the arteries of the heart where plaques of lipid material narrow blood vessels, which contributes to angina pectoris attacks and the formation of abnormal clots that go on to cause heart attacks and strokes). Currently, lipid-lowering drugs are generally only used where there is a family history of hyperlipidaemia, or clinical signs indicating the need for intervention. In most individuals, an appropriate low-fat diet can adequately do what is required.

Lipid-lowering drugs work in a number of ways: CHOLESTYRAMINE and COLESTIPOL HYDROCHLORIDE lower LDL-cholesterol production. The *clofibrate group* of drugs (BEZAFIBRATE, CIPROFIBRATE, CLOFIBRATE, FENOFIBRATE and GEMFIBROZIL) reduce triglycerides, increase LDL-cholesterol and raise HDL-cholesterol. The *nicotinic acid group* (ACIPIMOX and NICOTINIC ACID) can lower cholesterol and triglyceride levels by an action on enzymes in the liver. The *fish oils* (eg. OMEGA-3 MARINE TRIGLYCERIDES) are dietary supplements that may be useful in treating hypertriglyceridaemia. PROBUCOL can decrease both LDL-cholesterol and HDL-cholesterol, as well as having other beneficial properties. SIMVASTATIN, PRAVASTATIN and FLUVASTATIN are recently introduced drugs that inhibit an enzyme in the liver with the effect that LDL-cholesterol is lowered.

Lipostat

(Squibb) is a proprietary, prescription-only preparation of the LIPID-LOWERING DRUG pravastatin. It can be used in hyperlipidaemia to reduce the levels, or change the proportions, of various lipids in the bloodstream. It is

L

available as tablets.
✚▲ side-effects/warning: see PRAVASTATIN

liquid paraffin

is a traditional (*faecal softener*) LAXATIVE
that can be used to relieve constipation. It
is a constituent of a number of proprietary
laxatives and some non-proprietary
preparations. It is also incorporated into
many skin treatment preparations as an
EMOLLIENT.
✚ side-effects: because only a little of the
paraffin is absorbed in the intestines, seepage
may occur from the anus causing local
irritation. Prolonged use may interfere with
the internal absorption of fat-soluble
vitamins.
▲ warning: prolonged or continuous use of
liquid paraffin as a laxative is to be avoided.
**✪ Related entries: Agarol; Alcoderm;
Alpha Keri Bath; calamine cream,
aqueous, BP; calamine lotion, aqueous,
BP; Diprobase; Diprobath; E45 Cream;
Emmolate; Emulsiderm; Germoline
Ointment; Hydromol; Kamillosan; Keri;
Lacri-Lube; Lubrifilm; Mil-Par; Polytar
Emollient; Savlon Bath Oil; Unguentum
Merck**

Liquifilm Tears

(Allergan) is a proprietary, non-
prescription preparation of polyvinyl
alcohol. It can be used as artificial tears
where there is dryness of the eyes due to
disease. It is available as an ophthalmic
eye solution.
✚▲ side-effects/warning: see POLYVINYL
ALCOHOL

liquorice

is an extract from a leguminous plant. It
has a strong flavour and can be used in
medicines with unpleasant tastes.
Liquorice extract also has a weak
EXPECTORANT activity and is therefore
incorporated into a number of cough
remedies. There are certain preparations
of liquorice that are used to treat peptic
ulcers, some are prepared from

LIQUORICE, DEGLYCYRRHIZINISED and others
are a synthetic chemical derivative of
glycyrrhizinic acid (CARBENOXOLONE
SODIUM).
✪ Related entry: Caved-S

liquorice, deglycyrrhizinised

is a constituent of some preparations that
are used to treat peptic ulcers, particularly
in the stomach but also in the duodenum.
✪ Related entry: Caved-S

lisinopril

is an ACE INHIBITOR. It is a powerful
VASODILATOR that can be used in
ANTIHYPERTENSIVE treatment and is often
used in conjunction with other classes of
drug, particularly (THIAZIDE) DIURETICS. It
is available as tablets.
✚▲ side-effects/warning: see under
CAPTOPRIL
**✪ Related entries; Carace; Carace Plus;
Zestoretic; Zestril**

Liskonum

(SK&F) is a proprietary, prescription-only
preparation of the ANTIMANIA drug lithium
(as lithium carbonate). It can be used to
prevent and treat mania, manic-depressive
bouts and recurrent depression. It is
available as tablets.
✚▲ side-effects/warning: see LITHIUM

lisuride maleate

See LYSURIDE MALEATE

Litarex

(CP) is a proprietary, prescription-only
preparation of the ANTIMANIA drug lithium
(as lithium citrate). It can be used to treat
acute mania, manic-depressive bouts and
recurrent depression. It is available as
tablets.
✚▲ side-effects/warning: see
LITHIUM

lithium

in the form of lithium carbonate or lithium

citrate, is singularly effective as an ANTIMANIA drug to control or prevent the hyperactive manic episodes in manic-depressive illness.

It may also reduce the frequency and severity of depressive episodes. How it works remains imperfectly understood, but its use is so successful that the side-effects caused by its toxicity are deemed to be justified. Administration is oral in the form of tablets.

✚ side-effects: many long-term patients experience nausea, thirst and excessive urination, gastrointestinal disturbance, weakness and tremor. There may be fluid retention and consequent weight gain. Visual disturbances, worsening gastric problems, muscle weakness and lack of co-ordination indicate lithium intoxication.

▲ warning: it should not be administered to patients with certain heart or kidney disorders, or imperfect sodium balance in the bloodstream. It should be administered with caution to those who are pregnant or breast-feeding, who are elderly, taking diuretics, or have myasthenia gravis. Prolonged treatment may cause kidney and thyroid gland dysfunction; prolonged overdosage eventually causes serious effects on the brain. Consequently, blood levels of lithium must be regularly checked for toxicity, thyroid function must be monitored and there must be adequate intake of fluids and sodium.

۞ Related entries: Camcolit 250 Camcolit 400; Li-Liquid; Liskonum; Litarex; Phasal; Priadel

lithium succinate

is a constituent of an ointment for seborrhoeic dermatitis.
۞ Related entry: Efalith

Livial

(Organon) is a proprietary, prescription-only preparation of the drug tibolone, which has both OESTROGEN and PROGESTOGEN activity. It can be used in HRT and is available as tablets.

Lloyd's Cream

(Seton Healthcare) is a proprietary, non-prescription preparation of the COUNTER-IRRITANT, or RUBEFACIENT, agent diethylamine salicylate. It can be applied to the skin for symptomatic relief of underlying muscle or joint pain and is available as a cream.
✚▲ side-effects/warning: see DIETHYLAMINE SALICYLATE

Lobak

(Sanofi Winthrop) is a proprietary, prescription-only COMPOUND PREPARATION of the SKELETAL MUSCLE RELAXANT and ANXIOLYTIC drug chlormezanone and the NON-NARCOTIC ANALGESIC paracetamol. It can be used for the relief of muscle pain and is available as tablets.
✚▲ side-effects/warning: see CHLORMEZANONE; PARACETAMOL

Locabiotal

(Servier) is a proprietary, prescription-only preparation of the ANTI-INFLAMMATORY and ANTIBIOTIC drug fusafungine. It can be used to treat infection and inflammation in the nose and throat. It is available as an aerosol with a nose and mouth adapter and is not normally given to children under three years, except on medical advice.
✚▲ side-effects/warning: see FUSAFUNGINE

*local anaesthetic

drugs are used to reduce sensation (especially pain) in a specific, local area of the body and without loss of consciousness. GENERAL ANAESTHETIC drugs, in contrast, decrease sensation only because of a loss of consciousness. Local anaesthetics work by reversibly blocking the transmission of impulses in nerves. They can be administered by a number of routes and always close to their site of action. By local injection or infiltration, they can be used for dental and minor surgery (such as sutures). A more extensive loss of sensation with nerve

L

L block (eg. injected near to the nerve supplying a limb), or with spinal anaesthesia (eg. epidural injection in childbirth), or intrathecal block (for extensive procedures) produces a loss of sensation in whole areas of the body sufficient to allow major surgery (though with some, quickly reversible paralysis). Local anaesthetics are particularly valuable where the use of a general anaesthetic carries a high risk, or when the co-operation of the patient is required. When administered into a vascular region, ADRENALINE is co-injected and acts as a VASOCONSTRICTOR to limit the rate at which the anaesthetic is washed away. When applied topically, certain local anaesthetics are well absorbed from mucous membranes and abraded skin and can be used to treat discomfort at many sites. See: AMETHOCAINE HYDROCHLORIDE; BENZOCAINE; BUPIVACAINE HYDROCHLORIDE; CINCHOCAINE; COCAINE; LIGNOCAINE HYDROCHLORIDE; OXETHAZAINE; OXYBUPROCAINE HYDROCHLORIDE; PRILOCAINE HYDROCHLORIDE; PROCAINAMIDE HYDROCHLORIDE; PROCAINE; PROXYMETACAINE; TOCAINIDE HYDROCHLORIDE.

*local anaesthetic

is a term used to describe mediators that are released within the body to act at a site local to their point of release. In this respect, as mediators of body signals, they differ from blood-borne (*endocrine*) HORMONES that are released from specific glands and generally act remote to the point of release and NEUROTRANSMITTERS, which are released only from nerves and act very close to the point of release. Local hormones have many functions in the body.

One of their best-understood functions is their role in inflammation. It is known that local hormones are often released as a result of an injury to tissues or because of an allergic reaction and mediate responses in the body that are pro-

inflammatory (cause inflammation). Reactions such as these are generally intended to protect the body, but if too extreme or inappropriate they can cause adverse effects on health and need to be controlled with drugs. Many of the ANTI-INFLAMMATORY and ANTI-ALLERGIC drugs in common medical use work by preventing the formation, release, or actions of local hormones. Examples of pro-inflammatory local hormones are histamine and the members of the PROSTAGLANDIN family. ANTIHISTAMINES are drugs that inhibit the effects in the body of the local hormone histamine by blocking its RECEPTORS, whereas the NSAID drugs (eg. ASPIRIN and IBUPROFEN) work by preventing the formation and hence release, of the prostaglandin local hormones. CORTICOSTEROIDS and SODIUM CROMOGLYCATE-related drugs are also of value in treating allergic conditions where local hormones are released, for example, for asthma and skin conditions such as eczema and psoriasis.

Not all actions of local hormones are undesirable and many are a part of normal body function. For instance, the prostaglandins play a part in controlling the blood flow in the mucosal lining of the stomach and intestine and act as cytoprotectants and ULCER-HEALING DRUGS. Prostaglandins may also have a role in controlling motility and other functions of the intestine and uterus. The latter actions are used in obstetrics by the administration of synthetic preparations of the naturally occurring members of the prostaglandin family, such as prostaglandin E_2 (DINOPROSTONE), prostaglandin $F_2\alpha$ (DINOPROST) or prostacyclin (EPOPROSTENOL), or synthetic analogues (eg. MISOPROSTOL), which mimick the actions where prostaglandins are potent in contraction of the uterus, softening and dilation of the cervix and dilation of blood vessels. These actions can be used for abortion and in aiding labour.

There are many other local hormones and drugs that modify their actions are continually being developed. For example the recently introduced ANTINAUSEANT drug ONDANSETRON, blocks and mimicks some actions of SEROTONIN where it acts as a local hormone in the gastrointestinal tract.

Loceryl

(Roche) is a proprietary, prescription-only preparation of the ANTIFUNGAL drug AMOROLFINE. It can be used topically to treat fungal skin infections and is available as a cream and a nail lacquer.

Locoid

(Yamanouchi) is a proprietary, prescription-only preparation of the CORTICOSTEROID drug hydrocortisone (as butyrate). It can be used for serious inflammatory skin conditions, such as eczema and psoriasis and is available as a cream (*Lipocream*), an ointment and a scalp lotion.

+▲ side-effects/warning: see HYDROCORTISONE

Locoid C

(Yamanouchi) is a proprietary, prescription-only COMPOUND PREPARATION of the CORTICOSTEROID drug hydrocortisone (as butyrate) and the ANTIMICROBIAL drug chlorquinaldol. It can be used to treat inflammatory skin conditions, such as eczema and is available as a cream and an ointment.

+▲ side-effects/warning: see CHLORQUINALDOL; HYDROCORTISONE

Locorten-Vioform

(Zyma Healthcare) is a proprietary, prescription-only COMPOUND PREPARATION of the CORTICOSTEROID drug flumethasone pivalate and the ANTIMICROBIAL drug clioquinol. It can be be used to treat mild infections of the outer ear and is available as ear-drops.

+▲ side-effects/warning: see CLIOQUINOL

Lodine

(Wyeth) is a proprietary, prescription-only preparation of the (NSAID) NON-NARCOTIC ANALGESIC and ANTIRHEUMATIC drug etodolac. It can be used to treat the pain of osteoarthritis and rheumatoid arthritis and is available as capsules and tablets.

+▲ side-effects/warning: see ETODOLAC

Loestrin 20

(Parke-Davis) is a proprietary, prescription-only COMPOUND PREPARATION that can be used as a (*monophasic*) ORAL CONTRACEPTIVE (and also for certain menstrual problems) of the type that combines an OESTROGEN and a PROGESTOGEN, in this case ethinyloestradiol and norethisterone. It is available in the form of tablets in a calendar pack.

+▲ side-effects/warning: see ETHINYLOESTRADIOL; NORETHISTERONE

Loestrin 30

(Parke-Davis) is a proprietary, prescription-only COMPOUND PREPARATION that can be used as a (*monophasic*) ORAL CONTRACEPTIVE (and also for certain menstrual problems) of the type that combines an OESTROGEN and a PROGESTOGEN, in this case ethinyloestradiol and norethisterone. It is available in the form of tablets in a calendar pack.

+▲ side-effects/warning: see ETHINYLOESTRADIOL; NORETHISTERONE

Iofepramine

is an ANTIDEPRESSANT, one of the TRICYCLIC group, that is used to treat depressive illness. It has less SEDATIVE properties than other antidepressants and is therefore more suitable for the treatment of withdrawn and apathetic patients, rather than those who are agitated and restless. Administration is oral in the form of tablets.

+▲ side-effects/warning: see under AMITRIPTYLINE HYDROCHLORIDE; but is less

L

sedating. It should not be prescribed to patients with severe liver or kidney damage.
○ Related entry: Gamanil

lofexidine hydrochloride

is a recently introduced drug that is used to alleviate OPIOID withdrawal symptoms. It appears to have actions that are similar to those of the drug CLONIDINE, but is less effective. Administration is oral as tablets.
✚ side-effects: drowsiness, dry mouth, throat and nose, hypotension, slowing of the heart and hypertension on withdrawal.
▲ warning: use with caution in patients with certain heart disorders, kidney impairment, a history of depression; or who are pregnant or breast-feeding.
○ Related entry: BritLofex

Logynon

(Schering Health) is a proprietary, prescription-only COMPOUND PREPARATION that can be used as a (*triphasic*) ORAL CONTRACEPTIVE (and also for certain menstrual problems) of the type that combines an OESTROGEN and a PROGESTOGEN, in this case ethinyloestradiol and levonorgestrel. It is available in the form of tablets in a calendar pack.
✚▲ side-effects/warning: see ETHINYLOESTRADIOL; LEVONORGESTREL

Logynon ED

(Schering Health) is a proprietary, prescription-only COMPOUND PREPARATION that can be used as a (*triphasic*) ORAL CONTRACEPTIVE (and also for certain menstrual problems) of the type that combines an OESTROGEN and a PROGESTOGEN, in this case ethinyloestradiol and levonorgestrel. It is available in the form of tablets in a calendar pack.
✚▲ side-effects/warning: see ETHINYLOESTRADIOL; LEVONORGESTREL

Lomotil

(Searle) is a proprietary, prescription-only

COMPOUND PREPARATION of the ANTICHOLINERGIC drug atropine sulphate and the (OPIOID) ANTIDIARRHOEAL drug diphenoxylate hydrochloride, which is a combination called co-phenotrope. It can be used to treat chronic diarrhoea (eg. in mild chronic ulcerative colitis) and is available as a liquid and as tablets.
✚▲ side-effects/warning: see ATROPINE SULPHATE; DIPHENOXYLATE HYDROCHLORIDE

lomustine

is a CYTOTOXIC DRUG, which is used as an ANTICANCER treatment, particularly for Hodgkin's disease (cancer of the lymphatic tissues) and some solid tumours. It works by disrupting cellular DNA and so inhibiting cell replication. Administration is oral in the form of capsules.
✚▲ side-effects/warning: see under CYCTOTOXIC DRUGS. Nausea and vomiting can be quite severe.
○ Related entry: CCNU

Loniten

(Upjohn) is a proprietary, prescription-only preparation of the VASODILATOR drug minoxidil. It can be used as an ANTIHYPERTENSIVE to treat severe acute hypertension (usually in combination with a DIURETIC or BETA-BLOCKER). It is available as tablets.
✚▲ side-effects/warning: see MINOXIDIL

loperamide hydrochloride

is an (OPIOID) ANTIDIARRHOEAL drug. It acts on the nerves of the intestine to inhibit peristalsis (the waves of muscular activity that move along the contents of the intestines) so reducing motility and also decreases fluid loss from the intestines. Administration is oral in the form of syrup or capsules. (Preparations containing loperamide hydrochloride are available without prescription for the treatment of acute diarrhoea only.)
✚▲ side-effects/warning: see under OPIOID; but when used to treat acute diarrhoea there

is little or no risk of dependence and it is less sedative.

○ **Related entries: Arret; Imodium Capsules**

Lopid

(Parke-Davis) is a proprietary, prescription-only preparation of the LIPID-LOWERING DRUG gemfibrozil. It can be used in hyperlipidaemia to reduce the levels, or change the proportions, of various lipids in the bloodstream. It is available as capsules (*Lopid 300*) and tablets (*Lopid 600*).

✚▲ side-effects/warning: see GEMFIBROZIL

Lopidine

(Alcon) is a proprietary, prescription-only preparation of the SYMPATHOMIMETIC drug apraclonidine. It can be used to control or prevent postoperative elevation of intraocular pressure (pressure of the eyeball) after laser surgery. It is available as eye-drops.

✚▲ side-effects/warning: see APRACLONIDINE

loprazolam

is a BENZODIAZEPINE drug, which is used as a relatively short-acting HYPNOTIC for the short-term treatment of insomnia. Administration is oral in the form of tablets.

✚▲ side-effects/warning: see under BENZODIAZEPINE

○ **Related entry: Dormonoct**

Lopresor

(Geigy) is a proprietary, prescription-only preparation of the BETA-BLOCKER drug metoprolol tartrate. It can be used as an ANTIHYPERTENSIVE treatment for raised blood pressure, as an ANTI-ANGINA treatment to relieve symptoms and improve exercise tolerance and as an ANTI-ARRHYTHMIC to regularize heartbeat and to treat myocardial infarction. It can also be used as an ANTITHYROID drug for short-term treatment of thyrotoxicosis, or as an ANTIMIGRAINE treatment to prevent

attacks. It is available as tablets.

✚▲ side-effects/warning: see METOPROLOL TARTRATE

Lopresor SR

(Geigy) is a proprietary, prescription-only preparation of the BETA-BLOCKER drug metoprolol tartrate. It can be used as an ANTIHYPERTENSIVE treatment for raised blood pressure, as an ANTI-ANGINA treatment to relieve symptoms and improve exercise tolerance and as an ANTI-ARRHYTHMIC to regularize heartbeat and to treat myocardial infarction. It can also be used as an ANTITHYROID drug for short-term treatment of thyrotoxicosis, or as an ANTIMIGRAINE treatment to prevent attacks. It is available as modified-release tablets.

✚▲ side-effects/warning: see METOPROLOL TARTRATE

loratadine

is a recently developed ANTIHISTAMINE drug. It has less sedative side-effects than some older members of its class and can be used for the symptomatic relief of allergic symptoms such as hay fever and urticaria (itchy skin rash). Administration is oral as tablets or a syrup.

✚▲ side-effects/warning: see under ANTIHISTAMINE. But the incidence of sedative and anticholinergic effects is low; nevertheless, it may impair the performance of skilled tasks such as driving. It should not be given to patients who are pregnant.

○ **Related entry: Clarityn**

lorazepam

is a BENZODIAZEPINE drug with a number of applications. It is used as an ANXIOLYTIC in the short-term treatment of anxiety, as a HYPNOTIC for insomnia, as an ANTI-EPILEPTIC in status epilepticus and as a SEDATIVE in preoperative medication, because its ability to cause amnesia means that the patient forgets the unpleasant procedure. Administration is either oral as tablets or by injection.

L

+▲ side-effects/warning: see under
BENZODIAZEPINE
◘ Related entry: Ativan

lormetazepam

is a BENZODIAZEPINE drug, which is used
as a relatively short-acting HYPNOTIC for
the short-term treatment of insomnia.
Administration is oral in the form of
tablets.
+▲ side-effects/warning: see under
BENZODIAZEPINE

Loron

(Boehringer Mannheim) is a recently
introduced proprietary, prescription-only
preparation of the drug sodium
chlodronate. It can be used to treat high
calcium levels associated with malignant
tumours and bone lesions. It is available
in a form for intravenous infusion (*Loron
for infusion*), as capsules and as tablets
(*Loron 520*).
+▲ side-effects/warning: see SODIUM
CHLODRONATE

Losec

(Astra) is a proprietary, prescription-only
preparation of the PROTON-PUMP
INHIBITOR omeprazole. It can be used as
an ULCER-HEALING DRUG and for associated
conditions. It is available as capsules.
+▲ side-effects/warning: see OMEPRAZOLE

*lotions

are medicated liquids used to bathe or
wash skin, the hair and the eyes. In many
cases, lotions should be left wet after
application for as long as possible.

Lotriderm

(Schering-Plough) is a proprietary,
prescription-only COMPOUND PREPARATION
of the CORTICOSTEROID drug
betamethasone (as dipropionate) and
the ANTIFUNGAL drug clotrimazole. It
can be used to treat fungal infections,
particularly those associated with
inflammation. It is available as a
cream for topical application.
+▲ side-effects/warning: see
BETAMETHASONE; CLOTRIMAZOLE

Loxapac

(Novex) is a proprietary, prescription-only
preparation of the ANTIPSYCHOTIC drug
loxapine. It can be used to treat acute and
chronic psychoses and is available as
capsules.
+▲ side-effects/warning: see
LOXAPINE

loxapine

is an ANTIPSYCHOTIC drug. It is used to
treat acute and chronic psychoses and is
administered orally as capsules.
+▲ side-effects/warning: see under
CHLORPROMAZINE HYDROCHLORIDE; but there
is also nausea and vomiting, weight gain or
weight loss, shortness of breath, drooping of
the eyelids, raised body temperature, loss of
sensation in the extremities, flushing and
headache.
◘ Related entry: Loxapac

Luborant

(Antigen) is a proprietary, non-
prescription COMPOUND PREPARATION of
carmellose sodium, sorbitol, potassium
chloride and other salts. It can be used as
a form of ARTIFICIAL SALIVA for application
to the mouth and throat in conditions that
make the mouth abnormally dry. It is
available as an aerosol.
+▲ side-effects/warning: see CARMELLOSE
SODIUM; POTASSIUM CHLORIDE; SORBITOL

Lubrifilm

(Cusi) is a proprietary, non-prescription
preparation of liquid paraffin, yellow soft
paraffin and wool fat. It can be used as an
eye treatment both as a night-time eye
lubricant (in conditions that cause dry
eyes) and to soften the crusts of
inflammation of the eyelids (blepharitis).
It is available as an eye ointment.
+▲ side effects/warnings: see LIQUID
PARAFFIN; WOOL FAT; YELLOW SOFT PARAFFIN

Ludiomil

(Ciba) is a proprietary, prescription-only preparation of the TRICYCLIC-related ANTIDEPRESSANT drug maprotiline hydrochloride. It can be used to treat depressive illness, especially in cases where sedation is required and is available as tablets.

+▲ side-effects/warning: see MAPROTILINE HYDROCHLORIDE

Lugol's solution

See AQUEOUS IODINE ORAL SOLUTION

Lurselle

(Merrell) is a proprietary, prescription-only preparation of the LIPID-LOWERING DRUG probucol. It can be used in hyperlipidaemia to reduce the levels, or change the proportions, of various lipids in the bloodstream. It is available as tablets.

+▲ side-effects/warning: see PROBUCOL

Lustral

(Invicta) is a proprietary, prescription-only preparation of the (SSRI) ANTIDEPRESSANT drug sertraline. It has less sedative effects than some other antidepressants and is available as tablets.

+▲ side-effects/warning: see SERTRALINE

luteinizing hormone

(LH) is a HORMONE secreted by the anterior pituitary gland and (along with FOLLICLE-STIMULATING HORMONE; FSH) is a GONADOTROPHIN hormone. In women, in conjunction with FSH, it causes the monthly ripening in one ovary of a follicle and stimulates ovulation. In men, it facilitates the production of sperm in the testes (hence its alternative name interstitial cell-stimulating hormone, ICSH). It may be injected therapeutically, along with FSH, in infertility treatment to stimulate ovulation. It is available, in combination with FSH, as HUMAN MENOPAUSAL GONADOTROPHIN. See also CHORIONIC GONADOTROPHIN.

○ Related entries: Gonadotrophin LH; Humegon; Normegon; Pergonal

Lyclear

(Wellcome) is a proprietary, non-prescription preparation of the SCABICIDAL and PEDICULICIDAL drug permethrin. It can be used for the treatment of head-louse infestation. It is available as a cream rinse and a skin cream; the cream rinse is not normally used on infants under six months, except on medical advice.

+▲ side-effects/warning: see PERMETHRIN

lymecycline

is a broad-spectrum ANTIBACTERIAL and (TETRACYCLINE) ANTIBIOTIC drug. It can be used to treat infections of many kinds, for instance of the respiratory and genital tracts. Administration is oral in the form of capsules.

+▲ side-effects/warning: see under TETRACYCLINE

○ Related entry: Tetralysal 300

lypressin

is an analogue of the antidiuretic HORMONE vasopressin. It can be used as a DIABETES INSIPIDUS TREATMENT in pituitary-originated diabetes insipidus. Administration is topical in the form of a nasal spray.

+▲ side-effects/warning: see under VASOPRESSIN; but with less hypersensitivity. Also, with the nasal spray there may be ulceration of the nasal mucosa and nasal congestion.

○ Related entry: Syntopressin

lysuride maleate

(lisuride maleate) is a recently introduced ANTIPARKINSONISM drug that is an ERGOT ALKALOID derivative. It has actions that are similar to those of BROMOCRIPTINE and is particularly useful in patients who cannot tolerate levodopa. Administration is oral in the form of tablets.

+ side-effects: headache, nausea and vomiting, dizziness, lethargy, malaise,

lysuride maleate

drowsiness, psychotic reactions (including hallucinations), occasional hypotension, rashes, constipation and abdominal pain.
▲ warning: it should be administered with caution to patients with a history of psychosis, who have had a pituitary tumour; or are pregnant or breast-feeding. It should not be given to patients with certain, severe cardiovascular disorders, or porphyria. It may impair the performance of skilled tasks such as driving.
✪ Related entry: Revanil

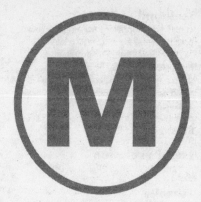

Maalox Plus Suspension

(Rhône-Poulenc Rorer) is a proprietary, non-prescription COMPOUND PREPARATION of the ANTACIDS magnesium hydroxide and aluminium hydroxide and the ANTIFOAMING AGENT dimethicone. It can be used for the symptomatic relief of dyspepsia, heartburn and flatulence and is available as a suspension.
+▲ side-effects/warning: see ALUMINIUM HYDROXIDE; DIMETHICONE; MAGNESIUM HYDROXIDE

Maalox Plus Tablets

(Rhône-Poulenc Rorer) is a proprietary, non-prescription COMPOUND PREPARATION of the ANTACIDS magnesium hydroxide and aluminium hydroxide and the ANTIFOAMING AGENT dimethicone. It can be used for the symptomatic relief of dyspepsia, heartburn and flatulence and is available as tablets. It is not normally given to children, except on medical advice.
+▲ side-effects/warning: see ALUMINIUM HYDROXIDE; DIMETHICONE; MAGNESIUM HYDROXIDE

Maalox Suspension

(Rhône-Poulenc Rorer) is a proprietary, non-prescription COMPOUND PREPARATION of the ANTACIDS magnesium hydroxide and aluminium hydroxide. It can be used for the symptomatic relief of dyspepsia, gastric hyperacidity and gastritis. It is available as a suspension and is not normally given to children under 14 years, except on medical advice.
+▲ side-effects/warning: see ALUMINIUM HYDROXIDE; MAGNESIUM HYDROXIDE

Maalox TC Suspension

(Rhône-Poulenc Rorer) is a proprietary, non-prescription COMPOUND PREPARATION of the ANTACIDS magnesium hydroxide and aluminium hydroxide. It can be used for the symptomatic relief of heartburn, gastric hyperacidity and gastritis. It is available as a suspension and is not normally given to children,

except on medical advice.
+▲ side-effects/warning: see ALUMINIUM HYDROXIDE; MAGNESIUM HYDROXIDE

Maclean Indigestion Tablets

(SmithKline Beecham) is a proprietary, non-prescription COMPOUND PREPARATION of the ANTACIDS calcium carbonate, magnesium carbonate and aluminium hydroxide. It can be used for the symptomatic relief of indigestion, flatulence and nausea and is available as tablets. It is not normally given to children, except on medical advice.
+▲ side-effects/warning: see ALUMINIUM HYDROXIDE; CALCIUM CARBONATE; MAGNESIUM CARBONATE

Macrobid

(Procter & Gamble) is a proprietary, prescription-only preparation of the ANTIBACTERIAL drug nitrofurantoin. It can be used to treat infections of the urinary tract and is available as capsules.
+▲ side-effects/warning: see NITROFURANTOIN

Macrodantin

(Procter & Gamble) is a proprietary, prescription-only preparation of the ANTIBACTERIAL drug nitrofurantoin. It can be used to treat infections of the urinary tract and is available as capsules.
+▲ side-effects/warning: see NITROFURANTOIN

macrolide

is the term used to describe a group of ANTIBIOTIC drugs that are used for their ANTIBACTERIAL action. They have a similar spectrum of action to penicillin, but a different mechanism of action; they work by inhibiting microbial protein synthesis – they are *bacteriostatic*. Their principal use is as an alternative antibiotic in patients who are allergic to penicillin. The original and best-known, member of the group is ERYTHROMYCIN, which is effective

M

against many Gram-positive bacteria including streptococci (which can cause soft tissue and respiratory tract infections), legionella (legionnaires' disease), chlamydia (urethritis) and is also used in the treatment of acne, chronic prostatitis, diphtheria and whooping cough. The macrolides are relatively non-toxic and serious side-effects are rare. See: AZITHROMYCIN; CLARITHROMYCIN

Madopar

(Roche) is a proprietary, prescription-only COMPOUND PREPARATION of the drugs levodopa and benserazide hydrochloride, which is a combination called co-beneldopa. It can be used to treat parkinsonism, but not the parkinsonian symptoms induced by drugs (see ANTIPARKINSONISM). It is available as tablets, capsules (both in several preparations of different strengths) and modified-release capsules called *Madopar CR*.
✚▲ side-effects/warning: see LEVODOPA

magaldrate

is an ANTACID complex that is used to treat severe dyspepsia. It is a combination of aluminium and magnesium hydroxides (with sulphuric acid).
✚▲ side-effects/warning: see ALUMINIUM HYDROXIDE; MAGNESIUM HYDROXIDE
✪ Related entries: Bisodol Heartburn; Dynese

Magnapen

(Beecham) is a proprietary, prescription-only COMPOUND PREPARATION of the broad-spectrum ANTIBACTERIAL (PENICILLIN) ANTIBIOTIC drug ampicillin and the *penicillinase-resistant*, antibacterial and (penicillin) antibiotic drug flucloxacillin, which is a combination called co-fluampicil. It can be used to treat severe infection where the causative organism has not been identified, but Gram-positive staphylococcal infection is suspected, or where penicillin-resistant bacterial

infection is probable. It is available as capsules, a syrup and in a form for injection.
✚▲ side-effects/warning: see AMPICILLIN; FLUCLOXACILLIN

Magnatol

(Sterling Health) is a proprietary, non-prescription COMPOUND PREPARATION of the ANTACIDS potassium bicarbonate, magnesium carbonate and alexitol sodium (with xanthan gum). It can be used for the symptomatic relief of heartburn and is available as a suspension. It is not normally given to children, except on medical advice.
✚▲ side-effects/warning: see ALEXITOL SODIUM; MAGNESIUM CARBONATE;

magnesium

is a metallic element necessary to the body and is ingested as a trace element in a well-balanced diet (a good source is green vegetables). It is essential to the bones and important for the proper functioning of nerves and muscles. Therapeutically, magnesium is used in the form of its salts: MAGNESIUM CARBONATE, MAGNESIUM HYDROXIDE, magnesium oxide (magnesia) and MAGNESIUM TRISILICATE are ANTACIDS; MAGNESIUM SULPHATE (Epsom salt/salts) is a LAXATIVE. Magnesium deficiency is usually treated with supplements of MAGNESIUM CHLORIDE.

magnesium carbonate

is an ANTACID that also has LAXATIVE properties. It is a mild antacid but fairly long-acting and is a constituent of many proprietary preparations that are used for the relief of hyperacidity and dyspepsia and for the symptomatic relief of heartburn or a peptic ulcer. Administration is oral in the form of a mixture or tablets.
✚ side-effects: there may be belching due to the internal liberation of carbon dioxide and diarrhoea.
▲ warning: it should be administered with

caution to patients with impaired function of the kidneys, or who are taking certain other drugs. It is not to be taken by those with low phosphate levels.

○ Related entries: Algicon; Aludrox Tablets; Andrews Antacid; Bismag Tablets; Bisodol Antacid Powder; Bisodol Antacid Tablets; Bisodol Extra Tablets; Caved-S; Dijex Tablets; Maclean Indigestion Tablets; Magnatol; Mooland Tablets; Nulacin Tablets; Original Andrews Salts; Rennie Tablets, Digestif; Topal

magnesium chloride

is the form of MAGNESIUM that is most commonly used to make up a magnesium deficiency in the body, which may result from prolonged diarrhoea or vomiting, or due to alcoholism.
○ Related entry: Balanced Salt Solution

magnesium hydroxide

or hydrated magnesium oxide (*magnesia*), is an ANTACID that also has LAXATIVE properties. As an antacid it is comparatively weak but fairly long-acting and is a constituent of many proprietary preparations that are used for the relief of hyperacidity and dyspepsia and for the symptomatic relief of heartburn or a peptic ulcer. It can also be used to treat constipation. Administration is oral in the form of tablets or as an aqueous suspension.
✚ side-effects: there may be diarrhoea.
▲ warning: it should be administered with caution to patients with impaired function of the kidneys, certain gastrointestinal conditions, or who are taking certain other drugs.
○ Related entries: Algicon; Aludrox Tablets; Asilone Liquid; Asilone Suspension; Caved-S; Dijex; Dijex Tablets; Diovol; Gastrocote; Gastron; Gaviscon 250; Kolanticon Gel; Maalox Plus Suspension; Maalox Plus Tablets; Maalox Suspension; Maalox TC Suspension; Maclean Indigestion Tablets; Milk of Magnesia Liquid; Milk of Magnesia Tablets; Mil-Par; Mucaine; Mucogel Suspension; Pyrogastrone; Topal

magnesium sulphate

or Epsom salt(s), is an *osmotic* LAXATIVE. It works by preventing the reabsorption of water within the intestines and can be used to facilitate rapid bowel evacuation. Occasionally, it can also be used as a MAGNESIUM supplement and to treat boils and carbuncles when it is applied topically as a paste with glycerol.
✚ side-effects: colitis when taken orally.
▲ warning: when administered orally, care must be taken in patients with renal or liver impairment and do not use in severe gastrointestinal impairment.
○ Related entry: Original Andrews Salts

magnesium trisilicate

is used as an ANTACID and has a long duration of action. It is a constituent of many proprietary preparations that are used to relieve hyperacidity and dyspepsia and for the symptomatic relief of heartburn or a peptic ulcer. Administration is oral in the form of tablets or as an aqueous suspension.
✚ side-effects: it may cause diarrhoea.
▲ warning: it should be administered with caution to patients with impaired function of the kidneys, or who are taking certain other drugs.
○ Related entries: Gastrocote; Gastron; Gaviscon 250; Moorland Tablets; Nulacin Tablets; Progastrone

major tranquillizer

See ANTIPSYCHOTIC

malathion

is an insecticidal drug that is used as a PEDICULICIDAL to treat infestations by head and pubic lice, or as a SCABICIDAL to treat skin infestation by mites (scabies). Administration is topical in the form of a liquid lotion or a shampoo.

✚ side-effects: skin irritation.

▲ warning: avoid contact with the eyes and do not use on broken or infected skin. It should not be used by asthmatics.

❍ Related entries: Derbac-M; Prioderm; Suleo-M

malic acid

is a weak organic acid found in apples and some fruits. It is incorporated into some medicinal preparations, such as ARTIFICIAL SALIVA and skin treatments, to adjust their acidity.

❍ Related entry: Aserbine.

Malix

(Lagap) is a proprietary, prescription-only preparation of the SULPHONYLUREA drug glibenclamide. It is used in DIABETIC TREATMENT for Type II diabetes (non-insulin-dependent diabetes mellitus; NIDDM; maturity-onset diabetes) and is available as tablets.

✚▲ side-effects/warning: see GLIBENCLAMIDE

Maloprim

(Wellcome) is a proprietary, prescription-only COMPOUND PREPARATION of the ANTIBACTERIAL and ANTIMALARIAL drug dapsone and the antimalarial drug pyrimethamine. It can be used to prevent visitors to tropical regions from contracting malaria and is available as tablets.

✚▲ side-effects/warning: see DAPSONE; PYRIMETHAMINE

Manerix

(Roche) is a proprietary, prescription-only preparation of the MONOAMINE-OXIDASE INHIBITOR (MAOI) ANTIDEPRESSANT drug moclobemide. It can be used to treat major depressive illness and is available as tablets.

✚▲ side-effects/warning: see MOCLOBEMIDE

Manevac

(Galen) is a proprietary, non-prescription COMPOUND PREPARATION of the (bulking agent) LAXATIVE ispaghula husk and the (*stimulant*) laxative senna. It can be used to treat a number of gastrointestinal disorders and is available as granules. It is not normally given to children under five years, except on medical advice.

✚▲ side-effects/warning: see ISPAGHULA HUSK; SENNA

mannitol

is one of the *osmotic diuretic* class of DIURETICS. It consists of substances secreted into the kidney proximal tubules, which are not resorbed and so carry water and mineral salts into the urine, therefore increasing the volume produced.

Therapeutically, it is used primarily to treat oedema (accumulation of fluid in the tissues), particularly cerebral (brain) oedema. It may also be used in GLAUCOMA TREATMENT to decrease pressure within the eyeball in acute attacks. Administration is by intravenous infusion.

✚ side-effects: there may be chills and fever.

▲ warning: treatment may, in the short term, expand the overall blood volume and therefore it should not be administered to patients with congestive heart failure or fluid on the lungs (pulmonary oedema). An escape of mannitol into the tissues from the site of infusion (vein) causes inflammation and thrombosis.

❍ Related entries: Dantrium; Min-I-Jet Mannitol (25%)

MAOI

See MONOAMINE-OXIDASE INHIBITORS

maprotiline hydrochloride

is a TRICYCLIC-related ANTIDEPRESSANT drug. It is used to treat depressive illness, particularly in cases where some degree of sedation is called for. Administration is oral in the form of tablets.

✚▲ side-effects/warning: see under

AMITRIPTYLINE HYDROCHLORIDE; but some anticholinergic actions are less marked. Rashes are common and there is a danger of convulsions and precipitated epileptic episodes; it is therefore not recommended for epileptics.

○ **Related entry: Ludiomil**

Marcain

(Astra) is a proprietary, prescription-only preparation of the LOCAL ANAESTHETIC drug bupivacaine hydrochloride. It can be used particularly when prolonged course of treatment is required. It is available in several forms for injection, for example *Marcain Heavy*.

+▲ side-effects/warning: see BUPIVACAINE HYDROCHLORIDE

Marcain with Adrenaline

(Astra) is a proprietary, prescription-only COMPOUND PREPARATION of the LOCAL ANAESTHETIC drug bupivacaine hydrochloride and the VASOCONSTRICTOR drug adrenaline, which prolongs its duration of action. It is available in a range of forms for injection.

+▲ side-effects/warning: see ADRENALINE; BUPIVACAINE HYDROCHLORIDE

Marevan

(Goldshield) is a proprietary, prescription-only preparation of the synthetic ANTICOAGULANT drug warfarin sodium. It can be used to prevent clot formation in heart disease, following heart surgery (especially following implantation of prosthetic heart valves), to prevent venous thrombosis and pulmonary embolism. It is available as tablets.

+▲ side-effects/warning: see WARFARIN SODIUM

Marplan

(Cambridge) is a proprietary, prescription-only preparation of the MONOAMINE-OXIDASE INHIBITOR (MAOI) ANTIDEPRESSANT drug isocarboxazid. It can be used to treat depressive illness and is

available in the form of tablets.

+▲ side-effects/warning: see ISOCARBOXAZID

M

Marvelon

(Organon) is a proprietary, prescription-only COMPOUND PREPARATION that can be used as a (*monophasic*) ORAL CONTRACEPTIVE (and also for certain menstrual problems) of the type that combines an OESTROGEN and a PROGESTOGEN, in this case ethinyloestradiol and desogestrel. It is available in the form of tablets.

+▲ side-effects/warning: see ETHINYLOESTRADIOL, DESOGESTREL

Masnoderm

(Cusi) is a proprietary, non-prescription preparation of the ANTIFUNGAL drug clotrimazole. It can be used to treat fungal (particularly *Candida*) skin infections and is available as a cream for topical application.

+▲ side-effects/warning: see CLOTRIMAZOLE

Massé Breast Cream

(Cilag) is a proprietary, non-prescription COMPOUND PREPARATION of arachis oil, wool fat, glycerol, glyceryl monostearate and other constituents. It can be used as an EMOLLIENT for sore nipples and is available as a cream.

+▲ side-effects/warning: see ARACHIS OIL; GLYCEROL; WOOL FAT

Matrex

(Pharmacia) is a proprietary, prescription-only preparation of the IMMUNOSUPPRESSANT and (CYTOTOXIC) ANTICANCER drug methotrexate. It can be used to treat rheumatoid arthritis and lymphoblastic leukaemia, other lymphomas and solid tumours. It is available in a form for injection.

+▲ side-effects/warning: see METHOTREXATE

Maxepa

(Innovex) is a proprietary, prescription-only preparation of the LIPID-LOWERING

M DRUG omega-3 marine triglycerides. It can be used in hyperlipidaemia to reduce the levels, or change the proportions, of various lipids. It is available as capsules, an emulsion and a liquid.
+▲ side-effects/warning: see OMEGA-3 MARINE TRIGLYCERIDES

Maxepa

(Alcon) is a proprietary, prescription-only COMPOUND PREPARATION of the CORTICOSTEROID and ANTI-INFLAMMATORY drug dexamethasone and the artificial tear medium hypromellose. It can be used to treat inflammation of the eye and is available as eye-drops.
+▲ side-effects/warning: see DEXAMETHASONE; HYPOMELLOSE

Maximum Strength Aspro Clear

(Roche) is a proprietary, non-prescription preparation of the (NSAID) NON-NARCOTIC ANALGESIC, ANTIRHEUMATIC and ANTIPYRETIC drug aspirin. It can be used to relieve pain, including headache, neuralgia, period and dental pain, for the relief of cold and flu symptoms, sore throats and to treat musculoskeletal pain. It is available in the form of effervescent tablets and is not normally given to children, except on medical advice.
+▲ side-effects/warning: see ASPIRIN

Maxitrol

(Alcon) is a proprietary, prescription-only COMPOUND PREPARATION of the ANTI-INFLAMMATORY and CORTICOSTEROID drug dexamethasone, the ANTIBACTERIAL and (AMINOGLYCOSIDE) ANTIBIOTIC drug neomycin sulphate and the antibacterial and (POLYMYXIN) antibiotic drug polymyxin B sulphate and hypromellose ('artificial tears'). It can be used to treat inflammation of the eye when infection is also present. It is available as eye-drops.
+▲ side-effects/warning: see DEXAMETHASONE; HYPROMELLOSE; NEOMYCIN SULPHATE; POLYMYXIN B SULPHATE

Maxivent

(Ashbourne) is a proprietary, prescription-only preparation of the BETA-RECEPTOR STIMULANT salbutamol. It can be used as a BRONCHODILATOR in reversible obstructive airways disease, as an ANTI-ASTHMATIC treatment in severe acute asthma and for the alleviation of symptoms of chronic bronchitis and emphysema. It is available in an aerosol inhalant.
+▲ side-effects/warning: see SALBUTAMOL

Maxolon

(Beecham) is a proprietary, prescription-only preparation of the ANTI-EMETIC and ANTINAUSEANT drug metoclopramide hydrochloride. It can be used for the treatment of nausea and vomiting, particularly when associated with gastrointestinal disorders and after treatment with radiation or cytotoxic drugs. It also has gastric MOTILITY STIMULANT actions and can be used in the treatment of non-ulcer dyspepsia, gastric stasis and to prevent reflux oesophagitis. It is available as tablets, a syrup, a liquid form (*Maxolon Paediatric Liquid*), as modified-release capsules (*Maxolon SR*) and in several forms for injection, for example, (*Maxolon High Dose*).
+▲ side-effects/warning: see METOCLOPRAMIDE HYDROCHLORIDE

MCR-50

(Pharmacia) (Mono-Cedocard Retard-50) is a proprietary, non-prescription preparation of the VASODILATOR and ANTI-ANGINA drug isosorbide mononitrate. It can be used to treat and prevent angina pectoris and in HEART FAILURE TREATMENT. It is available as modified-release capsules.
+▲ side-effects/warning: see ISOSORBIDE MONONITRATE

measles vaccine

is used for IMMUNIZATION, but has almost entirely been replaced by a combined measles/mumps/rubella vaccine (MMR)

and a measles/rubella (MR) vaccine for use in children. It is available as a single vaccine under special circumstances only.
✚▲ side-effects/warning: see under MMR VACCINE

mebendazole
is an (AZOLE) ANTHELMINTIC drug. It can be used in the treatment of infections by roundworm, threadworm, whipworm and hookworm. Administration is oral as tablets or a suspension.
✚ side-effects: side-effects are rare, but there may be diarrhoea and abdominal pain; hypersensitivity reactions (rash, urticaria and angio-oedema).
▲ warning: administer with caution to those who are pregnant or breast-feeding.
○ Related entries: Ovex Tablets; Pripsen Mebendazole; Vermox

mebeverine hydrochloride
is an ANTISPASMODIC drug. It is used to treat muscle spasm in the gastrointestinal tract, which causes abdominal pain and constipation, eg. irritable bowel syndrome. Administration is oral in the form of tablets, as a sugar-free liquid concentrate, or as soluble (dispersible) granules to be taken before food.
✚▲ side-effects/warning: it should not be taken by patients with paralytic ileus. Avoid in porphyria.
○ Related entries: Colofac; Fomac; Fybogel Mebeverine

meclozine hydrochloride
is an ANTIHISTAMINE drug. It is used primarily as an ANTINAUSEANT in the treatment or prevention of motion sickness and vomiting. Administration is oral in the form of tablets.
✚▲ side-effects/warning: see under CYCLIZINE
○ Related entry: Sea-Legs

Mectizan
(Merck, Sharp & Dohme) is a proprietary preparation of the ANTHELMINTIC drug

ivermectin, which (though not available in the UK) is effective in treating the tropical disease onchocerciasis (infestation by the filarial worm-parasite *Onchocerca volvulus*. It is administered orally.
✚▲ side-effects/warning: see IVERMECTIN

mecyteine hydrochloride
See METHYL CYSTEINE HYDROCHLORIDE

Mediclear 5 Acne Cream
(Boots) is a proprietary, non-prescription preparation of the KERATOLYTIC and ANTIMICROBIAL drug benzoyl peroxide (5%). It can be applied topically for the treatment of acne and spots and is available as a cream. It is not normally used on children under 12 years, except on medical advice.
✚▲ side-effects/warning: see BENZOYL PEROXIDE

Mediclear 10 Acne Cream
(Boots) is a proprietary, non-prescription preparation of the KERATOLYTIC and ANTIMICROBIAL drug benzoyl peroxide (5%). It can be applied topically for the treatment of acne and spots and is available as a cream. It is not normally used on children under 12 years, except on medical advice.
✚▲ side-effects/warning: see BENZOYL PEROXIDE

Mediclear Acne Lotion
(Boots) is a proprietary, non-prescription preparation of the KERATOLYTIC and ANTIMICROBIAL drug benzoyl peroxide (5%). It can be applied topically for the treatment of acne and spots and is available as a cream. It is not normally used on children under 12 years, except on medical advice.
✚▲ side-effects/warning: see BENZOYL PEROXIDE

Medicoal
(Torbet) is a proprietary, non-prescription preparation of activated charcoal. It can

M

be used to treat patients suffering from poisoning or a drug overdose. It is available as a granules.

Medihaler-epi

(3M Health Care) is a proprietary, prescription-only preparation of the SYMPATHOMIMETIC drug adrenaline acid tartrate. It can be used as a BRONCHODILATOR, in the form of an aerosol inhalant, for emergency treatment of acute and severe allergic reactions, cardiopulmonary resuscitation and angio-oedema.

➕▲ side-effects/warning: see ADRENALINE

Medihaler-Ergotamine

(3M Health Care) is a proprietary, prescription-only preparation of the VASOCONSTRICTOR drug ergotamine tartrate. It can be used as an ANTIMIGRAINE treatment for acute attacks and is available as an inhalant aerosol.

➕▲ side-effects/warning: see ERGOTAMINE TARTRATE

Medihaler-iso

(3M Health Care) is a proprietary, prescription-only preparation of the BETA-RECEPTOR STIMULANT isoprenaline (as isoprenaline sulphate). It can be used as a BRONCHODILATOR in reversible obstructive airways disease and as an ANTI-ASTHMATIC in severe acute asthma. It is available in a metered-dosage aerosol in two strengths (the stronger under the trade name *Medihaler-iso Forte*).

➕▲ side-effects/warning: see ISOPRENALINE

Medilave

(Martindale) is a proprietary, non-prescription COMPOUND PREPARATION of the ANTISEPTIC agent cetylpyridinium chloride and the LOCAL ANAESTHETIC drug benzocaine. It can be used to relieve pain of sores and ulcers in the mouth and is available as a gel for topical application. It is not normally used on children under 12 years, except on medical advice.

➕▲ side-effects/warning: see BENZOCAINE; CETYLPYRIDINIUM CHLORIDE

Medised

(Martindale) is a proprietary, non-prescription COMPOUND PREPARATION of the NON-NARCOTIC ANALGESIC drug paracetamol and the SEDATIVE ANTIHISTAMINE promethazine hydrochloride. It can be used for reducing temperature and relieving the symptoms of painful or feverish conditions, such as toothache, headache, sore throats, colds and flu. It is available as a suspension and is not normally given to children under one year, except on medical advice.

➕▲ side-effects/warning: see PARACETAMOL; PROMETHAZINE HYDROCHLORIDE

Medrone

(Upjohn) is a proprietary, prescription-only preparation of the CORTICOSTEROID and ANTI-INFLAMMATORY drug methylprednisolone. It can be used to treat allergic disorders, shock and cerebral oedema and is available as tablets.

➕▲ side-effects/warning: see METHYLPREDNISOLONE

medroxyprogesterone acetate

is a SEX HORMONE, a synthetic PROGESTOGEN. One of its uses is as an ORAL CONTRACEPTIVE, for a short period of time, or by deep intramuscular injection every three months for a longer duration of action. It can also be used as a hormonal supplement in women whose progestogen level requires boosting (such as in endometriosis or dysfunctional uterine bleeding). Additionally, it can be used in the treatment of cancer of the breast, uterine endometrium, and, less commonly, of the prostate gland in men. It is available in forms for taking by mouth and for injection.

➕ side-effects: fluid retention and weight gain, acne and urticaria, gastrointestinal disturbances, premenstrual syndrome and irregular periods, changes in libido, breast tenderness; also insomnia, depression and sleepiness; loss or growth of hair, and, rarely, jaundice.

▲ warning: it should not be administered to patients with certain liver disorders, undiagnosed vaginal haemorrhage, or sex hormone-linked cancer; who are pregnant; or have porphyria. Administer with caution to those with diabetes, certain heart or kidney disorders, or hypertension.

Related entries: Depo-Provera; Farlutal; Provera.

mefenamic acid

is a (NSAID) NON-NARCOTIC ANALGESIC and ANTIRHEUMATIC drug. It is used primarily to treat mild to moderate pain and inflammation in rheumatoid arthritis, osteoarthritis and other musculoskeletal disorders, including juvenile arthritis. It is also used to treat dysmenorrhoea. Administration is oral as capsules, tablets and as an oral suspension for children.

✚▲ side-effect/warning: see under NSAID. It has weaker anti-inflammatory properties than most drugs of this class and a higher incidence of diarrhoea. There may be blood disturbances.

❂ **Related entries: Contraflam; Dysman 250; Dysman 500; Ponstan**

mefloquine

is an ANTIMALARIAL drug. It is used to prevent and treat malaria infection by one of the three *Plasmodium* species that cause malaria, especially where there is resistance to the drug chloroquine. It is effective against the *Plasmodium falciparum* species of malaria and is used to treat infection from areas of the world where this species is common. It is available as tablets.

✚ side-effects: there may be nausea and vomiting with headache, visual disturbances, loss of balance, rash and itching; disturbances of the gastrointestinal tract and liver and

other disturbances. Susceptible patients may undergo psychotic episodes.

▲ warning: these depend on whether it is used to prevent or to treat malaria. It should not be used in patients with certain kidney, liver, or heart disorders. It should not be given to those who are breast-feeding, pregnant (and avoid getting pregnant for three months after treatment with mefloquine), or to those with a history of convulsions.

❂ **Related entry: Lariam**

Mefoxin

(Merck, Sharp & Dohme) is a proprietary, prescription-only preparation of the ANTIBACTERIAL and (CEPHALOSPORIN) ANTIBIOTIC drug cefoxitin. It can be used to treat many types of bacterial infection, including peritonitis and also to prevent infection following surgery. It is available in a form for injection or infusion.

✚▲ side-effects/warning: see CEFOXITIN

mefruside

is one of the THIAZIDE class of DIURETICS. It can be used in ANTIHYPERTENSIVE treatment, either alone or in conjunction with other types of drugs and can also be used in the treatment of oedema (accumulation of fluid in the tissues) associated with congestive heart failure. Administration is oral in the form of tablets.

✚▲ side-effects/warning: see under BENDROFLUAZIDE

❂ **Related entry: Baycaron**

Megace

(Bristol-Myers) is a proprietary, prescription-only preparation of the PROGESTOGEN megestrol acetate, which is a female SEX HORMONE. It can be used to treat oestrogen-linked cancers (such as cancer of the breast or of the endometrium of the uterus). It is available as tablets.

✚▲ side-effects/warning: see MEGESTROL ACETATE.

M

megestrol acetate

is a PROGESTOGEN, a female SEX HORMONE. It is used primarily as an ANTICANCER treatment when the presence of OESTROGENS is significant (eg. breast cancer or cancer of the endometrium of the uterus). Administration is oral in the form of tablets.

+▲ side-effects/warning: see under MEDROXYPROGESTERONE ACETATE

O Related entry: Megace

Meggezones

(Schering Plough) is a proprietary, non-prescription preparation of the aromatic oil menthol. It can be used for the symptomatic relief of sore throat, coughs, colds, catarrh and nasal congestion. It is available as pastilles.

+▲ side-effects/warning: see MENTHOL

Melleril

(Sandoz) is a proprietary, prescription-only preparation of the ANTIPSYCHOTIC drug thioridazine. It can be used to treat and tranquillize patients with psychotic disorders (such as schizophrenia), particularly manic forms of behavioural disturbance. It can also be used in the short-term treatment of anxiety. It is available as tablets, a suspension and a syrup.

+▲ side-effects/warning: see THIORIDAZINE

melphalan

is a CYTOTOXIC DRUG, which is used as an ANTICANCER drug in the treatment of various forms of cancers, especially cancer of the bone marrow (myelomatosis). It works by a direct action on the DNA of the cancer cells and so prevents cell replication. Administration is either oral in the form of tablets or by injection.

+▲ side-effects/warning: see under CYTOTOXIC DRUGS

O Related entry: Alkeran

Meltus Dry Cough Elixir, Adult

(Seton Healthcare) is a proprietary, non-prescription preparation of the SYMPATHOMIMETIC and DECONGESTANT drug pseudoephedrine hydrochloride and the NARCOTIC ANALGESIC and ANTITUSSIVE drug dextromethorphan hydrobromide. It can be used for the symptomatic relief of dry, painful, tickly cough and catarrh. It is available in the form of a liquid and is not to be given to children.

+▲ side-effects/warning: see DEXTROMETHORPHAN HYDROBROMIDE; PSEUDOEPHEDRINE HYDROCHLORIDE

Meltus Junior Dry Cough Elixir

(Seton Healthcare) is a proprietary, non-prescription preparation of the SYMPATHOMIMETIC and DECONGESTANT drug pseudoephedrine hydrochloride and the NARCOTIC ANALGESIC and ANTITUSSIVE drug dextromethorphan hydrobromide. It can be used for the symptomatic relief of unproductive coughs and congestion of the upper airways. It is available as a liquid and is not normally given to children under two years, except on medical advice.

+▲ side-effects/warning: see DEXTROMETHORPHAN HYDROBROMIDE; PSEUDOEPHEDRINE HYDROCHLORIDE

Meltus Junior Expectorant Linctus

(Seton Healthcare) is a proprietary, non-prescription preparation of the EXPECTORANT guaiphenesin, the ANTISEPTIC agent cetylpyridinium chloride, sucrose and honey. It can be used for the symptomatic relief of coughs and catarrh associated with flu, colds and mild cold infections. It is available as a liquid and is not normally given to children under two years, except on medical advice.

+▲ side-effects/warning: see CETYLPYRIDINIUM CHLORIDE; GUAIPHENESIN

M

menadiol sodium phosphate

(vitamin K₃) is a synthetic form of VITAMIN K. It is sometimes used in medicine in preference to vitamins K₃ and K₂, because these natural forms are only fat-soluble, whereas vitamin K₃ is water-soluble and is therefore effective when taken by mouth to treat vitamin deficiency caused by fat malabsorption syndromes (eg. due to obstruction of the bile ducts or in liver disease). In malabsorption syndromes it is important to make up a deficiency on a regular basis, because vitamin K is essential for maintaining the clotting factors in the blood and for calcification of bone. Administration is oral in the form of tablets.

+▲ side-effects/warning: see under
VITAMIN K
✺ Related entry: Synkavit

Mengivac (A+C)

(Merieux) is a proprietary, prescription-only preparation of a VACCINE that is used to give protection against the organism meningococcus (*Neisseria meningitidis* groups A and C), which can cause serious infections such as meningitis. It is available in a form for injection.

+▲ side-effects/warning: see
MENINGOCOCCAL POLYSACCHARIDE VACCINE

meningococcal polysaccharide vaccine

is a VACCINE that is used for IMMUNIZATION against infection from the organism meningococcus (*Neisseria meningitidis*), which can cause serious infection such as meningitis. It may be given to those intending to travel 'rough' through parts of the world where the risk of meningococcal infection is much higher than in the UK (eg. parts of India and much of Africa). Administration is by subcutaneous or intramuscular injection.

+▲ side-effects/warning: see VACCINE
✺ Related entries: AC Vax ; Mengivac (A+C)

menotropin

is a HORMONE preparation and is a collective name for combinations of the GONADOTROPHIN hormones – FOLLICLE-STIMULATING HORMONE (FSH) and LUTEINIZING HORMONE (LH) – in a particular activity ratio (1:1).

+▲ side-effects/warning: see under HUMAN MENOPAUSAL GONADOTROPHINS
✺ Related entries: Humegon; Normegon; Pergonal

menthol

is a white, crystalline substance derived from peppermint oil (an essential oil extracted from a plant of the mint family) and is chemically a TERPENE. It is commonly used, with or without the volatile substance eucalyptus oil, in inhalations intended to clear the nasal or catarrhal congestion associated with colds, rhinitis (inflammation of the nasal mucous membrane), or sinusitis. It is also included in some COUNTER-IRRITANT, or RUBEFACIENT, preparations that are rubbed into the skin to relieve muscle or joint pain and in preparations used to treat gallstones or kidney stones.

✺ Related articles: Aspellin; Balmosa Cream; Bengué's Balsam; Benylin Chesty Coughs Non-Drowsy; Benylin Dry Coughs Original; Benylin with Codeine; Copholco; Copholcoids Cough Pastilles; Covonia Bronchial Balsam; Fisherman's Friend; Karvol Decongestant Capsules; Meggezones; Mentholatum Deep Heat Massage Liniment; Mentholatum Deep Heat Rub; Merothol Lozenges; Nirolex; Penetrol Catarrh Lozenges; Penetrol Inhalant; Radian B Heat Spray; Radian B Muscle Lotion; Radian B Muscle Rub; Ralgex Stick; Tixylix Inhalant; Rowachol; Vicks Sinex Decongestant Nasal Spray.

Mentholatum Deep Heat Massage Liniment

(Mentholatum) is a proprietary, non-prescription COMPOUND PREPARATION of

M

menthol and methyl salicylate, which both have COUNTER-IRRITANT, or RUBEFACIENT, actions. It can be applied to the skin for symptomatic relief of underlying muscle or joint pain. It is available as a liquid emulsion for topical application and is not normally used for children under five years, except on medical advice.

✚▲ side-effects/warning: see MENTHOL; METHYL SALICYLATE

Mentholatum Deep Heat Rub

(Mentholatum) is a proprietary, non-prescription COMPOUND PREPARATION of turpentine oil, eucalyptus oil, menthol and methyl salicylate, which all have COUNTER-IRRITANT, or RUBEFACIENT, actions. It can be applied to the skin for symptomatic relief of underlying muscle or joint pain. It is available as an emulsion cream for topical application and is not normally used for children under five years, except on medical advice.

✚▲ side-effects/warning: see MENTHOL; METHYL SALICYLATE; TURPENTINE OIL. Avoid inflamed, broken skin and mucous membranes.

Menzol

(Swarz) is a proprietary, prescription-only preparation of the PROGESTOGEN norethisterone. It can be used to treat uterine bleeding, abnormally heavy menstruation, premenstrual tension, endometriosis and other menstrual problems and for contraception. It is available as tablets.

✚▲ side-effects/warning: see NORETHISTERONE

mepacrine hydrochloride

is a drug with ANTIPROTOZOAL properties. It is used primarily to treat infection of the small intestine by the intestinal protozoan *Giardia lamblia*. Giardiasis (lambliasis) occurs throughout the world, particularly in children and is contracted by eating contaminated food. However, mepacrine

has largely been superseded by METRONIDAZOLE, which is now the drug of choice. It is still sometimes used to treat discoid lupus erythematosus. Administration is oral as tablets.

✚ side-effects: gastrointestinal disturbances, nausea and vomiting; headache and dizziness; stimulation of the central nervous system and psychoses; discolouration of the skin and dermatitis (with prolonged use); blood disturbances; discolouration of nails, palate and cornea (with vision disturbances). warning: it should not be administered to patients with psoriasis; and with care to those with liver impairment or psychosis.

mepenzolate bromide

is an ANTICHOLINERGIC drug, which can be used as an ANTISPASMODIC for the symptomatic relief of smooth muscle spasm in the gastrointestinal tract. It is available as tablets.

✚▲ side-effects/warning: see under ATROPINE SULPHATE

◉ Related entry: Cantil

Mepranix

(Ashbourne) is a proprietary, prescription-only preparation of the BETA-BLOCKER drug metoprolol tartrate. It can be used as an ANTIHYPERTENSIVE treatment for raised blood pressure, as an ANTI-ANGINA treatment to relieve symptoms and improve exercise tolerance and as an ANTI-ARRHYTHMIC to regularize heartbeat and to treat myocardial infarction. It can also be used as an ANTITHYROID drug for short-term treatment of thyrotoxicosis, or as an ANTIMIGRAINE treatment to prevent attacks. It is available as tablets.

✚▲ side-effects/warning: see METOPROLOL TARTRATE

meprobamate

is an ANXIOLYTIC drug, which is used in the short-term treatment of anxiety. It is also used in some SKELETAL MUSCLE RELAXANT and COMPOUND ANALGESIC preparations. It is potentially more hazardous than the

BENZODIAZEPINES in overdose and can
cause dependence (addiction).
Administration is oral in the form of
tablets. Preparations containing
meprobamate are on the Controlled
Drugs List.

✛ side-effects: see under BENZODIAZEPINE;
but there are also gastrointestinal
disturbances, hypotension, disturbed
peripheral nerve function, weakness,
headache, disturbances of vision and blood
changes. Drowsiness is a very common side-
effect.

▲ warning: it should not be administered to
patients with porphyria, who have certain
lung and breathing disorders, or who are
breast-feeding. It should be administered with
caution to those with respiratory difficulties,
epilepsy, or impaired liver or kidney function,
drug or alcohol abuse, personality disorders,
or who are pregnant. Withdrawal of treatment
must be gradual otherwise convulsions may
occur.

✪ **Related entries: Equagesic; Equanil**

meptazinol

is a powerful, synthetic (OPIOID)
NARCOTIC ANALGESIC drug. It is used to
treat moderate to severe pain, including
pain in childbirth, renal colic, or
following surgery. Administration is
either oral in the form of tablets, or
by injection.

✛▲ side-effects/warning: see under OPIOID;
but less respiratory depression.

✪ **Related entry: Meptid**

Meptid

(Monmouth) is a proprietary,
prescription-only preparation of the
(OPIOID) NARCOTIC ANALGESIC drug
meptazinol (as hydrochloride). It can be
used to treat moderate to severe pain,
particularly during or following surgical
procedures and also in childbirth. It is
available as tablets and in a form for
injection.

✛▲ side-effects/warning: see
MEPTAZINOL

mequitazine

is an ANTIHISTAMINE drug. It is used to
treat the symptoms of allergic conditions
such as hay fever and urticaria (itchy skin
rash). Administration is oral in the form of
tablets.

✛▲ side-effects/warning: see under
ANTIHISTAMINE. It may increase appetite
and cause weight gain. Because of its
sedative properties, the performance
of skilled tasks such as driving may
be impaired.

✪ **Related entry: Primalan**

Merbentyl

(Merrell) is a proprietary, prescription-
only preparation of the ANTICHOLINERGIC
drug dicyclomine hydrochloride. It can be
used as an ANTISPASMODIC for the
symptomatic relief of smooth muscle
spasm in the gastrointestinal tract. It is
available as tablets and a syrup. (There
are preparations available without
prescription, but they are subject to
certain limitations.)

✛▲ side-effects/warning: see DICYCLOMINE
HYDROCHLORIDE

Merbentyl 20

(Merrell) is a proprietary, prescription-
only preparation of the ANTICHOLINERGIC
drug dicyclomine hydrochloride. It can be
used as an ANTISPASMODIC for the
symptomatic relief of muscle spasm in the
gastrointestinal tract. It is available as
tablets.

✛▲ side-effects/warning: see DICYCLOMINE
HYDROCHLORIDE

mercaptopurine

is a CYTOTOXIC DRUG, which is used as an
ANTICANCER drug in the treatment of acute
leukaemias. It works by preventing cell
replication. Administration is oral in the
form of tablets.

✛▲ side-effects/warning: see under
CYTOTOXIC DRUGS. Avoid its use in patients
with porphyria.

✪ **Related entry: Puri-Nethol**

M

Mercilon

(Organon) is a proprietary, prescription-only COMPOUND PREPARATION that can be used as a (*monophasic*) ORAL CONTRACEPTIVE (and also for certain menstrual problems) of the type that combines an OESTROGEN and a PROGESTOGEN, in this case ethinyloestradiol and desogestrel. It is available in the form of tablets.

✚▲ warning/side-effects: see DESOGESTREL; ETHINYLOESTRADIOL

Merocaine Lozenges

(Merrell) is a proprietary, non-prescription COMPOUND PREPARATION of the ANTISEPTIC agent cetylpyridinium chloride and the LOCAL ANAESTHETIC drug benzocaine. It can be used for the temporary relief of the pain and discomfort of a sore throat and superficial, minor mouth infections. It is not normally given to children under 12 years, except on medical advice.

✚▲ side-effects/warning: see BENZOCAINE; CETYLPYRIDINIUM CHLORIDE

Merocets Gargle/Mouthwash

(Marion Merrell Dow) is a proprietary, non-prescription preparation of the ANTISEPTIC agent cetylpyridinium chloride. It can be used for the symptomatic relief of sore throat and minor irritations of the throat and mouth. It is available as an oral solution for use as a gargle or mouthwash.

✚▲ side-effects/warning: see CETYLPYRIDINIUM CHLORIDE

Merothol Lozenges

(Marion Merrell Dow) is a proprietary, non-prescription COMPOUND PREPARATION of the ANTISEPTIC agent cetylpyridinium chloride and the DECONGESTANT drugs cineole and menthol. It can be used for the symptomatic relief of sore throat and nasal congestion.

It is available as lozenges.

✚▲ side-effects/warning: see CETYLPYRIDINIUM CHLORIDE; CINEOLE; MENTHOL

Merovit Lozenges

(Marion Merrell Dow) is a proprietary, non-prescription preparation of the ANTISEPTIC agent cetylpyridinium chloride (with vitamin C). It can be used for the symptomatic relief of a minor sore throat due to colds. It is available as lozenges and is not normally given to children under six years, except on medical advice.

✚▲ side-effects/warning: see CETYLPYRIDINIUM CHLORIDE

mersalyl

is a DIURETIC drug that is now almost never used, except when all other methods of treating fluid retention have failed or are not tolerated. The drug is toxic and can be administered only by intramuscular injection: an intravenous injection may cause a severe fall in blood pressure.

✚ side-effects: there may be gastrointestinal disturbances; some patients experience allergic reactions. This drug is very toxic to the renal system.

▲ warning: it should not be administered to patients with certain kidney disorders, or who are pregnant; and with caution to those who have recently had a heart attack, or who suffer from certain heartbeat irregularities.

mesalazine

is an AMINOSALICYLATE drug. It can be used in the treatment of ulcerative colitis, particularly in patients sensitive to the sulphonamide content of sulphasalazine. Administration can be oral as tablets or by suppositories or a foam enema.

✚ side-effects: nausea, diarrhoea, abdominal pain, headache, exacerbated colitis symptoms, kidney, liver and pancreas problems and blood disorders.

▲ warning: it should not be administered to patients who have kidney impairment, or who are allergic to aspirin or other salicylates; it

should be administered with caution to those who are pregnant or breast-feeding.
○ **Related entries: Asacol; Pentasa; Salofalk**

mesna

is a synthetic drug that has the property of combating the haemorrhagic cystitis that is a toxic complication caused by CYTOTOXIC DRUGS (eg. CYCLOPHOSPHAMIDE and IFOSFAMIDE). It works by reacting with a toxic metabolite (break down product) produced by the cytotoxic drugs and which is the cause of the haemorrhagic cystitis. Mesna is therefore used as an adjunct in the treatment of certain forms of cancer. Administration is either oral or by injection.
✚ side-effects: overdosage may cause gastrointestinal disturbances and headache, tiredness, limb pains, depression, irritability, rash and lack of energy.
○ **Related entry: Uromitexan**

mesterolone

is an ANDROGEN, a male SEX HORMONE, which is produced mainly in the testes that, with other androgens and promotes the development of the secondary male sexual characteristics. Therapeutically, it may be administered to treat hormonal deficiency, for instance for delayed puberty in boys. Administration is oral in the form of tablets.
✚▲ side-effects/warning: see under ANDROGEN; but there is no effect on sperm production.
○ **Related entry: Pro-Viron**

Mestinon

(Roche) is a proprietary, prescription-only preparation of the ANTICHOLINESTERASE and PARASYMPATHOMIMETIC drug pyridostigmine (as bromide). It can be used to treat myasthenia gravis and also to stimulate intestinal activity. It is available as tablets and in a form for injection.
✚▲ side-effects/warning: see PYRIDOSTIGMINE

mestranol

is a synthetic OESTROGEN, a female SEX HORMONE, that is a constituent in several *combined* ORAL CONTRACEPTIVES and is also used in HRT (hormone replacement therapy). Administration is oral in the form of tablets in a calendar pack.
✚▲ side-effects/warning: see under OESTROGEN
○ **Related entries: Norinyl-1; Ortho-Novin 1/50; Syntex Menophase**

Metalpha

(Ashbourne) is a proprietary, prescription-only preparation of the ANTISYMPATHETIC drug methyldopa. It can be used in ANTIHYPERTENSIVE treatment and is available as tablets.
✚▲ side-effects/warning: see METHYLDOPA

Metamucil

(Procter & Gamble) is a proprietary, non-prescription preparation of the (*bulking agent*) LAXATIVE ispaghula husk. It can be used for the relief of constipation and is available as a powder. It is not normally used for children under six years, except on medical advice.
✚▲ side-effects/warning: see ISPAGHULA HUSK

Metanium

(Bengué) is a proprietary, non-prescription preparation of titanium dioxide (and other titanium salts) in a silicone base. It can be used as a BARRIER CREAM for nappy rash and related skin conditions and is available as an ointment.
✚▲ side-effects/warning: see TITANIUM DIOXIDE

metaraminol

is a SYMPATHOMIMETIC and VASOCONSTRICTOR drug. It can be used to treat cases of acute hypotension, particularly in emergency situations as a temporary measure while preparations are made for a blood transfusion.

M

Administration is by injection or infusion.

+▲ side-effects/warning: see under
NORADRENALINE

☉ Related entry: Aramine

Metenix 5

(Hoechst) is a proprietary, prescription-only preparation of the (THIAZIDE-like)
DIURETIC drug metolazone. It can be used,
either alone or in conjunction with other
drugs, in the treatment of oedema and as
an ANTIHYPERTENSIVE. It is available as
tablets.

+▲ side-effects/warning: see
METOLAZONE

Meterfolic

(Sinclair) is a proprietary, non-prescription COMPOUND PREPARATION of
ferrous fumarate and folic acid. It can be
used as an IRON and folic acid supplement
during pregnancy and is available as
tablets.

+▲ side-effects/warning: see FERROUS
FUMARATE; FOLIC ACID

metformin hydrochloride

is a BIGUANIDE drug that is used in
DIABETIC TREATMENT of Type II diabetes
(non-insulin-dependent diabetes mellitus;
NIDDM; maturity-onset diabetes),
particularly in patients who are not totally
dependent on additional supplies of
INSULIN. It works by increasing the
utilization and decreasing the formation of
glucose, to make up for the reduction in
insulin available from the pancreas.
Administration is oral in the form of
tablets.

+ side-effects: there may be nausea and
vomiting, with diarrhoea and weight loss.
Body uptake of CYANOCOBALAMIN (vitamin
B_{12}) or its analogues may be reduced.

▲ warning: it should not be administered to
patients with certain heart, liver, or kidney
disorders, who are dehydrated, alcoholics,
have severe infection, trauma, or are pregnant
or breast-feeding.

☉ Related entry: Glucophage

methadone hydrochloride

is a NARCOTIC ANALGESIC drug (an OPIOID)
and is on the Controlled Drugs List. It is
used primarily for the relief of severe pain,
but is less effective and less SEDATIVE than
morphine and acts for a longer time. It is
also used as a substitute for addictive
opioids in detoxification therapy.
Administration is oral in the form of
tablets, a tolu-flavoured linctus for cough
in the terminally ill, or by injection.

+▲ side-effects/warning: see under OPIOID

☉ Related entry: Physeptone

methenamine hippurate

See HEXAMINE HIPPURATE

methicillin

is an ANTIBACTERIAL and (PENICILLIN)
ANTIBIOTIC drug, which was the first of its
type to be resistant to the penicillinase
enzyme secreted by penicillin-resistant
strains of *Staphylococcus aureus*. It has
been superseded by orally active,
penicillinase-resistant penicillins (eg.
FLUCLOXACILLIN) and is no longer used. In
recent years the occurrence of
methicillin-resistant strains of
Staphylococcus has created major
problems in hospitals throughout the
world. The similar antibiotic
pivmecillinam hydrochloride is present in
some COMPOUND PREPARATIONS.

methionine

is an ANTIDOTE to poisoning caused by an
overdose of the NON-NARCOTIC ANALGESIC
drug paracetamol. The initial symptoms of
poisoning usually settle within 24 hours,
but are followed by a serious toxic effect
on the liver that takes several days to
develop. The purpose of treatment is to
prevent these latter effects and must start
immediately after the overdose has been
taken. Methionine is used until the drug
ACETYLCYSTEINE can be given by
intravenous infusion. Administration is
oral in the form of tablets.

☉ Related entry: Methionine Tablets

Methionine Tablets

(Evans) is a proprietary, prescription-only preparation of the ANTIDOTE methionine. It can be used for emergency treatment of overdose poisoning by the NON-NARCOTIC ANALGESIC drug paracetamol. It is available as tablets.

methocarbamol

is a SKELETAL MUSCLE RELAXANT drug. It is used for the symptomatic relief of muscle spasm and works by an action on the central nervous system. Administration is either oral as tablets or by injection.
✚ side-effects: light-headedness, lassitude, dizziness, confusion, restlessness, anxiety, drowsiness, nausea, allergic rash, angio-oedema and convulsions.
▲ warning: it should not be administered to patients with brain damage, epilepsy, or myasthenia gravis. Administer with care to those with impaired liver or kidney function. Drowsiness may impair the performance of skilled tasks such as driving; avoid alcohol as its effects are enhanced.
◐ Related entries: Robaxin; Robaxisal Forte

methohexital

See METHOHEXITONE SODIUM

methohexitone sodium

(methohexital) is a BARBITURATE drug. It can be used as a GENERAL ANAESTHETIC for induction and maintenance of anaesthia during short operations. Administration is by injection.
✚▲ side-effects/warning: see under BARBITURATE
◐ Related entry: Brietal Sodium

Methotrexate

(Lederle) is a proprietary, prescription-only preparation of the IMMUNOSUPPRESSANT and CYTOTOXIC DRUG methotrexate. It can be used to treat rheumatoid arthritis and as an ANTICANCER drug for lymphoblastic leukaemia, other lymphomas and some solid tumours. It is

available in forms to be taken orally and by injection.
✚▲ side-effects/warning: see METHOTREXATE

methotrexate

is a CYTOTOXIC DRUG, which is used primarily as an ANTICANCER treatment of childhood acute lymphoblastic leukaemia, but also to treat other lymphomas, choriocarcinoma and some solid tumours. It works by inhibiting the activity of an enzyme essential to the DNA metabolism in cells. It is also used as an IMMUNOSUPPRESSANT to treat rheumatoid arthritis and (under specialist supervision) severe resistant psoriasis. Administration is either oral or by injection.
✚▲ side-effects/warning: see under CYTOTOXIC DRUGS. It should not be given to patients with severe kidney impairment; and avoid its use in those with porphyria.
◐ Related entries: Matrex; Methotrexate

methotrimeprazine

(levomepromazine) is chemically a PHENOTHIAZINE DERIVATIVE. It is used as an ANTIPSYCHOTIC drug to tranquillize patients suffering from psychotic disorders such as schizophrenia and also to calm and soothe patients with a terminal illness. Administration is either oral in the form of tablets or by injection.
✚▲ side-effects/warning: see under CHLORPROMAZINE HYDROCHLORIDE; but there is more of a sedative effect and a risk of postural hypotension.
◐ Related entry: Nozinan

methoxamine hydrochloride

is a SYMPATHOMIMETIC and VASOCONSTRICTOR drug. It is used primarily to raise lowered blood pressure caused by the induction of anaesthesia. Administration is by infusion or injection.
✚▲ side-effects/warning: see under NORADRENALINE. It is not used where there is

M

severe cardiovascular disease; there may be hypertension.

○ Related entry: Vasoxine

methylcellulose

is a *bulking agent* LAXATIVE. It works by increasing the overall mass of faeces and also retaining a lot of water and so stimulating bowel movement. However, the full effect may not be achieved for many hours. It can be used in patients who cannot tolerate bran when treating a range of bowel conditions, including diverticular disease and irritable bowel syndrome. Administration is oral in the form of tablets.

✚▲ side-effects/warning: see under ISPAGHULA HUSK

○ Related entry: Celevac

methyl cysteine hydrochloride

(mecyteine hydrochloride) is a MUCOLYTIC drug that is used to reduce the viscosity of sputum and so acts as an EXPECTORANT in patients with disorders of the upper respiratory tract (e.g chronic asthma or bronchitis). Administration is oral in the form of tablets.

○ Related entry: Visclair

methyldopa

is an ANTISYMPATHETIC drug. It acts in the brain to reduce the activity of the sympathetic nervous system. It can be used in ANTIHYPERTENSIVE treatment (commonly in combination with a DIURETIC drug) of moderate to severe hypertension. Administration can be oral as capsules, tablets, or a suspension, or in a form for injection or infusion.

✚ side-effects: there may be dry mouth, drowsiness, fluid retention, diarrhoea; sedation, depression, impaired liver function, skin and blood disorders and nasal stuffiness; parkinsonian symptoms and failure to ejaculate.

▲ warning: it should not be administered to patients with certain blood or liver disorders,

phaeochromocytoma, or a history of depression. Administer with care when there is kidney damage. Regular blood counts and tests on liver function are necessary during treatment. The drug may cause drowsiness and impair the ability to drive or operate machinery; and the effects of alcohol may be enhanced.

○ Related entries: Aldomet; Dopamet; Hydromet; Metalpha

methyldopate hydrochloride

is the form of the ANTIHYPERTENSIVE drug methyldopa that is used for injection.

✚▲ side-effects/warning: see METHYLDOPA

methyl nicotinate

is a drug with mild, local pain-relieving properties, which are principally due to its COUNTER-IRRITANT, or RUBEFACIENT, action. It can be used in the mouth or ears to relieve the pain of teething, ulcers, or minor scratches. Administration is as a cream for topical application.

○ Related entries: Algipan Rub; Cremalgin Balm; Dubam; Ralgex Cream

methylphenobarbitone

(methyphenobarbital) is a BARBITURATE drug, which is used as an ANTICONVULSANT and ANTI-EPILEPTIC to treat all forms of epilepsy (except absence seizures). It is largely converted in the liver to PHENOBARBITONE and therefore has similar actions and effects. Administration is oral in the form of tablets. Preparations containing methylphenobarbitone are on the Controlled Drugs List.

✚▲ side-effects/warning: see under BARBITURATE

○ Related entry: Prominal

methylprednisolone

is a CORTICOSTEROID with ANTI-INFLAMMATORY properties. It is used to relieve the inflammation of allergic reaction, to treat cerebral oedema (fluid retention in the brain), shock, rheumatic

disease and inflammatory skin disorders such as eczema. Administration (as methylprednisolone, methylprednisolone acetate, or methylprednisolone sodium succinate) can be oral in the form of tablets, by topical application as a cream, or by injection or intravenous infusion.
✚▲ side-effects/warning: see under CORTICOSTEROIDS
✪ Related entries: Depo-Medrone; Depo-Medrone with Lidocaine; Medrone; Neo-Medrone; Solu-Medrone

methylrosanilium chloride
See CRYSTAL VIOLET

methyl salicylate
is used as a COUNTER-IRRITANT, or RUBEFACIENT, for local pain relief of underlying muscle or joint pains (though how it acts is not clear). It is administered topically to the skin and is available as a non-proprietary liniment and ointment and in several proprietary preparations as a cream or a balsam.
✚ side-effects: there may be local irritation.
▲ warning: it should not be used on broken or inflamed skin. It can cause sensitivity to bright sunlight; systemic effects may occur with prolonged or excessive use.
✪ Related entries: Algipan Rub; Aspellin; Balmosa Cream; Bengué's Balsam; Dubam; Germoline Ointment; Mentholatum Deep Heat Massage Liniment; Mentholatum Deep Heat Rub; Monphytol; Radian B Muscle Rub; Ralgex Cream; Ralgex Stick

methyl valerate
is a constituent of a proprietary COMPOUND PREPARATION, which contains several aromatic substances, that is used during withdrawal from smoking tobacco products. Administration is in the form of capsules.
✪ Related entry: Nicobrevin

methyl violet
See CRYSTAL VIOLET

methylphenobarbital
See METHYLPHENOBARBITONE

methysergide
is a potentially dangerous drug that is used, under strict medical supervision in hospital, as an ANTIMIGRAINE treatment to prevent severe recurrent migraine and similar headaches in patients for whom other forms of treatment have failed. Administration is oral in the form of tablets.
✚ side-effects: nausea, vomiting, abdominal discomfort, heartburn, insomnia, weight gain, rashes, mental disturbences, hair loss, cramps, effects on the cardiovascular system, drowsiness and dizziness.
▲ warning: it is not to be used in patients with certain kidney, lung, liver, or cardiovascular disorders; severe hypertension, urinary tract disorders, collagen disease, cellulitis; or who are pregnant or breast-feeding. Administer with caution to those with peptic ulcer. Withdrawal of treatment should be gradual.
✪ Related entry: Deseril

metipranolol
is a BETA-BLOCKER that can be used as a GLAUCOMA TREATMENT for chronic simple glaucoma. It is thought to work by slowing the rate of production of the aqueous humour in the eye and is available as eye-drops.
✚ side-effects: there may be some systemic absorption after using eye-drops, so some of the side-effects listed under propranolol hydrochloride may be seen. Dry eyes and some local allergic reactions, including conjunctivitis of the eyelids, may also occur. It does not contain the preservative benzalkonium chloride, found in several eye-drops for glaucoma, so it can be used by patients who are allergic to this preservative and those wearing soft contact lenses.
▲ warning: in view of possible absorption, dangerous side-effects should be borne in mind, particularly the danger of bronchospasm in asthmatics and interactions

M

with calcium-channel blockers.
○ Related entry: Minims Metipranolol

metirosine

is an ANTISYMPATHETIC drug. It inhibits the
enzymes that produce NORADRENALINE and
is used in the preoperative treatment of
phaeochromocytoma. Administration is
oral in the form of capsules.
✚ side-effects: sedation, severe diarrhoea,
sensitivity reactions and extrapyramidal
symptoms (muscle tremor and rigidity).
▲ warning: increased fluid intake during
treatment is essential. Regular checks on
overall blood volume are advisable. Sedation
may effect the ability to drive or operate
machinery.
○ Related entry: Demser

metoclopramide hydrochloride

is an effective ANTI-EMETIC and
ANTINAUSEANT drug with useful MOTILITY
STIMULANT properties. It can be used to
prevent vomiting caused by
gastrointestinal disorders or by
chemotherapy or radiotherapy (in the
treatment of cancer). It works both by a
direct action on the vomiting centre of the
brain (where it is an ANTAGONIST of
dopamine) and by actions within the
intestine. It enhances the strength of
oesophageal sphincter contraction
(preventing the passage of stomach
contents up into the gullet), stimulates
emptying of the stomach and increases the
rate at which food is moved along the
intestine. These last actions lead to its use
in non-ulcer dyspepsia, for gastric stasis
and to prevent reflux oesophagitis.
Administration is either oral in the form of
tablets, capsules or syrups, or by injection.
✚ side-effects: there may be extrapyramidal
effects (muscle tremor and rigidity),
especially in the young and elderly; tardive
dyskinesia (involuntary motor movements),
raised levels of the hormone prolactin in the
blood. Drowsiness, restlessness, depression and
diarrhoea have been reported.

▲ warning: it should be administered with
caution to those with impaired kidney or liver
function, porphyria, or who are pregnant,
breast-feeding, or under 20 years old.
○ Related entries: Gastrobid Continus;
Gastroflux; Gastromax; Maxolon;
Migravess; Paramax; Parmid; Primperan

metolazone

is one of the THIAZIDE class of DIURETICS.
It can be used in ANTIHYPERTENSIVE
treatment, either alone or in conjunction
with other types of drugs and can also be
used in the treatment of oedema
(accumulation of fluid in the tissues)
associated with congestive heart failure.
Administration is oral in the form of
tablets.
✚▲ side-effects/warning: see under
BENDROFLUAZIDE. There can be marked
diuresis (urine production) when given with
frusemide.
○ Related entries: Metenix 5; Xuret

Metopirone

(Ciba) is a proprietary, prescription-only
preparation of the ENZYME INHIBITOR
metyrapone. It can be used to treat
conditions that result from the excessive
secretion of corticosteroids into the
bloodstream (eg. Cushing's syndrome)
and also to treat postmenopausal breast
cancer. Administration is oral in the form
of capsules.
✚▲ side-effects/warning: see METYRAPONE

metoprolol tartrate

is a BETA-BLOCKER that can be used as an
ANTIHYPERTENSIVE treatment for raised
blood pressure, as an ANTI-ANGINA
treatment to relieve symptoms and
improve exercise tolerance, as an ANTI-
ARRHYTHMIC to regularize heartbeat and to
treat myocardial infarction, as an
ANTIMIGRAINE treatment to prevent
migraine attacks and as an ANTITHYROID
for short-term treatment of thyrotoxicosis.
Administration can be oral as tablets or
modified-release tablets, or by injection. It

is also available, as an antihypertensive treatment, in the form of COMPOUND PREPARATIONS with DIURETICS.
+▲ side-effect/warning: see under PROPRANOLOL HYDROCHLORIDE
○ Related entries: Arbralene; Betaloc; Betaloc-SA; Co-Betaloc; Co-Betaloc SA; Lopresor; Lopresor SR; Mepranix

Metosyn

(Zeneca) is a proprietary, prescription-only preparation of the CORTICOSTEROID and ANTI-INFLAMMATORY drug fluocinonide. It can be used to treat severe, acute inflammatory skin disorders, such as eczema, that are unresponsive to less powerful drugs and also psoriasis. Administration is by topical application in the form of a cream, ointment, or scalp lotion.
+▲ side-effects/warning: see FLUOCINONIDE

metriphonate

is an organophosphorus ANTHELMINTIC compound that destroys the blood fluke *Schistosoma haematobium*, which causes a form of bilharzia that is common in North Africa and the Middle East. The disease is contracted by bathing in water contaminated by fluke larvae. Adult flukes then infest the veins of the bladder, ureter and other pelvic organs, causing severe inflammation. Metriphonate has largely been superseded by PRAZIQUANTEL. Administration is oral and it is not available in the UK.

Metrodin High Purity

(Serono) is a proprietary, prescription-only preparation of urofollitrophin, which is a form of the pituitary HORMONE follicle-stimulating hormone (FSH) and is prepared from human menopausal urine that contains FSH. It can be used primarily to treat women suffering from specific hormonal deficiencies in infertility treatment and in assisted conception (eg. in *in vitro* fertilization). It is available in a form for injection.

+▲ side-effects/warning: see UROFOLLITROPHIN

Metrogel

(Sandoz) is a proprietary, prescription-only preparation of the ANTIMICROBIAL drug metronidazole, which has ANTIBACTERIAL and ANTIPROTOZOAL actions. It can be applied topically as a gel to treat acute acne rosacea outbreaks.
+▲ side-effects/warning: see METRONIDAZOLE

Metrolyl

(Lagap) is a proprietary, prescription-only preparation of the ANTIMICROBIAL drug metronidazole, which has ANTIBACTERIAL and ANTIPROTOZOAL actions. It can be used to treat bacterial infections such as vaginitis, dental infections and infections that may occur following surgery. The antiprotozoal activity is effective against the organisms that cause amoebic dysentery, giardiasis and trichomoniasis. It is available as tablets.
+▲ side-effects/warning: see METRONIDAZOLE

metronidazole

is an (AZOLE) ANTIMICROBIAL drug with ANTIBACTERIAL and ANTIPROTOZOAL actions. As an antibacterial agent its spectrum is narrow, being limited to activity against anaerobic bacteria, including bacterial vaginal infections caused by *Gardnerella vaginalis*, dental infections, leg ulcers, pressure sores and during surgery. It acts by interfering with bacterial DNA replication. As an antiprotozoal drug it is specifically active against the protozoa *Entamoeba histolytica* (which causes dysentery), *Giardia lamblia* (giardiasis; an infection of the small intestine) and *Trichomonas vaginalis* (vaginitis). It is also used to treat outbreaks of acne rosacea and to deodorize fungating, malodorous tumours. Additionally, it has been used to treat guinea worms (*Dracunculus*

M

medinensis). Administration can be oral as tablets or a suspension (as metronidazole benzoate), or topical in the form of anal suppositories or vaginal pessaries, or by injection or infusion.
✚ side-effects: these include nausea and vomiting with drowsiness, headache, rashes and itching. Some patients experience a discolouration of the urine. Prolonged treatment may eventually cause neuromuscular disorders or seizures.
▲ warning: it should be administered with caution to patients with impaired liver function, or who are pregnant or breast-feeding. During treatment patients must avoid alcohol, which would cause very unpleasant side-effects.
❍ Related entries: Dentomycin; Elyzol; Flagyl; Flagyl Compak; Flagyl S; Metrogel; Metrolyl; Metrotop; Vaginyl; Zadstat

Metrotop

(Pharmacia) is a proprietary, prescription-only preparation of the ANTIMICROBIAL drug metronidazole, which has both ANTIPROTOZOAL and ANTIBACTERIAL properties. It can be used to deodorize and treat fungating, malodorous tumours. It is available as a gel for topical application.
✚▲ side-effects/warning: see METRONIDAZOLE

metyrapone

is an ENZYME INHIBITOR that inhibits the production of both *glucocorticoid* and *mineralocorticoid* CORTICOSTEROIDS by the adrenal glands. It can therefore be used to treat conditions that result from the excessive secretion of corticosteroids into the bloodstream (such as Cushing's syndrome). It can also be used as an ANTICANCER treatment of postmenopausal breast cancer. Administration is oral in the form of capsules.
✚ side-effects: occasional nausea and vomiting, dizziness, headache, hypotension and allergic reactions.

▲ warning: it is not to be used in patients with adrenal insufficiency; or who are pregnant or breast-feeding. Administer with care to those with hypopituitary function.
❍ Related entry: Metopirone

mexiletine hydrochloride

is an ANTI-ARRHYTHMIC drug which is used to reduce heartbeat irregularities, particularly after a heart attack. Administration is by injection, infusion, or capsules.
✚ side-effects: slowing of the heart and low blood pressure; nausea and vomiting; constipation; tremor, eye-twitch, confusion; jaundice and hepatitis; blood disorders.
▲ warning: it should not be administered to patients who have a slow heart rate, heart block; and used with care in those with certain liver disorders.
❍ Related entries: Mexitil; Mexitil PL

Mexitil

(Boehringer Ingelheim) is a proprietary, prescription-only preparation of the ANTI-ARRHYTHMIC drug mexiletine hydrochloride. It can be used to treat irregularities of the heartbeat and is available as capsules and in a form for injection or infusion.
✚▲ side-effects/warning: see MEXILETINE HYDROCHLORIDE

Mexitil PL

(Boehringer Ingelheim) is a proprietary, prescription-only preparation of the ANTI-ARRHYTHMIC drug mexiletine hydrochloride. It can be used to treat irregularities of the heartbeat and is available as modified-release capsules (*Perlongets*).
✚▲ side-effects/warning: see MEXILETINE HYDROCHLORIDE

Miacalcic

(Sandoz) is a proprietary, prescription-only preparation of the THYROID HORMONE calcitonin, in the form of

salcatonin. It can be used to lower blood levels of calcium when they are abnormally high (hypercalaemia) and to treat Paget's disease of the bone. It is available in the form for subcutaneous, intramuscular, or intravenous injection.
+▲ side-effects/warning: see SALCATONIN

mianserin hydrochloride
is a TRICYCLIC-related ANTIDEPRESSANT drug. It is used to treat depressive illness, especially in cases where a degree of SEDATION may be useful. Administration is oral in the form of tablets.
+▲ side-effects/warning: see under AMITRIPTYLINE HYDROCHLORIDE; but potentially serious blood disorders may be seen (a regular full blood count is necessary). Flu-like symptoms may occur with painful joints and jaundice.
❍ Related entries: Bolvidon; Norval

Micolette Micro-enema
(Cusi) is a proprietary, non-prescription preparation of sodium citrate, sodium alkylsulphoacetate, sorbic acid and glycerol. It can be used as a LAXATIVE and is administered as an enema.
+▲ side-effects/warning: see GLYCEROL; SODIUM CITRATE

miconazole
is an (AZOLE) ANTIFUNGAL drug. It can be used to treat and prevent many forms of fungal infection, including athlete's foot, oropharyngial infections such as aspergillosis, candiasis, acne and intestinal infection. In solution, the drug can be used for irrigation of the bladder. It is available as an oral gel, a spray powder, a cream, tablets, and, for systemic infections, in a form for injection.
+ side-effects: nausea and vomiting, pruritus and rashes. The injection form contains a derivative of castor that may cause sensitivity reactions.
▲ warning: it is not to be used in patients

with porphyria; administer with care to those who are pregnant.
❍ Related entries: Acnidazil; Benoxyl 5 Cream; Benoxyl 10 Lotion; Benzagel; Daktacort; Daktarin; Daktarin Cream; Daktarin Oral Gel; Daktarin Powder; Daktarin Spray Powder; Femeron; Femeron Soft Pessary; Gyno-Daktarin; Nericur

Micralax Micro-enema
(Evans) is a proprietary, non-prescription preparation of sodium citrate, sodium alkylsulphoacetate and sorbic acid. It can be used as a LAXATIVE and is administered as an enema.
+▲ side-effects/warning: see SODIUM CITRATE;

Microgynon 30
(Schering Health) is a proprietary, prescription-only COMPOUND PREPARATION that can be used as a (*monophasic*) ORAL CONTRACEPTIVE (and also for certain menstrual problems) of the type that combines an OESTROGEN and a PROGESTOGEN, in this case ethinyloestradiol and levonorgestrel. It is available in the form of tablets in a calendar pack.
+▲ side-effects/warning: see ETHINYLOESTRADIOL; LEVONORGESTREL

Micronor
(Ortho) is a proprietary, prescription-only preparation that can be used as a ORAL CONTRACEPTIVE of the PROGESTOGEN-only pill (POP) type and contains norethisterone. It is available in the form of tablets in a calendar pack.
+▲ side-effects/warning: see NORETHISTERONE

Micronor HRT
(Cilag) is a proprietary, prescription-only preparation of the PROGESTOGEN norethisterone. It can be used in HRT and is available as tablets.

M ✚▲ side-effects/warning: see
NORETHISTERONE

Microval

(Wyeth) is a proprietary, prescription-only
preparation that can be used as an ORAL
CONTRACEPTIVE of the PROGESTOGEN-only
pill (POP) type and contains
levonorgestrel. It is available in the form
of tablets in a calendar pack.
✚▲ side-effects/warning: see
LEVONORGESTREL

Mictral

(Sanofi Winthrop) is a proprietary,
prescription-only preparation of the
ANTIBACTERIAL and (QUINOLONE)
ANTIBIOTIC drug nalidixic acid. It can be
used to treat infections, particularly of the
urinary tract and including cystitis. It is
available as granules.
✚▲ side-effects/warning: see NALIDIXIC ACID

Midamor

(Morson) is a proprietary, prescription-
only preparation of the (*potassium-
sparing*) DIURETIC drug amiloride
hydrochloride. It can be used to treat
oedema, ascites in cirrhosis or the liver,
congestive heart failure (in conjunction
with other diuretics) and as an
ANTIHYPERTENSIVE. It is available as
tablets.
✚▲ side-effects/warning: see AMILORIDE
HYDROCHLORIDE

midazolam

is a BENZODIAZEPINE drug, which can be
used as an ANXIOLYTIC and SEDATIVE in
preoperative medication, because its
ability to cause amnesia means that the
patient forgets the unpleasant procedure.
Administration is by injection.
✚▲ side-effects/warning: see under
BENZODIAZEPINE; but the incidence of side-
effects is lower than in some other
benzodiazepines; it may cause respiratory
depression after injection.
✪ Related entry: Hypnovel

Midrid

(Shire) is a proprietary, non-prescription
COMPOUND PREPARATION of the
SYMPATHOMIMETIC and VASOCONSTRICTOR
drug isometheptene mucate and the NON-
NARCOTIC ANALGESIC drug paracetamol. It
can be used to relieve acute migraine
attacks and other headaches. It is available
as capsules and is not to be given to
children.
✚▲ side-effects/warning: see
ISOMETHEPTENE MUCATE; PARACETAMOL

Mifegyne

(Roussel) is a proprietary, prescription-
only preparation of the uterine stimulant
mifepristone. It is used for termination of
pregnancy at up to 63 days of
gestation,and is available as tablets.
✚▲ side-effects/warnings: see MIFEPRISTONE

mifepristone

is a uterine stimulant that is used for
termination of uterine pregnancy at up to
63 days of gestation. It is taken by mouth
as tablets and under medical supervision
with monitoring and followed, if
necessary, with GEMEPROST vaginal
pessaries.
✚ side-effects: vaginal bleeding (which can
be severe), uterine pain, nausea and
vomiting, faintness, hypotension, rashes;
infections of the uterus and urinary tract.
▲ warning: to be used to terminate ectopic
pregnancy; not to be used with certain adrenal
gland disorders, certain blood disorders, or by
smokers over 35 years. Administer with
caution to patients with certain
cardiovascular diseases, asthma, liver or
kidney disorders, with a history of heart
infection (endocarditis), or who have
artificial heart valves.
✪ Related entry: Mifegyne

Migraleve

(Charwell) is a proprietary, non-
prescription COMPOUND PREPARATION that
is used for acute migraine attacks, not for
preventing them (prophylactically). It is

available in the form of two types of tablets wrapped in different colours: a pink pack containing the ANTIHISTAMINE drug buclizine hydrochloride, the NON-NARCOTIC ANALGESIC drug paracetamol and the (OPIOID) NARCOTIC ANALGESIC drug codeine phosphate; and a yellow pack containing tablets without buclizine hydrochloride. The preparations are not normally given to children under ten years, except on medical advice.
+▲ side-effects/warning: see BUCLIZINE HYDROCHLORIDE; CODEINE PHOSPHATE; PARACETAMOL

Migravess
(Bayer) is a proprietary, prescription-only COMPOUND PREPARATION of the ANTI-EMETIC and ANTINAUSEANT drug metoclopramide hydrochloride and the (NSAID) NON-NARCOTIC ANALGESIC drug aspirin. It can be used as an ANTIMIGRAINE treatment for acute migraine attacks. It is available as effervescent tablets and also as a stronger preparation called *Migravess Forte*.
+▲ side-effects/warning: see ASPIRIN; METOCLOPRAMIDE HYDROCHLORIDE. Note the side-effects of metoclopramide hydrochloride in young people.

Migril
(Wellcome) is a proprietary, prescription-only COMPOUND PREPARATION of the ergot VASOCONSTRICTOR drug ergotamine tartrate, the ANTINAUSEANT drug cyclizine (as hydrochloride) and the STIMULANT caffeine (as hydrate). It can be used as an ANTIMIGRAINE treatment and also for some other vascular headaches. It is available as tablets.
+▲ side-effects/warning: see CAFFEINE; CYCLIZINE; ERGOTAMINE TARTRATE

Mildison
(Yamanouchi) is a proprietary, prescription-only preparation of the CORTICOSTEROID and ANTI-INFLAMMATORY drug hydrocortisone. It can be used to

treat mild inflammatory skin conditions such as eczema and is available as a cream.
+▲ side-effects/warning: see HYDROCORTISONE

Milk of Magnesia Liquid
(Sterling Health) is a proprietary, non-prescription preparation of the ANTACID magnesium hydroxide. It can be used for the relief of stomach discomfort, indigestion, hyperacidity, heartburn, flatulence and constipation. It is available as a suspension and is not normally given to children under one year, except on medical advice.
+▲ side-effects/warning: see MAGNESIUM HYDROXIDE

Milk of Magnesia Tablets
(Sterling Health) is a proprietary, non-prescription preparation of the ANTACID magnesium hydroxide. It can be used for the relief of indigestion, nausea, biliousness, acid stomach, heartburn and flatulence. It is available as tablets and is not normally given to children under one year, except on medical advice.
+▲ side-effects/warning: see MAGNESIUM HYDROXIDE

Mil-Par
(Sterling Health) is a proprietary, non-prescription COMPOUND PREPARATION of the LAXATIVES liquid paraffin and magnesium hydroxide. It can be used for the temporary relief of constipation and is available as a liquid suspension.
+▲ side-effects/warning: see LIQUID PARAFFIN; MAGNESIUM HYDROXIDE

milrinone
is a PHOSPHODIESTERASE INHIBITOR. It is used, in the short term, in congestive HEART FAILURE TREATMENT (especially where other drugs have been unsuccessful) and in acute heart failure. Administration is by intravenous injection or infusion.

M

+▲ side-effects/warning: see under
ENOXIMONE. Blood potassium should be
controlled and kidney function monitored. It
may cause chest pain.
○ Related entry: Primacor

*mineral supplement

is the term used to describe the salts of
essential (required in the diet) dietary
minerals, which may be taken, usually by
mouth, to make up deficiencies in the diet,
or where there are problems with
absorption of the minerals into the body
from normal foodstuffs. Examples include:
CALCIUM, IRON, sodium, phosphorus,
potassium and zinc.

Minihep

(Leo) is a proprietary, prescription-only
preparation of the ANTICOAGULANT drug
heparin (as heparin sodium). It can be
used to treat various forms of thrombosis
and is available in a form for injection.
+▲ side-effects/warning: see HEPARIN

Minihep Calcium

(Leo) is a proprietary, prescription-only
preparation of the ANTICOAGULANT drug
heparin (as heparin calcium). It can be
used to treat various forms of thrombosis
and is available in a form for injection.
+▲ side-effects/warning: see HEPARIN

Min-I-Jet Adrenaline

(IMS) is a proprietary, prescription-only
preparation of the natural HORMONE
adrenaline (as adrenaline hydrochloride).
It is used as a SYMPATHOMIMETIC drug to
treat acute and severe bronchial asthma
attacks, in the emergency treatment of
acute allergic reactions and for angio-
oedema and cardiopulmonary
resuscitation. It is available in a form for
intramuscular, subcutaneous, or
intravenous injection.
+▲ side-effects/warning: see ADRENALINE

Min-I-Jet Aminophylline

(IMS) is a proprietary, prescription-only

preparation of the BRONCHODILATOR drug
aminophylline. It can be used to treat
severe acute asthma attacks and is
available in a form for intravenous
injection.
+▲ side-effects/warning: see
AMINOPHYLLINE

Min-I-Jet Bretylate Tosylate

(IMS) is a proprietary, prescription-only
preparation of the ADRENERGIC NEURONE
BLOCKER drug bretylium tosylate. It can be
used in resuscitation and as an ANTI-
ARRHYTHMIC treatment of ventricular
arrhythmias where other treatments have
not been successful. It is available in a
form for injection.
+▲ side-effects/warning: see BRETYLIUM
TOSYLATE

Min-I-Jet Frusemide

(IMS) is a proprietary, prescription-only
preparation of the (*loop*) DIURETIC drug
frusemide. It can be used to treat oedema,
particularly pulmonary (lung) oedema in
patients with chronic heart failure and low
urine production due to kidney failure
(oliguria). It is available in a form for
injection or infusion.
+▲ side-effects/warning: see FRUSEMIDE

Min-I-Jet Isoprenaline

(IMS) is a proprietary, prescription-only
preparation of the BETA-RECEPTOR
STIMULANT and SYMPATHOMIMETIC drug
isoprenaline (as isoprenaline
hydrochloride). It can be used to treat
acute heart block and severe bradycardia
and is available in a form for intravenous
injection.
+▲ side-effects/warning: see ISOPRENALINE

Min-I-Jet Lignocaine

(IMS) is a proprietary, prescription-only
preparation of the LOCAL ANAESTHETIC drug
lignocaine hydrochloride. It can be used
as an ANTI-ARRHYTHMIC drug to treat
irregularities in the heartbeat, especially
after a heart attack. It is available in a

form for injection.
+▲ side-effects/warning: see LIGNOCAINE
HYDROCHLORIDE

Min-I-Jet Lignocaine Hydrochloride with Adrenaline

(IMS) is a proprietary, prescription-only
COMPOUND PREPARATION of the LOCAL
ANAESTHETIC drug lignocaine
hydrochloride and adrenaline. It can be
used for dental anaesthesia and a variety
of surgical procedures after local
injection. It is available in a form for
injection.
+▲ side-effects/warning: see ADRENALINE;
LIGNOCAINE HYDROCHLORIDE

Min-I-Jet Mannitol (25%)

(IMS) is a proprietary, prescription-only
preparation of the (*osmotic*) DIURETIC
drug mannitol. It can be used in
GLAUCOMA TREATMENT and to treat
oedema. It is available as a 25% solution
for intravenous infusion.
+▲ side-effects/warning: see MANNITOL

Min-I-Jet Morphine Sulphate

(IMS) is a proprietary, prescription-only
preparation of the (OPIOID) NARCOTIC
ANALGESIC drug morphine sulphate and is
on the Controlled Drugs List. It can be
used to treat severe pain, for example in
the terminally ill and is available in
disposable syringes ready for use.
+▲ side-effects/warning: see under OPIOID

Min-I-Jet Naloxone

(IMS) is a proprietary, prescription-only
preparation of the OPIOID ANTAGONIST drug
naloxone hydrochloride. It can be used to
treat overdosage with opioids and
postoperative respiratory depression
(caused by opioid analgesia during
operations). It is available in syringes
ready for use.
+▲ side-effects/warning: see NALOXONE
HYDROCHLORIDE

Min-I-Jet Sodium Bicarbonate

(IMS) is a proprietary, prescription-only
preparation of sodium bicarbonate. It can
be used to treat metabolic acidosis and is
available in a form for injection.
+▲ side-effects/warning: see SODIUM
BICARBONATE

Minims Amethocaine Hydrochloride

(Smith & Nephew) is a proprietary,
prescription-only preparation of the LOCAL
ANAESTHETIC drug amethocaine
hydrochloride. It can be used by topical
application for ophthalmic procedures
and is available as eye-drops.
+▲ side-effects/warning: see AMETHOCAINE
HYDROCHLORIDE

Minims Artificial Tears

(Smith & Nephew) is a proprietary, non-
prescription preparation of
hydroxyethylcellulose. It is used as
artificial tears where there is dryness of
the eyes due to disease and is available as
eye-drops.
+▲ side-effects/warning: see
HYDROXYETHYLCELLULOSE

Minims Atropine Sulphate

(Smith & Nephew) is a proprietary,
prescription-only preparation of the
ANTICHOLINERGIC drug atropine sulphate.
It can be used to dilate the pupils and so
facilitate inspection of the eyes. It is
available as eye-drops.
+▲ side-effects/warning: see ATROPINE
SULPHATE

Minims Benoxinate (Oxybuprocaine) Hydrochloride

(Smith & Nephew) is a proprietary,
prescription-only preparation of the LOCAL
ANAESTHETIC drug oxybuprocaine
hydrochloride. It can be used by topical
application for ophthalmic procedures
and is available as eye-drops.

M

+▲ side-effects/warning: see
OXYBUPROCAINE HYDROCHLORIDE

Minims Chloramphenicol
(Smith & Nephew) is a proprietary,
prescription-only preparation of the
ANTIBACTERIAL and ANTIBIOTIC drug
chloramphenicol. It can be used to treat
bacterial infections in the eye and is
available as eye-drops.
+▲ side-effects/warning: see
CHLORAMPHENICOL

Minims Cyclopentolate
(Smith & Nephew) is a proprietary,
prescription-only preparation of the
ANTICHOLINERGIC drug cyclopentolate
hydrochloride. It can be used to dilate the
pupil and paralyse focusing and so
facilitate inspection of the eyes. It is
available as eye-drops.
+▲ side-effects/warning: see
CYCLOPENTOLATE HYDROCHLORIDE

Minims Fluorescein Sodium
(Smith & Nephew) is a proprietary, non-
prescription preparation of the dye
fluorescein sodium. It can be used on the
surface of the eye in ophthalmic diagnostic
procedures and is available as eye-drops.
+▲ side-effects/warning: see FLUORESCEIN
SODIUM

Minims Gentamicin
(Smith & Nephew) is a proprietary,
prescription-only preparation of the
ANTIBACTERIAL and (AMINOGLYCOSIDE)
ANTIBIOTIC drug gentamicin (as sulphate).
It can be used to treat many forms of
infection, particularly serious infections
caused by Gram-negative bacteria. It is
available as an eye ointment.
+▲ side-effects/warning: see
GENTAMICIN

Minims Homatropine
(Smith & Nephew) is a proprietary,
prescription-only preparation of the
ANTICHOLINERGIC drug homatropine

hydrobromide. It can be used as a
mydriatic agent to dilate the pupils and
paralyse certain eye muscles to allow
ophthalmic examination. It is available as
eye-drops.

Minims Lignocaine and Fluorescein
(Smith & Nephew) is a proprietary,
prescription-only preparation of the LOCAL
ANAESTHETIC drug lignocaine
hydrochloride (with the diagnostic dye
fluorescein). It is used in ophthalmic
diagnostic procedures and is available as
eye-drops.
+▲ side-effects/warning: see LIGNOCAINE
HYDROCHLORIDE

Minims Metipranolol
(Smith & Nephew) is a proprietary,
prescription-only preparation of the BETA-
BLOCKER metipranolol. It can be used for
GLAUCOMA TREATMENT and is available as
eye-drops.
+▲ side-effects/warning: see
METIPRANOLOL. It is used by patients allergic
to the preservative benzalkonium chloride,
which is found in several other similar eye-
drops and can be used by those wearing soft
contact lenses.

Minims Neomycin Sulphate
(Smith & Nephew) is a proprietary,
prescription-only preparation of the
ANTIBACTERIAL and (AMINOGLYCOSIDE)
ANTIBIOTIC drug neomycin sulphate. It can
be used to treat bacterial infections in the
eye and is available as eye-drops.
+▲ side-effects/warning: see NEOMYCIN
SULPHATE

Minims Phenylephrine Hydrochloride
(Smith & Nephew) is a proprietary, non-
prescription preparation of the
SYMPATHOMIMETIC drug phenylephrine
hydrochloride. It can be used to dilate the
pupils for ophthalmic examination and is
available as eye-drops.

+▲ side-effects/warning: see
PHENYLEPHRINE HYDROCHLORIDE

Minims Pilocarpine Nitrate

(Smith & Nephew) is a proprietary,
prescription-only preparation of the
PARASYMPATHOMIMETIC drug pilocarpine.
It can be used to constrict the pupil and
treat glaucoma and is available as eye-
drops.
+▲ side-effects/warning: see PILOCARPINE

Minims Prednisolone

(Smith & Nephew) is a proprietary,
prescription-only preparation of the
CORTICOSTEROID and ANTI-INFLAMMATORY
drug prednisolone (as sodium
phosphate). It can be used to treat
conditions in and around the eye and is
available as eye-drops.
+▲ side-effects/warning: see PREDNISOLONE

Minims Rose Bengal

(Smith & Nephew) is a proprietary, non-
prescription preparation of the dye rose
bengal. It can be used on the surface of
the eye for ophthalmic diagnostic
procedures and is available as eye-drops.
+▲ side-effects/warning: see ROSE BENGAL

Minims Sodium Chloride

(Smith & Nephew) is a proprietary,
non-prescription preparation of saline
solution (sodium chloride). It can
be used for the irrigation of the eyes
and to facilitate the removal of
harmful substances. It is available as
eye-drops.
+▲ side-effects/warning: see SODIUM
CHLORIDE

Minims Tropicamide

(Smith & Nephew) is a proprietary,
prescription-only preparation of
tropicamide. It can be used to dilate the
pupils to facilitate inspection of the eyes
and is available as eye-drops.
+▲ side-effects/warning: see
TROPICAMIDE

Minitran

(3M Health Care) is a proprietary, non-
prescription preparation of the
VASODILATOR and ANTI-ANGINA drug glyceryl
trinitrate. It can be used to treat and
prevent angina pectoris. It is available as a
self-adhesive dressing (patch), which,
when placed on the chest wall, is
absorbed through the skin and helps to
give lasting relief.
+▲ side-effects/warning: see GLYCERYL
TRINITRATE

Minocin

(Lederle) is a proprietary, prescription-
only preparation of the ANTIBACTERIAL and
(TETRACYCLINE) ANTIBIOTIC drug
minocycline. It can be used to treat a wide
range of infections and is available as
tablets.
+▲ side-effects/warning: see
MINOCYCLINE

Minocin MR

(Lederle) is a proprietary, prescription-
only preparation of the ANTIBACTERIAL and
(TETRACYCLINE) ANTIBIOTIC drug
minocycline. It can be used to treat a wide
range of infections (including acne) and is
available as capsules.
+▲ side-effects/warning: see
MINOCYCLINE

minocycline

is a broad-spectrum ANTIBACTERIAL and
(TETRACYCLINE) ANTIBIOTIC. It has a wider
range of action than most other
tetracyclines, because it is also effective in
preventing certain forms of meningitis
(caused by *Neisseria meningitidis*).
Administration is oral as tablets or
capsules.
+▲ side-effects/warning: see under
TETRACYCLINE. It may cause dizziness and
vertigo, rashes and pigmentation. There have
been reports of liver damage. It can be used in
patients with impaired kidney function.
**✪ Related entries: Aknemin; Blemix;
Minocin; Minocin MR**

M

Minodiab

(Pharmacia) is a proprietary, prescription-only preparation of the SULPHONYLUREA drug glipizide. It is used in DIABETIC TREATMENT of Type II diabetes (non-insulin-dependent diabetes mellitus; NIDDM; maturity-onset diabetes) and is available as tablets.

+▲ side-effects/warning: see GLIPIZIDE

minor tranquilliser

See ANXIOLYTIC

minoxidil

is a VASODILATOR drug. It can be used in ANTIHYPERTENSIVE treatment (often combined with a DIURETIC or BETA-BLOCKER) and is administered in the form of tablets. It can also be used, as a lotion, to treat male-pattern baldness (in men and women).

+ side-effects: there are gastrointestinal disturbances and weight gain; there may also be fluid retention, a rise in the heart rate and breast tenderness. When used topically to the scalp, there may be itching and dermatitis.

▲ warning: it should not be administered to patients with phaeochromocytoma or porphyria. Administer with care to those who are pregnant, or have certain heart disorders. When used as a lotion, avoid contact with the eyes and mucous membranes.

O Related entries: Loniten; Regaine

Mintec

(Innovex) is a proprietary, non-prescription preparation of the ANTISPASMODIC drug peppermint oil. It can be used to relieve the discomfort of abdominal colic and distension, particularly in irritable bowel syndrome. It is available as capsules.

+▲ side-effects/warning: see peppermint oil.

Mintezol

(Merck, Sharp & Dohme) is a proprietary, non-prescription preparation of the ANTHELMINTIC drug thiabendazole. It can be used to treat intestinal infestations,

especially by the *Strongyloides* species and to assist in the treatment of resistant infections by hookworm, whipworm and roundworm. It is available as chewable tablets.

+▲ side-effects/warning: see THIABENDAZOLE

Minulet

(Wyeth) is a proprietary, prescription-only COMPOUND PREPARATION that can be used as a (*monophasic*) ORAL CONTRACEPTIVE (and also for certain menstrual problems) of the type that combines an OESTROGEN and a PROGESTOGEN, in this case ethinyloestradiol and gestodene. It is available in the form of tablets in a calendar pack.

+▲ side-effects/warning: see DESOGESTREL; ETHINYLOESTRADIOL

Miochol

(Ciba Vision) is a proprietary, prescription-only preparation of the PARASYMPATHOMIMETIC drug acetylcholine chloride. It is used mainly to contract the pupils prior to surgery on the iris, the cornea, or other sections of the exterior of the eye. It is available as a solution for intraocular irrigation.

+▲ side-effects/warning: see ACETYLCHOLINE CHLORIDE

misoprostol

is a synthetic analogue of the PROSTAGLANDIN E_1 (ALPROSTADIL). It can be used as an ULCER-HEALING DRUG, because it inhibits acid secretion and promotes protective blood flow to the mucosal layer of the intestine. It cannot be used to treat dyspepsia, but can be very useful in protecting against ulcers caused by non-steroidal anti-inflammatory drugs (NSAIDs) and for this reason is now available in combination with some (NSAID) NON-NARCOTIC ANALGESIC and ANTIRHEUMATIC drugs (eg. Arthrotec and Napratec) in the treatment of rheumatic disease. It is available as tablets.

M

✚ side-effects: diarrhoea (which may be severe), nausea, flatulence and vomiting, abdominal pain, dyspepsia, abnormal vaginal bleeding, dizziness and rashes.

▲ warning: it should not be administered to women who are pregnant or planning pregnancy; and used with caution in patients with severe hypotension.

○ Related entries: Arthrotec; Cytotec; Napratec

Mithracin

(Pfizer) is a proprietary, prescription-only preparation of the drug plicamycin. It is used in the emergency treatment of hypercalcaemia (excessive levels of calcium in the bloodstream) caused by malignant disease. It is available in a form for injection.

✚▲ side-effects/warning: see PLICAMYCIN

mithramycin
See PLICAMYCIN

mitomycin

is a CYTOTOXIC DRUG (of ANTIBIOTIC origin), which is used as an ANTICANCER treatment of cancers of the upper gastrointestinal tract, recurrent superficial bladder tumours and breast tumours. Administration is by injection or bladder instillation.

✚▲ side-effects/warning: see under CYTOTOXIC DRUGS. It can cause lung fibrosis and kidney damage.

○ Related entry: Mitomycin C Kyowa

Mitomycin C Kyowa

(Kyowa Hakko) is a proprietary, prescription-only preparation of the (CYTOTOXIC) ANTICANCER drug mitomycin. It can be used in the treatment of upper gastrointestinal cancer, breast cancer and some superficial bladder tumours. It is available in forms for injection and for bladder instillation.

✚▲ side-effects/warning: see MITOMYCIN

Mitoxana

(ASTA Medica) is a proprietary, prescription-only preparation of the (CYTOTOXIC) ANTICANCER drug ifosamide, which can be used in the treatment of cancer. It is available in a form for injection.

✚▲ side-effects/warning: see IFOSAMIDE

mitoxantrone
See MITOZANTRONE

mitozantrone

(mitoxantrone) is a CYTOTOXIC DRUG that is chemically related to doxorubicin. It is used as an ANTICANCER treatment for several types of cancer, for example, breast cancer. Administration is by intravenous infusion.

✚▲ side-effects/warning: see under CYTOTOXIC DRUGS; there are also effects on the heart.

○ Related entry: Novantrone

Mivacron

(Wellcome) is a proprietary, prescription-only preparation of the (*non-depolarizing*) SKELETAL MUSCLE RELAXANT drug mivacurium chloride. It can be used to induce muscle paralysis during surgery. It is available in a form for injection.

✚▲ side-effects/warning: see MIVACURIUM CHLORIDE

mivacurium chloride

is a (*non-depolarizing*) SKELETAL MUSCLE RELAXANT drug. It is used to induce muscle paralysis during surgery. Administration is by injection.

✚▲ side-effects/warning: see under TUBOCURARINE CHLORIDE. It may cause the release of histamine.

○ Related entry: Mivacron

Mixtard 30/70

(Novo Nordisk, Wellcome) is a proprietary, non-prescription preparation of (mixed) BIPHASIC ISOPHANE INSULIN, highly purified porcine insulins and is

M

used as a DIABETIC TREATMENT to treat and maintain diabetic patients. It is a preparation of both neutral (30%) and isophane (70%) insulins. It is available in vials for injection and has an intermediate duration of action. HUMAN MIXTARD 30/70 is also available.

➕▲ side-effects/warning: see INSULIN

MMR

(District Health Authorities) is a proprietary, prescription-only preparation of a VACCINE that can be used for the prevention of measles, mumps and rubella (German measles) in children. It is available in a form for injection.

➕▲ side-effects/warning: see MMR VACCINE

MMR II

(Merck, Sharp & Dohme) is a proprietary, prescription-only preparation of a VACCINE that can be used for the prevention of measles, mumps and rubella (German measles) in children. It is available in a form for injection.

➕▲ side-effects/warning: see MMR VACCINE

MMR vaccine

is a combined VACCINE used for IMMUNIZATION against measles, mumps and rubella. It uses live but weakened (attenuated) strains of the viruses and was introduced with the objective of eliminating rubella (German measles) through universal vaccination of children before they began school. The vaccine is available from District Health Authorities under a number of names that include 'MMR II'.

➕▲ side-effects/warning: see under VACCINE. There may be fever, malaise, and/or rash about a week after administration; there may be a swelling of the parotid gland (salivary gland in the jaw) after two to three weeks.

○ **Related entry: MMR II**

Mobiflex

(Roche) is a proprietary, prescription-only preparation of the (NSAID) NON-NARCOTIC ANALGESIC and ANTIRHEUMATIC drug tenoxicam. It can be used to treat the pain and inflammation of rheumatism and other musculoskeletal disorders. It is available as tablets, effervescent tablets, granules for solution, or in a form for injection.

➕▲ side-effects/warning: see TENOXICAM

Mobilan

(Galen) is a proprietary, prescription-only preparation of the (NSAID) NON-NARCOTIC ANALGESIC and ANTIRHEUMATIC drug indomethacin. It can be used to treat the pain and inflammation of rheumatism and other musculoskeletal disorders. It is available as capsules.

➕▲ side-effects/warning: see INDOMETHACIN

moclobemide

is a recently introduced type of MONOAMINE-OXIDASE INHIBITOR (MAOI) ANTIDEPRESSANT drug and is used to treat major depressive illness. It is a reversible inhibitor of the monoamine oxidase type A (therefore termed RIMA) and reported to show less potentiation of dangerous side-effects of tyramine found in foodstuffs (a common side-effect of other MAOIs). Interactions with other medicines is also claimed to be less. It should not be used in conjunction with conventional MAO inhibitors, but in view of its short duration of action the switch to other forms of antidepressant may be quicker than is usual. However, there may be a more STIMULANT action than with most other MAOIs, making it less suitable for agitated patients. Administration is oral in the form of tablets.

➕ side-effects: there is some stimulation resulting in restlessness, agitation, sleep disturbances; also dizziness, nausea, confusion, changes in liver enzymes and lowered blood sodium.

▲ warnings: avoid its use in patients who are agitated or confused; those with severe liver disorders, thyroid imbalance, phaeochromocytoma; or who are

pregnant or breast-feeding.
○ Related entry: Manerix

Modalim

(Sanofi Winthrop) is a proprietary,
prescription-only preparation of the LIPID-
LOWERING DRUG ciprofibrate. It can be
used in hyperlipidaemia to reduce the
levels, or change the proportions, of
various lipids in the bloodstream. It is
available as tablets.
✛▲ side-effects/warning: CIPROFIBRATE

Modecate

(Sanofi Winthrop) is a proprietary,
prescription-only preparation of the
ANTIPSYCHOTIC drug fluphenazine
decanoate. It can be used in the long-term
maintenance of tranquillization for
patients with psychotic disorders
(including schizophrenia). It is available
in two strengths for depot deep
intramuscular injection; the stronger
preparation is called *Modecate
Concentrate*.
✛▲ side-effects/warning: see FLUPHENAZINE
DECANOATE

Moditen

(Sanofi Winthrop) is a proprietary,
prescription-only preparation of the
ANTIPSYCHOTIC drug fluphenazine. It can
be used in the long-term maintenance of
tranquillization for patients suffering from
psychotic disorders (including
schizophrenia) and for the short-term
control of severe manic or violent agitated
states. It is available as tablets (as
fluphenazine hydrochloride) and in a form
for depot deep intramuscular injection (as
fluphenazine decanoate).
✛▲ side-effects/warning: see FLUPHENAZINE
HYDROCHLORIDE

Modrasone

(Schering-Plough) is a proprietary,
prescription-only preparation of the
CORTICOSTEROID and ANTI-INFLAMMATORY
drug alclometasone dipropionate. It can

be used to treat inflammatory skin
conditions such as eczema. It is available
as a cream and an ointment for topical
application.
✛▲ side-effects/warning: see
ALCLOMETASONE DIPROPIONATE

Modrenal

(Sterling Research) is a proprietary,
prescription-only preparation of the
ENZYME INHIBITOR trilostane. It can be
used to treat conditions that result from
the excessive secretion of corticosteroids
into the bloodstream (eg. Cushing's
syndrome). It can also be used in the
ANTICANCER treatment of postmenopausal
breast cancer. It is available as capsules.
✛▲ side-effects/warning: see TRILOSTANE

Moducren

(Morson) is a proprietary, prescription-
only COMPOUND PREPARATION of the BETA-
BLOCKER drug timolol maleate and the
DIURETIC drugs hydrochlorothiazide and
amiloride hydrochloride. It can be used as
an ANTIHYPERTENSIVE treatment for raised
blood pressure and is available as
capsules.
✛▲ side-effects/warning: see AMILORIDE
HYDROCHLORIDE; HYDROCHLOROTHIAZIDE;
TIMOLOL MALEATE

Moduret-25

(Du Pont) is a proprietary, prescription-
only COMPOUND PREPARATION of the
(*potassium-sparing*) DIURETIC drug
amiloride hydrochloride and the
(THIAZIDE) diuretic hydrochlorothiazide
(a combination called co-amilozide
2.5/25). It can be used to treat oedema
and as an ANTIHYPERTENSIVE. It is available
as tablets.
✛▲ side-effects/warning: see AMILORIDE
HYDROCHLORIDE; HYDROCHLOROTHIAZIDE

Moduretic

(Du Pont) is a proprietary, prescription-
only COMPOUND PREPARATION of the
(*potassium-sparing*) DIURETIC drug

M

M amiloride hydrochloride and the (THIAZIDE) diuretic hydrochlorothiazide (a combination called co-amilozide 5/50). It can be used to treat oedema and as an ANTIHYPERTENSIVE. It is available as tablets and an oral solution.

+▲ side-effects/warning: see AMILORIDE HYDROCHLORIDE; HYDROCHLOROTHIAZIDE

Mogadon

(Roche) is a proprietary, prescription-only preparation of the BENZODIAZEPINE drug nitrazepam. It can be used as a relatively long-acting HYPNOTIC for the short-term treatment of insomnia, where a degree of sedation during the daytime is acceptable. It is available as tablets.

+▲ side-effects/warning: see NITRAZEPAM

Molcer

(Wallace) is a proprietary, non-prescription preparation of docusate sodium. It can be used for the dissolution and removal of earwax and is available as ear-drops.

+▲ side-effects/warning: see DOCUSATE SODIUM

Molipaxin

(Roussel) is a proprietary, prescription-only preparation of the TRICYCLIC-related ANTIDEPRESSANT drug trazodone hydrochloride. It can be used to treat depressive illness, especially in anxious patients where a degree of sedation may be useful. It is available as tablets, capsules and a sugar-free liquid.

+▲ side-effects/warning: see TRAZODONE HYDROCHLORIDE

Monit

(Lorex) is a proprietary, non-prescription preparation of the VASODILATOR and ANTI-ANGINA drug isosorbide mononitrate. It can be used for HEART FAILURE TREATMENT and to treat and prevent angina pectoris. It is available as tablets.

+▲ side-effects/warning: see ISOSORBIDE MONONITRATE

Monit SR

(Lorex) is a proprietary, non-prescription preparation of the VASODILATOR and ANTI-ANGINA drug isosorbide mononitrate. It can be used to treat and prevent angina pectoris and is available as modified-release tablets.

+▲ side-effects/warning: see ISOSORBIDE MONONITRATE

*monoamine-oxidase inhibitors

or MAOIs, are ENZYME-INHIBITOR drugs and one of the three major classes of ANTIDEPRESSANT drugs that are used to relieve the symptoms of depressive illness. Chemically, they are usually hydrazine derivatives and include ISOCARBOXAZID, TRANYLCYPROMINE and PHENELZINE. Although they are well established, having been used for many years, they are nowadays used much less often than TRICYCLIC antidepressants, largely because of the dangers of interactions with foodstuffs and other drugs. However, they may be used when other classes of antidepressant have not proved useful, or for some reason cannot be used. Their action is said to be better suited for use in patients with hypochondria, phobias, or hysterical episodes. Treatment often takes some weeks to show maximal beneficial effects. If a monoamine-oxidase inhibitor is used after certain other antidepressants, including tricyclics and SSRIs (or vice versa), a suitably long wash-out period must be allowed for to minimize interactions. MAOIs work by inhibiting the enzyme that metabolizes monoamines (including noradrenaline and serotonin), which, in the brain, results in a change in mood. However, this same enzyme detoxifies the amine tyramine in the body, so when certain foodstuffs that contain this amine (eg. cheese, fermented soya bean products, meat or yeast extracts and some alcoholic beverages) are ingested, or medicines that contain sympathomimetic amines are taken (eg. cough and cold 'cures' that contain ephedrine hydrochloride or pseudoephedrine hydrochloride) the outcome may be a hypertensive crisis. A patient-guidance treatment card is provided that should be carried at all times.

See PHENELZINE for principal actions and side-effects.

Mono-Cedocard

(Pharmacia) is a proprietary, non-prescription preparation of the VASODILATOR and ANTI-ANGINA drug isosorbide mononitrate. It can be used for HEART FAILURE TREATMENT and to treat and prevent angina pectoris. It is available as tablets.

+▲ side-effects/warning: see ISOSORBIDE MONONITRATE

Mono-Cedocard Retard-50

See MCR-50

Monoclate-P

(Armour) is a proprietary, prescription-only preparation of dried human factor VIII fraction, which acts as a HAEMOSTATIC drug to reduce or stop bleeding in the treatment of disorders in which bleeding is prolonged and potentially dangerous (mainly haemophilia A). It is available in a form for infusion or injection.

+▲ side-effects/warning: see FACTOR VIII FRACTION, DRIED

Monocor

(Cyanamid) is a proprietary, prescription-only preparation of the BETA-BLOCKER drug bisoprolol fumarate. It can be used as an ANTIHYPERTENSIVE treatment for raised blood pressure and as an ANTI-ANGINA treatment to relieve symptoms and improve exercise tolerance. It is available as tablets.

+▲ side-effects/warning: see BISOPROLOL FUMARATE

monoethanolamine oleate

See ETHANOLAMINE OLEATE

Mononine

(Armour) is a recently introduced, proprietary, prescription-only preparation of factor IX fraction, dried, prepared from human blood plasma. It can be used to treat patients with a deficiency in factor IX (haemophilia B),and is available in a form for infusion.

+▲ side-effects/warning: FACTOR IX FRACTION, DRIED

Monoparin

(CP Pharmaceuticals) is a proprietary, prescription-only preparation of the ANTICOAGULANT drug heparin (as heparin sodium). It can be used to treat various forms of thrombosis and is available in a form for injection.

+▲ side-effects/warning: see HEPARIN

Monoparin Calcium

(CP Pharmaceuticals) is a proprietary, prescription-only preparation of the ANTICOAGULANT drug heparin (as heparin calcium). It can be used to treat various forms of thrombosis and is available in a form for injection.

+▲ side-effects/warning: see HEPARIN

Monotrim

(Duphar) is a proprietary, prescription-only preparation of the ANTIBACTERIAL drug trimethoprim. It can be used to treat infections of the upper respiratory tract and the urinary tract. It is available as tablets, a sugar-free suspension and in a form for injection.

+▲ side-effects/warning: see TRIMETHOPRIM

Monovent

(Lagap) is a proprietary, prescription-only preparation of the BETA-RECEPTOR STIMULANT terbutaline sulphate. It can be used as a BRONCHODILATOR in reversible obstructive airways disease, as an ANTI-ASTHMATIC treatment in severe acute asthma and for the alleviation of symptoms of chronic bronchitis and emphysema. It may also be used to prevent premature

M

labour. It is available as a syrup.
+▲ side-effects/warning: see TERBUTALINE
SULPHATE

Monozide 10

(Lederle) is a proprietary, prescription-
only COMPOUND PREPARATION of the BETA-
BLOCKER drug bisoprolol fumarate and the
(THIAZIDE) DIURETIC drug
hydrochlorothiazide. It can be used as an
ANTIHYPERTENSIVE treatment for raised
blood pressure and is available as tablets.
+▲ side-effects/warning: see BISOPROLOL
FUMARATE; HYDROCHLOROTHIAZIDE

Monphytol

(LAB) is a proprietary, non-prescription
COMPOUND PREPARATION of a number of
ANTISEPTIC and KERATOLYTIC agents,
including methyl undecenoate, methyl
salicylate, salicylic acid, propyl salicylate
and chlorbutol. It can be used to treat skin
infections, particularly of the nails, caused
by *Tinea* fungi (eg. athlete's foot). It is
available as a paint for topical application.
+▲ side-effects/warning: CHLORBUTOL;
METHYL SALICYLATE; SALICYLIC ACID

Monuril

(Pharmax) is a proprietary, prescription-
only preparation of the ANTIBACTERIAL and
ANTIBIOTIC drug fosfomycin. It can be used
to treat infections of the urinary tract,
including uncomplicated infections of the
lower urinary tract. It is available as oral
granules in adult and paediatric strengths.
+▲ side-effects/warning: see FOSFOMYCIN

Moorland Tablets

(Seton) is a proprietary, non-prescription
COMPOUND PREPARATION of the ANTACID
drugs calcium carbonate, aluminium
hydroxide, magnesium carbonate,
magnesium trisilicate and bismuth
aluminate with KAOLIN. It can be used to
relieve indigestion, heartburn and
flatulence and is available as tablets. It is
not normally given to children under six
years, except on medical advice.

+▲ side-effects/warning: see ALUMINIUM
HYDROXIDE; CALCIUM CARBONATE; MAGNESIUM
CARBONATE; MAGNESIUM TRISILICATE

moracizine hydrochloride

is an ANTI-ARRHYTHMIC drug. It can be
used to reduce certain heartbeat
irregularities, particularly after a heart
attack. Administration is oral in the form
of tablets
+ side-effects: gastrointestinal disturbances;
headache, fatigue, palpitations; heart failure;
jaundice; blood disorders, dizziness, chest
pain and changes in liver function.
▲ warning: it should be avoided in a wide
variety of heart disturbances; in patients with
certain kidney or liver disorders; or who are
pregnant or breast-feeding.
○ Related entry: Ethmozine

Morhulin Ointment

(Seton Healthcare) is a proprietary, non-
prescription COMPOUND PREPARATION of
zinc oxide and COD-LIVER OIL. It can be
used as an EMOLLIENT for minor wounds,
pressure sores, skin ulcers, eczema and
nappy rash. It is available as a cream.
+▲ side-effects/warning: see ZINC OXIDE.

morphine hydrochloride

See MORPHINE SULPHATE

morphine sulphate

is a powerful (OPIOID) NARCOTIC
ANALGESIC and is the principal alkaloid of
opium. It is widely used to treat severe
pain and to relieve the associated stress
and anxiety. It is used during operations as
an analgesic and to enhance GENERAL
ANAESTHESIA; to relieve cough in the
terminally ill; as an ANTITUSSIVE (though it
may cause nausea and vomiting); and for
reducing secretion and peristalsis in the
intestine, so it has a powerful
ANTIDIARRHOEAL and ANTIMOTILITY action
and is used in some antidiarrhoeal
mixtures. Tolerance occurs extremely
readily and dependence (addiction) may
follow. Administration may be oral as

granules for dissolving, as oral solutions, as tablets, or by suppositories or injection (morphine is more active when given by injection). Proprietary preparations that contain morphine (in the form of morphine tartrate, hydrochloride, or sulphate) are all on the Controlled Drugs List. It is sometimes available as a COMPOUND PREPARATION with atropine (when used in general anaesthesia) and with an ANTI-EMETIC (eg. CYCLIZINE).
+▲ side-effects/warning: see under OPIOID. It may also cause itching and a rash.
✪ Related entries: Aspav; Cyclimorph; Diocalm; Gee's Linctus; ipecacuanha and morphine mixture, BP; ✪ Collis Browne's Mixture; kaolin and morphine mixture, BP; Min-I-Jet Morphine Sulphate; MST Continus; Oramorph; papaveretum; Sevredol

Motens

(Boehringer Ingelheim) is a proprietary, prescription-only preparation of the CALCIUM-CHANNEL BLOCKER drug lacidipine. It can be used as an ANTIHYPERTENSIVE treatment and is available as tablets.
+▲ side-effects/warning: SEE LACIDIPINE

Motifene 75 mg

(Panpharma) is a proprietary, prescription-only preparation of the (NSAID) NON-NARCOTIC ANALGESIC and ANTIRHEUMATIC drug diclofenac sodium. It can be used to treat the pain and inflammation of arthritis and rheumatism and other musculoskeletal disorders, including juvenile arthritis. It is available as modified-release capsules.
+▲ side-effects/warning: SEE DICLOFENAC SODIUM

*motility stimulants

are a class of drugs that stimulate stomach emptying and the rate of passage of food along the intestine. They can also enhance closure of the oesophageal sphincter, thereby reducing reflux passage of stomach contents up into the oesophagus

and may have ANTI-EMETIC properties. Older drugs of this class (eg. METOCLOPRAMIDE HYDROCHLORIDE) have undesirable effects on the brain. Some recently introduced motility stimulants, such as CISAPRIDE, do not have this action and are thought to work by acting at receptors for 5-HT (serotonin) to cause release of acetylcholine (see NEUROTRANSMITTER) from nerves within the gut wall.

Motilium

(Sanofi Winthrop) is a proprietary, prescription-only preparation of the ANTINAUSEANT and ANTI-EMETIC drug domperidone. It can be used to treat drug-induced nausea and vomiting, especially during treatment with cytotoxic drugs and for Parkinson's disease. It is available as tablets, a sugar-free suspension and as suppositories.
+▲ side-effects/warning: see DOMPERIDONE

Motipress

(Sanofi Winthrop) is a proprietary, prescription-only COMPOUND PREPARATION of the ANTIPSYCHOTIC drug fluphenazine hydrochloride and the (TRICYCLIC) ANTIDEPRESSANT drug nortriptyline hydrochloride, in the ratio 1:20. It can be used to treat depressive illness with anxiety and is available as tablets.
+▲ side-effects/warning: SEE FLUPHENAZINE HYDROCHLORIDE; NORTRIPTYLINE HYDROCHLORIDE

Motival

(Sanofi Winthrop) is a proprietary, prescription-only COMPOUND PREPARATION of the ANTIPSYCHOTIC drug fluphenazine hydrochloride and the (TRICYCLIC) ANTIDEPRESSANT drug nortriptyline hydrochloride, in the ratio 1:20. It can be used to treat depressive illness with anxiety and is available as tablets.
+▲ side-effects/warning: see FLUPHENAZINE HYDROCHLORIDE; NORTRIPTYLINE HYDROCHLORIDE

M

Motrin

(Upjohn) is a proprietary, prescription-only preparation of the (NSAID) NON-NARCOTIC ANALGESIC and ANTIRHEUMATIC drug ibuprofen. It can be used to relieve pain, particularly the pain and inflammation of rheumatic disease and other musculoskeletal disorders. It is available as tablets.

+▲ side-effects/warning: see IBUPROFEN

Movelat Cream

(Panpharma) is a proprietary, non-prescription COMPOUND PREPARATION of salicylic acid and mucopolysaccharide polysulphate, which both have COUNTER-IRRITANT, or RUBEFACIENT, actions. It can be applied to the skin for symptomatic relief of underlying muscle or joint pain. It is available as a cream and a gel and is not normally used for children, except on medical advice.

+▲ side-effects/warning: see MUCOPOLYSACCHARIDE POLYSULPHATE; SALICYLIC ACID

moxisylyte

See THYMOXAMINE

MR vaccine

is a combined VACCINE for IMMUNIZATION against measles and rubella. It uses live but weakened (attenuated) strains of the viruses and was introduced with the objective of eliminating rubella (German measles) through universal vaccination of children before they began school. The intention is to immunize all children irrespective of previous history of vaccination and this policy will allow discontinuation of the previous single-antigen rubella immunization programme. MR vaccine is available from District Health Authorities under a number of names, including Eolarix MR Vaccine and Merieux MR Vaccine.

+▲ side-effects/warning: see under VACCINE

MST Continus

(Napp) is a proprietary, prescription-only preparation of the (OPIOID) NARCOTIC ANALGESIC drug morphine sulphate, which is on the Controlled Drugs List. It can be used primarily to relieve pain following surgery and the pain experienced during the final stages of a terminal malignant disease. It is available as modified-release tablets and as an oral suspension.

+▲ side-effects/warning: see under OPIOID

Mucaine

(Wyeth) is a proprietary, prescription-only COMPOUND PREPARATION of the ANTACIDS aluminium hydroxide and magnesium hydroxide and the LOCAL ANAESTHETIC drug oxethazaine. It can be used to relieve reflux oesophagitis and hiatus hernia and is available as an oral suspension.

+▲ side-effects/warning: see ALUMINIUM HYDROXIDE; MAGNESIUM HYDROXIDE; OXETHAZAINE

Mucodyne

(Rhône-Poulenc Rorer) is a proprietary, prescription-only preparation of the MUCOLYTIC and EXPECTORANT drug carbocisteine. It can be used to reduce the viscosity of sputum and thus facilitate expectoration in patients with chronic asthma or bronchitis. It is available as capsules and a syrup.

+▲ side-effects/warning: see CARBOCISTEINE

Mucogel Suspension

(Pharmax) is a proprietary, non-prescription COMPOUND PREPARATION of the ANTACIDS aluminium hydroxide and magnesium hydroxide. It can be used to relieve indigestion, dyspepsia, heartburn, reflux oesophagitis and hiatus hernia. It is available as an oral suspension.

+▲ side-effects/warning: see ALUMINIUM HYDROXIDE; MAGNESIUM HYDROXIDE

*mucolytic

describes a drug that dissolves, or breaks down, mucus. Mucolytic drugs are generally used in an effort to reduce the viscosity of sputum in the upper airways and thus facilitate expectoration (coughing up sputum) and so they may also be regarded as EXPECTORANTS. It is not clear how they work, though mucolytic agents are commonly prescribed to treat such conditions as asthma and chronic bronchitis. They can also be used to increase tear secretion (lacrimation) in chronic conditions where this is reduced, causing sore, dry eyes. The best-known and most-used mucolytic agents are ACETYLCYSTEINE, CARBOCISTEINE and METHYL CYSTEINE HYDROCHLORIDE.

mucopolysaccharide polysulphate
See HEPARINOID

Mu-Cron Tablets
(Zyma Healthcare) is a proprietary, non-prescription, COMPOUND PREPARATION of the NON-NARCOTIC ANALGESIC drug paracetamol and the SYMPATHOMIMETIC and DECONGESTANT drug phenylpropanolamine hydrochloride. It can be used for the symptomatic relief of sinus pain, nasal congestion (including hay fever), colds and flu. It is available as capsules and is not normally given to children under 12 years, except on medical advice.
+▲ side-effects/warning: see PARACETAMOL; PHENYLPROPANOLAMINE HYDROCHLORIDE

Multiparin
(CP Pharmaceuticals) is a proprietary, prescription-only preparation of the ANTICOAGULANT drug heparin (as heparin sodium). It can be used to treat various forms of thrombosis and is available in a form for injection.
+▲ side-effects/warning: see HEPARIN

*multivitamin
preparations contain a selection of various VITAMINS. There are a large number of such preparations available and are mostly used as dietary supplements and for making up vitamin deficiencies. The choice of a particular multivitamin depends on its content. They are not normally available from the National Health Service, except when used in infusion solutions. However, Children's Vitamin Drops (vitamins A, C and D) is recommended by the Department of Health for routine supplement to the diet of young children and is available without prescription direct to families under the Welfare Food Scheme.
○ Related entry: Children's Vitamin Drops

mumps vaccine
is a VACCINE used for IMMUNIZATION and is made from a suspension of live, attenuated mumps viruses cultured in chick embryo tissue. Administration is by injection. (Combined with measles and rubella vaccine it constitutes MMR VACCINE.)
+▲ side-effects/warning: see under VACCINE. As these vaccines are prepared from virus strains grown in chicken embryos, the vaccines should be used with caution in individuals known to be sensitive to eggs.
○ Related entry: Mumpsvax

Mumpsvax
(Morson) is a proprietary, prescription-only preparation of a VACCINE (Jeryl Lynn strain, made from live, attenuated viruses). It can be used for IMMUNIZATION against mumps and is available in a form for injection.
+▲ side-effects/warning: see under MUMPS VACCINE

mupirocin
is an ANTIBACTERIAL and ANTIBIOTIC drug, which is unrelated to any other antibiotic. It can be used to treat bacterial skin infection and is of value in treating infections caused by bacteria resistant to other antibacterials, for instance, in and around the nostrils (eg. methoxycillin-resistant *Staphylococcus aureus*).

M

Administration is in the form of a cream for topical application.

✚ side-effects: it may sting at the site of application.

▲ warning: it is not to be used on patients with known hypersensitivity to mupirocin (or any of the constituents of the ointment preparation).

❍ Related entries: Bactroban; Bactroban Nasal

Muripsin

(Norgine) is a proprietary, non-prescription preparation of glutamic acid hydrochloride, which is the equivalent of hydrochloric acid in the stomach. It can be used to treat hypochlorhydria and achlorhydria (deficiency of hydrochloric acid) and is available as tablets.

✚▲ side-effects/warning: see under HYDROCHLORIC ACID

Mustine hydrochloride

(Boots) is a proprietary, prescription-only preparation of the (CYTOTOXIC) ANTICANCER drug mustine hydrochloride. It can be used in the treatment of Hodgkin's disease and is available in a form for intravenous infusion.

✚▲ side-effects/warning: see MUSTINE HYDROCHLORIDE

mustine hydrochloride

(chlormethine hydrochloride) is a CYTOTOXIC DRUG, which is used as an ANTICANCER drug in the treatment of the lymphatic cancer Hodgkin's disease. Administration is by intravenous infusion.

✚▲ side-effects/warning: see under CYTOTOXIC DRUGS

❍ Related entry: Mustine Hydrochloride

Myambutol

(Lederle) is a proprietary, prescription-only preparation of the ANTIBACTERIAL drug ethambutol hydrochloride. It can be used as an ANTITUBERCULAR treatment and is available as tablets.

✚▲ side-effects/warning: see ETHAMBUTOL HYDROCHLORIDE

Mycardol

(Sanofi Winthrop) is a proprietary, non-prescription preparation of the VASODILATOR and ANTI-ANGINA drug pentaerythritol tetranitrate. It can be used to prevent angina pectoris and is available as tablets.

✚▲ side-effects/warning: see PENTAERYTHRITOL TETRANITRATE

Mycifradin

(Upjohn) is a proprietary, prescription-only preparation of the ANTIBACTERIAL and (AMINOGLYCOSIDE) ANTIBIOTIC drug neomycin sulphate. It can be used to reduce bacterial levels in the intestines before surgery and is available as tablets.

✚▲ side-effects/warning: see NEOMYCIN SULPHATE

Mycil Athlete's Foot Ointment

(Crookes Healthcare) is a proprietary, non-prescription preparation of the ANTIFUNGAL drug tolnaftate. It can be used to treat fungal infections responsible for athlete's foot (tinea pedis), dhobie itch (tinea cruris) and prickly heat (miliaria). It is available as an ointment for topical application.

✚▲ side-effects/warning: see TOLNAFTATE

Mycil Athlete's Foot Spray

(Crookes Healthcare) is a proprietary, non-prescription preparation of the ANTIFUNGAL drug tolnaftate. It can be used to treat fungal infections responsible for athlete's foot (tinea pedis), dhobie itch (tinea cruris) and prickly heat (miliaria). It is available as a spray for topical application.

✚▲ side-effects/warning: see TOLNAFTATE

Mycil Powder

(Crookes Healthcare) is a proprietary, non-prescription COMPOUND PREPARATION of the ANTIFUNGAL drug tolnaftate and the ANTISEPTIC agent chlorhexidine (as hydrochloride). It can be used to treat fungal infections responsible for athlete's foot (tinea pedis), dhobie itch (tinea cruris) and prickly heat (miliaria). It is available as a powder for topical application.

+▲ side-effects/warning: see CHLORHEXIDINE, TOLNAFTATE

Mycobutin

(Pharmacia) is a proprietary, prescription-only preparation of the ANTIBACTERIAL, ANTITUBERCULAR and ANTIBIOTIC drug rifabutin. It can be used in the prevention of *Mycobacterium avium* infection in immunocompromised patients and for the treatment of pulmonary tuberculosis and mycobacterial disease. It is available as capsules.

+▲ side-effects/warning: see RIFABUTIN

Mycota Cream

(Seton Healthcare) is a proprietary, non-prescription, preparation of the ANTIFUNGAL agents zinc undecenoate and UNDECENOIC ACID. It can be used to treat athlete's foot and is available as a cream for topical application.

Mycota Powder

(Seton Healthcare) is a proprietary, non-prescription preparation of the ANTIFUNGAL agents zinc undecenoate and UNDECENOIC ACID. It can be used to treat athlete's foot and is available as a dusting powder for topical application.

Mycota Spray

(Seton Healthcare) is a proprietary, non-prescription preparation of the ANTIFUNGAL agents zinc undecenoate and UNDECENOIC ACID. It can be used to treat athlete's foot and is available as a spray for topical application.

Mydriacyl

(Alcon) is a proprietary, prescription-only preparation of the ANTICHOLINERGIC drug tropicamide. It can be used to dilate the pupil to facilitate inspection of the eyes and is available as eye-drops.

+▲ side-effects/warning: see TROPICAMIDE

Mydrilate

(Boehringer Ingelheim) is a proprietary, prescription-only preparation of the ANTICHOLINERGIC drug cyclopentolate hydrochloride. It can be used to dilate the pupils and paralyse focusing of the eye to allow ophthalmic examination. It is available as eye-drops.

+▲ side-effects/warning: see CYCLOPENTOLATE HYDROCHLORIDE

Myleran

(Wellcome) is a proprietary, prescription-only preparation of the (CYTOTOXIC) ANTICANCER drug busulphan. It can be used in the treatment of chronic myeloid leukaemias and is available as tablets.

+▲ side-effects/warning: see BUSULPHAN

Myocrisin

(Rhône-Poulenc Rorer) is a proprietary, prescription-only preparation of the ANTI-INFLAMMATORY and ANTIRHEUMATIC drug sodium aurothiomalate. It can be used to treat rheumatoid arthritis and juvenile arthritis and is available in a form for injection.

+▲ side-effects/warning: see SODIUM AUROTHIOMALATE

Myotonine

(Glenwood) is a proprietary, prescription-only preparation of the PARASYMPATHOMIMETIC drug bethanechol chloride. It can be used to stimulate motility in the intestines or to treat urinary retention, particularly following surgery. It is available as tablets.

+▲ side-effects/warning: see BETHANECHOL CHLORIDE

Mysoline

(Zeneca) is a proprietary, prescription-

M

only preparation of the ANTICONVULSANT and ANTI-EPILEPTIC, drug primidone. It can be used in the treatment of all forms of epilepsy (except absence seizures) and of essential tremor. It is available as tablets and as an oral suspension.

+▲ side-effects/warning: see PRIMIDONE

Mysteclin

(Squibb) is a proprietary, prescription-only COMPOUND PREPARATION of the ANTIBACTERIAL and (TETRACYCLINE) ANTIBIOTIC drug tetracycline (as hydrochloride) and the ANTIFUNGAL and antibiotic drug nystatin. It can be used to treat a variety of infections and is available as tablets.

+▲ side-effects/warning: see TETRACYCLINE; NYSTATIN.

nabilone

is a synthetic cannabinoid (a drug derived from cannabis). It is used as an ANTI-EMETIC and ANTINAUSEANT to relieve toxic side-effects, particularly the nausea and vomiting associated with chemotherapy. However, it too has significant side-effects. Administration is oral in the form of capsules.

✚ side-effects: euphoria, drowsiness, vertigo, dry mouth, visual and sleep disturbances, difficulty in concentrating, nausea, headache, confusion, psychosis, depression, movement disorders, decreased appetite and abdominal pain.

▲ warning: administer with care to patients with severe liver impairment, heart disease, hypertension, or psychiatric disorders. The effect of alcohol may be enhanced and it may impair the performance of skilled tasks such as driving.

⊕ Related entry: Cesamet

nabumetone

is a (NSAID) NON-NARCOTIC ANALGESIC and ANTIRHEUMATIC drug. It is used primarily to relieve pain and inflammation, particularly in osteoarthritis and rheumatoid arthritis. Administration is oral in the form of tablets and an oral suspension.

✚▲ side-effects/warning: see under NSAID.

⊕ Related entry: Relifex

Nacton

(Pharmark) is a proprietary, prescription-only preparation of the ANTICHOLINERGIC drug poldine methylsulphate. It can be used as an ANTISPASMODIC for the symptomatic relief of smooth muscle spasm in the gastrointestinal tract. It is available as tablets.

✚▲ side-effects/warning: see POLDINE METHYLSULPHATE.

nadolol

is a BETA-BLOCKER that can be used as an ANTIHYPERTENSIVE treatment for raised blood pressure, as an ANTI-ANGINA treatment to relieve symptoms and improve exercise tolerance and as an ANTI-ARRHYTHMIC to regularize heartbeat and to treat myocardial infarction. It can also be used as an ANTITHYROID drug for short-term treatment of thyrotoxicosis,and as an ANTIMIGRAINE treatment to prevent attacks. Administration is oral in the form of tablets. It is also available, as an antihypertensive treatment, in the form of COMPOUND PREPARATIONS with DIURETICS.

✚▲ side-effect/warning: see under PROPRANOLOL HYDROCHLORIDE

⊕ Related entries: Corgard; Corgaretic 40; Corgaretic 80

nafarelin

is an analogue of the hypothalamic HORMONE GONADORELIN (gonadothrophin-releasing hormone; GnRH). It reduces the secretion of gonadotrophin by the pituitary gland, which results in the reduced secretion of SEX HORMONES by the ovaries. It is used to treat endometriosis (a growth of the lining of the uterus at inappropriate sites) and for pituitary desensitization before induction of ovulation for *in vitro* fertilization. Administration is by topical application as a nasal spray.

✚▲ side-effects/warning: see under BUSERELIN

⊕ Related entry: Synarel

naftidrofuryl oxalate

is a VASODILATOR drug. It dilates the blood vessels of the extremities and so can be used to treat peripheral vascular disease (Raynaud's phenomenon). Administration can be oral as capsules or in a form for infusion.

✚ side-effects: there may be nausea and pain in the abdomen.

▲ warning: it should be administered with care to patients with certain heart, kidney, or liver disorders.

⊕ Related entry: Praxilene

nalbuphine hydrochloride

is a NARCOTIC ANALGESIC, an OPIOID, that is

N very similar to morphine in relieving pain, but with fewer side-effects and possibly less abuse potential. Like morphine, it is used primarily to relieve moderate to severe pain, especially during or after surgery. Administration is by injection.

✚▲ side-effects/warning: see under OPIOID; it is reported to cause less nausea and vomiting than morphine.

◯ Related entry: Nubain

Nalcrom

(Fisons) is a proprietary, prescription-only preparation of the ANTI-ALLERGIC drug sodium cromoglycate. It can be used to treat allergy to certain foodstuffs and is available as capsules.

✚▲ side-effects/warning: see SODIUM CROMOGLYCATE

nalidixic acid

is an ANTIBACTERIAL and ANTIBIOTIC drug, which is one of the original members of the QUINOLONE family. It is used primarily to treat Gram-negative infections of the urinary tract and works by inhibiting DNA replication in the bacterial cell. Administration is oral in the form of tablets, as a dilute suspension, or as an effervescent solution.

✚▲ side-effects/warning: see under ACROSOXACIN. It is not to be used by patients with porphyria or a history of convulsive disorders. Avoid strong sunlight. Additiona✚ side-effects include certain psychoses, weakness and tingling in the extremities.

◯ Related entries: Mictral; Negram; Uriben

Nalorex

(Du Pont) is a proprietary, prescription-only preparation of the OPIOID ANTAGONIST naltrexone hydrochloride. It can be used to reverse the effects of (OPIOID) NARCOTIC ANALGESIC drugs. Pharmacologically, it is an opioid and is used in detoxification therapy for formerly opioid-dependent individuals to help prevent relapse. It is available in the form of tablets.

✚▲ side-effects/warning: see NALTREXONE HYDROCHLORIDE

naloxone hydrochloride

is a powerful OPIOID ANTAGONIST drug. It is used primarily as an antidote to an overdose of (OPIOID) NARCOTIC ANALGESICS. It is quick but short-acting and effectively reverses the respiratory depression, coma, or convulsions that follow overdosage of opioids. Administration is by intramuscular or intravenous injection and may be repeated at short intervals until there is some response. It is also used at the end of operations to reverse respiratory depression caused by (opioid) narcotic analgesics and in newborn babies where mothers have been administered large amounts of opioid (such as pethidine) for pain relief during labour. Administration is by injection.

▲ warning: it should not be administered to patients who are physically dependent on narcotics.

◯ Related entries: Min-I-Jet Naloxone; Narcan

naltrexone hydrochloride

is an OPIOID ANTAGONIST of (OPIOID) NARCOTIC ANALGESIC drugs. It is used in detoxification treatment for formerly opioid-dependent individuals to help prevent relapse. Since it is an antagonist of dependence-forming opioids (such as heroin), it will precipitate withdrawal symptoms in those already taking opioids. During naltrexone treatment, the euphoric effects of habit-forming opioids are blocked, so helping prevent re-addiction. It should only be used in specialist clinics. (For overdose with opioids the related drug naloxone is normally used.) Administration is oral in the form of tablets.

✚ side-effects: there may be nausea, vomiting, abdominal pain, anxiety, nervousness, difficulty in sleeping, headache and pain in the joints and muscles. There may also be diarrhoea or constipation, sweating, dizziness, chills, irritability, rash, lethargy and decreased sexual potency. There have been reports of liver and blood abnormalities.

▲ warning: administer with care to patients with certain kidney or liver disorders (function tests before and during treatment are advisable).

○ Related entry: Nalorex

nandrolone

is an *anabolic* STEROID that has similar actions to the male SEX HORMONE TESTOSTERONE (though it has far fewer masculinizing effects). It can be used to treat osteoporosis and aplastic anaemia. Administration (in the form of nandrolone decanoate or nandrolone phenylpropionate) is by injection.

✚ side-effects: acne, sodium retention with oedema (fluid accumulation in the tissues), virilization (voice changes in women, with amenorrhoea (absence of periods)), inhibition of sperm production, effects on the bones and liver function.

▲ warning: it is not to be administered to patients with severe liver function disorders, cancer of the prostate gland, male breast cancer, porphyria; or who are pregnant. Administer with caution to those with impaired heart or kidney or liver function, hypertension, diabetes, epilepsy, or migraine. When treating young patients, bone growth should be monitored.

○ Related entry: Deca-Durabolin

naphazoline hydrochloride

is a SYMPATHOMIMETIC and VASOCONSTRICTOR drug, which is used for the symptomatic relief of conjunctivitis. Administration is by topical application in the form of eye-drops.

✚▲ side-effects/warning: see under XYLOMETAZOLINE HYDROCHLORIDE

○ Related entry: Clearine Eye Drops

Napratec

(Searle) is a proprietary, prescription-only COMPOUND PREPARATION of the powerful (NSAID) NON-NARCOTIC ANALGESIC and ANTIRHEUMATIC drug naproxen and the ulcer-healing drug the PROSTAGLANDIN misoprostol. It is used to treat the pain and inflammation of rheumatoid and osteoarthritis. This combination represents a novel approach to minimizing the gastrointestinal side-effects of the NSAID by supplementing the local hormone whose production has been inhibited and which is necessary for unimpaired blood circulation in the gastrointestinal lining. It is available in the form of tablets.

✚▲ side-effects/warning: see NAPROXEN; MISOPROSTOL

Naprosyn

(Syntex) is a proprietary, prescription-only preparation of the (NSAID) NON-NARCOTIC ANALGESIC and ANTIRHEUMATIC drug naproxen. It can be used to relieve pain and inflammation, particularly rheumatic and arthritic pain, acute gout and other musculoskeletal disorders. It is available as tablets, enteric-coated tablets (*Naprosyn EC*), modified-release tablets (*Naprosyn S/R*), an oral suspension, granules for oral solution and as suppositories.

✚▲ side-effects/warning: see NAPROXEN

naproxen

is a (NSAID) NON-NARCOTIC ANALGESIC and ANTIRHEUMATIC drug. It is used to relieve pain and inflammation, particularly rheumatic and arthritic pain, gout, juvenile arthritis and other musculoskeletal disorders and period pain. Administration (as naproxen or naproxen sodium) is oral in the form of tablets, as a dilute suspension, or by suppositories.

✚▲ side-effects/warning: see under NSAID. The risk of gastrointestinal side-effects is intermediate for this group. Suppositories may cause rectal irritation and bleeding.

○ Related entries: Arthrosin; Arthroxen;

N Laraflex; Napratec; Naprosyn; Nycopren; Prosaid; Synflex; Timpron; Valrox

Narcan

(Du Pont) is a proprietary, prescription-only preparation of the OPIOID ANTAGONIST drug naloxone hydrochloride, which is used to treat acute overdosage of (OPIOID) NARCOTIC ANALGESICS such as morphine. It is available in ampoules for injection and as a weaker form (*Narcan Neonatal*) for the treatment of respiratory depression in babies born to mothers who have been given narcotic analgesics during labour or who are drug addicts.

➕▲ side-effects/warning: see NALOXONE HYDROCHLORIDE

*narcotic

is a description applied to drugs that induce stupor and insensibility. Commonly, the term is applied to the OPIOIDS (such as MORPHINE SULPHATE and DIAMORPHINE HYDROCHLORIDE), but it can also be used to describe SEDATIVES, HYPNOTIC drugs and alcohol, which act directly on the brain centres to depress their functioning. In law, certainly in the USA, the term tends to be used to describe any *addictive* drug that is used illegally and is the subject of abuse, even if it is a stimulant (eg. cocaine or amphetamine). See also NARCOTIC ANALGESIC

*narcotic analgesic

drugs, such as MORPHINE SULPHATE, are OPIOIDS and have powerful actions on the central nervous system and alter the perception of pain. Because of the numerous possible side-effects, the most important of which is drug dependence (habituation, or addiction), this class is usually used under strict medical supervision and normally the drugs are only available on prescription. Other notable side-effects include depression of respiration, nausea and vomiting, sometimes hypotension, constipation

(therefore they can be used as ANTIDIARRHOEAL and ANTIMOTILITY drugs), inhibition of coughing (ANTITUSSIVE) and constriction of the pupils (miosis). Other narcotic analgesics are DIAMORPHINE HYDROCHLORIDE (heroin), PENTAZOCINE, METHADONE HYDROCHLORIDE, PETHIDINE HYDROCHLORIDE and CODEINE PHOSPHATE. Narcotic analgesics are used for different types and severities of pain. For example, pethidine is used during labour, since it produces prompt, short-lasting analgesia and causes less respiratory depression to the baby. It is now recognized that the characteristic pharmacology of the narcotic analgesics follows from their acting as mimics of natural opioid neurotransmitters (enkephalins, endorphins, dynorphins) in the brain. Most effects of the opioid narcotic analgesics (eg. respiratory depression) may be reversed with an OPIOID ANTAGONIST (eg. naloxone hydrochloride). See also NON-NARCOTIC ANALGESIC; NSAID.

narcotic antagonist

See OPIOID ANTAGONIST

Nardil

(Parke-Davis) is a proprietary, prescription-only preparation of the (MONOAMINE-OXIDASE INHIBITOR) ANTIDEPRESSANT drug phenelzine. It can be used to treat depressive illness and is available as tablets.

➕▲ side-effects/warning: see PHENELZINE

Narphen

(Napp) is a proprietary, prescription-only preparation of the (OPIOID) NARCOTIC ANALGESIC drug phenazocine hydrobromide, which is on the Controlled Drugs List. It can be used to relieve severe pain or biliary pain and is available as tablets.

➕▲ side-effects/warning: see PHENAZOCINE HYDROBROMIDE

*nasal decongestants

are drugs that relieve or reduce the symptoms of congestion of the nose. They are generally and most safely, administered in the form of nose-drops or as a nasal spray, which avoids the tendency of such drugs to cause side-effects such as raised blood pressure, though some are administered orally. Most nasal decongestants are SYMPATHOMIMETIC drugs, which work by constricting blood vessels in general, including those within the mucous membranes of the nasal cavity, so reducing the thickness of the membranes, improving drainage and possibly also decreasing mucous and fluid secretions. However, rhinitis (inflammation of the mucous membrane of the nose), especially when caused by allergy (eg. hay fever), is usually dealt with by using ANTIHISTAMINES, which inhibit the detrimental and congestive effects of histamine released by the allergic response, or by drugs which inhibit the allergic response itself and so effectively reduce inflammation (eg. CORTICOSTEROIDS and SODIUM CROMOGLYCATE). Nasal decongestant drugs are often included in COMPOUND PREPARATIONS intended for the relief of cold symptoms.

Naseptin

(Zeneca) is a proprietary, prescription-only COMPOUND PREPARATION of the ANTIBACTERIAL and (AMINOGLYCOSIDE) ANTIBIOTIC drug neomycin sulphate and the ANTISEPTIC agent chlorhexidine (as hydrochloride). It can be used to treat staphylococcal infections in and around the nostrils and is available as a cream for topical application.
+▲ side-effects/warning: see CHLORHEXIDINE; NEOMYCIN SULPHATE

Natrilix

(Servier) is a proprietary, prescription-only preparation of the (THIAZIDE-like) DIURETIC drug indapamide. It can be used, either alone or in conjunction with other drugs, as an ANTIHYPERTENSIVE treatment. It is available as tablets .
+▲ side-effects/warning: see INDAPAMIDE

Natulan

(Roche) is a proprietary, prescription-only preparation of the (CYTOTOXIC) ANTICANCER drug procarbazine. It can be used in the treatment of the lymphatic cancer Hodgkin's disease and is available as capsules.
+▲ side-effects/warning: see PROCARBAZINE

Navidrex

(Ciba) is a proprietary, prescription-only preparation of the (THIAZIDE) DIURETIC cyclopenthiazide. It can be used to treat oedema and as an ANTIHYPERTENSIVE. It is available as tablets.
+▲ side-effects/warning: see CYCLOPENTHIAZIDE

Navispare

(Ciba) is a proprietary, prescription-only COMPOUND PREPARATION of the (*potassium-sparing*) DIURETIC drug amiloride hydrochloride and the (THIAZIDE) diuretic cyclopenthiazide. It can be used as an ANTIHYPERTENSIVE and is available as tablets.
+▲ side-effects/warning: see AMILORIDE HYDROCHLORIDE; CYCLOPENTHIAZIDE

Navoban

(Sandoz) is a proprietary, prescription-only preparation of the ANTI-EMETIC and ANTINAUSEANT drug tropisetron. It can be used to give relief from nausea and vomiting, especially in patients receiving radiotherapy or chemotherapy and where other drugs are ineffective. It is available as capsules or in a form for injection.
+▲ side-effects/warning: see TROPISETRON

Nebcin

(Lilly) is a proprietary, prescription-only preparation of the ANTIBACTERIAL and (AMINOGLYCOSIDE) ANTIBIOTIC drug

N

tobramycin. It can be used to treat a range of serious bacterial infections and is available in a form for injection.
✚▲ side-effects/warning: see TOBRAMYCIN

nedocromil sodium

is used as an ANTI-ASTHMATIC drug to prevent recurrent attacks of asthma. Administration is by inhalation from an aerosol.
✚ side-effects: nausea, headache, vomiting, dyspepsia and abdominal pain.
○ Related entry: Tilade

nefopam hydrochloride

is a NON-NARCOTIC ANALGESIC drug, which is used to treat moderate pain. Administration is either oral in the form of tablets or by injection.
✚ side-effects: there may be nausea, nervous agitation, dizziness, headache, insomnia or drowsiness; dry mouth, difficulty in urination, blurred vision, increased heart rate and sweating. Confusion and hallucinations have been reported and it may colour the urine pink.
▲ warning: it should not be administered to patients who suffer from convulsive disorders.
○ Related entry: Acupan

Negram

(Sanofi Winthrop) is a proprietary, prescription-only preparation of the ANTIBACTERIAL and (QUINOLONE) ANTIBIOTIC drug nalidixic acid. It can be used to treat various infections, particularly those of the urinary tract and is available as tablets and an oral suspension.
✚▲ side-effects/warning: see NALIDIXIC ACID

Neocon-1/35

(Ortho) is a proprietary, prescription-only COMPOUND PREPARATION that can be used as a (*monophasic*) ORAL CONTRACEPTIVE (and also for certain menstrual problems) of the type that combines an OESTROGEN and a PROGESTOGEN, in this case ethinyloestradiol and norethisterone. It is

available as tablets in a calendar pack.
✚▲ side-effects/warning: see ETHINYLOESTRADIOL; NORETHISTERONE

Neo-Cortef

(Cusi) is a proprietary, prescription-only COMPOUND PREPARATION of the ANTI-INFLAMMATORY and CORTICOSTEROID drug hydrocortisone (as acetate) and the ANTIBACTERIAL and (AMINOGLYCOSIDE) ANTIBIOTIC drug neomycin sulphate. It can be used to treat bacterial infections in the outer ear and inflammation in the eye. It is available as ear-drops, eye-drops and an ointment.
✚▲ side-effects/warning: see HYDROCORTISONE; NEOMYCIN SULPHATE

Neo-Cytamen

(Evans) is a proprietary, prescription-only preparation of the VITAMIN hydroxocobalamin. It can be used to correct diagnosed clinical deficiency of vitamin B_{12}, including pernicious anaemia. It is available in a form for injection.
✚▲ side-effects/warning: see HYDROXOCOBALAMIN

Neogest

(Schering Health) is a proprietary, prescription-only preparation that can be used as an ORAL CONTRACEPTIVE of the PROGESTOGEN-only pill (POP) type and contains norgestrel. It is available in the form of tablets in a calendar pack.
✚▲ side-effects/warning: see NORGESTREL

Neo-Medrone

(Upjohn) is a proprietary, prescription-only COMPOUND PREPARATION of the ANTI-INFLAMMATORY and CORTICOSTEROID drug methylprednisolone (as acetate) and the ANTIBACTERIAL and (AMINOGLYCOSIDE) ANTIBIOTIC drug neomycin sulphate. It can be used to treat inflammatory skin conditions, particularly those resulting from allergy, that may be infected (eg. eczema). It is available as a cream for

topical application.
+▲ side-effects/warning: see
METHYLPREDNISOLONE; NEOMYCIN SULPHATE

Neo-Mercazole

(Roche) is a proprietary, prescription-only
preparation of the drug carbimazole. It
can be used to treat the effects of an
excess of thyroid hormones in the
bloodstream (thyrotoxicosis) and is
available as tablets.
+▲ side-effects/warning: see CARBIMAZOLE

neomycin sulphate

is a broad-spectrum ANTIBACTERIAL and
ANTIBIOTIC drug, which is an original
member of the AMINOGLYCOSIDE family. It
is effective in treating some superficial
bacterial infections and has quite a
widespread use when used topically (in
the eyes, ears, or on the skin). However, it
is too toxic to be administered by
intravenous or intramuscular injection. It
is occasionally taken by mouth to reduce
the levels of bacteria in the colon prior to
intestinal surgery or examination, or in
liver failure.

When administered orally it is not
absorbed from the gastrointestinal tract.
Administration can be oral as tablets, or
topical as a solution, nose-,
ear-, or eye-drops, as an ear or eye
ointment, or by nasal spray.
+▲ side-effects/warning: see under
GENTAMICIN. Prolonged or widespread topical
application may eventually lead to sensitivity
reactions.
**✪ Related entries: Adcortyl with
Graneodin; Audicort; Betnesol-N;
Betnovate-N; Cicatrin; Dermovate-NN;
Dexa-Rhinaspray; Eumovate-N;
FML-Neo; Graneodin; Gregoderm;
Maxitrol; Minims Neomycin Sulphate;
Mycifradin; Naseptin; Neo-Cortef;
Neo-Medrone; Neosporin; Nivemycin;
Otomize; Otosporin; Predsol-N;
Synalar N; Tri-Adcortyl;
Tri-Adcortyl Otic; Tribiotic;
Vista-Methasone; Vista-Methasone-N**

Neo-NaClex

(Goldshield) is a proprietary,
prescription-only preparation of the
(THIAZIDE) DIURETIC drug bendrofluazide.
It can be used in HEART FAILURE
TREATMENT, to treat oedema and as an
ANTIHYPERTENSIVE. It is available as
tablets.
+▲ side-effects/warning: see
BENDROFLUAZIDE

Neo-NaClex-K

(Goldshield) is a proprietary,
prescription-only COMPOUND PREPARATION
of the (THIAZIDE) DIURETIC drug
bendrofluazide and the potassium
supplement potassium chloride. It can be
used in HEART FAILURE TREATMENT, to treat
oedema and as an ANTIHYPERTENSIVE. It is
available as tablets, which should be
swallowed whole with plenty of fluid at
mealtimes or when in an upright posture.
+▲ side-effects/warning see
BENDROFLUAZIDE; POTASSIUM CHLORIDE

Neosporin

(Cusi) is a proprietary, prescription-only
COMPOUND PREPARATION of the
ANTIBACTERIAL and ANTIBIOTIC drug
neomycin sulphate, the antibacterial and
(polymyxin) antibiotic polymyxin B
sulphate and gramicidin. It can be used to
treat infections and inflammation of the
eye and is available as eye-drops.
+▲ side-effects/warning: see GRAMICIDIN;
NEOMYCIN SULPHATE; POLYMYXIN B SULPHATE

neostigmine

is an ANTICHOLINESTERASE drug, which
enhances the effects of the
NEUROTRANSMITTER acetylcholine (and of
certain cholinergic drugs). Because of this
property, it has PARASYMPATHOMIMETIC
actions and can be used to stimulate the
bladder to treat urinary retention and the
intestine to treat paralytic ileus. It can also
be used to treat the neuromuscular
transmission disorder myasthenia gravis.
Administration is either oral as tablets (as

N neostigmine bromide) or by injection (as neostigmine methylsulphate).

✚ side-effects: nausea and vomiting, increased salivation, diarrhoea and abdominal cramps.

▲ warning: it should not be administered to patients with intestinal or urinary blockage; it should be administered with caution to those with asthma, epilepsy, myocardial infarction, peptic ulcer, parkinsonism, hypotension, slow heart rate, or who are pregnant or breast-feeding.

❍ Related entries: Prostigmin; Robinul-Neostigmine

Neotigason

(Roche) is a proprietary, prescription-only preparation of acitretin. It can be used as a systemic treatment of long-term, severe psoriasis and certain other skin disorders. It is available as a capsules.

✚▲ side-effects/warning: see ACITRETIN

Nephril

(Pfizer) is a proprietary, prescription-only preparation of the (THIAZIDE) DIURETIC drug polythiazide. It can be used, either alone or in conjunction with other drugs, in the treatment of oedema and as an ANTIHYPERTENSIVE. It is available as tablets.

✚▲ side-effects/warning: see POLYTHIAZIDE

Nericur

(Schering Health) is a proprietary, non-prescription COMPOUND PREPARATION of the ANTIFUNGAL drug miconazole (as nitrate) and the KERATOLYTIC and ANTIMICROBIAL drug benzoyl peroxide. It can be used in the treatment of acne and is available as a gel for topical application.

✚▲ side-effects/warning: see BENZOYL PEROXIDE; MICONAZOLE

Nerisone

(Schering Health) is a proprietary, prescription-only preparation of the CORTICOSTEROID and ANTI-INFLAMMATORY drug diflucortolone valerate. It can be used to treat severe, acute inflammatory skin disorders such as eczema and psoriasis. It is available as a cream and an ointment for topical application (a stronger preparation, *Nerisone Forte*, is also available).

✚▲ side-effects/warning: see DIFLUCORTOLONE VALERATE

Netillin

(Schering-Plough) is a proprietary, prescription-only preparation of the ANTIBACTERIAL and (AMINOGLYCOSIDE) ANTIBIOTIC drug netilmicin (as sulphate). It can be used to treat a range of serious bacterial infections and is available in a form for injection.

✚▲ side-effects/warning: see NETILMICIN

netilmicin

is a broad-spectrum (AMINOGLYCOSIDE) ANTIBIOTIC drug. It can be used, alone or in combination with other antibiotics, to treat serious bacterial infections caused by Gram-negative bacteria, especially those that are resistant to the more commonly used aminoglycoside drug gentamicin. Administration is by injection.

✚▲ side-effects/warning: see under GENTAMICIN

❍ Related entry: Netillin

Neulactil

(Rhône-Poulenc Rorer) is a proprietary, prescription-only preparation of the ANTIPSYCHOTIC drug pericyazine. It can be used to treat psychotic disorders, such as schizophrenia and also severe anxiety in the short term. It is available as tablets and a syrup.

✚▲ side-effects/warning: see PERICYAZINE

neuroleptic

See ANTIPSYCHOTIC

Neurontin

(Parke-Davis) is a proprietary, prescription-only preparation of the ANTICONVULSANT and ANTI-EPILEPTIC drug gabapentin. It can be used to assist in the control of seizures that have not responded to other drugs and is available as capsules.

+▲ side-effects/warning: see GABAPENTIN

*neurotransmitter

is a chemical messenger that is released from a nerve ending to act near to where it is released, to excite or inhibit either other nerves or the cells within organs innervated by the nerves (such as the heart, intestine, skeletal muscle and glands). Neurotransmitters are therefore rather like HORMONES, but unlike the latter they act locally rather than reaching their target tissue via the blood. Such mediators work by interacting with specific recognition sites on cells, called RECEPTORS, that 'recognize' only that mediator (or chemically similar analogues). They may be blocked by drugs called receptor antagonists (see BETA-BLOCKERS and ALPHA-ADRENOCEPTOR BLOCKERS). Examples of neurotrensmitters include acetylcholine (see ACETYLCHOLINE CHLORIDE), DOPAMINE, NORADRENALINE and SEROTONIN (5-HT).

neutral insulin

See SOLUBLE INSULIN

Neutrogena Dermatological Cream

(Neutrogena) is a proprietary, non-prescription EMOLLIENT preparation of glycerol. It can be used for dry skin and is available as a cream.

+▲ side-effects/warning: see GLYCEROL

niacin

is another name for NICOTINIC ACID, which is a form of VITAMIN B.

Nicabate

(Merrell) is a proprietary, non-prescription preparation of nicotine. It can be used to alleviate the withdrawal

symptoms experienced when giving up smoking tobacco products. It is available in the form of a skin patch for transdermal delivery (absorbed through the skin).

+▲ side-effects/warning: see NICOTINE

nicardipine hydrochloride

is a CALCIUM-CHANNEL BLOCKER drug. It can be used as an ANTI-ANGINA drug to treat and prevent attacks and as an ANTIHYPERTENSIVE. Administration is oral in the form of capsules.

+ side-effects: there may be nausea and headache; dizziness, flushing, palpitations and increased heart rate; drowsiness or insomnia; hypotension, oedema (accumulation of fluid in the tissues), gastrointestinal disturbances; increased salivation; rashes; increased frequency of urination; blood upsets.

▲ warning: administer with care to those with certain heart, aortic, kidney, or liver disorders and in the elderly. Do not use in pregnancy. Treatment should be stopped if ischaemic heart pain occurs.

✪ Related entries: Cardene; Cardene SR

niclosamide

is a synthetic ANTHELMINTIC drug, which is used to treat infestation by tapeworms. Administration is oral in the form of tablets.

+ side-effects: there may be gastrointestinal disturbances (nausea, retching and abdominal pain), light-headedness and skin itching.

✪ Related entry: Yomesan

Nicobrevin

(Intercare Products) is a proprietary, non-prescription COMPOUND PREPARATION of methyl valerate, quinine and camphor (with eucalyptus oil). It can be used to alleviate the withdrawal symptoms experienced when giving up smoking tobacco products. It is available as a chewing gum (which must be kept out of the reach of children).

N

+▲ side-effects/warning: see CAMPHOR; METHYL VALERATE; QUININE

Niconil

(Elan) is a proprietary, non-prescription preparation of nicotine. It can be used to alleviate the withdrawal symptoms experienced when giving up smoking tobacco products. It is available in the form of a skin patch for transdermal delivery (absorbed through the skin).
+▲ side-effects/warning: see NICOTINE

Nicorette

(Pharmacia) is a proprietary, non-prescription preparation of nicotine (as resin). It can be used to alleviate the withdrawal symptoms experienced when giving up smoking tobacco products. It is available as a chewing gum (which must be kept out of the reach of children).
+▲ side-effects/warning: see NICOTINE

Nicorette Patch

(Pharmacia) is a proprietary, non-prescription preparation of nicotine. It can be used to alleviate the withdrawal symptoms experienced when giving up smoking tobacco products. It is available in the form of a skin patch for transdermal delivery (absorbed through the skin).
+▲ side-effects/warning: see NICOTINE

Nicorette Plus

(Pharmacia) is a proprietary, non-prescription preparation of nicotine (as resin). It can be used to alleviate the withdrawal symptoms experienced when giving up smoking tobacco products. It is available as a chewing gum (which must be kept out of the reach of children).
+▲ side-effects/warning: see NICOTINE

nicotinamide

is a derivative (the amide) of the B complex vitamin NICOTINIC ACID. It is used primarily as a constituent in vitamin supplements, especially in cases where a large dose is required because it does not have as great a VASODILATOR effect as nicotinic acid.

nicotine

is an ALKALOID found in tobacco products and is absorbed into the body whether the tobacco is smoked or chewed. It causes a SYMPATHOMIMETIC effect on the cardiovascular system with a rise in blood pressure and heart rate and stimulation of the central nervous system. Like many habituating drugs there is tolerance to its action so bigger doses are required on continued usage and there is a marked psychological and physical withdrawal syndrome if an individual abruptly stops using it, in other words drug-dependence becomes established. It is available in various replacement forms to help those trying to give it up, including as chewing gum and skin patches for continuous transdermal delivery (absorbed through the skin).
+ side-effects: cold and flu-like symptoms, with headache, nausea, dizziness, insomnia, dreaming, muscle ache, swelling of tongue, palpitations, acid stomach and skin reaction (with patches).
▲ warning: do not use when pregnant or breast-feeding; use with care if there is cardiovascular disease, hyperthyroidism, diabetes, liver or kidney impairment, phaeochromocytoma, gastric ulcers, or skin disorders (with patches). Patients should not smoke or use other nicotine products while receiving any kind of treatment.
✪ Related entries: Nicabate; Nicobrevin; Nicorette; Nicorette Nasal Spray; Nicorette Patch; Nicorette Plus; Niconil; Nicotinell TTS

Nicotinell TTS

(Zyma Healthcare) is a proprietary, non-prescription preparation of nicotine. It can be used to alleviate the withdrawal symptoms experienced when giving up smoking tobacco products. It is available in the form of a skin patch for transdermal delivery (absorbed through the skin).

✚▲ side-effects/warning: see NICOTINE

nicotinic acid

or niacin, is a B complex VITAMIN. It is a derivative of pyridine and is required in the diet, but is also synthesized in the body to a small degree from the amino acid tryptophan. Dietary deficiency results in the disease pellagra, but deficiency is rare. Good food sources include meat, cereals and yeast extract.

Nicotinic acid may be administered therapeutically as a vitamin supplement (as tablets), but its effect as a VASODILATOR precludes high dosage. It is, indeed, commonly used as a vasodilator, especially in symptomatic relief of peripheral vascular disease (Raynaud's phenomenon).

It is also used as a LIPID-LOWERING DRUG because it reduces blood levels of lipids by inhibiting their synthesis in the liver. Derivatives such as inositol nicotinate and nicotinyl alcohol (both available as tablets and a suspension) are mainly used for their vasodilator actions and nicotinamide (as tablets) for vitamin actions.

✚ side-effects: there may be nausea and vomiting, flushing, dizziness and headache; palpitations. Itching, rashes and some other side-effects may be reduced by taking with food. Sensitivity reactions and actions on the liver may occur.

▲ warning: it should not be administered to patients who are pregnant or breast-feeding; and administered with caution to those with diabetes, certain liver disorders, peptic ulcers, or gout.

✪ Related entries: Hexopal; Ronicol

nicotinyl alcohol

is a VASODILATOR drug. It can be used to help improve blood circulation to the hands and feet when this is impaired, for

example in peripheral vascular disease (Raynaud's phenomenon). Administration is by tablets or as a suspension.

✚▲ side-effects/warning: see under NICOTINIC ACID

✪ Related entry: Ronicol

nicoumalone

(acenocoumarol) is a synthetic ANTICOAGULANT drug. It can be used to prevent the formation of clots in heart disease, after heart surgery (especially following implantation of prosthetic heart valves) and to prevent venous thrombosis and pulmonary embolism. Administration is oral in the form of tablets.

✚▲ side-effects/warning: see under WARFARIN SODIUM

✪ Related entry: Sinthrome

nifedipine

is a CALCIUM-CHANNEL BLOCKER drug. It is used as an ANTI-ANGINA drug to treat and prevent attacks, as an ANTIHYPERTENSIVE treatment and as a VASODILATOR in peripheral vascular disease (Raynaud's phenomenon). Administration is oral as capsules or tablets (several in modified-release formulations).

✚ side-effects: there may be nausea and headache; dizziness, flushing, palpitations; drowsiness, lethargy and insomnia; hypotension, oedema (accumulation of fluid in the tissues); gastrointestinal disturbances; increased salivation; rashes; increased frequency of urination; blood upsets; depression and excessive growth of gums have been reported.

▲ warning: administer with care to those with certain heart, aortic, kidney, or liver disorders, in cardiac shock, or who are breast-feeding. Do not use in patients who are pregnant or who have porphyria. Treatment should be stopped if heart pain occurs.

✪ Related entries: Adalat; Adalat LA; Adalat Retard: Angiopine; Beta-Adalat; Calcilat; Cardilate MR; Coracten; Nifensar XL; Tenif

N | ## Nifensar XL
(Rhône-Poulenc Rorer) is a proprietary, prescription-only preparation of the CALCIUM-CHANNEL BLOCKER drug nifedipine. It can be used as an ANTIHYPERTENSIVE treatment and is available as tablets.
✚▲ side-effects/warning: see NIFEDIPINE

Night Cold Comfort Capsules
(Boots) is a proprietary, non-prescription COMPOUND PREPARATION of the SYMPATHOMIMETIC and VASOCONSTRICTOR drug pseudoephedrine hydrochloride, the NON-NARCOTIC ANALGESIC and ANTIPYRETIC drug paracetamol, the ANTITUSSIVE pholcodine and the ANTIHISTAMINE drug diphenhydramine hydrochloride. It can be used to relieve nasal congestion during colds and flu, aches, cough and fever. It should not be given to children.
✚▲ side-effects/warning: see DIPHENHYDRAMINE HYDROCHLORIDE; PARACETAMOL; PSEUDOEPHEDRINE HYDROCHLORIDE

Night Nurse Capsules
(SmithKline Beecham) is a proprietary, non-prescription COMPOUND PREPARATION of the NON-NARCOTIC ANALGESIC and ANTIPYRETIC drug paracetamol, the ANTITUSSIVE dextromethorphan hydrobromide and the SEDATIVE and ANTIHISTAMINE drug promethazine hydrochloridethe. It can be used for the symptomatic relief of colds, chills and flu at night. It is available as capsules and is not normally given to children under six years, except on medical advice.
✚▲ side-effects/warning: see DEXTROMETHORPHAN HYDROBROMIDE; PARACETAMOL; PROMETHAZINE HYDROCHLORIDE

Night Nurse Liquid
(SmithKline Beecham) is a proprietary, non-prescription COMPOUND PREPARATION of the NON-NARCOTIC ANALGESIC and ANTIPYRETIC drug paracetamol, the

ANTITUSSIVE dextromethorphan hydrobromide and the SEDATIVE and ANTIHISTAMINE drug promethazine hydrochloride. It can be used for the symptomatic relief of colds, chills and flu at night. It is available as a liquid and is not normally given to children under six years, except on medical advice.
✚▲ side-effects/warning: see DEXTROMETHORPHAN HYDROBROMIDE; PARACETAMOL; PROMETHAZINE HYDROCHLORIDE

nimodipine
is a CALCIUM-CHANNEL BLOCKER drug. It is used to treat and prevent ischaemic (lack of blood supply) damage following subarachnoid haemorrhage (bleeding from blood vessels supplying the outer surface of the brain). Administration can be oral as tablets or in a form for intravenous infusion.
✚ side effects: changes in heart rate; hypotension, headaches, gastrointestinal disorders, flushes, nausea, feeling of warmth, blood disorders and changes in liver enzymes.
▲ warning: administer with care because of cerebral oedema (accumulation of fluid in the brain) and greatly raised intracranial pressure; and with caution to patients with impaired kidney function, or who are pregnant.
⊙ Related entry: Nimotop

Nimotop
(Bayer) is a proprietary, prescription-only preparation of the CALCIUM-CHANNEL BLOCKER drug nimodipine. It can be used to treat and prevent ischaemic damage following subarachnoid haemorrhage. It is available as tablets and in a form for infusion.
✚▲ side-effects/warning: see NIMODIPINE

Nipride
(Roche) is a proprietary, prescription-only preparation of the VASODILATOR drug sodium nitroprusside. It can be used as an

acute ANTIHYPERTENSIVE (i.e. in a crisis), in HEART FAILURE TREATMENT and as a HYPOTENSIVE for controlling blood pressure in surgery. It is available in a form for infusion.
✚▲ side-effects/warning: see SODIUM NITROPRUSSIDE

Nirolex

(Boots) is a proprietary, non-prescription COMPOUND PREPARATION of the EXPECTORANT guaiphenesin, the SYMPATHOMIMETIC and DECONGESTANT drug ephedrine hydrochloride, glycerin, sucrose and menthol. It can be used for the symptomatic relief of chesty coughs and is avaialble as a liquid. It is not normally given to children under five years, except on medical advice.
✚▲ side-effects/warning: see GUAIPHENESIN; EPHEDRINE HYDROCHLORIDE

Nirolex for Children

(Boots) is a proprietary, non-prescription preparation of the EXPECTORANT guaiphenesin. It can be used for the relief of chesty coughs and is available as a sugar-free liquid. It is not normally given to children under one year, except on medical advice.
✚▲ side-effects/warning: see GUAIPHENESIN

Nirolex Lozenges

(Boots) is a proprietary, non-prescription preparation of the (OPIOID) NARCOTIC ANALGESIC and ANTITUSSIVE drug dextromethorphan hydrobromide. It can be used for the symptomatic relief of dry and ticklish coughs and is available as lozenges. It is not normally given to children under six years.
✚▲ side-effects/warning: see DEXTROMETHORPHAN HYDROBROMIDE

Nitoman

(Roche) is a proprietary, prescription-only preparation of the drug tetrabenazine. It can be used to assist a patient to regain voluntary control of movement in Huntington's chorea and related disorders. It is available as tablets.
✚▲ side-effects/warning: see TETRABENAZINE

nitrates

are powerful SMOOTH MUSCLE RELAXANTS. They are mainly used as VASODILATORS to relax the walls of blood vessels in the treatment or prevention of angina pectoris (heart pain) and in HEART FAILURE TREATMENT. The best-known and most-used nitrates include GLYCERYL TRINITRATE, ISOSORBIDE DINITRATE, ISOSORBIDE MONONITRATE and PENTAERYTHRITOL TETRANITRATE. Administration is commonly as tablets to be held under the tongue (sublingual) until dissolved, but aerosol sprays (directed into the mouth) are also used. Other preparations available are modified-release tablets, impregnated dressings, ointment for topical application on the chest and in a form for injection.

nitrazepam

is a BENZODIAZEPINE drug, which is used as a relatively long-acting HYPNOTIC for the short-term treatment of insomnia. Administration is oral in the form of tablets or an oral suspension.
✚▲ side-effects/warning: see under BENZODIAZEPINE
○ **Related entries: Mogadon; Remnos; Somnite; Unisomnia**

Nitrocine

(Schwarz) is a proprietary, prescription-only preparation of the VASODILATOR and ANTI-ANGINA drug glyceryl trinitrate. It can be used in HEART FAILURE TREATMENT and to treat and prevent angina pectoris. It is available in a form for injection.
✚▲ side-effects/warning: see GLYCERYL TRINITRATE

Nitrocontin Continus

(ASTA Medica) is a proprietary, non-

N prescription preparation of the VASODILATOR and ANTI-ANGINA drug glyceryl trinitrate. It can be used to treat and prevent angina pectoris and is available as modified-release tablets.
✚▲ side-effects/warning: see GLYCERYL TRINITRATE

Nitro-Dur

(Schering-Plough) is a proprietary, non-prescription preparation of the VASODILATOR and ANTI-ANGINA drug glyceryl trinitrate. It can be used to treat and prevent angina pectoris. It is available as a self-adhesive dressing (patch), which, when placed on the chest wall, is absorbed through the skin and helps to give lasting relief.
✚▲ side-effects/warning: see GLYCERYL TRINITRATE

nitrofurantoin

is an ANTIBACTERIAL drug. It is used particularly to treat infections of the urinary tract and to prevent infection during surgery on the genitourinary tract. It is especially useful in treating kidney infections that prove to be resistant to other forms of therapy. Administration is oral as tablets, capsules, or a suspension.
✚ side-effects: there may be loss of appetite, nausea, vomiting and diarrhoea; impaired lung function; peripheral neuropathy, causing tingling and other sensory disorders in the fingers and toes (patients should report such symptoms). Rarely, there is liver damage, allergic skin reactions and blood disorders.
▲ warning: it should not be administered to patients with impaired kidney function, porphyria, or with G6PD deficiency. Administer with caution to those with diabetes, anaemia and certain lung and kidney disorders. Lung, liver and peripheral nerve function should be monitored in long-term treatment. Urine may be coloured yellow or brown.
❍ Related entries: Furadantin; Macrobid; Macrodantin

Nitrolingual Spray

(Lipha) is a proprietary, non-prescription preparation of the VASODILATOR and ANTI-ANGINA drug glyceryl trinitrate. It can be used to treat and prevent angina pectoris. It is available as an aerosol spray (directed into the mouth) in metered doses.
✚▲ side-effects/warning: see GLYCERYL TRINITRATE

Nitronal

(Lipha) is a proprietary, prescription-only preparation of the VASODILATOR and ANTI-ANGINA drug glyceryl trinitrate. It can be used in HEART FAILURE TREATMENT and to treat and prevent angina pectoris. It is available in a form for injection.
✚▲ side-effects/warning: see GLYCERYL TRINITRATE

nitrous oxide

is a gas that is used as an inhalant GENERAL ANAESTHETIC for both induction and maintenance of general anaesthesia. It also has analgesic properties and is used in subanaesthetic concentrations, for instance, in childbirth. Administration is by inhalation.
✚ side-effects: nausea and vomiting and effects on the blood.

Nivaquine

(Rhône-Poulenc Rorer) is a proprietary, prescription-only preparation of the ANTIMALARIAL drug chloroquine (as sulphate). It can be used to prevent or suppress certain forms of malaria and also as an ANTIRHEUMATIC to treat rheumatoid disease. It is available as tablets, a syrup and in a form for injection. (This product also appears in a non-prescription preparation, as tablets or a syrup, labelled for use in the prevention of malaria.)
✚▲ side-effects/warning: see CHLOROQUINE

Nivemycin

(Boots) is a proprietary, prescription-only preparation of the ANTIBACTERIAL and

(AMINOGLYCOSIDE) ANTIBIOTIC drug neomycin sulphate. It can be used to reduce bacterial levels in the intestines before surgery and is available as tablets and an elixir.

➕▲ side-effects/warning: see NEOMYCIN SULPHATE

nizatidine

is an effective H_2-ANTAGONIST and ULCER-HEALING DRUG. It can be used to assist in the treatment of benign peptic (gastric and duodenal) ulcers, to relieve heartburn in cases of reflux oesophagitis (caused by regurgitation of acid and enzymes into the oesophagus), Zollinger-Ellison syndrome and a variety of conditions where reduction of acidity is beneficial. It works by reducing the secretion of gastric acid (by acting as a histamine receptor H_2-receptor antagonist), so reducing erosion and bleeding from peptic ulcers and allowing them a chance to heal. However, nizatidine should not be used until a full diagnosis of gastric bleeding or serious pain has been made, because its action in restricting gastric secretions may possibly mask the presence of stomach cancer. Administration is either oral in the form of capsules or by intravenous injection or infusion.

➕▲ side-effects/warning: see under CIMETIDINE; but it does not significantly inhibit microsomal drug-metabolizing enzymes.

✪ Related entry: Axid

Nizoral

(Janssen) is a proprietary, prescription-only preparation of the (IMIDAZOLE) ANTIFUNGAL drug ketoconazole. It can be used to treat serious systemic and skin-surface fungal infections. It is available as tablets, an oral suspension, a cream for topical application and as a shampoo.

➕▲ side-effects/warning: see KETOCONAZOLE

Noctec

(Squibb) is a proprietary, prescription-only preparation of the HYPNOTIC drug chloral hydrate. It can be used in the short-term treatment of insomnia in children and the elderly. It is available as capsules.

➕▲ side-effects/warning: see CHLORAL HYDRATE

NODS Tropicamide

(Smith & Nephew) is a proprietary, prescription-only preparation of the ANTICHOLINERGIC drug tropicamide. It can be used to dilate pupils and facilitate inspection of the eyes and is available as ophthalmic applicator strips.

➕▲ side-effects/warning: see TROPICAMIDE

Noltam

(Lederle) is a proprietary, prescription-only preparation of the sex HORMONE ANTAGONIST tamoxifen, which, because it inhibits the effect of OESTROGENS, is used primarily as an ANTICANCER treatment for cancers that depend on the presence of oestrogen in women, particularly breast cancer. It can also be used to treat certain conditions of infertility. It is available as tablets.

➕▲ side-effects/warning: see TAMOXIFEN

Nolvadex

(Zeneca) is a proprietary, prescription-only preparation of the sex HORMONE ANTAGONIST tamoxifen, which, because it inhibits the effect of OESTROGENS, is used primarily as an ANTICANCER treatment for cancers that depend on the presence of oestrogen in women, particularly breast cancer. It can also be used to treat certain conditions of infertility. It is available as tablets in three strengths (the stronger ones under the trade names *Nolvadex-D* and *Nolvadex-Forte*).

➕▲ side-effects/warning: see TAMOXIFEN

non-narcotic analgesic

is a drug that relieves pain. The term non-narcotic distinguishes them from the NARCOTIC ANALGESICS, though they are

N

referred to by many names, including *weak analgesics* and, in medical circles, a very large number are referred to as *non-steroidal anti-inflammatory drugs* or NSAIDs. The latter term refers to the valuable ANTI-INFLAMMATORY action of some members of the class. Non-narcotic analgesics are drugs that have no tendency to produce dependence (addiction), but are by no means free of side-effects. For example, ASPIRIN-like drugs can cause gastrointestinal upsets ranging from dyspepsia to serious haemorrhage. However, they can be used for a wide variety of purposes, from mild aches and pains (at a lower range of dosage) to the treatment of rheumatoid arthritis (at higher dosages: see ANTIRHEUMATIC). PARACETAMOL does not have strong anti-inflammatory actions, but is non-narcotic and, along with other non-narcotic analgesics, has valuable ANTIPYRETIC action. These drugs work by altering the synthesis of prostaglandins (natural local hormones within the body) that induce pain. Often drugs in this class are used in combination with other ANALGESICS (eg. codeine) or with drugs of other classes (eg. caffeine). See also IBUPROFEN and INDOMETHACIN.

non-steroidal anti-inflammatory drug

See NSAID

nonoxinol

is a SPERMICIDAL drug that is used to assist barrier methods of contraception (such as the condom). Administration is by topical application as a jelly.

○ Related entries: C-Film; Delfen; Double Check; Duracreme; Duragel; Gynol II Creme; Ortho-Cream; Orthoforms; Staycept

Nootropil

(UCB Pharma) is a proprietary, prescription-only preparation of the recently introduced drug piracetam. It can

be used in the treatment of cortical myoclonus (involuntary spasmic contractions of muscles of the body) and is available as tablets and an oral solution.
+▲ side-effects/warning: see PIRACETAM

noradrenaline

is both a HORMONE and a NEUROTRANSMITTER and is chemically a catecholamine. (In the USA, it is called *norepinephrine* or *levarterenol*.) It is produced and secreted (along with the closely related substance ADRENALINE) as a hormone into the bloodstream by the adrenal gland (from the region called the medulla, which is the central core of the adrenal gland – hence the term *adrenomedullary hormone*). The adrenal gland constitutes an important part of the sympathetic nervous system. Noradrenaline also acts as a neurotransmitter. It is released from nerve endings by electrical signals travelling from the central nervous system via nerves in the body, in order to activate or inhibit a wide variety of muscles, glands and metabolic processes. The responses of the body to stimulation of the sympathetic nervous system are primarily concerned with reactions to stress. In the face of stress, or the need for exertion, the body uses adrenaline and noradrenaline to cause constriction of some blood vessels while dilating others, with the net effect of the two catecholamines increasing blood flow to the skeletal muscles and heart. The heart rate is raised and there is relaxation of the smooth muscles of the intestine and bronchioles. There is also a rise in concentration of energy supplying glucose and free fatty-acids in the bloodstream. The actions of noradrenaline and adrenaline are similar, though noradrenaline causes a more marked rise in blood pressure, whereas adrenaline stimulates the heart more. In order to bring about one or more of these responses SYMPATHOMIMETIC drugs that mimic certain of these actions (eg.

adrenaline, ISOPRENALINE and PHENYLEPHRINE) are administered therapeutically. Noradrenaline itself is not widely used because its actions are so widespread. But in emergencies it may be used as a vasoconstrictor in acute hypotension and cardiac arrest (when it is injected in the form of noradrenaline acid tartrate).

✚ side-effects: there may be palpitation of the heart with slowed and irregular heartbeat; and headache.

▲ warning: it should not be administered to patients who are undergoing a myocardial infarction, or who are pregnant. Leakage of the hormone into the tissues at the site of injection may cause tissue damage.

✪ Related entry: Levophed

noradrenaline acid tartrate

is the chemical form of the naturally occurring NORADRENALINE that is used in medicine.

Norcuron

(Organon-Teknika) is a proprietary, prescription-only preparation of the (*non-depolarizing*) SKELETAL MUSCLE RELAXANT drug vecuronium bromide. It can be used to induce muscle paralysis during surgery and is available in a form for injection.

✚▲ side-effects/warning: see VECURONIUM BROMIDE

Norditropin

(Novo Nordisk) is a proprietary, prescription-only preparation of somatropin (the biosynthetic form of the pituitary HORMONE human growth hormone). It can be used to treat hormonal deficiency and associated symptoms (in particular, short stature). It is available in various forms for injection.

✚▲ side-effects/warning: see SOMATROPIN

Nordox

(Panpharma) is a proprietary,

prescription-only preparation of the ANTIBACTERIAL and (TETRACYCLINE) ANTIBIOTIC drug doxycycline. It can be used to treat a range of infections and is available as capsules.

✚▲ side-effects/warning: see DOXYCYCLINE

norepinephrine

See NORADRENALINE

norethisterone

is a PROGESTOGEN. It is used primarily as a constituent in ORAL CONTRACEPTIVES that combine an OESTROGEN with a progestogen, in implant contraception, in HRT (hormone replacement therapy) and as an ANTICANCER drug to assist in the treatment of sex-hormone linked cancers (eg. breast cancer). Administration can be oral as tablets or topical as skin patches.

✚▲ side-effects/warning: see under PROGESTOGEN

✪ Related entries: BiNovum; Brevinor; Climagest; Estracombi; Estrapak 50; Evorel Pak; Loestrin 20; Loestrin-30; Menzol; Micronor; Micronor HRT; Neocon-1/35; Norimin; Norinyl-1; Noristerat; Ortho-Novin 1/50; Ovysmen; Primolut N; Synphase; Syntex Menophase; TriNovum; TriNovum ED; Trisequens; Utovlan

Norflex

(3M Health Care) is a proprietary, prescription-only preparation of the SKELETAL MUSCLE RELAXANT drug orphenadrine citrate. It can be used for short-term, symptomatic relief of skeletal muscle spasm and is available in a form for injection.

✚▲ side-effects/warning: see ORPHENADRINE CITRATE

norfloxacin

is an ANTIBACTERIAL and (QUINOLONE) ANTIBIOTIC drug. It can be used to treat infections in patients who are allergic to penicillin, or whose strain of bacterium is resistant to more commonly used

N

antibacterials. Administration can be oral in the form of tablets or by eye-drops.
+▲ side-effects/warning: see under ACROSOXACIN; but it may also include depression, anorexia and tinnitus (ringing in the ears).
O Related entry: Utinor

Norgalex Micro-enema

(Norgine) is a proprietary, non-prescription preparation of the (*stimulant*) LAXATIVE docusate sodium. It can be used to relieve constipation and also to evacuate the rectum prior to abdominal procedures. It is available as an enema.
+▲ side-effects/warning: see DOCUSATE SODIUM

Norgeston

(Schering Health) is a proprietary, prescription-only preparation that can be used as a ORAL CONTRACEPTIVE of the PROGESTOGEN-only pill (POP) type and contains levonorgestrel. It is available in the form of tablets in a calendar pack.
+▲ side-effects/warning: see LEVONORGESTREL

norgestrel

is a female SEX HORMONE, a PROGESTOGEN, which is used in *progesterone-only* ORAL CONTRACEPTIVES and also, in combination with OESTROGEN, in HRT (hormone replacement therapy). Administration is oral as tablets. (LEVONORGESTREL is a stronger form of norgestrel.)
+▲ side-effects/warning: see under PROGESTOGEN
O Related entries: Cyclo-Progynova; Neogest; Prempak-C

Noriday

(Syntex) is a proprietary, prescription-only preparation that can be used as a ORAL CONTRACEPTIVE of the PROGESTOGEN-only pill (POP) type and contains levonorgestrel. It is available in the form of tablets in a calendar pack.

+▲ side-effects/warning: see NORETHISTERONE

Norimin

(Syntex) is a proprietary, prescription-only COMPOUND PREPARATION that can be used as a (*monophasic*) ORAL CONTRACEPTIVE (and also for certain menstrual problems) of the type that combines an OESTROGEN and a PROGESTOGEN, in this case ethinyloestradiol and norethisterone. It is available in the form of tablets in a calendar pack.
+▲ side-effects/warning: see ETHINYLOESTRADIOL; NORETHISTERONE

Norinyl-1

(Syntex) is a proprietary, prescription-only COMPOUND PREPARATION that can be used as a (*monophasic*) ORAL CONTRACEPTIVE (and also for certain menstrual problems) of the type that combines an OESTROGEN and a PROGESTOGEN, in this case mestranol and norethisterone. It is available in the form of tablets in a calendar pack.
+▲ side-effects/warning: see MESTRANOL; NORETHISTERONE

Noristerat

(Schering Health) is a proprietary, prescription-only preparation that can be used as a parenteral CONTRACEPTIVE of the PROGESTOGEN-only pill type and contains norethisterone (as enanthate). It is available in a form for intramuscular depot implant injection.
+▲ side-effects/warning: see NORETHISTERONE

Normacol

(Norgine) is a proprietary, non-prescription preparation of the (*bulking agent*) LAXATIVE sterculia. It can be used to relieve constipation and is available as a powder. It is not normally given to children under six years, except on

medical advice.
+▲ side-effects/warning: see STERCULIA

Normacol Plus

(Norgine) is a proprietary, non-
prescription preparation of the (*bulking
agent*) LAXATIVE sterculia (with added
frangula bark). It can be used to relieve
constipation and is available as a powder.
+▲ side-effects/warning: see STERCULIA

normal immunoglobulin

(gamma globulin; human normal
immunoglobulin; HNIG) is used in
IMMUNIZATION to give *passive immunity*
by the injection of immunoglobulin
prepared from the pooled blood plasma
donated by individuals with antibodies to
viruses prevalent in the general
population, including hepatitis A virus,
rubeola (measles) and rubella (German
measles).

It is commonly given to patients at risk,
such as infants who cannot tolerate
vaccines that incorporate live (though
weakened) viruses (active immunity).
Administration is normally by
intramuscular injection. (There are also
special forms for intravenous infusion,
including formulations for patients
undergoing a bone-marrow transplant, or
patients with certain congenital blood
component deficiencies, eg.
agammaglobulinaemia,
hypogammaglobulinaemia, idiopathic
thrombocytopenic purpurea and Kawasaki
syndrome.)
+▲ side-effects/warning: see IMMUNIZATION
○ Related entries: Gammabulin:
Kabiglobulin

Normax

(Evans) is a proprietary, prescription-only
preparation of co-danthramer 50/60,
which is a (*stimulant*) LAXATIVE based on
danthron and docusate sodium. It can be
used to relieve constipation and to
prepare patients for abdominal
procedures. It is available as capsules.

+▲ side-effects/warning: see DANTHRON;
DOCUSATE SODIUM

Normegon

(Organon) is a proprietary, prescription-
only HORMONE preparation of a form of
the human menopausal gonadotrophins,
which contains FOLLICLE-STIMULATING
HORMONE (FSH) and LUTEINIZING
HORMONE (LH). It can be used to treat
infertile women with proven
hypopituitarism and who do not respond
to CLOMIPHENE CITRATE (another drug
commonly used to treat infertility) and
also in superovulation treatment in
assisted conception (as with *in vitro*
fertilization). It is available in a form for
intramuscular injection.
+▲ side-effects/warning: see HUMAN
MENOPAUSAL GONADOTROPHINS

Norplant

(Roussel) is a proprietary, prescription-
only preparation that can be used as a
parenteral CONTRACEPTIVE of the
PROGESTOGEN-only type and contains
levonorgestrel. It is available in the form
of a capsules for implantation.
+▲ side-effects/warning: see
LEVONORGESTREL. Prolonged bleeding and
amenorrhagia is common.

nortriptyline hydrochloride

is an ANTIDEPRESSANT drug of the
TRICYCLIC group. It has mild SEDATIVE
properties and is used primarily to
treat depressive illness. Like several other
drugs of its type, it may also be used to
prevent bed-wetting by children.
Administration is oral in the form of
tablets, capsules, or a sugar-free dilute
liquid.
+▲ side-effects/warning: see under
AMITRIPTYLINE HYDROCHLORIDE; but is less
sedating.
○ Related entries: Allegron; Motival

Norval

(Bencard) is a proprietary, prescription-

N

only preparation of the TRICYCLIC-related ANTIDEPRESSANT drug mianserin hydrochloride. It is used to treat depressive illness, especially where some sedation is required, for instance when depression is associated with anxiety. It is available in as tablets.

✚▲ side-effects/warning: see MIANSERIN HYDROCHLORIDE

Novantrone

(Lederle) is a proprietary, prescription-only preparation of the (CYTOTOXIC) ANTICANCER drug mitozantrone. It can be used in the treatment of certain types of cancer, including breast cancer and is available in a form for intravenous infusion.

✚▲ side-effects/warning: see MITOZANTRONE

Nozinan

(Link) is a proprietary, prescription-only preparation of the ANTIPSYCHOTIC drug methotrimeprazine (as hydrochloride). It can be used to tranquillize patients with psychotic disorders such as schizophrenia and to calm and soothe those with terminal illness. It is available as tablets or in a form for injection.

✚▲ side-effects/warning: see METHOTRIMEPRAZINE

*NSAID

is an abbreviation for *non-steroidal anti-inflammatory drug*, which is used to describe a large group of drugs, of which ASPIRIN is an original member. Although they are all acidic compounds of different chemical structures, they have several important actions in common. They can be used as ANTI-INFLAMMATORY drugs (to the extent that some may be used as ANTIRHEUMATIC treatments), as NON-NARCOTIC ANALGESICS (particularly when the pain is associated with inflammation) and as ANTIPYRETIC drugs (with the added advantage that they lower body temperature only when it is raised in fever). Additionally, some NSAIDs may be

used as ANTIPLATELET drugs, because they can be used to beneficially reduce platelet aggregation. All these actions are thought to be due to the ability of NSAIDs to change the synthesis and metabolism of the natural LOCAL HORMONES the PROSTAGLANDINS. In practice, the side-effects of NSAIDs are so extensive that the use of individual members depends on the ability of individual patients to tolerate their side-effects. Some with the least side-effects are regarded as safe enough for non-prescription, over-the-counter sale, such as aspirin and IBUPROFEN. Although PARACETAMOL shares some of the NSAIDs' properties, it is only very weakly anti-inflammatory and is not normally classified with them. See also ANALGESIC.

✚ side-effects: gastrointestinal upsets, dyspepsia, nausea, diarrhoea, bleeding and ulceration. There may be hypersensitivity reactions, including rash, bronchospasm, oedema, headache, blood disorders, ringing in the ears, dizziness and fluid retention. Reversible kidney failure particularly in renal impairment. Liver damage is rare. The gastrointestinal upsets may be minimized by taking the drug with milk or food.

▲ warning: use with care in patients with allergic disorders (especially asthma and skin conditions), in the elderly and where there are certain liver or kidney disorders. They should not be used where there is a tendency to, or active, peptic ulceration; but different NSAIDs vary in the severity of their gastrointestinal side-effects (eg. azaprolazone is high-risk, whereas ibuprofen has a lower risk). NSAIDs should not be taken by pregnant women and some are best avoided when breast-feeding (eg. aspirin).

✪ **Related entries: acemetacin; azapropazone; benorylate; diclofenac sodium; diflunisal; etodolac; fenbufen; fenoprofen; flurbiprofen; indomethacin; ketoprofen; mefenamic acid; nabumetone; naproxen; phenylbutazone; piroxicam; salicylate; sulindac; tenoxicam; tiaprofenic acid; tolmetin**

Nubain
(Du Pont) is a proprietary, prescription-only preparation of the (OPIOID) NARCOTIC ANALGESIC drug nalbuphine hydrochloride. It can be used to treat moderate to severe pain, particularly during or following surgical procedures or a heart attack. It is available in a form for injection.

✚▲ side-effects/warning: see NALBUPHINE HYDROCHLORIDE

Nuelin
(3M Health Care) is a proprietary, non-prescription preparation of the BRONCHODILATOR drug theophylline. It can be used as an ANTI-ASTHMATIC (including severe acute asthma) and to treat chronic bronchitis. It is available as tablets and as a liquid.

✚▲ side-effects/warning: see THEOPHYLLINE

Nuelin SA
(3M Health Care) is a proprietary, non-prescription preparation of the BRONCHODILATOR drug theophylline. It can be used as an ANTI-ASTHMATIC (including severe acute asthma) and to treat chronic bronchitis. It is available as tablets and modified-release tablets (including *Nuelin SA 250*).

✚▲ side-effects/warning: see THEOPHYLLINE

Nulacin Tablets
(Goldshield) is a proprietary, non-prescription COMPOUND PREPARATION of the ANTACIDS calcium carbonate, magnesium carbonate, magnesium oxide and magnesium trisilicate. It can be used for the relief of indigestion, heartburn, acid indigestion and hiatus hernia. It is available as tablets and is not normally given to children, except on medical advice.

✚▲ side-effects/warning: see CALCIUM CARBONATE; MAGNESIUM CARBONATE; MAGNESIUM TRISILICATE

Nurofen
(Crookes Healthcare) is a proprietary, non-prescription preparation of the (NSAID) NON-NARCOTIC ANALGESIC, ANTIRHEUMATIC and ANTIPYRETIC drug ibuprofen. It can be used for the relief of headache, period pain, muscular pain, dental pain and feverishness. It is available as tablets and is not normally given to children under 12 years, except on medical advice.

✚▲ side-effects/warning. see IBUPROFEN

Nurofen Soluble
(Crookes Healthcare) is a proprietary, non-prescription preparation of the (NSAID) NON-NARCOTIC ANALGESIC, ANTIRHEUMATIC and ANTIPYRETIC drug ibuprofen. It can be used for the relief of pain, including headache, period pain, muscular pain, dental pain and feverishness. It is available as soluble tablets.

✚▲ side-effects/warning: see IBUPROFEN

Nurse Sykes Powders
(Rosmarine) is a proprietary, non-prescription COMPOUND PREPARATION of the (NSAID) NON-NARCOTIC ANALGESIC and ANTIRHEUMATIC drug aspirin, the non-narcotic analgesic drug paracetamol and the STIMULANT caffeine. It can be used to relieve cold and flu symptoms, mild to moderate pain and aches and pains. It is available as a powder and is not normally given to children under 12 years, except on medical advice.

✚▲ side-effects/warning: see aspirin; caffeine; PARACETAMOL

Nu-Seals Aspirin
(Lilly) is a proprietary, non-prescription preparation of the (NSAID) NON-NARCOTIC ANALGESIC and ANTIRHEUMATIC drug aspirin. It can be used to treat chronic pain such as that of arthritis and rheumatism and also as an ANTIPLATELET aggregation (antithrombotic) drug. It is available as tablets.

✚▲ side-effects/warning: see ASPIRIN

N

Nutraplus

(Novex) is a proprietary, non-prescription preparation of the HYDRATING AGENT urea. It can be used to treat dry, scaling and itching skin. It is available as a cream.

✚▲ side-effects/warning: see
UREA

*nutritional preparations

(nutritional supplements) are primarily used in medicine for the nutrition of patients who cannot tolerate normal foods for some reason. Their use is only seen as essential under certain circumstances, such as after major bowel surgery, serious stomach and intestinal disorders, for those allergic to certain food products such as cows' milk or gluten (gluten-intolerance) and for those unable to metabolize certain sugars and amino-acids (eg. phenylketonuria).

Nutrizym 10

(Merck) is a proprietary, non-prescription preparation of the digestive enzyme pancreatin. It can be used to treat deficiencies of digestive juices that are normally supplied by the pancreas. It is available as capsules.

✚▲ side-effects/warning: see PANCREATIN

Nutrizym 22

(Merck) is a proprietary, non-prescription preparation of the digestive enzyme pancreatin. It can be used to treat deficiencies of digestive juices that are normally supplied by the pancreas. It is available as capsules, which are at a higher strength than *Nutrizym 10*.

✚▲ side-effects/warning: see PANCREATIN

Nutrizym GR

(Merck) is a proprietary, non-prescription preparation of the digestive enzyme pancreatin. It can be used to treat deficiencies of digestive juices that are normally supplied by the pancreas. It is available as capsules.

✚▲ side-effects/warning: see PANCREATIN

Nuvelle

(Schering Health) is a proprietary, prescription-only COMPOUND PREPARATION of the female SEX HORMONES oestradiol (as valerate; an OESTROGEN) and levonorgestrel (a PROGESTOGEN). It can be used to treat menopausal problems in HRT and is available as tablets.

✚▲ side-effects/warning: see
LEVONORGESTREL; OESTRADIOL

Nycopren

(Nycomed) is a proprietary, prescription-only preparation of the (NSAID) NON-NARCOTIC ANALGESIC and ANTIRHEUMATIC drug naproxen. It can be used to relieve pain and inflammation, particularly rheumatic and arthritic pain, acute gout and to treat other musculoskeletal disorders. It is available as tablets.

✚▲ side-effects/warning: see NAPROXEN

Nylax Tablets

(Crookes Healthcare) is a proprietary, non-prescription COMPOUND PREPARATION of the (*stimulant*) LAXATIVES bisacodyl, phenolphthalein and senna. It can be used for the short-term relief of constipation and is available as tablets. It is not normally given to children, except on medical advice.

✚▲ side-effects/warning: see BISACODYL; PHENOLPHTHALEIN; SENNA

Nystadermal

(Squibb) is a proprietary, prescription-only COMPOUND PREPARATION of the ANTIFUNGAL and ANTIBIOTIC drug nystatin and the CORTICOSTEROID drug triamcinolone acetonide. It can be used to treat serious fungal infections with inflammation. It is available as a cream for topical application.

✚▲ side-effects/warning: see NYSTATIN; TRIAMCINOLONE ACETONIDE

Nystaform

(Bayer) is a proprietary, prescription-only COMPOUND PREPARATION of the ANTIFUNGAL

and ANTIBIOTIC drug nystatin and the ANTISEPTIC agent chlorhexidine. It can be used to treat *Candida* fungal infections of the skin and is available as a cream for topical application.
✚▲ side-effects/warning: see CHLORHEXIDINE; NYSTATIN

Nystaform-HC

(Bayer) is a proprietary, prescription-only COMPOUND PREPARATION of the ANTIFUNGAL and ANTIBIOTIC drug nystatin and the ANTI-INFLAMMATORY and CORTICOSTEROID drug hydrocortisone. It can be used to treat fungal infections with inflammation of the skin, such as nappy rash. It is available as a cream for topical application.
✚▲ side-effects/warning: see HYDROCORTISONE; NYSTATIN

Nystan

(Squibb) is a range of proprietary, prescription-only preparations of the ANTIFUNGAL and ANTIBIOTIC drug nystatin. They can be used to treat fungal infections (eg. candidiasis; thrush) and are available in a variety of forms. Preparations for oral administration include tablets, a suspension, a gluten-, lactose- and sugar-free suspension, granules for solution and pastilles (for treating mouth infections). For vaginal and vulval infections there is a vaginal cream, a gel and pessaries (vaginal inserts). A cream, a gel, an ointment and dusting powder are available for topical application.
✚▲ side-effects/warning: see NYSTATIN

nystatin

is an ANTIFUNGAL and ANTIBIOTIC drug, which is effective when administered topically or orally. When taken orally, it is not absorbed into the blood and its antifungal action is restricted to the mouth and gastrointestinal tract. It is primarily used to treat the yeast infection candidiasis (thrush) of the skin, mucous membranes and intestinal tract. Administration is by many forms: tablets, a suspension, a

solution, pastilles, vaginal inserts (pessaries), creams, a gel, an ointment and a mouthwash.
✚ side-effects: there may be nausea, vomiting or diarrhoea, local irritation, sensitization of the mouth and a rash.
❂ **Related entries: Dermovate-NN; Flagyl Compak; Gregoderm; Mysteclin; Nystadermal; Nystaform; Nystaform-HC; Nystan; Nystatin-Dome; Terra-Cortril Nystatin; Timodine; Tinaderm-M; Tri-Adcortyl; Tri-Adcortyl Otic; Trimovate**

Nystatin-Dome

(Lagap) is a proprietary, prescription-only preparation of the ANTIFUNGAL and ANTIBIOTIC drug nystatin. It can be used to treat intestinal candidiasis (thrush) and oral infections and is available as a suspension.
✚▲ side-effects/warning: see NYSTATIN.

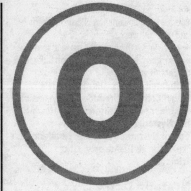

O

Occlusal

(Euroderma) is a proprietary, non-prescription preparation of the KERATOLYTIC agent salicylic acid (with lactic acid). It can be used to remove warts and hard skin, and is available as a liquid paint.

✚▲ side-effects/warning: see SALICYLIC ACID

octoxinol

is a SPERMICIDAL drug that is used to assist barrier methods of contraception. It is produced as a jelly.

✪ Related entry: Staycept

octreotide

is a long-lasting analogue of the hypothalamic HORMONE somatostatin (hypothalamic release-inhibiting hormone). It is used as an ANTICANCER drug for the relief of symptoms caused by the release of hormones from carcinoid tumours of the endocrine system, including VIPomas and glucagonomas, and for the short-term treatment of acromegaly. It is administered by subcutaneous or intravenous injection.

✚ side-effects: gastrointestinal upsets including nausea and vomiting, anorexia, bloating, pain, flatulence, fatty faeces and diarrhoea. Kidney dysfunction, gall stone formation and pain at injection site have been reported.

▲ warning: it should not be administered to patients who are pregnant or breast-feeding. In diabetes there may be a reduction in antidiabetic drug requirement. Gall bladder and thyroid function should be monitored. Withdrawal of treatment should be gradual.

✪ Related entry: Sandostatin

Ocufen

(Allergan) is a proprietary, prescription-only preparation of the (NSAID) NON-NARCOTIC ANALGESIC drug flurbiprofen (with polyvinyl alcohol). It can be used by topical application to inhibit constriction of the pupil during an operation on the eye. It is available as eye-drops.

+▲ side-effects/warning: see FLURBIPROFEN

Ocusert Pilo

(Rhône-Poulenc Rorer) is a proprietary, prescription-only preparation of the PARASYMPATHOMIMETIC drug pilocarpine. It can be used to constrict the pupil and treat glaucoma. It is available as plastic inserts (*Pilo-20* and *Pilo-40*) that are placed under the eyelid.

+▲ side-effects/warning: see PILOCARPINE

Odrik

(Roussel) is a proprietary, prescription-only preparation of the ACE INHIBITOR trandolapril. It can be used as an ANTIHYPERTENSIVE treatment in conjunction with other classes of drug. It is available as capsules.

+▲ side-effects/warning: see TRANDOLAPRIL

oestradiol

is the main female SEX HORMONE produced and secreted by the ovaries. It is an OESTROGEN and is used therapeutically to make up hormonal deficiencies, for instance, in HRT (hormone replacement therapy). Administration is oral in the form of tablets, or by injection or implants.

+▲ side-effects/warning: see under OESTROGEN

✪ Related entries: Climagest; Climaval; Cyclo-Progynova; Estracombi; Estraderm TTS; Estrapak 50; Estring; Evorel; Evorel Pak; Hormonin; Nuvelle; Oestradiol Implants; Progynova; Trisequens; Vagifem; Zumenon

Oestradiol Implants

(Organon) is a proprietary, prescription-only preparation of the OESTROGEN oestradiol. It can be used in HRT, and is available in the form of an implant.

+▲ side-effects/warning: see OESTRADIOL

Oestrifen

(Ashbourne) is a proprietary,

prescription-only preparation of the sex HORMONE ANTAGONIST tamoxifen, which, because it inhibits the effect of OESTROGENS, is used primarily as an ANTICANCER treatment for cancers that depend on the presence of oestrogen in women, particularly breast cancer. Additionally, it can be used to treat certain conditions of infertility. It is available as of tablets.

+▲ side-effects/warning: see TAMOXIFEN

oestriol

is a female SEX HORMONE produced and secreted by the ovary. An OESTROGEN. It is used therapeutically to make up hormonal deficiencies (sometimes in combination with a PROGESTOGEN) and to treat menstrual, menopausal, or other gynaecological problems (such as infertility). Administration is either oral as tablets or by topical application as an intravaginal cream or pessaries.

+▲ side-effects/warning: see under OESTROGEN

✪ Related entries: Hormonin; Ortho-Gynest; Ovestin; Trisequens

oestrogen

is the name given to the group of (STEROID) SEX HORMONES that promote the growth and functioning of the female sex organs and the development of female sexual characteristics. In their natural forms, they are produced and secreted mainly by the ovary (and to a small extent the placenta of pregnant women, the adrenal cortex, and – in men – the testes). Natural and synthesized oestrogens are used therapeutically, sometimes in combination with PROGESTOGENS, to treat menstrual, menopausal (HRT), or other gynaecological problems, and as ORAL CONTRACEPTIVES (in combination with progesterones). Some synthetic oestrogens are also used to treat certain cancers (eg. prostate and breast cancer). The best-known and most-used oestrogens

O

are OESTRADIOL, OESTRIOL, ETHINYLOESTRADIOL, MESTRANOL and STILBOESTROL.

✚ side-effects: depending on the dose, route of administration and the particular preparation used; there may be nausea, vomiting, weight gain and oedema (fluid accumulation in the tissues), tender and enlarged breasts, premenstrual syndrome-like symptoms, headache, depression; sometimes rash and changes in liver function.

▲ warning: they should not be administered to patients with certain oestrogen-dependent cancers, a history of thrombosis, inflamed endometrial lining of the uterus, or impaired liver function. Prolonged treatment (without oestrogen) increases the risk of cancer of the endometrium. Administer with caution to patients who are diabetic or epileptic, have certain heart or kidney disorders, multiple sclerosis, porphyria, who are pregnant or breast-feeding, or who have hypertension or migraine.

ofloxacin

is a broad-spectrum ANTIBACTERIAL and (QUINOLONE) ANTIBIOTIC drug. It is used to treat infections in patients who are allergic to penicillin, or who have infections resistant to more commonly used antibacterials. It can be used to treat infections of the genitourinary tract, including both gonorrhoea and non-gonorrhoeal infections, some respiratory infections, infections of the cervix, and septicaemia. Administration is either oral in the form of tablets or by intravenous infusion.

✚▲ side-effects/warning: see under NALIDIXIC ACID. Administer with caution to patients with a history of psychiatric illness or G6PD deficiency. It should not be used in epileptics. Other possible side-effects include inflamed tendons, anxiety, unsteady gait, tremor, tingling in the extremities, psychotic reactions, and effects on the blood and cardiovascular system.

420 ✪ Related entries: Exocin, Tarivid

Oilatum

(Stiefel) is a proprietary, non-prescription preparation of the the EMOLLIENT arachis oil. It can be used to soften skin and is available as an ointment, a shower emollient and a bath emulsion.

✚▲ side-effects/warning: see ARACHIS OIL

*ointments

is a general term that is used to describe a group of essentially greasy preparations which are insoluble in water and so do not wash off. They are used as bases for many therapeutic preparations for topical application (particularly in the treatment of dry lesions or ophthalmic complaints). Most ointments have a form of PARAFFIN as their base, but a few contain LANOLIN and WOOL ALCOHOLS, which may cause sensitivity reactions in a some people.

Olbetam

(Pharmacia) is a proprietary, prescription-only preparation of the the LIPID-LOWERING DRUG acipimox. It can be used in hyperlipidaemia to reduce the levels, or change the proportions, of various lipids (eg. cholesterol and LDL) in the bloodstream. It is available as capsules.

✚▲ side-effects/warning: see ACIPIMOX

olive oil

can be used therapeutically to soften earwax prior to syringing the ears, or to treat the yellow-brown, flaking skin that commonly appears on the heads of young infants (cradle cap) prior to shampooing.

olsalazine sodium

is an AMINOSALICYLATE drug. It is used primarily to induce and maintain remission of the symptoms of ulcerative colitis – often in patients who are sensitive to the more commonly prescribed drug sulphasalazine. Administration is oral in the form of capsules.

✚ side-effects: nausea, watery diarrhoea,

abdominal cramps, headaches, dyspepsia, joint pain and rashes.

▲ warning: it should not be administered to patients who are allergic to aspirin or other salicylates, or where there is impaired kidney function; administer with caution to those who are pregnant or breast-feeding.

○ Related entry: Dipentum

omega-3 marine triglycerides

are derived from fish oils and used as LIPID-LOWERING DRUGS in hyperlipidaemia to reduce the levels, or change the proportions, of various lipids (eg. cholesterol and LDL) in the bloodstream. They are available as capsules and a liquid.

✚▲ side-effects/warning: there may be belching and nausea.

○ Related entry: Maxepa

omeprazole

is an ULCER-HEALING DRUG. It works by being a PROTON-PUMP INHIBITOR and so interferes with the secretion of gastric acid from the parietal (acid-producing) cells of the stomach lining. It is used for the treatment of benign gastric and duodenal ulcers (including those that complicate NSAID therapy), Zollinger-Ellison syndrome and reflux oesophagitis (inflammation of the oesophagus caused by regurgitation of acid and enzymes). It can also be used in conjunction with antibiotics to treat gastric *Helicobacter pylori* infection. Omeptazole may be tried in cases where there has been a poor response to conventional therapies, especially H$_2$-ANTAGONISTS.

Administration is oral in the form of capsules.

✚ side-effects: these include diarrhoea or constipation, nausea, flatulence; dizziness, headaches, sleep disorders, disturbances of vision, oedema (accumulation of fluid in the tissues), hair loss, liver dysfunction, gynaecomasia and sometimes impotence in males, blood, skin and mood disorders

(some of these last side-effects occur only in the very ill).

▲ warning: administer only when the ulcer has been established to be benign; avoid its use in patients who are pregnant or breast-feeding.

○ Related entry: Losec

Omnopon

(Roche) is a proprietary, prescription-only preparation of the (OPIOID) NARCOTIC ANALGESIC drug papaveretum, which is on the Controlled Drugs List. It is used primarily prior to, during, or following surgery to relieve severe pain. It is available in a form for injection.

✚▲ side-effects/warning: see PAPAVERETUM

Oncovin

(Lilly) is a proprietary, prescription-only preparation of the (CYTOTOXIC) ANTICANCER drug vincristine sulphate. It can be used in the treatment of acute leukaemias, lymphomas and certain solid tumours. It is available in a form for injection.

✚▲ side-effects/warning: see VINCRISTINE SULPHATE

ondansetron

is a recently introduced ANTI-EMETIC and ANTINAUSEANT drug. It gives relief from nausea and vomiting, especially in patients receiving radiotherapy or chemotherapy and where other drugs are ineffective. It acts by blocking the action of the naturally occurring mediator SEROTONIN. Administration is either oral as tablets or by injection or infusion.

✚ side-effects: headache, constipation, warmth or flushing in the head and over stomach. Hypersensitivity reactions, effects on liver enzymes and chest pain have been reported.

▲ warning: administer with caution to patients with liver impairment, or who are pregnant or breast-feeding.

○ Related entry: Zofran

O

One-A-Day Antihistamine Tablets

(Boots) is a proprietary, non-prescription preparation of the ANTIHISTAMINE drug terfenadine. It can be used to treat the symptoms of allergic disorders such as hay fever and urticaria. It is available as tablets.

✚▲ side-effects/warning: see TERFENADINE

One-Alpha

(Leo) is a proprietary, prescription-only preparation of the VITAMIN D analogue alfacalcidol. It can be used to treat a deficiency of vitamin D and is available as capsules, a solution and in a form for injection.

✚▲ side-effects/warning: see ALFACALCIDOL

Operidine

(Janssen) is a proprietary, prescription-only preparation of the (OPIOID) NARCOTIC ANALGESIC drug phenoperidine hydrochloride, which is on the Controlled Drugs List. It is used primarily during surgery and is available in a form for injection.

✚▲ side-effects/warning: see PHENOPERIDINE HYDROCHLORIDE

Ophthaine

(Squibb) is a proprietary, prescription-only preparation of the LOCAL ANAESTHETIC drug proxymetacaine (as hydrochloride). It can be used during ophthalmic procedures and is available as eye-drops.

✚▲ side-effects/warning: see PROXYMETACAINE

*opiate

refers to the members of a group of drugs that are chemically ALKALOIDS, similar to constituents of opium and which influence functions of the central nervous system. Because of this property they can be used as NARCOTIC ANALGESICS to relieve pain. They also have two other actions: they can be used as ANTITUSSIVES to reduce coughing and, because of an ANTIMOTILITY action, as powerful ANTIDIARRHOEAL drugs. Therapeutically, the most important opiate is probably morphine. They are all potentially habituating (addictive), especially the synthetic derivative of heroin, diamorphine. Today, the term OPIOID is increasingly used to embrace all drugs irrespective of chemical structure, including naturally occuring peptide NEUROTRANSMITTERS, that share this common pharmacology.

Opilon

(Parke-Davis) is a proprietary, prescription-only preparation of ALPHA-ADRENOCEPTOR BLOCKER drug thymoxamine, which has VASODILATOR properties. It can be used to treat peripheral vascular disease (primary Raynaud's phenomenon) and is available as tablets.

✚▲ side-effects/warning: see THYMOXAMINE

*opioid

is a term that has superseded OPIATE. Opioids influence the central nervous system and so they can be used as NARCOTIC ANALGESICS to relieve pain. They can also be used therapeutically for their ANTITUSSIVE and ANTIDIARRHOEAL, or ANTIMOTILITY, actions. It is now recognized that the characteristic actions of opioids are due to their ability to mimic natural NEUROTRANSMITTERS (enkephalins, endorphins, dynorphins) and because of this the term opioid is used for any chemical (synthetic or natural) that acts on opioid RECEPTORS.

Opioid drugs have similar pharmacological actions and potential side-effects. But the severity of these effects, and the strength of their analgesic and other therapeutic actions, varies with individual drugs, the dose and route of administration. The risk of habituation (addiction) is also much greater with the stronger drugs (eg. morphine and diamorphine) than with the weaker ones (eg. dextromethorphan, codeine and dihydrocodeine).

See: ALFENTANIL; BUPRENORPHINE; CO-CODAMOL; CO-DYDRAMOL; CO-PHENOTROPE; CO-PROXAMOL; CODEINE PHOSPHATE; DEXTROMETHORPHAN HYDROBROMIDE; DEXTROMORAMIDE; DEXTROPROPOXYPHENE HYDROCHLORIDE; DIAMORPHINE HYDROCHLORIDE; DIPIPANONE; FENTANYL; LOPERAMIDE HYDROCHLORIDE; MEPTAZINOL; METHADONE HYDROCHLORIDE; MORPHINE SULPHATE; NALBUPHINE HYDROCHLORIDE; NALOXONE HYDROCHLORIDE; NALTREXONE HYDROCHLORIDE; PAPAVERETUM; PENTAZOCINE; PETHIDINE HYDROCHLORIDE; PHENAZOCINE HYDROBROMIDE; PHENOPERIDINE HYDROCHLORIDE; PHOLCODINE; TRAMADOL HYDROCHLORIDE.

✚ side-effects: there may be nausea and vomiting, loss of appetite, urinary retention and constipation. There is commonly sedation and euphoria, which may lead to a state of mental detachment or confusion. Also, there may be a dry mouth, flushing of the face, sweating, headache, palpitations, slowed heart rate, postural hypotension (a lowering of blood pressure on standing, causing dizziness), miosis (pupil constriction), mood change and hallucinations.

▲ warning: opioids (even the weaker ones) should not be administered to patients with depressed breathing or asthma, who have raised intracranial pressure, or a head injury. They should be administered with caution to those with hypotension, certain liver or kidney disorders, or hypothyroidism (under-activity of the thyroid gland); or who are pregnant or breast-feeding. Dosage should be reduced for the elderly or debilitated. Treatment by injection may cause pain and tissue damage at the site of the injection.

*opioid antagonist

is a term used to describe a drug that opposes the actions of OPIOID drugs, which are used for a number of purposes, including as NARCOTIC ANALGESICS for pain relief, ANTITUSSIVES and as ANTIDIARRHOEAL or ANTIMOTILITY treatments. It is now recognized that opioids achieve their characteristic actions by mimicking naturally occurring peptide NEUROTRANSMITTERS (enkephalins, endorphins and dynorphins), so now the term opioid is used to describe any chemical, synthetic or natural, that acts on *opioid* RECEPTORS.

Opioid antagonist drugs occupy these receptors without stimulating them and so can reverse the actions of a wide range of opioid drugs. This is an extremely beneficial action, because an opioid antagonist such as NALOXONE HYDROCHLORIDE can effectively reverse the respiratory depression, coma, or convulsions that result from an overdose of opioids. Administration of naloxone hydrochloride is by intramuscular or intravenous injection and may be repeated at short intervals until there is some response. It is also used at the end of operations to reverse respiratory depression caused by narcotic analgesics, and in newborn babies where mothers have been given large amounts of opioid (such as pethidine) for pain relief during labour. It is also very effective in reviving individuals who have overdosed on heroin.

NALTREXONE HYDROCHLORIDE, another opioid antagonist, is used in detoxification therapy to help prevent relapse of formerly opioid-dependent patients. It is able to do this because as an antagonist of dependence-forming opioids (such as heroin), it will precipitate withdrawal symptoms in those already taking opioids.

Opticrom

(Fisons) is a proprietary, prescription-only preparation of the ANTI-ALLERGIC drug sodium cromoglycate. It can be used to treat allergic conjunctivitis and is available as eye-drops (called *Opticrom Aqueous*) and an eye ointment. It is also available without a prescription subject to certain conditions of quantity and use.

✚▲ side-effects/warning: see sodium CROMOGLYCATE

O

Opticrom Allergy Eye Drops

(Fisons) is a proprietary, non-prescription preparation of the ANTI-ALLERGIC drug sodium cromoglycate. It can be used to treat allergic conjunctivitis and is available as eye-drops.

+▲ side-effects/warning: see SODIUM CROMOGLYCATE

Optimax

(Merck) is a proprietary, prescription-only preparation of the ANTIDEPRESSANT drug tryptophan. It can be used to treat long-standing depressive illness where no other treatment is suitable. It is available as tablets.

+▲ side-effects/warning: see TRYPTOPHAN

Optimine

(Schering-Plough) is a proprietary, non-prescription preparation of the ANTIHISTAMINE drug azatadine maleate. It can be used to relieve the symptoms of allergic reactions such as hay fever and urticaria. It is available as tablets and a syrup for dilution.

+▲ side-effects/warning: SEE AZATADINE MALEATE

Optrex Hayfever Allergy Eye Drops

(Crookes Healthcare) is a proprietary, non-prescription preparation of the ANTI-ALLERGIC drug sodium cromoglycate. It can be used to treat allergic conjunctivitis and is available as eye-drops.

+▲ side-effects/warning: see SODIUM CROMOGLYCATE

Orabase

(ConvaTec) is a proprietary, non-prescription preparation of CARMELLOSE SODIUM (with pectin and gelatin). It can be used for the mechanical protection of oral and perioral lesions and is available as an oral paste .

Orahesive

(ConvaTec) is a proprietary, non-prescription preparation of CARMELLOSE SODIUM (with pectin and gelatin). It can be used for the mechanical protection of oral and perioral lesions and is available as a powder.

Oralcer

(Vitabiotics) is a proprietary, non-prescription preparation of the ANTIMICROBIAL drug clioquinol (and vitamin C). It can be used to treat infections and ulcers in the mouth and is available as lozenges.

+▲ side-effects/warning: see CLIOQUINOL

*oral contraceptives

are prophylactic (preventive) SEX HORMONE preparations, which are taken by women to prevent conception following sexual intercourse and are commonly referred to as the *pill*. The majority of oral contraceptives contain both an OESTROGEN and a PROGESTOGEN. The oestrogen inhibits the release of FOLLICLE-STIMULATING HORMONE (FSH) and prevents egg development; the progestogen inhibits release of LUTEINIZING HORMONE (LH), prevents ovulation and makes the cervix mucus unsuitable for sperm. Their combined action is to alter the uterine lining (endometrium) and prevent any fertilized eggs from implanting. This type of preparation is known as the *combined oral contraceptive* (COC), or *combined pill*, and is taken daily for three weeks and stopped for one week during which menstruation occurs.

Two forms of the combined pill (the phased formulations) are the biphasic and triphasic pills. In these the hormonal content varies according to the time of the month at which each pill is to be taken (and are produced in a 'calendar pack') and the dose is reduced to the bare minimum. Another type of pill is the progestogen-only pill (POP) and this is thought to work by making the cervical mucus inhospitable to sperm and by preventing implantation. This form has the advantage that it can be used by breast-feeding women.

An alternative to the progesterone-only pill is to administer the progestogen as an injection or an implant (which is renewed every three months). Post-coital contraception is also available in an emergency and involves the use of a high dose combined preparation – the morning-after pill. All the oral contraceptive preparations produce side-effects and a form that is suited to each patient requires expert advice. Various oral contraceptive preparations are also used in the treatment of certain menstrual problems.

+▲ side-effects/warning: see under OESTROGEN; PROGESTOGEN. Adverse effects are more pronounced with the combined pill; thromboembolism, weight gain, nausea, flushing, irritability, depression, dizziness, increased blood pressure, impaired liver function and glucose tolerance, amenorrhoea after coming off the pill. Slight changes in cervical and breast cancer rates (depending on dose and preparation).

○ Related entries: BiNovum; Brevinor; Conova 30; Eugynon 30; Femodene; Femodene ED; Femulen; Loestrin 20; Loestrin 30; Logynon; Logynon ED; Marvelon; Mercilon; Microgynon 30; Micronor; Microval; Minulet; Neocon-1/35; Neogest; Norgeston; Noriday; Norimin; Norinyl-1; Ortho-Novin 1/50; Ovran; Ovran 30; Ovranette; Ovysmen; Schering PC4; Synphase; Tri-Minulet; TriNovum; TriNovum ED; Triadene; Trinordiol

Oraldene

(Warner-Wellcome) is a proprietary, non-prescription preparation of the ANTISEPTIC agent hexetidine. It can be used to treat minor mouth infections, including thrush and sores and ulcers in the mouth. It is available as a mouthwash.

+▲ side-effects/warning: see HEXETIDINE

*oral hypoglycaemic

drugs are synthetic agents taken by mouth to reduce the levels of glucose (sugar) in the bloodstream and are used mainly in the treatment of Type II diabetes (non-insulin-dependent diabetes mellitus; NIDDM; maturity-onset diabetes) when there is some residual capacity in the pancreas to produce the HORMONE insulin. The main type of oral hypoglycaemic drug is the SULPHONYLUREA group (eg. CHLORPROPAMIDE and GLIBENCLAMIDE), but the (BIGUANIDE) METFORMIN HYDROCHLORIDE and the drug ACARBOSE are also effective. Additionally, GUAR GUM can be administered in the diet. However, INSULIN, which is mainly used in Type I diabetes (insulin-dependent diabetes mellitus; IDDM; juvenile-onset diabetes), can not be taken by mouth and must be injected.

Oramorph

(Boehringer Ingelheim) is a proprietary, prescription-only preparation of the (OPIOID) NARCOTIC ANALGESIC drug morphine sulphate. It can be used primarily to relieve pain following surgery, or the pain experienced during the final stages of terminal malignant disease. It is available as oral solutions, oral unit-dose vials and as modified-release tablets called *Oramorph SR*. The more concentrated unit-dose vials and the SR tablets are on the Controlled Drugs List and the SR tablets are not administered to children.

+▲ side-effects/warning: see MORPHINE SULPHATE

Orap

(Janssen) is a proprietary, prescription-only preparation of the ANTIPSYCHOTIC drug pimozide. It can be used (with care) to treat and tranquillize patients with psychotic disorders, particularly those with schizophrenia and also to treat Gilles de la Tourette syndrome. It is available as tablets.

+▲ side-effects/warning: see PIMOZIDE

O

Orbenin

(Forley) is a proprietary, prescription-only preparation of the ANTIBACTERIAL and (PENICILLIN) ANTIBIOTIC drug cloxacillin. It can be used to treat bacterial infections, particularly staphylococcal infections that prove to be resistant to penicillin. It is available as capsules and in a form for injection.

✚▲ side-effects/warning: SEE CLOXACILLIN

orciprenaline sulphate

is a SYMPATHOMIMETIC and BETA-RECEPTOR STIMULANT that has some beta$_2$-receptor selectivity (though much less than SALBUTAMOL and is therefore more likely to cause side-effects). It is mainly used as a BRONCHODILATOR in reversible obstructive airways disease and as an ANTI-ASTHMATIC treatment in severe acute asthma. It can also be used for the alleviation of symptoms of chronic bronchitis and emphysema. Administration is by aerosol.

✚▲ side-effects/warning: see under SALBUTAMOL; but it is more likely to cause cardiac problems such as arrhythmias.

○ Related entry: Alupent

Orelox

(Roussel) is a proprietary, prescription-only preparation of the ANTIBACTERIAL and (CEPHALOSPORIN) ANTIBIOTIC drug cefpodoxime. It can be used to treat infections of the respiratory tract (including bronchitis and pneumonia) and tonsillitis and is usually reserved for infections that are recurrent, chronic, or resistant to other drugs. It is available as tablets.

✚▲ side-effects/warning: see CEFPODOXIME

Orgafol

(Organon) is a proprietary, prescription-only preparation of a pituitary HORMONE called urofollitrophin, which is prepared from human menopausal urine containing FOLLICLE-STIMULATING HORMONE (FSH). It is used primarily as an INFERTILITY TREATMENT for women suffering from specific hormonal deficiencies. It is available in a form for injection.

✚▲ side-effects/warning: see UROFOLLITROPHIN

Orgaran

(Organon) is a proprietary, prescription-only preparation of (the heparinoid) danaparoid sodium. It can be used as an ANTICOAGULANT for the prevention of deep vein thrombosis, particularly in orthopaedic surgery. It is available in a form for injection.

✚▲ side-effects/warning: see DANAPAROID SODIUM

Original Andrews Salts

(Sterling Health) is a proprietary, non-prescription COMPOUND PREPARATION of the ANTACID sodium bicarbonate, the (*osmotic*) LAXATIVE magnesium sulphate and citric acid. It can be used for the relief of upset stomach, indigestion, symptoms of overindulgence and constipation. It is available as an effervescent powder and is not normally given to children under three years, except on medical advice.

✚▲ side-effects/warning: SEE MAGNESIUM CARBONATE; MAGNESIUM SULPHATE; SODIUM BICARBONATE

Orimeten

(Ciba) is a proprietary, prescription-only preparation of the sex HORMONE ANTAGONIST aminoglutethimide. It can be used as an ANTICANCER treatment for Cushing's syndrome caused by cancer of the thyroid gland. It is available as tablets.

✚▲ side-effects/warning: see AMINOGLUTETHIMIDE

Orlept

(CP Pharmaceuticals) is a proprietary, prescription-only preparation of the ANTICONVULSANT and ANTI-EPILEPTIC drug sodium valproate. It can be used to treat all forms of epilepsy and is available as tablets and a liquid.

✚▲ side-effects/warning: see SODIUM VALPROATE

orphenadrine citrate

is an ANTICHOLINERGIC drug, which is also used as a SKELETAL MUSCLE RELAXANT for short-term, symptomatic relief of skeletal muscle spasm. It works by an action on the central nervous system and is administered by injection. See also ORPHENADRINE HYDROCHLORIDE.
✚▲ side-effects/warning: see under BENZHEXOL HYDROCHLORIDE. Avoid its use in patients with porphyria.
⚙ Related entry: Norflex

orphenadrine hydrochloride

is an ANTICHOLINERGIC drug, which is used in the treatment of some types of parkinsonism (see ANTIPARKINSONISM). It increases mobility and decreases rigidity and tremor, but has only a limited effect on bradykinesia and also the tendency to produce an excess of saliva is reduced. It is thought to work by correcting the over-effectiveness of the NEUROTRANSMITTER ACETYLCHOLINE (cholinergic excess), which is caused by the deficiency of dopamine that occurs in parkinsonism. It also has the capacity to treat these conditions, in some cases, where they are produced by drugs. Administration is oral in the form of tablets or an elixir.
✚▲ side-effects/warning: see under BENZHEXOL HYDROCHLORIDE; but it is more euphoric and may cause insomnia. Avoid its use in patients with porphyria.
⚙ Related entries: Biorphen; Disipal

Ortho-Creme

(Ortho) is a proprietary, non-prescription SPERMICIDAL CONTRACEPTIVE for use in combination with barrier methods of contraception (such as a condom). It is available as a cream containing nonoxinol in a water-soluble basis.
✚▲ side-effects/warning: see NONOXINOL

Ortho Dienoestrol

(Cilag) is a proprietary, prescription-only preparation of the OESTROGEN dienoestrol, which is a SEX HORMONE. It can be used to treat infection and irritation of the membranous surface of the vagina, including vaginal atrophy in HRT (hormone-replacement therapy). It is available as a vaginal cream.
✚▲ side-effects/warning: see DIENOESTROL

Ortho-Gynest

(Cilag) is a proprietary, prescription-only preparation of the OESTROGEN oestriol, a SEX HORMONE, which can be used to treat infection and irritation of the membranous surface of the vagina, including vaginal atrophy in HRT. It is available as an intravaginal cream and pessaries.
✚▲ side-effects/warning: see OESTRIOL

Ortho-Gynol

(Ortho) is a proprietary, non-prescription SPERMICIDAL CONTRACEPTIVE for use in combination with barrier methods of contraception (such as a condom). It is available as a jelly containing *p*-di-isobutylphenoxypolyethoxyethanol.
✚▲ side-effects/warning: see under NONOXINOL

Orthoforms

(Ortho) is a proprietary, non-prescription SPERMICIDAL CONTRACEPTIVE for use in combination with barrier methods of contraception (such as a condom). It is availabe as a pessary containing nonoxinol.
✚▲ side-effects/warning: see NONOXINOL

Ortho-Novin 1/50

(Cilag) is a proprietary, prescription-only COMPOUND PREPARATION that can be used as a (*monophasic*) ORAL CONTRACEPTIVE (and also for certain menstrual problems) of the type that combines an OESTROGEN and a PROGESTOGEN, in this case mestranol and norethisterone. It is available in the form of tablets in a calendar pack.

O

427

O ✚▲ side-effects/warning: see MESTRANOL; NORETHISTERONE

Orudis

(Rhône-Poulenc Rorer) is a proprietary, prescription-only preparation of the (NSAID) NON-NARCOTIC ANALGESIC and ANTIRHEUMATIC drug ketoprofen. It can be used to relieve arthritic and rheumatic pain and inflammation, to treat other musculoskeletal disorders, pain and inflammation following orthopaedic surgery and period pain. It is available as capsules and suppositories.
✚▲ side-effects/warning: see KETOPROFEN

Oruvail Gel 2.5%

(Rhône-Poulenc Rorer) is a proprietary, prescription-only preparation of the (NSAID) NON-NARCOTIC ANALGESIC and ANTIRHEUMATIC drug ketoprofen, which also has COUNTER-IRRITANT, or RUBEFACIENT, actions. It can be applied to the skin for symptomatic relief of underlying muscle or joint pain. It is available as a gel for topical application to the skin. It is not normally used for children, except on medical advice.
✚▲ side-effects/warning: see KETOPROFEN; but adverse effects on topical application are limited.

Osmolax

(Ashbourne) is a proprietary, non-prescription preparation of the (*osmotic*) LAXATIVE lactulose. It can be used to relieve constipation and is available as an oral solution.
✚▲ side-effects/warning: see LACTULOSE

Ossopan

(Sanofi Winthrop) is a proprietary, non-prescription preparation of calcium carbonate. It can be used as a MINERAL SUPPLEMENT for calcium in cases of calcium deficiency. It is available as tablets and granules to be taken by mouth.
✚▲ side-effects/warning: see CALCIUM CARBONATE

Otex

(DDD) is a proprietary, non-prescription preparation of the ANTISEPTIC and ANTIFUNGAL agent hydrogen peroxide in a complex with urea in glycerol. It can be used to dissolve and wash out earwax and is available as ear-drops.
✚▲ side-effects/warning: see GLYCEROL; HYDROGEN PEROXIDE; UREA

Otomize

(Stafford-Miller) is a proprietary, prescription-only COMPOUND PREPARATION of the CORTICOSTEROID drug dexamethasone and the ANTIBACTERIAL and (AMINOGLYCOSIDE) ANTIBIOTIC drug neomycin sulphate (and acetic acid). It can be used to treat bacterial infections in the outer ear and is available as an ear-spray.
✚▲ side-effects/warning: see DEXAMETHASONE; NEOMYCIN SULPHATE

Otosporin

(Wellcome) is a proprietary, prescription-only COMPOUND PREPARATION of the CORTICOSTEROID drug hydrocortisone, the ANTIBACTERIAL and (AMINOGLYCOSIDE) ANTIBIOTIC drug neomycin sulphate and the antibacterial and (POLYMYXIN) antibiotic drug polymyxin B sulphate. It can be used to treat infections and inflammation in the outer ear and is available as ear-drops.
▲ warning: see HYDROCORTISONE; NEOMYCIN SULPHATE; POLYMYXIN B SULPHATE

Otrivine Adult Formula Drops

(Zyma Healthcare) is a proprietary, non-prescription preparation of the SYMPATHOMIMETIC and VASOCONSTRICTOR drug xylometazoline hydrochloride. It can be used as a NASAL DECONGESTANT for the symptomatic relief of nasal congestion, allergic and other forms of rhinitis (including hay fever) and sinusitis. It is available as drops and is not normally given to children under 12 years, except on medical advice.

+▲ side-effects/warning: see
XYLOMETAZOLINE HYDROCHLORIDE

Otrivine Adult Formula Spray

(Zyma Healthcare) is a proprietary, non-prescription preparation of the SYMPATHOMIMETIC and VASOCONSTRICTOR drug xylometazoline hydrochloride. It can be used as a NASAL DECONGESTANT for the symptomatic relief of nasal congestion, allergic and other forms of rhinitis (including hay fever) and sinusitis. It is available as a spray and is not normally given to children under 12 years, except on medical advice.

+▲ side-effects/warning: see
XYLOMETAZOLINE HYDROCHLORIDE

Otrivine-Antistin

(CIBA Vision) is a proprietary, non-prescription COMPOUND PREPARATION of the ANTIHISTAMINE antazoline (as antazoline sulphate) and the SYMPATHOMIMETIC and VASOCONSTRICTOR drug xylometazoline hydrochloride. It can be used for the relief of allergic conjunctivitis and is available as eye-drops.

+▲ side-effects/warning: see ANTAZOLINE;
XYLOMETAZOLINE HYDROCHLORIDE

Otrivine Children's Formula Drops

(Zyma Healthcare) is a proprietary, non-prescription preparation of the SYMPATHOMIMETIC and VASOCONSTRICTOR drug xylometazoline hydrochloride. It can be used as a NASAL DECONGESTANT for the symptomatic relief of nasal congestion, allergic and other forms of rhinitis (including hay fever) and sinusitis. It is available as a spray and is not normally given to children under two years, except on medical advice.

+▲ side-effects/warning: see
XYLOMETAZOLINE HYDROCHLORIDE

Ovestin

(Organon) is a proprietary, prescription-only preparation of the OESTROGEN oestriol. It can be used in HRT and is available as tablets.

+▲ side-effects/warning: see OESTRIOL

Ovex Tablets

(Janssen) is a proprietary, non-prescription preparation of the ANTHELMINTIC drug mebendazole. It can be used to treat infection by threadworms and is available as chewable tablets. It is not normally given to children under two years, except on medical advice.

+▲ side-effects/warning: see MEBENDAZOLE

Ovran

(Wyeth) is a proprietary, prescription-only COMPOUND PREPARATION that can be used as a (*monophasic*) ORAL CONTRACEPTIVE (and also for certain menstrual problems) of the type that combines an OESTROGEN and a PROGESTOGEN, in this case ethinyloestradiol and levonorgestrel. It is available in the form of tablets in a calendar pack.

+▲ side-effects/warning: see
ETHINYLOESTRADIOL; LEVONORGESTREL

Ovran 30

(Wyeth) is a proprietary, prescription-only COMPOUND PREPARATION that can be used as a (*monophasic*) ORAL CONTRACEPTIVE (and also for certain menstrual problems) of the type that combines an OESTROGEN and a PROGESTOGEN, in this case ethinyloestradiol and levonorgestrel. It is available in the form of tablets in a calendar pack.

+▲ side-effects/warning: see
ETHINYLOESTRADIOL; LEVONORGESTREL

Ovranette

(Wyeth) is proprietary, prescription-only COMPOUND PREPARATION that can be used as a (*monophasic*) ORAL CONTRACEPTIVE (and also for certain menstrual problems) of the type that combines an OESTROGEN

O

and a PROGESTOGEN, in this case ethinyloestradiol and levonorgestrel. It is available in the form of tablets in a calendar pack.

+▲ side-effects/warning: see ETHINYLOESTRADIOL; LEVONORGESTREL

Ovysmen

(Ortho) is a proprietary, prescription-only COMPOUND PREPARATION that can be used as a (*monophasic*) ORAL CONTRACEPTIVE (and also for certain menstrual problems) of the type that combines an OESTROGEN and a PROGESTOGEN, in this case ethinyloestradiol and norethisterone. It is available in the form of tablets in a calendar pack.

+▲ side-effects/warning: see NORETHISTERONE; ETHINYLOESTRADIOL

Owbridge's for Dry Tickly and Allergy Coughs

(Chefaro) is a proprietary, non-prescription preparation of the (OPIOID) NARCOTIC ANALGESIC and ANTITUSSIVE drug dextromethorphan hydrobromide with glycerine. It can be used for the symptomatic relief of dry, ticklish unproductive coughs. It is available as an oral liquid and is not normally given to children, except on medical advice.

+▲ side-effects/warning: see DEXTROMETHORPHAN HYDROBROMIDE

oxatomide

is an ANTIHISTAMINE drug, which can be used to relieve the symptoms of hay fever, urticaria (itchy skin rash) and food allergy. Administration is oral in the form of tablets.

+▲ side-effects/warning: see under ANTIHISTAMINE. It may increase appetite and cause weight gain. Because of its sedative property, the performance of skilled tasks such as driving may be impaired.

◎ Related entry: Tinset

oxazepam

is a BENZODIAZEPINE drug, which is used

as an ANXIOLYTIC in the short-term treatment of anxiety. Administration is oral in the form of capsules or tablets.

+▲ side-effects/warning: see under BENZODIAZEPINE

oxerutins

are mixtures of RUTOSIDES that are thought to reduce the fragility and the permeability of capillary blood vessels. They are used to treat disorders of the veins, for example cramp in the legs and for oedema (accumulation of fluid in the tissues). Administration is oral as capsules.

+ side-effects: flushing, headache, rashes and gastrointestinal disturbances.

◎ Related entry: Paroven

oxethazaine

is a LOCAL ANAESTHETIC drug, which is used by topical application for the relief of local pain. It is a constituent of a proprietary ANTACID that is administered as an oral suspension.
Related entry: MUCAINE

oxitropium bromide

is an ANTICHOLINERGIC drug that has the properties of a BRONCHODILATOR. It is primarily used to treat chronic bronchitis, but it can also be used as an ANTI-ASTHMATIC. Administration is by aerosol.

+▲ side-effects/warning: see under IPRATROPIUM BROMIDE. There may be blurring of vision.

◎ Related entry: Oxivent

Oxivent

(Boehringer Ingelheim) is a proprietary, prescription-only preparation of the ANTICHOLINERGIC drug oxitropium bromide, which also has BRONCHODILATOR properties. It can be used to treat chronic bronchitis and other disorders of the upper respiratory tract. It is available as an aerosol spray administered from a breath-activated *Autohaler* and as a

metered aerosol.
+▲ side-effects/warning: see OXITROPIUM
BROMIDE

oxpentifylline

(pentoxifylline) is a VASODILATOR drug. It
dilates the blood vessels of the extremities
and can be used to treat peripheral
vascular disease (Raynaud's
phenomenon). Administration is oral in
the form of tablets.
+ side-effects: gastrointestinal disturbances;
headache, dizziness; sometimes flushing and
a speeding of the heart.
▲ warning: it should not be used in patients
with brain haemorrhage, or with certain heart
disorders.
❂ Related entry: Trental

oxprenolol hydrochloride

is a BETA-BLOCKER that can be used as an
ANTIHYPERTENSIVE treatment for raised
blood pressure, as an ANTI-ANGINA
treatment to relieve symptoms and
improve exercise tolerance and as an
ANTI-ARRHYTHMIC to regularize heartbeat
and to treat myocardial infarction. It can
also be used as an ANXIOLYTIC treatment,
particularly for symptomatic relief of
tremor and palpitations. Administration
is oral in the form of tablets and
modified-release tablets. It is also
available, as an antihypertensive
treatment, in the form of COMPOUND
PREPARATIONS with a DIURETIC.
+▲ side-effects/warnings: see under
PROPRANOLOL HYDROCHLORIDE
**❂ Related entries: Apsolox;
Slow-Trasicor; Trasicor; Trasidrex**

Oxy 5 Lotion

(SK&F) is a proprietary, non-prescription
preparation of the KERATOLYTIC and
ANTIMICROBIAL drug benzoyl peroxide
(5%). It can be used for the treatment of
acne and spots and is available as a lotion
for topical application.
+▲ side-effects/warning: see BENZOYL
PEROXIDE

Oxy 10 Lotion

(SK&F) is a proprietary, non-prescription
preparation of the KERATOLYTIC and
ANTIMICROBIAL drug benzoyl peroxide
(10%). It can be used for the treatment of
acne and spots and is available as a lotion
for topical application.
+▲ side-effects/warning: SEE BENZOYL
PEROXIDE

oxybuprocaine hydrochloride

is a LOCAL ANAESTHETIC drug, which is
used by topical application in ophthalmic
procedures. Aministration is by eye-drops.
+ side-effects: there may be initial stinging
on application.
**❂ Related entry: Minims Benoxinate
(Oxybuprocaine) Hydrochloride**

oxybutynin hydrochloride

is an ANTICHOLINERGIC drug. It can be used
as an ANTISPASMODIC to treat urinary
frequency, incontinence and bladder
spasms. Administration is oral in the form
of tablets or an elixir.
+ side-effects: these include dry mouth,
blurred vision, constipation, nausea,
abdominal discomfort, difficulty in urination,
flushing of the face, headache, dizziness,
diarrhoea, dry skin and heart irregularities.
▲ warning: it should not be administered to
patients with intestinal obstruction, severe
ulcerative colitis, toxic megacolon, glaucoma,
or bladder obstruction. Administer with care
to those with certain heart, liver, or kidney
disorders, hyperthyroidism, prostatic
hypertrophy, hiatus hernia with reflux
oesophagitis (inflammation of the
oesophagus caused by regurgitation of acid
and enzymes), porphyria; or who are
pregnant or breast-feeding.
❂ Related entries: Cystrin; Ditropan

oxymetazoline hydrochloride

is a SYMPATHOMIMETIC, an alpha-
adrenoreceptor stimulant, generally used
for its VASOCONSTRICTOR properties which

O

O make it an effective NASAL DECONGESTANT. It is applied topically to the nasal passages where it constricts the blood vessels of the nose, reducing congestion in the nasal mucous membranes and possibly also reducing secretions. Administration is in the form of nose-drops or a nasal spray.

✚▲ side-effects/warning: see under XYLOMETAZOLINE HYDROCHLORIDE

✚ Related entries: Afrazine; Dristan Nasal Spray; Sudafed Nasal Spray; Vicks Sinex Decongestant Nasal Spray

oxymetholone

is an *anabolic* STEROID, which is used to treat aplastic anaemia. Administration is oral in the form of tablets.

✚ side-effects: nausea, vomiting, diarrhoea, sleeplessness, excitement, muscle cramps, chills, acne, jaundice and liver toxicity, pruritus, oedema (accumulation of fluid in the tissues), congestive heart failure, effects on bones; with high doses, masculinization in women and children, amenorrhoea, changes in fertility, raised blood calcium and changes in blood lipids.

▲ warning: it is not to be administered to patients with severe impairment of liver function, certain cancers, who are pregnant, or with porphyria. Administer with caution to those with heart, kidney, or liver disorders, hypertension, diabetes, epilepsy, or migraine. Bone growth should be monitored when treating young people or children.

✚ Related entry: Anapolon 50

Oxymycin

(DDSA Pharmaceuticals) is a proprietary, prescription-only preparation of the ANTIBACTERIAL and (TETRACYCLINE) ANTIBIOTIC drug oxytetracycline. It can be used to treat a wide range of infections and is available as tablets.

✚▲ side-effects/warning: see OXYTETRACYCLINE

Oxypertine

(Sterwin) is a proprietary, prescription-only preparation of the ANTIPSYCHOTIC drug oxypertine. It can be used to treat and tranquillize patients with psychotic disorders such as schizophrenia. It may also be used in the short-term treatment of severe anxiety. It is available as tablets and capsules.

✚▲ side-effects/warning: see OXYPERTINE

oxypertine

is an ANTIPSYCHOTIC drug, which is used to treat and tranquillize patients with psychotic disorders such as schizophrenia. The drug may also be used in the short-term treatment of severe anxiety. Administration is oral in the form of capsules or tablets.

✚▲ side-effects/warning: see under CHLORPROMAZINE HYDROCHLORIDE; but with less extrapyramidal symptoms (muscle tremor and rigidity) and occasional photophobia. There may be excitation or sedation depending on dose.

✚ Related entry: Oxypertine

oxyphenisatin

(oxyphenisatine) is a (*stimulant*) LAXATIVE, which is used to promote defecation and relieve constipation. It seems to work by stimulating motility in the intestine and can be used to evacuate the colon prior to rectal examination or surgery. Administration is in the form of an enema.

✚ side-effects: abdominal cramps.

▲ warning: avoid repeated use as it can damage the liver; do not use in patients with intestinal obstruction.

✚ Related entry: Veripaque

oxyphenisatine

See OXYPHENISATIN

Oxyprenix SR

(Ashbourne) is a proprietary, prescription-only preparation of the BETA-BLOCKER drug oxprenolol hydrochloride. It can be used as an ANTIHYPERTENSIVE treatment for raised blood pressure, as an ANTI-ANGINA treatment to relieve symptoms

and improve exercise tolerance and as an
ANTI-ARRHYTHMIC to regularize heartbeat
and to treat myocardial infarction. It can
also be used as an ANXIOLYTIC treatment,
particularly for symptomatic relief of
tremor and palpitations. It is available as
modified-release tablets.
✚▲ side-effects/warning: see OXPRENOLOL
HYDROCHLORIDE

oxytetracycline

is a broad-spectrum ANTIBACTERIAL and
(TETRACYCLINE) ANTIBIOTIC drug. It can be
used to treat many serious infections,
particularly those of the urinogenital and
respiratory tracts and of the skin (such as
acne). Administration is oral in the form
of tablets or capsules.
✚▲ side-effects/warning: see under
TETRACYCLINE. It should not be administered
to patients with porphyria.
✪ Related entries: Berkmycen;
Oxymycin; Oxytetramix; Terra-Cortril;
Terra-Cortril Nystatin; Terramycin;
Trimovate

Oxytetramix

(Ashbourne) is a proprietary,
prescription-only preparation of the
ANTIBACTERIAL and (TETRACYCLINE)
ANTIBIOTIC drug oxytetracycline. It can be
used to treat a wide range of infections
and is available as tablets.
✚▲ side-effects/warning: see
OXYTETRACYCLINE

oxytocin

is a natural pituitary HORMONE
produced and secreted by the posterior
pituitary gland. It increases the
contractions of the womb during normal
labour and stimulates lactation.
Therapeutically, it may be administered by
injection or infusion to induce or assist
labour (or abortion), to speed up the
third stage of labour (delivery of the
placenta) and it is also used in
conjunction with ERGOMETRINE
MALEATE to help stop bleeding

following childbirth and abortion.
✚ side-effects: high doses may lead to violent
contractions of the uterus, which may rupture
the uterine wall and/or cause foetal distress.
In the mother, there may be hypertension,
haemorrhage in the subarachnoid space,
water retention, oedema of the lungs and
pain.
▲ warning: it should not be administered to
patients who suffer from certain
abnormalities of the uterus, or where there is
a mechanical obstruction to delivery, where
the foetus is in evident distress, in placenta
praevia, or where there is a risk of embolism.
Administer with caution to those who suffer
from hypertension and certain other
cardiovascular disorders, who are about to
undergo a multiple birth, or who have
previously had a Caesarean section.
✪ Related entries: Syntocinon;
Syntometrine

P

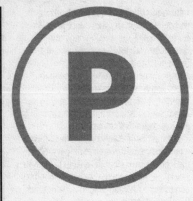

Pacifene

(Sussex Pharmaceuticals) is a proprietary, non-prescription preparation of the (NSAID) NON-NARCOTIC ANALGESIC, ANTIRHEUMATIC and ANTIPYRETIC drug ibuprofen. It can be used for the relief of pain, including headache, period pain, muscular pain, dental pain and feverishness and also to relieve cold and flu symptoms. It is available as tablets and is not normally given to children under 12 years, except on medical advice.

+▲ side-effects/warning: see IBUPROFEN

Pacifene Maximum Strength

(Sussex Pharmaceuticals) is a proprietary, non-prescription preparation of the (NSAID) NON-NARCOTIC ANALGESIC, ANTIRHEUMATIC and ANTIPYRETIC drug ibuprofen. It can be used for the relief of pain, including headache, period pain, muscular pain, dental pain, and feverishness, and also to relieve cold and flu symptoms. It is available as tablets, and is not normally given to children under 12 years, except on medical advice.

+▲ side-effects/warning: see IBUPROFEN

paclitaxel

is a CYTOTOXIC DRUG, which is used as an ANTICANCER drug in the treatment of ovarian cancer. Administration is by intravenous infusion.

+▲ side-effects/warning: see under CYTOTOXIC DRUGS.

○ Related entry: Taxol

Paldesic

(RP Drugs) is a proprietary, non-prescription preparation of the NON-NARCOTIC ANALGESIC and ANTIPYRETIC drug paracetamol. It is available as a paediatric oral solution, which, on medical advice, can be used to reduce fever in infants over three months (or temperature following vaccination at two months).

+▲ side-effects/warning: see PARACETAMOL

Palfium

(Boehringer Mannheim) is a proprietary, prescription-only preparation of the (OPIOID) NARCOTIC ANALGESIC drug dextromoramide, which is on the Controlled Drugs List. It can be used to relieve severe pain, especially during the final stages of terminal malignant disease. It is available as tablets and suppositories.
+▲ side-effects/warning: see DEXTROMORAMIDE

Paludrine

(Zeneca) is a proprietary, non-prescription preparation of the ANTIMALARIAL drug proguanil hydrochloride. It can be used in the prevention of malaria, and is available as tablets.
+▲ side-effects/warning: see PROGUANIL HYDROCHLORIDE

Pamergan P100

(Martindale) is a proprietary, prescription-only COMPOUND PREPARATION of the (OPIOID) NARCOTIC ANALGESIC drug pethidine hydrochloride and the SEDATIVE and HYPNOTIC (and ANTIHISTAMINE) drug promethazine hydrochloride, which is on the Controlled Drugs List. It can be used to relieve pain, especially during childbirth, and is available in a form for injection.
+▲ side-effects/warning: see PETHIDINE HYDROCHLORIDE; PROMETHAZINE HYDROCHLORIDE

Pameton

(Sterling Health) is a proprietary, non-prescription COMPOUND PREPARATION of the NON-NARCOTIC ANALGESIC and ANTIPYRETIC drug paracetamol and the amino acid methionine (an antidote to paracetamol overdose). It can be used to provide relief from painful and feverish conditions, such as period pain, toothache, cold and flu symptoms, and to reduce high body temperature (especially for patients likely to overdose). It is available as capsule-shaped tablets

(*Caplets*), and is not normally given to children under six years, except on medical advice.
+▲ side-effects/warning: see METHIONINE; PARACETAMOL

Panadeine Tablets

(Sterling Health) is a proprietary, non-prescription COMPOUND ANALGESIC preparation of the NON-NARCOTIC ANALGESIC and ANTIPYRETIC drug paracetamol and the NARCOTIC ANALGESIC codeine phosphate (a combination known as co-codamol 8/500). It can be used to treat pain, such as toothache, sore throat, period pain, arthritis and rheumatic pain, and to reduce high body temperature. It is available as tablets, and is not normally given to children under seven years, except on medical advice.
+▲ side-effects/warning: see CODEINE PHOSPHATE; PARACETAMOL

Panadol Baby and Infant Suspension

(Sterling Health) is a proprietary, non-prescription preparation of the NON-NARCOTIC ANALGESIC and ANTIPYRETIC drug paracetamol. It can be used to relieve pain, such as teething pain and toothache, to reduce high body temperature and fever in babies and infants with colds, flu, or childhood infections (eg. chicken pox). It is available as a suspension, and should not be given to babies under two months.
+▲ side-effects/warning: see PARACETAMOL

Panadol Capsules

(Sterling Health) is a proprietary, non-prescription preparation of the NON-NARCOTIC ANALGESIC and ANTIPYRETIC drug paracetamol. It can be used to treat mild pain and to reduce high body temperature, such as musculoskeletal pain, toothache, period pain, and to relieve cold and flu symptoms. It is available as capsules, and is not normally given to children under 12 years, except

P on medical advice.

✚▲ side-effects/warning: see PARACETAMOL

Panadol Extra Soluble Tablets

(Sterling Health) is a proprietary, non-prescription COMPOUND PREPARATION of the NON-NARCOTIC ANALGESIC and ANTIPYRETIC drug paracetamol and the STIMULANT caffeine. It can be used to treat mild pain and to reduce high body temperature, such as musculoskeletal pain, toothache, period pain, and to relieve cold and flu symptoms. It is available as soluble tablets, and is not normally given to children under 12 years, except on medical advice.

✚▲ side-effects/warning: see CAFFEINE; PARACETAMOL

Panadol Extra Tablets

(Sterling Health) is a proprietary, non-prescription COMPOUND PREPARATION of the NON-NARCOTIC ANALGESIC and ANTIPYRETIC drug paracetamol and the STIMULANT caffeine. It can be used to treat mild pain, such as musculoskeletal pain, toothache and period pain, to reduce high body temperature and to relieve cold and flu symptoms. It is available as tablets and is not normally given to children under 12 years, except on medical advice.

✚▲ side-effects/warning: see CAFFEINE; PARACETAMOL

Panadol Junior

(Sterling Health) is a proprietary, non-prescription preparation of the NON-NARCOTIC ANALGESIC and ANTIPYRETIC drug paracetamol. It can be used to treat pain, reduce high body temperature and to relieve cold and flu symptoms, sore throat, headache and toothache. It is available as an orange powder sachets and is not normally given to children under three years, except on medical advice.

✚▲ side-effects/warning: see PARACETAMOL

Panadol Soluble

(Sterling Health) is a proprietary, non-prescription preparation of the NON-NARCOTIC ANALGESIC and ANTIPYRETIC drug paracetamol. It can be used to treat pain such as musculoskeletal pain, toothache and period pain, to reduce high body temperature and to relieve cold and flu symptoms. It is available as effervescent tablets and is not normally given to children under six years, except on medical advice.

✚▲ side-effects/warning: see PARACETAMOL

Panadol Tablets

(Sterling Health) is a proprietary, non-prescription preparation of the NON-NARCOTIC ANALGESIC and ANTIPYRETIC drug paracetamol. It can be used to treat pain such as musculoskeletal pain, toothache and period pain, to reduce high body temperature and to relieve cold and flu symptoms. It is available as effervescent tablets and is not normally given to children under six years, except on medical advice.

✚▲ side-effects/warning: see PARACETAMOL

Panadol Ultra

(Sterling Health) is a proprietary, non-prescription COMPOUND PREPARATION of the NON-NARCOTIC ANALGESIC and ANTIPYRETIC drug paracetamol and the STIMULANT caffeine. It can be used to treat pain such as musculoskeletal pain, sciatica, strains, toothache and period pain, to reduce high body temperature, to relieve cold and flu symptoms and sore throat. It is available as tablets and is not to be given to children under 12 years, except on medical advice.

✚▲ side-effects/warning: see CAFFEINE; PARACETAMOL

Pancrease

(Cilag) is a proprietary, non-prescription preparation of the digestive ENZYME pancreatin. It can be used to treat a deficiency of the digestive juices that are normally supplied by the pancreas. It is available as capsules.

+▲ side-effects/warning: see pancreatin

Pancrease HL

(Cilag) is a proprietary, non-prescription preparation of the digestive enzyme pancreatin. It can be used to treat a deficiency of the digestive juices that are normally supplied by the pancreas. It is available as capsules (at a higher strength than *Pancrease*).

+▲ side-effects/warning: see PANCREATIN

pancreatin

is the term used to describe extracts of the pancreas that contain pancreatic enzyme. It can be given by mouth to treat deficiencies due to impaired natural secretion by the pancreas, such as in cystic fibrosis and also following operations involving removal of pancreatic tissue, such as panreatectomy and gastrectomy. The enzymes are inactivated by the acid in the stomach and so preparations should be taken with food or with certain other drugs, such as H₂-ANTAGONIST drugs, that reduce acid secretion. Alternatively, pancreatin is available as enteric-coated capsules, which overcome some of these problems, but are destroyed by heat and should be mixed with food after its preparation. The majority of pancreatin preparations are of porcine origin and administered as capsules or granules.

+ side-effects: irritation of the skin around the mouth and anus; there may be gastrointestinal upsets, including nausea, vomiting, abdominal discomfort; and at high dose there may be raised uric acid levels in the blood and urine.

▲ warning: there may be hypersensitivity reactions in those that handle the powder. There are particular problems (fibrotic structures in the bowel) that seem to be associated with high-dose preparations and these should only be taken with specialist advice.

✪ Related entries: Creon; Creon 25 000; Nutrizym 10; Nutrizym 22; Nutrizym GR; Pancrease; Pancrease HL; Pancrex; Pancrex V; Panzytrat 25 000

Pancrex

(Paines & Byrne) is a proprietary, non-prescription preparation of the digestive enzyme pancreatin. It can be used to treat a deficiency of the digestive juices that are normally supplied by the pancreas. It is available as granules.

+▲ side-effects/warning: see PANCREATIN

Pancrex V

(Paines & Byrne) is a proprietary, non-prescription preparation of the digestive enzyme pancreatin. It can be used to treat a deficiency of the digestive juices that are normally supplied by the pancreas. It is available as capsules (one preparation is called *Pancrex V 125*), tablets and a powder.

+▲ side-effects/warning: see PANCREATIN

pancuronium bromide

is a *non-depolarizing* SKELETAL MUSCLE RELAXANT drug. It is used to induce muscle paralysis during surgery and is administered by injection.

+▲ side-effects/warning: see under TUBOCURARINE CHLORIDE

✪ Related entry: Pavulon

Panda Baby Cream & Castor Oil Cream with Lanolin

(Thornton & Ross) is a proprietary, non-prescription COMPOUND PREPARATION of zinc oxide, castor oil, wool fat (lanolin) and several other minor constituents. It can be used as an EMOLLIENT and a BARRIER CREAM for nappy rash and to protect chapped skin.

+▲ side-effects/warning: see CASTOR OIL; WOOL FAT; ZINC OXIDE

PanOxyl 5 Gel

(Stiefel) is a proprietary, non-prescription

P preparation of the KERATOLYTIC and ANTIMICROBIAL drug benzoyl peroxide (5%). It can be used to treat acne and is available as a gel for topical application. It is not normally used on children, except on medical advice.

✚▲ side-effects/warning: see BENZOYL PEROXIDE

PanOxyl 10 Gel

(Stiefel) is a proprietary, non-prescription preparation of the KERATOLYTIC and ANTIMICROBIAL drug benzoyl peroxide (10%). It can be used to treat acne and is available as a gel for topical application. It is not normally used on children, except on medical advice.

✚▲ side-effects/warning: see BENZOYL PEROXIDE

PanOxyl Aquagel 5

(Stiefel) is a proprietary, non-prescription preparation of the KERATOLYTIC and ANTIMICROBIAL drug benzoyl peroxide (2.5%). It can be used to treat acne and is available as a gel for topical application.

✚▲ side-effects/warning: see BENZOYL PEROXIDE

PanOxyl Aquagel 10

(Stiefel) is a proprietary, non-prescription preparation of the KERATOLYTIC and ANTIMICROBIAL drug benzoyl peroxide (10%). It can be used to treat acne and is available as a gel for topical application.

✚▲ side-effects/warning: see BENZOYL PEROXIDE

PanOxyl Aquagel 25

(Stiefel) is a proprietary, non-prescription preparation of the KERATOLYTIC and ANTIMICROBIAL drug benzoyl peroxide (5%). It can be used to treat acne and is available as a gel for topical application.

✚▲ side-effects/warning: see BENZOYL PEROXIDE; MICONAZOLE

PanOxyl Wash

(Stiefel) is a proprietary, non-prescription

preparation of the KERATOLYTIC and ANTIMICROBIAL drug benzoyl peroxide (10%). It can be used to treat acne and is available as a lotion for topical application. It is not normally used on children, except on medical advice.

✚▲ side-effects/warning: see BENZOYL PEROXIDE

Panzytrat 25 000

(Knoll) is a proprietary, non-prescription preparation of the digestive ENZYME pancreatin. It can be used to treat a deficiency of the digestive juices that are normally supplied by the pancreas. It is available as higher-strength capsules.

✚▲ side-effects/warning: see PANCREATIN

papaveretum

is a COMPOUND PREPARATION of alkaloids of opium, most of which is made up of morphine with the rest largely consisting of codeine and papaverine. It is used as an (OPIOID) NARCOTIC ANALGESIC drug primarily during or following surgery, but can also be used as a sedative prior to an operation. Administration is either oral as tablets or by injection. All proprietary preparations containing papaveretum are on the Controlled Drugs List because the drug is potentially addictive.

✚▲ side-effects/warning: see under OPIOID

✪ Related entry: Omnopon

papaverine

is a SMOOTH MUSCLE RELAXANT drug that is rarely used any more, though it is included in a proprietary pain remedy. There have been some recent trials of its use for impotence by direct injection into the corpus cavernosum. Administration is either oral as tablets or in a form for injection.

✚ side-effects: local burning pain and haematoma (swelling) at the site of injection.

▲ warning: administer with care to patients with certain cardiovascular disorders.

✪ Related entry: Aspav

paracetamol

(called acetaminophen in the USA) is a NON-NARCOTIC ANALGESIC drug, which can be used to treat all forms of mild to moderate pain. It also has ANTIPYRETIC properties and can be used to reduce fever and raised body temperature. In many ways it is similar to aspirin, except that it does not cause gastric irritation or relieve inflammation. Many proprietary preparations are COMPOUND ANALGESICS that combine paracetamol and aspirin. Administration is oral in the form of tablets, capsules, suppositories, or a liquid.

✚ side-effects: there are few side-effects if dosage is low, though there may be rashes, acute pancreatitis and blood disorders; high overdosage or prolonged use may result in liver dysfunction.

▲ warning: it should be administered with caution to patients with impaired liver function or who suffer from alcoholism (which causes liver damage).

◐ Related articles: Actron; Anadin Extra Soluble Tablets; Anadin Paracetamol Tablets; Andrews Answer; Beechams Hot Blackcurrant; Benylin Day and Night; Calpol Infant Suspension; Calpol Infant Suspension, Sugar-Free; Calpol Six Plus; Catarrh-Ex; Codanin Tablets; Cold Relief Capsules; Coldrex Powders, Blackcurrant; Coldrex Tablets; Cosalgesic; Cupanol Over 6 Paracetamol Oral Suspension; Cupanol Under 6 Paracetamol Oral Suspension; Day Cold Comfort Capsules; Day Nurse Capsules; Day Nurse Liquid; Disprin Extra; Disprol; Disprol Infant; Disprol Junior; Distalgesic; Doan's Backache Pills' Fennings Children's Cooling Powders; Flurex Cold/Flu Capsules with Cough Suppressant; Flurex Tablets; Fortagesic; Fynnon Calcium Aspirin; Galake; Hedex Extra Tablets; Hedex Tablets; Kapake; Lemsip; Lemsip Cold Relief Capsules; Lemsip Flu Strength; Lemsip, Junior; Lemsip Night-Time; Lobak; Medised; Midrid; Migraleve; Mu-Cron Tablets; Night Cold Comfort Capsules; Night Nurse Capsules; Night Nurse Liquid; Nurse Sykes Powders; Paldesic; Pameton; Panadeine Tablets; Panadol Baby and Infant Suspension; Panadol Capsules; Panadol Extra Soluble Tablets; Panadol Extra Tablets; Panadol Junior; Panadol Soluble; Panadol Ultra; Paracets; Paracets Capsules; Paraclear Extra Strength; Paraclear Junior; Paracodol Capsules; Paracodol Tablets; Parake; Paramol Tablets; Powerin Analgesic Tablets; Propain Tablets; Remedeine; Resolve; Salzone; Solpadeine Capsules; Solpadeine Soluble Tablets; Solpadeine Tablets; Solpadol; Sudafed-Co Tablets; Syndol; Tramil 500 Analgesic Capsules; Triogesic Tablets; Tylex; Veganin Tablets; Vicks Coldcare Capsules.

Paracets

(Sussex Pharmaceuticals) is a proprietary, non-prescription preparation of the NON-NARCOTIC ANALGESIC and ANTIPYRETIC drug paracetamol. It can be used to treat mild to moderate pain, such as toothache and period pain, to reduce high body temperature and to relieve cold and flu symptoms. It is available as tablets and is not normally given to children under six years, except on medical advice.

✚▲ side-effects/warning: see PARACETAMOL

Paracets Capsules

(Sussex Pharmaceuticals) is a proprietary, non-prescription preparation of the NON-NARCOTIC ANALGESIC and ANTIPYRETIC drug paracetamol. It can be used to treat mild to moderate pain, such as toothache and period pain, to reduce high body temperature and to relieve cold and flu symptoms. It is available as capsules and is not normally given to children under six years, except on medical advice.

✚▲ side-effects/warning: see PARACETAMOL

Paraclear

(Roche) is a proprietary, non-prescription

P preparation of the NON-NARCOTIC ANALGESIC and ANTIPYRETIC drug paracetamol. It can be used to treat mild to moderate pain, such as toothache and period pain, to reduce high body temperature and to relieve cold and flu symptoms. It is available as effervescent tablets and is not normally given to children under six years, except on medical advice.

✚▲ side-effects/warning: see PARACETAMOL

Paraclear Extra Strength

(Roche) is a proprietary, non-prescription COMPOUND PREPARATION of the NON-NARCOTIC ANALGESIC and ANTIPYRETIC drug paracetamol and the STIMULANT caffeine. It can be used to treat mild to moderate pain, such as toothache and period pain, to reduce high body temperature and to relieve cold and flu symptoms. It is available as tablets and is not to be given to children under six years, except on medical advice.

✚▲ side-effects/warning: see CAFFEINE; PARACETAMOL

Paraclear Junior

(Roche) is a proprietary, non-prescription preparation of the NON-NARCOTIC ANALGESIC and ANTIPYRETIC drug paracetamol. It can be used to relieve teething pain, headache, sore throat and cold and flu symptoms. It is available as effervescent tablets and is not normally given to babies under three months, except on medical advice.

✚▲ side-effects/warning: see PARACETAMOL

Paracodol Capsules

(Roche) is a proprietary, non-prescription COMPOUND PREPARATION of the NON-NARCOTIC ANALGESIC and ANTIPYRETIC drug paracetamol and the (OPIOID) NARCOTIC ANALGESIC codeine phosphate (a combination known as co-codamol 8/500). It can be used to treat mild to moderate pain and to reduce high body temperature. It is available as tablets and

is not normally given to children under 12 years, except on medical advice.

✚▲ side-effects/warning: see CODEINE PHOSPHATE; PARACETAMOL

Paracodol Tablets

(Roche) is a proprietary, non-prescription COMPOUND ANALGESIC preparation of the NON-NARCOTIC ANALGESIC and ANTIPYRETIC drug paracetamol and the (OPIOID) NARCOTIC ANALGESIC drug codeine phosphate (a combination known as co-codamol 8/500). It can be used to relieve mild to moderate pain and to reduce high body temperature. It is available as tablets and is not normally given to children under six years, except on medical advice.

✚▲ side-effects/warning: see CODEINE PHOSPHATE; PARACETAMOL

paraffin

is a hydrocarbon derived from petroleum. Its main therapeutic use is as a base for ointments as either YELLOW SOFT PARAFFIN or WHITE SOFT PARAFFIN. As a mineral oil, LIQUID PARAFFIN is used as a LAXATIVE and is also incorporated into many preparations as an EMOLLIENT.

Parake

(Galen) is a proprietary, non-prescription COMPOUND ANALGESIC preparation of the NON-NARCOTIC ANALGESIC and ANTIPYRETIC drug paracetamol and the (OPIOID) NARCOTIC ANALGESIC drug codeine phosphate (a combination known as co-codamol 8/500). It can be used to relieve pain and to reduce high body temperature. It is available as tablets and is not normally given to children under seven years, except on medical advice.

✚▲ side-effects/warning: see CODEINE PHOSPHATE; PARACETAMOL

paraldehyde

is a drug that is used mainly as an ANTICONVULSANT and ANTI-EPILEPTIC in the treatment of status epilepticus (severe and continuous epileptic seizures).

Administration is by injection or enema.
✚ side-effects: rash, pain and abscess after injections, rectal irritation after enema.
▲ warning: administer with caution to patients with lung disease or impaired liver function.

Paramax

(Lorex) is a proprietary, prescription-only COMPOUND PREPARATION of the ANTI-EMETIC and ANTINAUSEANT drug metoclopramide hydrochloride and the NON-NARCOTIC ANALGESIC drug paracetamol. It can be used as an ANTIMIGRAINE treatment for acute migraine attacks and is available as tablets and an effervescent powder.
✚▲ side-effects/warning: see ASPIRIN; METOCLOPRAMIDE HYDROCHLORIDE. Note the side-effects in young people.

Paramol Tablets

(Napp) is a proprietary non-prescription COMPOUND ANALGESIC preparation of the NON-NARCOTIC ANALGESIC drug paracetamol and the (OPIOID) NARCOTIC ANALGESIC and ANTITUSSIVE drug dihydrocodeine tartrate. It can be used for general pain relief, including period pains, headache, toothache and muscular aches and for cough relief. It is available as tablets and is not normally given to children under 12 years, except on medical advice. (The proprietary name *Paramol* was formerly used for a prescription-only combination known as co-dydramol.)
✚▲ side-effects/warning: see DIHYDROCODEINE TARTRATE; PARACETAMOL

Paraplatin

(Bristol-Myers) is a proprietary, prescription-only preparation of the (CYTOTOXIC) ANTICANCER drug carboplatin. It can be used specifically in the treatment of ovarian cancer, and is available in a form for injection.
✚▲ side-effects/warning: see CARBOPLATIN

*parasympathomimetic

drugs have effects similar to those of the parasympathetic nervous system. They work by mimicking the actions of the natural neurotransmitter acetylcholine (eg. PILOCARPINE and CARBACHOL). The ANTICHOLINESTERASE drugs (eg. NEOSTIGMINE) are *indirect parasympathomimetics* because they prolong the duration of action of the naturally released acetylcholine. *Direct parasympathomimetics* act at (so-called 'muscarinic') receptors for acetylcholine. Important parasympathomimetic actions include slowing of the heart, vasodilation, constriction of the bronchioles of the lung, stimulation of the muscles of the intestine and bladder and constriction of the pupil and altered focusing of the eye. ANTICHOLINERGIC drugs oppose some of these actions.

parathormone
See CALCITONIN

Parathyroid Hormone
See CALCITONIN

Parlodel

(Sandoz) is a proprietary, prescription-only preparation of the drug bromocriptine. It is used primarily to treat parkinsonism, but not the parkinsonian symptoms caused by certain drug therapies (see ANTIPARKINSONISM). It can also be used to treat a number of other hormonal disorders. It is available as tablets and capsules.
✚▲ side-effects/warning: see BROMOCRIPTINE

Parmid

(Lagap) is a proprietary, prescription-only preparation of the ANTI-EMETIC and ANTINAUSEANT drug metoclopramide hydrochloride. It can be used for the treatment of nausea and vomiting, particularly when associated with gastrointestinal disorders and after

P

treatment with radiation or cytotoxic drugs. It also has gastric MOTILITY STIMULANT actions and can be used in the treatment of non-ulcer dyspepsia, gastric stasis and for prevention of reflux oesophagitis. It is available as tablets and an oral solution.

+▲ side-effects/warning: see METOCLOPRAMIDE HYDROCHLORIDE. Note the side-effects in young people.

Parnate

(SK&F) is a proprietary, prescription-only preparation of the MONOAMINE-OXIDASE INHIBITOR (MAOI) ANTIDEPRESSANT drug tranylcypromine. It is available as tablets.

+▲ side-effects/warning: see TRANYLCYPROMINE

Paroven

(Zyma Healthcare) is a proprietary, non-prescription preparation of oxerutins. It can be used to treat cramp and other manifestations of poor circulation in the veins, such as oedema. It is available as capsules.

+▲ side-effects/warning: see OXERUTINS

paroxetine

is an ANTIDEPRESSANT drug of the recently developed SSRI group. It can be used to treat depressive illness and has the advantage over some other antidepressant drugs because it has less sedative and ANTICHOLINERGIC side-effects. It is available as tablets.

+▲ side-effects/warning: see under FLUOXETINE. There may be spasm of facial muscles and withdrawal symptoms may be marked.

✪ Related entry: Seroxat

Parstelin

(SK&F) is a proprietary, prescription-only COMPOUND PREPARATION of the MONOAMINE-OXIDASE INHIBITOR (MAOI) ANTEDEPRESSANT drug tranylcypromine and the ANTIPSYCHOTIC drug trifluoperazine. It can be used to treat

depressive illness, particularly in association with anxiety and is available as tablets.

+▲ side-effects/warning: see TRANYLCYPROMINE; TRIFLUOPERAZINE

Partobulin

(Immuno) is a proprietary, prescription-only preparation of ANTI-D RH$_0$ IMMUNOGLOBIN. It can be used to prevent rhesus-negative mothers from making antibodies against foetal rhesus-positive cells that may pass into the mother's circulation during childbirth, so protecting a future child from haemolytic disease of the newborn. It should be injected within a few days of birth.

+▲ side-effects/warning: see ANTI-D RH$_0$ IMMUNOGLOBULIN

Parvolex

(Evans) is a proprietary, prescription-only preparation of the ANTIDOTE drug acetylcysteine. It can be used to treat overdose poisoning by the NON-NARCOTIC ANALGESIC drug paracetamol. It is available in a form for injection.

+▲ side-effects/warning: see ACETYLCYSTEINE

Pavacol-D

(Boehringer Ingelheim) is a proprietary, non-prescription preparation of the (OPIOID) ANTITUSSIVE drug pholcodine. It can be used for dry or painful coughs and is available as a linctus.

+▲ side-effects/warning: see PHOLCODINE

Pavulon

(Organon-Teknika) is a proprietary, prescription-only preparation of the (*non-depolarizing*) SKELETAL MUSCLE RELAXANT drug pancuronium bromide. It can be used to induce muscle paralysis during surgery and is available in a form for injection.

+▲ side-effects/warning: see PANCURONIUM BROMIDE

Pecram

(Zyma Healthcare) is a proprietary, non-prescription preparation of the BRONCHODILATOR drug aminophylline (as aminophylline hydrate). It can be used as an ANTI-ASTHMATIC and in bronchitis treatment and is available as modified-release tablets.

✚▲ side-effects/warning: see AMINOPHYLLINE

*pediculicidal

treatments are used to kill lice of the genus *Pediculus*, which infest either the body or the scalp, or both and cause intense itching. Scratching tends to damage the skin surface and may eventually cause weeping lesions with bacterial infection as well. The best-known and most-used pediculicides include MALATHION and CARBARYL. LINDANE, which was once commonly administered, is now no longer used for lice on the scalp because resistant strains of lice have developed. Administration is topical, usually as a lotion and contact between the drug and the skin should be as long as possible (at least 12 hours or overnight) and repeated after seven days.

pemoline

is a drug that is used to treat hyperkinesis (hyperactivity) in children, but, in contrast, in adults it acts as a weak STIMULANT. Administration is oral in the form of tablets.

✚▲ side-effects/warning: see under DEXAMPHETAMINE SULPHATE; but also mania, depression, muscle twitches and movement disorders, blood changes and liver abnormalities.

✪ Related entry: Volital

Penbritin

(Beecham) is a proprietary, prescription-only preparation of the broad-spectrum ANTIBACTERIAL and (PENICILLIN) ANTIBIOTIC drug ampicillin. It can be used to treat systemic bacterial infections, infections of the upper respiratory tract, the ear, nose and throat and of the urinogenital tracts. It is available as capsules, a syrup, a paediatric suspension and in a form for injection.

✚▲ side-effects/warning: see AMPICILLIN

Pendramine

(ASTA Medica) is a proprietary, prescription only preparation of the CHELATING AGENT penicillamine. It can be used as an ANTIDOTE to copper or lead poisoning, to reduce copper levels in Wilson's disease and as a long-term treatment for rheumatoid arthritis. It is available as tablets.

✚▲ side-effects/warning: see PENICILLAMINE

Penetrol Catarrh Inhalant

(Seton Healthcare) is a proprietary, non-prescription COMPOUND PREPARATION of the aromatics oils MENTHOL and peppermint. It can be used for the symptomatic relief of nasal congestion associated with catarrh, hay fever and colds. It is available as lozenges and is not normally given to children under three months, except on medical advice.

✚▲ side-effects/warning: see PEPPERMINT OIL

Penetrol Catarrh Lozenges

(Seton Healthcare) is a proprietary, non-prescription COMPOUND PREPARATION of the EXPECTORANT drug AMMONIUM CHLORIDE and the SYMPATHOMIMETIC and DECONGESTANT drug phenylephrine hydrochloride with MENTHOL and peppermint oil. It can be used for the symptomatic relief of nasal congestion associated with catarrh, hay fever and colds. It is available as an inhalant and is not normally given to children under ten years, except on medical advice.

✚▲ side-effects/warning: see PEPPERMINT OIL; PHENYLEPHRINE HYDROCHLORIDE

Penetrol Inhalant

(Seton Healthcare) is a proprietary, non-

P prescription preparation of MENTHOL and peppermint oil. It can be used for the symptomatic relief of catarrh, hay fever and nasal congestion. It is available as an inhalant and is not normally given to children under three months, except on medical advice.

✚▲ side-effects/warning: see PEPPERMINT OIL

penicillamine
is a derivative of penicillin and is an extremely effective CHELATING AGENT. It binds various metal ions within the body, so facilitating their excretion (elimination from the body). It can be used as an ANTIDOTE to various types of metallic poisoning (eg. copper and lead) and to reduce copper levels in Wilson's disease. It is also used in the long-term treatment of severe rheumatoid arthritis or juvenile chronic arthritis, where it has ANTI-INFLAMMATORY and ANTIRHEUMATIC actions. Administration is oral in the form of tablets.

✚ side-effects: nausea, anorexia, fever, rashes, taste impairment, blood and kidney disturbances, lupus-like syndrome, or muscle weakness.

▲ warning: it should not be used in patients known to have sensitivity to penicillins, or with lupus erythematus. Administer with care to those with kidney impairment, who are pregnant and with known sensitivity to certain other drugs. Regular monitoring of body functions is required.

❍ Related entries: Distamine; Pendramine

penicillin G
See BENZYLPENICILLIN

penicillin V
See PHENOXYMETHYLPENICILLIN

*penicillinases
are enzymes that are produced by some bacteria and which inhibit, or completely neutralize, the antibacterial activity of many PENICILLIN drugs. Consequently, treatment of infections caused by such bacteria has usually involved the administration of either *penicillinase-resistant penicillins*, such as FLUCLOXACILLIN, or entirely different types of antibiotic. Some preparations combine a *penicillinase-sensitive* drug with an inhibitor of the enzyme, which then artificially gives that antibiotic penicillinase-resistance (for example CLAVULANIC ACID is a beta-lactamase inhibitor). Therapeutically, however, penicillinases themselves can be used (in a purified form) to treat sensitivity reactions to penicillin, or in tests to identify micro-organisms in blood samples taken from patients who are taking penicillin.

penicillins
are ANTIBACTERIAL and ANTIBIOTIC drugs that work by interfering with the synthesis of bacterial cell walls. The early penicillins were mainly effective against Gram-positive bacteria, though they could be used against the Gram-negative organisms that caused gonorrhoea and meningitis, as well as the organism causing syphilis. Later penicillins (eg. AMPICILLIN and PIPERACILLIN) expanded the spectrum to include a greater range of Gram-negative organisms. They are absorbed rapidly by most (but not all) body tissues and fluids and are excreted in the urine. One great disadvantage of penicillins is that many patients are allergic to them – allergy to one, means allergy to all of them – and may have reactions that range from a minor rash right up to anaphylactic shock, which occasionally can be fatal. Otherwise they are remarkably non-toxic. Rarely, very high dosage may cause convulsions, haemolytic anaemia, or abnormally high levels of sodium or potassium in the body with consequent symptoms. Those taken orally tend to cause diarrhoea and there is also a risk with broad-spectrum penicillins of allowing a superinfection to

develop. The best-known and most-used penicillins include BENZYLPENICILLIN (penicillin G; the first of the penicillins), PHENOXYMETHYLPENICILLIN (penicillin V), FLUCLOXACILLIN, ampicillin and AMOXICILLIN.

See also: AZLOCILLIN; BACAMPICILLIN HYDROCHLORIDE; CARBENICILLIN; CLOXACILLIN; METHICILLIN; PHENOXYMETHYLPENICILLIN; PIVAMPICILLIN; PROCAINE PENICILLIN; TEMOCILLAN; TICARCILLIN.

PenMix 10/90

(Novo Nordisk) is a proprietary, non-prescription preparation of human BIPHASIC ISOPHANE INSULIN (10% soluble/90% isophane). It is used as a DIABETIC TREATMENT to treat and maintain diabetic patients and is available in cartridges for injection with *Novopen* devices and in prefilled, disposable injectors. It has an intermediate duration of action.
✚▲ side-effects/warning: see INSULIN

PenMix 20/80

(Novo Nordisk) is a proprietary, non-prescription preparation of human BIPHASIC ISOPHANE INSULIN (20% soluble/80% isophane). It is used as a DIABETIC TREATMENT to treat and maintain diabetic patients and is available in cartridges (*Penfill*) for injection with *Novopen* devices and as prefilled, disposable injectors. It has an intermediate duration of action.
✚▲ side-effects/warning: see INSULIN

PenMix 30/70

(Novo Nordisk) is a proprietary, non-prescription preparation of human BIPHASIC ISOPHANE INSULIN (30% soluble/70% isophane). It is used as a DIABETIC TREATMENT to treat and maintain diabetic patients and is available in cartridges (*Penfill*) for injection with *Novopen* devices and as prefilled, disposable injectors. It has an

intermediate duration of action.
✚▲ side-effects/warning: see INSULIN

PenMix 40/60

(Novo Nordisk) is a proprietary, non-prescription preparation of human BIPHASIC ISOPHANE INSULIN (40% soluble/60% isophane). It is used as a DIABETIC TREATMENT to treat and maintain diabetic patients and is available in cartridges (*Penfill*) for injection with *Novopen* devices and as prefilled, disposable injectors. It has an intermediate duration of action.
✚▲ side-effects/warning: see INSULIN

PenMix 50/50

(Novo Nordisk) is a proprietary, non-prescription preparation of human BIPHASIC ISOPHANE INSULIN (50% soluble/50% isophane). It is used as a DIABETIC TREATMENT to treat and maintain diabetic patients and is available in cartridges (*Penfill*) for injection with *Novopen* devices and as prefilled, disposable injectors. It has an intermediate duration of action.
✚▲ side-effects/warning: see INSULIN

Pentacarinat

(Rhône-Poulenc Rorer) is a proprietary, prescription-only preparation of the ANTIPROTOZOAL drug pentamidine isethionate. It can be used to treat pneumonia caused by the protozoan micro-organism *Pneumocystis carinii* in patients whose immune system has been suppressed (either following transplant surgery or because of a condition such as AIDS). It is available only for specialist use and is administered either by injection or inhalation.
✚▲ side-effects/warning: see PENTAMIDINE ISETHIONATE

pentaerythritol tetranitrate

is a short-acting VASODILATOR and ANTI-ANGINA drug. It is used to prevent attacks

P

of angina pectoris (ischaemic heart pain) when it is taken before exercise. It works by dilating the blood vessels returning blood to the heart and so reducing the heart's workload. Administration is oral in the form of tablets.

+▲ side-effects/warning: see under GLYCERYL TRINITRATE

✪ Related entry: Mycardol

pentamidine isethionate

(pentamidine isetionate) is an ANTIPROTOZOAL drug, which is used to treat pneumonia caused by the protozoan micro-organism *Pneumocystis carinii* in patients whose immune system has been suppressed (either following transplant surgery or because of a condition such as AIDS). It has also been used as an antiprotozoal drug to treat a form of leishmaniasis. It is available only for specialist use and is administered either by injection or inhalation.

+ side-effects: it can cause severe hypotension while being administered or immediately after. There may also be serious pancreatitis, hypoglycaemia, arrhythmias, blood disorders, kidney failure and various other potentially serious side-effects.

▲ warning: administer with care to patients with certain liver, kidney and blood disorders. Careful monitoring is required.

✪ Related entry: Pentacarinat

pentamidine isetionate

See PENTAMIDINE ISETHIONATE

Pentasa

(Yamanouchi) is a proprietary, prescription-only preparation of the AMINOSALICYLATE drug mesalazine. It can be used to treat patients who suffer from ulcerative colitis and is available as modified-release tablets, suppositories and as a retention enema.

+▲ side-effects/warning: see MESALAZINE

pentazocine

is a powerful NARCOTIC ANALGESIC drug,

which can be used to treat moderate to severe pain. It is an OPIOID and is like morphine sulphate in effect and action, but is less likely to cause dependence. However, it can precipitate withdrawal symptoms if used in patients dependent on opioids. Administration can be oral in the form of capsules and tablets, or topical in the form of suppositories, or by injection. The proprietary form is on the Controlled Drugs List. It is also available as COMPOUND PREPARATIONS in combination with PARACETAMOL.

+▲ side-effect/warning: see under OPIOID. Disturbances and hallucinations are thought to occur. It is not suitable for use in patients with certain heart complications and should be avoided in patients with porphyria.

✪ Related entries: Fortagesic; Fortral

Pentostam

(Wellcome) is a proprietary, prescription-only preparation of the drug sodium stibogluconate, which has ANTIPROTOZOAL properties. It can be used to treat skin infections by protozoal micro-organisms of the genus *Leishmania* (eg. leishmaniasis). It is available in a form for injection.

+▲ side-effects/warning: see SODIUM STIBOGLUCONATE

pentoxifylline

See OXPENTIFYLLINE

Pentran

(Berk) is a proprietary, prescription-only preparation of the ANTICONVULSANT and ANTI-EPILEPTIC drug phenytoin. It can be used to treat and prevent most forms of seizure and also trigeminal (facial) neuralgia. It is available as tablets.

+▲ side-effects/warning: see PHENYTOIN

Pentrax

(Euroderma) is a proprietary, non-prescription preparation of coal tar. It can be used to treat skin conditions such as dandruff (seborrhoeic dermatitis) and psoriasis of the scalp. It is available as a liquid scalp preparation.

+▲ side-effects/warning: see COAL TAR

Pepcid

(Morson) is a proprietary, prescription-only preparation of the H₂-ANTAGONIST drug famotidine. It can be used as an ULCER-HEALING drug for benign peptic ulcers (in the stomach or duodenum), gastro-oesophagial reflux, dyspepsia and associated conditions. It is available as tablets.

+▲ side-effects/warning: see FAMOTIDINE

Pepcid AC

(Morson) is a proprietary, non-prescription preparation of the H₂-ANTAGONIST famotidine. It can be used for the short-term relief of heartburn, dispepsia and excess stomach acid. It is available as tablets in a limited amount for short-term uses only.

+▲ side-effects/warning: see FAMOTIDINE

peppermint oil

is used to relieve the discomfort of abdominal colic and distension, particularly in irritable bowel syndrome. It is thought to act as an ANTISPASMODIC by directly relaxing the smooth muscle of the intestinal walls. It is also incorporated into preparations for the relief of catarrh and nasal congestion. Administration is oral in the form of capsules.

+ side-effects: there may be heartburn and rarely allergic reactions such as rash, headache, muscle tremor, slowing of the heart and unsteady gait.

✪ Related entries: Colpermin; ✪ Collis Browne's Mixture; KLN Suspension; Mintec; Penetrol Inhalant

Peptimax

(Ashbourne) is a proprietary preparation of the H2-ANTAGONIST drug cimetidine. It is available on prescription or without a prescription in a limited amount and for short-term uses only. It can be used as an ULCER-HEALING DRUG for benign peptic ulcers (in the stomach or duodenum), gastro-oesophageal reflux, dyspepsia and associated conditions. It is available as tablets.

+▲ side-effects/warning: see CIMETIDINE

Percutol

(Cusi) is a proprietary, non-prescription preparation of the VASODILATOR and ANTI-ANGINA drug glyceryl trinitrate. It can be used to treat and prevent angina pectoris. It is available in the form of an ointment for use on a dressing secured to the skin surface (usually on the chest, abdomen, or thigh).

+▲ side-effects/warning: see GLYCERYL TRINITRATE

Perfan

(Merrell) is a proprietary, prescription-only preparation of the PHOSPHODIESTERASE INHIBITOR drug enoximone. It can be used, in the short term, in HEART FAILURE TREATMENT, especially where other drugs have not been successful. It is available in a form for infusion or injection.

+▲ side-effects/warning: see ENOXIMONE

pergolide

is a recently introduced ANTIPARKINSONISM drug, an ERGOT ALKALOID derivative and is similar to BROMOCRIPTINE in that it is useful in reducing 'off' periods in the disease. It is available in the form of tablets.

+ side-effects: hallucinations, confusion, impaired muscle movements, somnolence, nausea and abdominal pain, dyspepsia, double vision, rhinitis, laboured breathing, insomnia, constipation or diarrhoea, hypotension and charges in heart rate or rhythm.

▲ warning: administer with care to patients with certain heart disorders, dyskinesias, history of confusion or hallucinations, porphyria; or who are

P

pregnant or breast-feeding.
○ **Related entry: Celance**

Pergonal

(Serono) is a proprietary, prescription-only HORMONE preparation of human menopausal gonadotrophins, which contains FOLLICLE-STIMULATING HORMONE (FSH) and LUTEINIZING HORMONE (LH). It can be used in infertility treatment in women with proven hypopituitarism and who do not respond to CLOMIPHENE CITRATE (another drug commonly used to treat infertility) and also in superovulation treatment in assisted conception (as with *in vitro* fertilization). It is available in a form for intramuscular injection.
+▲ side-effects/warning: see HUMAN MENOPAUSAL GONADOTROPHINS

Periactin

(Merck, Sharp & Dohme) is a proprietary, non-prescription preparation of cyproheptadine hydrochloride, which is a drug with ANTIHISTAMINE activity. It can be used for the symptomatic relief of allergic disorders such as hay fever and urticaria. It is available as tablets and a syrup.
+▲ side-effects/warning: see CYPROHEPTADINE HYDROCHLORIDE

pericyazine

is chemically a PHENOTHIAZINE DERIVATIVE. It is used as an ANTIPSYCHOTIC drug to treat patients suffering from schizophrenia and other psychoses, particularly during behavioural disturbances. It can also be used in the short-term treatment of severe anxiety. Administration is oral in the form of tablets or a syrup.
+▲ side-effects/warning: see under CHLORPROMAZINE HYDROCHLORIDE; but is more sedating and initially hypotension may occur.
○ **Related entry: Neulactil**

Perinal

(Demal) is a proprietary, prescription-only COMPOUND PREPARATION of the CORTICOSTEROID and ANTI-INFLAMMATORY drug hydrocortisone (as acetate) and the LOCAL ANAESTHETIC drug lignocaine hydrochloride. It can be used to treat haemorrhoids and inflammation in the anal region and is available as a spray for topical application.
+▲ side-effects/warning: see HYDROCORTISONE; LIGNOCAINE HYDROCHLORIDE

perindopril

is an ACE INHIBITOR. It is a powerful VASODILATOR that can be used as an ANTIHYPERTENSIVE and in HEART FAILURE TREATMENT. It is often used in conjunction with other classes of drugs, particularly (THIAZIDE) DIURETICS. Administration is oral as tablets.
+▲ side-effects/warning: see under CAPTOPRIL
○ **Related entry: Coversyl**

permethrin

is a PEDICULICIDAL drug. It can be used to treat infestations by lice and as a SCABICIDAL to treat skin infestation by mites (scabies). Administration is topical in the form of a cream rinse and a skin cream.
+ side-effects: skin irritation, including itching, reddening and stinging; rarely, there may be swelling and rashes.
▲ warning: avoid contact with the eyes and do not use on broken or infected skin. Administer with caution to patients who are pregnant or breast-feeding.
○ **Related entry: Lyclear**

Permitabs

(Bioglan) is a proprietary, non-prescription preparation of the ANTISEPTIC agent potassium permanganate. It can be used for cleaning and deodorizing suppurating eczematous reactions and wounds. It is available as tablets for solution for topical application.
+▲ side-effects/warning: see POTASSIUM PERMANGANATE

perphenazine

is chemically a PHENOTHIAZINE DERIVATIVE. It is used as an ANTIPSYCHOTIC drug in patients suffering from schizophrenia and other psychoses, in the short-term treatment of severe anxiety and as an ANTINAUSEANT and ANTI-EMETIC to relieve nausea and vomiting. Administration is oral in the form of tablets.
✚▲ side-effects/warning: see under CHLORPROMAZINE HYDROCHLORIDE; but is less sedating and extrapyramidal symptoms (muscle tremor and rigidity) are more likely.

Persantin

(Boehringer Ingelheim) is a proprietary, prescription-only preparation of the ANTIPLATELET drug dipyridamole. It can be used to prevent thrombosis and is available as tablets and in a form for injection.
✚▲ side-effects/warning: see DIPYRIDAMOLE

Pertofran

(Ciba) is a proprietary, prescription-only preparation of the (TRICYCLIC) ANTIDEPRESSANT drug desipramine hydrochloride. It is available as tablets.
✚▲ side-effects/warning: see DESIPRAMINE HYDROCHLORIDE

pertussis vaccine

(whooping-cough) is a VACCINE used for IMMUNIZATION and is a suspension of dead pertussis bacteria *Bordetella pertussis*. When injected, it causes the body's immune system to form antibodies against the bacteria and so provide *active immunity*. Administration of the vaccine is normally by three injections one month apart and is combined with diphtheria and tetanus vaccine (*triple vaccine*) or adsorbed diphtheria, tetanus and pertussis vaccine (DTPer/Vac/Ads).
✚▲ side-effects/warning: see under VACCINE. Administer with particular care to children with a history of febrile convulsions and with caution to children whose relatives have a history of seizures or who appear to have any form of neurological disorder.
○ Related entries: Adsorbed Diphtheria, Tetanus and Pertussis Vaccine; Trivax-AD

Per/Vac

is an abbreviation for PERTUSSIS VACCINE (whooping cough vaccine), which is usually administered in combination with diphtheria and tetanus vaccine (*triple vaccine*) as DTPer/Vac/Ads.
✚▲ side-effects/warning: see PERTUSSIS VACCINE

pethidine hydrochloride

is an (OPIOID) NARCOTIC ANALGESIC drug, which is used primarily for the relief of moderate to severe pain, especially during labour and operations. It is less effective than morphine and not suitable for relieving severe, chronic pain. Its effect is rapid and short-lasting, so its SEDATIVE properties are made use of only as a premedication prior to surgery, or to enhance the effects of other anaesthetic drugs during or following surgery. Administration is either oral in the form of tablets or by injection. Its proprietary preparation is on the Controlled Drugs List.
✚▲ side-effects/warning: see under OPIOID; but, compared to many opioids, it is less likely to cause constipation and there is less depression of respiration in the newborn when used to relieve pain during labour. It should not be used in patients with severe kidney damage. Overdose can cause convulsions.
○ Related entry: Pamergan P100

Pevaryl

(Cilag) is a proprietary, non-prescription preparation of the ANTIFUNGAL drug econazole nitrate. It can be used to treat fungal infections on the skin, such as nail infections and in the genital areas. It is available as a cream, a lotion and a dusting powder for topical application.
✚▲ side-effects/warning: see ECONAZOLE

P

P NITRATE; but side-effects are limited with
topical application.

Pevaryl TC

(Cilag) is a proprietary, non-prescription
COMPOUND PREPARATION of the
CORTICOSTEROID drug triamcinolone and
the ANTIFUNGAL drug econazole nitrate. It
can be used to treat fungal infections of
the skin, such as nail infections and in the
genital areas. It is available as a cream for
topical application.
✚▲ side-effects/warning: ECONAZOLE
NITRATE; TRIAMCINOLONE; but side-effects are
limited with topical application.

Pharmalgen

(Allerayde) is a proprietary, prescription-
only preparation of DESENSITIZING VACCINE.
It is available in a version for bee venom
or for wasp venom and can be used in
diagnosing and desensitizing patients who
are allergic to one or the other. It is
available in a form for injection.
✚▲ side-effects/warning: see
DESENSITIZING VACCINES

Pharmorubicin Rapid Dissolution

(Pharmacia) is a proprietary,
prescription-only preparation of the
(CYTOTOXIC) ANTICANCER drug epirubicin
hydrochloride. It can be used to treat
several types of cancer, including breast
cancer, and is available in a form for
injection.
✚▲ side-effects/warning: see EPIRUBICIN
HYDROCHLORIDE

Pharmorubicin Solution for Injection

(Pharmacia) is a prescription-only,
proprietary preparation of the (CYTO-
TOXIC) ANTICANCER drug epirubicin hydrochloride. It can be used to treat several
types of cancer, including breast cancer,
and is available in a form for injection.
✚▲ side-effects/warning: see EPIRUBICIN
HYDROCHLORIDE

Phasal

(Lagap) is a proprietary, prescription-only
preparation of the ANTIMANIA drug lithium
(as lithium carbonate). It is used to treat
acute mania, manic-depressive bouts and
recurrent depression. It is available as
tablets.
✚▲ side-effects/warning: see LITHIUM

phenazocine hydrobromide

is an (OPIOID) NARCOTIC ANALGESIC drug,
which is used primarily for the relief
of severe pain, especially pain arising
from disorders of the bile ducts.
Administration is oral in the form of
tablets and sublingual tablets. Its
proprietary preparation is on the
Controlled Drugs List.
✚▲ side-effect/warning: see under OPIOID.
✪ Related entry: Narphen

phenelzine

is an ANTIDEPRESSANT drug, one of the
MONOAMINE-OXIDASE INHIBITOR (MAOI)
group. It is used particularly when
treatment with TRICYCLIC antidepressants
(eg. AMITRIPTYLINE HYDROCHLORIDE or
IMIPRAMINE HYDROCHLORIDE) has failed
and is one of the safer, less STIMULANT MAO
inhibitors. However, a suitably long wash-
out period is necessary before switching
between different groups of
antidepressant. Administration (as
phenelzine sulphate) is oral in the form of
tablets. Treatment with the drug requires a
strict dietary regime (for example, a
patient must avoid eating cheese, meat or
yeast extracts, or drinking alcoholic
beverages) and extreme care must be
taken if using certain other forms of
medication.
✚ side-effects: drowsiness, fatigue, headache;
there may be weakness and dizziness,
particularly on standing up from lying or
sitting (postural hypotension). There may be
dry mouth and blurred vision, difficulty in
urinating, constipation, sweating, oedema,
rash, nervousness and sexual disturbances.
There may be changes in appetite and weight

gain. Susceptible patients may experience agitation, confusion, hallucinations, tremor, or even psychotic episodes. There are rare reports of jaundice and liver disorders, of severely lowered blood sodium and of peripheral nerve disease.

▲ warning: it should not be administered to patients with certain liver disorders, vascular disease of the brain, or abnormal secretion of hormones by the adrenal glands (phaeochromocytoma). Administer with caution to patients with certain cardiovascular diseases, epilepsy, diabetes, blood disorders, or who are agitated or elderly. Counselling, or supervision, over diet and any other medication is essential. Withdrawal of treatment should be gradual.

◐ Related entry: Nardil

Phenergan

(Rhône-Poulenc Rorer) is a proprietary, non-prescription preparation of the ANTIHISTAMINE drug promethazine hydrochloride. It can be used for the symptomatic relief of allergic conditions of the upper respiratory tract and skin, including hay fever, allergic rhinitis, urticaria and for the treatment of anaphylactic reaction. It has marked SEDATIVE actions and can be used in treating temporary sleep disorders and as an ANTINAUSEANT to prevent motion sickness. It is available as tablets and an elixir (for motion sickness) and is not normally given to children under two years, except on medical advice. It is also available on a prescription-only basis in a form for injection.

✚▲ side-effects/warning: see PROMETHAZINE HYDROCHLORIDE

phenindamine tartrate

is an ANTIHISTAMINE drug. It can be used for the symptomatic relief of allergic symptoms such as hay fever and urticaria (itchy skin rash). Administration is oral in the form of tablets.

✚▲ side-effects/warning: see under ANTIHISTAMINE. But it differs from most other antihistamines because it may cause mild stimulation.

◐ Related entry: Thephorin

phenindione

is an ANTICOAGULANT drug. It is effective when taken orally (though it is not as commonly used as warfarin sodium) and is used in the treatment and prevention of thrombosis, such as after insertion of prosthetic heart valves. Administration is oral in the form of tablets.

✚▲ side-effects/warning: see under WARFARIN SODIUM. There may also be hypersensitivity reactions, including rashes and fever; blood disorders; diarrhoea; kidney and liver damage. Avoid when breast-feeding. Related entry: Dindevan.

pheniramine maleate

is an ANTIHISTAMINE drug. It can be used for the symptomatic relief of allergic symptoms such as hay fever and urticaria (itchy skin rash). It is also a constituent of several cough and decongestant preparations. Administration is oral in the form of tablets.

✚▲ side-effects/warning: see under ANTIHISTAMINE. Because of its sedative property, the performance of skilled tasks such as driving may be impaired.

◐ Related entries: Daneral SA; Triominic Tablet

phenobarbital

See PHENOBARBITONE

phenobarbitone

(phenobarbital) is a BARBITURATE drug. It is used as an ANTICONVULSANT and ANTI-EPILEPTIC in the prevention of most types of recurrent epileptic seizures (except absence seizures). Administration is either oral as tablets or an elixir, or by injection. Preparations containing phenobarbitone are on the Controlled Drugs List.

✚▲ side-effects/warning: see under BARBITURATE. The doses administered in the prevention of epileptic attacks are calculated

P

to minimize drowsiness and sedation. There may be additional side-effects such as lethargy, drowsiness, unsteady gait, skin reactions, mental depression (or paradoxical excitement, restlessness and confusion – especially in the elderly – or overactivity in children). Administer with care to patients with impaired liver or kidney function, respiratory depression, or who are pregnant or breast-feeding. It should not be given to those with porphyria. Withdrawal of treatment should be gradual.

❍ Related entry: see Gardenal Sodium

phenol

or carbolic acid, is a DISINFECTANT and ANTISEPTIC agent. It is used for cleaning wounds or inflammation (such as boils and abscesses), for mouth, throat or ear hygiene and to inject into haemorrhoids. Administration is topical as solutions, lotions, creams, ointments, or a mouthwash.

✚ side-effects: there may be skin irritation.
▲ warning: it is toxic if swallowed in concentrated form.

❍ Related entries: Blisteze; Chloraseptic; Germoline Cream; Germoline Ointment; Secaderm; TCP Antiseptic Throat Pastilles; TCP Liquid Antiseptic

phenolphthalein

is a *stimulant* LAXATIVE, which works by having an irritant action on the gastrointestinal tract. It is not used as much as it once was due to its side-effects and long-lasting action, which may continue for several days because the drug is recycled through the liver. Proprietary preparations that contain phenolphthalein usually contain other laxatives as well.

✚▲ side-effects/warning: the laxative effects may continue for several days; there may be discolouration of the urine and skin rashes.

❍ Related entries: Agarol; Alophen Pills; Bonomint; Brooklax; Correctol; Ex-Lax Chocolate; Ex-Lax Pills; Nylax Tablets; Reguletts.

phenoperidine hydrochloride

is an (OPIOID) NARCOTIC ANALGESIC drug. It is used to relieve pain during surgery, particularly in combination with GENERAL ANAESTHETICS to enhance their effects. Its additional property as a respiratory depressant is sometimes made use of in the treatment of patients who undergo prolonged assisted respiration. Administration is by injection.

✚▲ side-effects/warning: see under OPIOID
❍ Related entry: Operidine

phenothiazine derivatives

or phenothiazines, are a group of drugs that all have a similar chemical structure. Many of them are used as ANTIPSYCHOTIC drugs, eg. CHLORPROMAZINE HYDRO-CHLORIDE, FLUPHENAZINE HYDROCHLORIDE, PROMAZINE HYDROCHLORIDE, THIORIDAZINE and TRIFLUOPERAZINE and it is thought that their ability to block DOPAMINE receptors in the brain is the reason for their usefulness in treating psychoses. A number of them are also powerful ANTINAUSEANT or ANTI-EMETIC drugs and others (eg. PIPERAZINE) are ANTHELMINTICS.

See also: METHOTRIMEPRAZINE; PERICYAZINE; PERPHENAZINE; PIPOTHIAZINE PALMITATE; PROCHLORPERAZINE.

phenothrin

is a PEDICULICIDAL drug that is used to treat infestations by head and pubic lice (crabs). Administration is topical as a lotion.

✚ side-effects: there may be skin irritation.
▲ warning: avoid contact with the eyes and do not use on broken or infected skin. It may cause wheezing in asthmatics.

❍ Related entry: Full Marks Lotion

phenoxybenzamine hydrochloride

is an ALPHA-ADRENOCEPTOR BLOCKER drug. It is used, in combination with BETA-BLOCKERS, as a short-term

ANTIHYPERTENSIVE treatment and for severe hypertensive crises in phaeochromocytoma (a carcinoid syndrome involving cells, such as those in the adrenal medulla gland, that secrete ADRENALINE and NORADRENALINE). It can also be used to manage severe shock that is unresponsive to conventional treatment. Administration can be oral as capsules or in a form for injection.

✚ side-effects: the heart rate increases; there may be postural hypotension (dizziness, particularly on standing up from a lying or sitting position) and lethargy. There is sometimes nasal congestion and contraction of the pupils. There may be gastrointestinal disturbances, or a failure to ejaculate.

▲ warning: it should be administered with caution to patients with certain heart conditions, severe arteriosclerosis, impaired kidney function, or who are elderly.

✪ Related entry: Dibenyline

phenoxymethylpenicillin

(penicillin V) is a widely used ANTIBACTERIAL and ANTIBIOTIC drug. It is particularly effective in treating tonsillitis, infection of the middle ear, certain skin infections and to prevent recurrent streptococcal throat infection, which can lead to episodes of rheumatic fever. Administration is oral as tablets or liquids.

✚▲ side-effects/warning: see under BENZYLPENICILLIN

✪ Related entry: Apsin

Phensedyl Plus

(Rhône-Poulenc Rorer) is a proprietary, non-prescription COMPOUND PREPARATION of the ANTIHISTAMINE drug promethazine hydrochloride, the (OPIATE) ANTITUSSIVE drug pholcodine and the SYMPATHOMIMETIC drug pseudoephedrine hydrochloride. It can be used for the symptomatic relief of coughs and colds and is available as a syrup. It is not normally given to children, except on medical advice.

✚▲ warning/side-effects: see PHOLCODINE; PROMETHAZINE HYDROCHLORIDE; PSEUDOEPHEDRINE HYDROCHLORIDE

Phensic

(SmithKline Beecham) is a proprietary, non-prescription COMPOUND PREPARATION of the (NSAID) NON-NARCOTIC ANALGESIC and ANTIRHEUMATIC drug aspirin and the STIMULANT caffeine. It can be used to treat mild to moderate pain and to provide relief of mild upper airways infections such as colds and flu. It is available as capsule-shaped tablets and is not normally given to children under 12 years, except on medical advice.

✚▲ side-effects/warning: see ASPIRIN; CAFFEINE

phentermine

is an APPETITE SUPPRESSANT drug, which is used under medical supervision and on a short-term basis, to aid weight loss in severe obesity. It is a STIMULANT and potentially subject to abuse and so its proprietary preparations are on the Controlled Drugs List. There is growing doubt among experts over the medical value of such treatment. Administration is in the form of modified-release capsules.

✚▲ side-effects/warning: see under FENFLURAMINE HYDROCHLORIDE

✪ Related entries: Duromine; Ionamin

phentolamine mesylate

is an ALPHA-ADRENOCEPTOR BLOCKER drug. It is used, in combination with BETA-BLOCKERS, as an ANTIHYPERTENSIVE treatment of hypertensive crises in phaeochromocytoma (it is also used in the diagnosis of this condition) and may have some use in the treatment of impotence. Administration is by injection.

✚ side-effects: postural hypotension (fall in blood pressure on standing); dizziness; dry mouth and nasal congestion; decreased sweating, gastrointestinal upsets, chest pains in the elderly.

▲ warning: it should not be used in certain heart disorders. Administer with care to

P patients with kidney impairment, who are pregnant, or have various vascular or blood disorders.

○ Related entry: Rogitine

phenylbutazone

is a (NSAID) NON-NARCOTIC ANALGESIC and ANTIRHEUMATIC drug, which, because of its sometimes severe side-effects, is used solely in the treatment of ankylosing spondylitis under special conditions of medical supervision in hospitals. Even for that purpose it is used only when all other therapies have failed and treatment may then be prolonged. Administration is oral in the form of tablets.

✚ side-effects: there may be gastrointestinal disturbances, nausea, vomiting and allergic reactions such as a rash. Less often there is inflammation of the salivary glands of the mouth, throat and neck; and visual disturbances. Rarely, there is severe fluid retention (which in susceptible patients may eventually precipitate heart failure) and serious and potentially dangerous blood disorders.

▲ warning: it should not be administered to patients with certain cardiovascular diseases, thyroid disease, impaired liver or kidney function; who are pregnant; who have a history of stomach or intestinal haemorrhaging, or who have Sjögren's syndrome (wasting of the salivary glands). It should be administered with caution to those who are elderly or breast-feeding. Regular and frequent blood counts are essential.

○ Related entry: Butacote

phenylephrine hydrochloride

is a VASOCONSTRICTOR and SYMPATHOMIMETIC drug administered by injection or infusion to increase blood pressure (sometimes in emergency situations until plasma transfusion is available). It is also incorporated into a number of proprietary cold cures as a vasoconstrictor and DECONGESTANT and in eye-drops to dilate the pupil to facilitate ophthalmic examination.

✚ side-effects: hypertension and headache; changes in heart rate; vomiting, tingling and coolness of the skin.

▲ warning: see under NORADRENALINE. It should not be given to patients with hyperthyroidism or severe hypertension.

○ Related entries: Beechams Hot Blackcurrant; Beechams Hot Lemon; Beechams Hot Lemon and Honey; Beechams Powders Capsules; Betnovate; Catarrh-Ex; Coldrex Powders, Blackcurrant; Coldrex Tablets; Dimotapp Elixir; Dimotapp Elixir Paediatric; Dimotapp LA Tablets; Dristan Decongestant Tablets; Fenox Nasal Drops; Fenox Nasal Spray; Flurex Cold/Flu Capsules with Cough Suppressant; Flurex Tablets; Isopto Frin; Lemsip; Lemsip Cold Relief Capsules; Lemsip Flu Strength; Lemsip, Junior; Lemsip Menthol Extra; Minims Phenylephrine Hydrochloride; Phenylephrine Injection 1%

Phenylephrine Injection 1%

(Boots) is a proprietary, prescription-only preparation of the SYMPATHOMIMETIC and VASOCONSTRICTOR drug phenylephrine hydrochloride. It can be used to treat cases of acute hypotension (low blood pressure), particularly in emergency situations as a temporary measure while preparations are made for blood transfusion. It is available in a form for injection.

✚▲ side-effects/warning: see under PHENYLEPHRINE HYDROCHLORIDE

phenylpropanolamine hydrochloride

is a SYMPATHOMIMETIC and VASOCONSTRICTOR drug. It is used systemically as an upper airways DECONGESTANT in the symptomatic relief of allergic disorders, such as asthma and hay fever, (when it is often administered with an antihistamine) and also for the symptomatic relief of colds and flu (often

in combination with ANALGESIC drugs).
Administration can be by several routes,
including orally as tablets, modified-
release tablets, capsules, a syrup, or an
elixir.

+▲ side-effects/warning: see under
EPHEDRINE HYDROCHLORIDE

**✪ Related entries: Aller-eze Plus;
Benylin Day and Night; Contac 400; Day
Nurse Capsules; Day Nurse Liquid;
Dimotapp Elixir; Dimotapp Elixir
Paediatric; Dimotapp LA Tablets;
Eskornade Capsules; Eskornade Syrup;
Lemsip Night-Time; Mu-Cron Tablets;
Night Nurse Capsules; Triogesic Tablets;
Triominic Tablet; Vicks Coldcare
Capsules; Vicks Vaposyrup for Chesty
Coughs; Vicks Vaposyrup for Chesty
Coughs and Nasal Congestion; Vicks
Vaposyrup for Dry Coughs and Nasal
Congestion**

phenytoin

is an ANTICONVULSANT and ANTI-EPILEPTIC
drug. It is used to treat most forms of
epilepsy (except absence seizures) and
trigeminal (facial) neuralgia. It has also
been used as an ANTI-ARRHYTHMIC drug.
Administration (as phenytoin or phenytoin
sodium) is either oral as tablets, chewable
tablets, capsules or a suspension, or by
injection.

+ side-effects: nausea, vomiting, confusion,
headache, dizziness, nervousness, insomnia;
rarely, movement disorders, peripheral nerve
disorders, unsteady gait, slurred speech, eye-
flicker and blurred vision, rashes, acne,
enlargement of the gums, growth of excess
hair and blood disorders

▲ warning: administer with caution to
patients with liver impairment, or who are
pregnant or breast-feeding; avoid its use in
those with porphyria. Withdrawal of treatment
should be gradual.

**✪ Related entries: Epanutin; Epanutin
Ready Mixed Parenteral; Pentran**

Phimetin

(BHR) is a proprietary preparation of the

H₂-ANTAGONIST drug cimetidine. It is
available on prescription or without a
prescription in a limited amount and for
short-term uses only. It can be used as an
ULCER-HEALING DRUG for benign peptic
ulcers (in the stomach or duodenum),
gastro-oesophageal reflux, dyspepsia and
associated conditions. It is available as
tablets.

+▲ side-effects/warning: see CIMETIDINE

Phiso-med

(Sanofi Winthrop) is a proprietary, non-
prescription preparation of the ANTISEPTIC
agent chlorhexidine (as gluconate). It can
be used as a soap or shampoo substitute
in acne and seborrhoeic conditions and
for bathing babies in maternity units to
prevent cross infection. It is available as a
solution.

+▲ side-effects/warning: see
CHLORHEXIDINE

pholcodine

is a weak OPIOID drug that is used as a
cough treatment (in preference to
stronger opioids of the NARCOTIC
ANALGESIC type) and as an ANTITUSSIVE
constituent in many cough linctuses or
syrups. Although its action resembles that
of other opioids it has no appreciable
analgesic effect or addictive liability.

+▲ side-effects/warning: see under CODEINE
PHOSPHATE

**✪ Related entries: Copholco;
Copholcoids Cough Pastilles; Davenol;
Day Cold Comfort Capsules; Expulin
Children's Cough Linctus – Sugar Free;
Expulin Cough Linctus – Sugar Free;
Expulin Dry Cough Linctus; Famel
Linctus; Galenphol Linctus; Galenphol
Linctus, Strong; Galenphol Paediatric
Linctus; Night Cold Comfort Capsules;
Pavacol-D; Phensedyl Plus; Pholcomed;
Pholcomed Diabetic Forte; Tixylix
Cough and Cold**

Pholcomed D

(Medo) is a proprietary, non-prescription

P preparation of the (OPIOID) ANTITUSSIVE drug pholcodine. It can be used as a cough treatment for dry or painful coughs and is available as a sugar-free linctus.
✚▲ warning/side-effects: see PHOLCODINE

Pholcomed Diabetic Forte

(Medo) is a proprietary, non-prescription preparation of the (OPIOID) ANTITUSSIVE drug pholcodine. It can be used as a cough treatment in dry or painful coughs and is available as a sugar-free linctus.
✚▲ warning/side-effects: see PHOLCODINE

PhorPain

(Goldshield) is a proprietary, non-prescription preparation of the (NSAID) NON-NARCOTIC ANALGESIC, ANTIRHEUMATIC and ANTIPYRETIC drug ibuprofen. It can be used for the relief of headache, backache, muscular pain, dental pain and cold and flu symptoms. It is available as tablets and is not normally given to children under 12 years, except on medical advice.
✚▲ side-effects/warning: see IBUPROFEN

PhorPain Double Strength

(Goldshield) is a proprietary, non-prescription preparation of the (NSAID) NON-NARCOTIC ANALGESIC, ANTIRHEUMATIC and ANTIPYRETIC drug ibuprofen. It can be used for the relief of headache, backache, muscular pain, dental pain and cold and flu symptoms. It is available as tablets and is not normally used in children under 12 years, except on medical advice.
✚▲ side-effects/warning: see IBUPROFEN

Phosphate-Sandoz

(Sandoz) is a proprietary, non-prescription COMPOUND PREPARATION of potassium bicarbonate, sodium acid phosphate and sodium bicarbonate. It can be used as a MINERAL SUPPLEMENT to provide phosphate, which may be required in addition to vitamin D in patients with vitamin D-resistant rickets. It is available as tablets.

✚▲ side-effects/warning: see SODIUM ACID PHOSPHATE; SODIUM BICARBONATE

*phosphodiesterase inhibitors

are a relatively new class of drugs, which have so far been used in short-term congestive HEART FAILURE TREATMENT, especially where other drugs have been unsuccessful. They work by inhibiting certain enzymes and so effect the heart in ways that mimic SYMPATHOMIMETICS acting at beta-adrenoceptors. Examples of these drugs include ENOXIMONE and MILRINONE.

Phyllocontin Continus

(Napp) is a proprietary, non-prescription preparation of the BRONCHODILATOR drug aminophylline. It can be used as an ANTI-ASTHMATIC and to treat bronchitis and is available as modified-release tablets.
✚▲ warning/side-effects: see AMINOPHYLLINE

Physeptone

(Wellcome) is a proprietary, prescription-only preparation of the (OPIOID) NARCOTIC ANALGESIC drug methadone hydrochloride, which is on the Controlled Drugs List. It can be used to treat severe pain and is available as tablets and in a form for injection.
✚▲ side-effects/warning: see METHADONE HYDROCHLORIDE

physostigmine sulphate

(eserine) is a vegetable ALKALOID and is an ANTICHOLINESTERASE drug that enhances the effects of the NEUROTRANSMITTER acetylcholine (and of certain cholinergic drugs). Because of this property, it has PARASYMPATHOMIMETIC actions and can be used to stimulate the pupil of the eye in GLAUCOMA TREATMENT (when it is usually given with PILOCARPINE). Administration is topical in the form of eye-drops.
✚▲ side-effects/warning: there can be parasympathomimetic side-effects if a

sufficient amount is absorbed into the eye (see under NEOSTIGMINE).

Phytex

(Pharmax) is a proprietary, non-prescription COMPOUND PREPARATION of several ANTIFUNGAL and KERATOLYTIC drugs, including salicylic acid, tannic acid and boric acid (with ethyl acetate and alcohol). It can be used to treat fungal infections of the skin and nails and is available as a paint for topical application.

+▲ side-effects/warning: see SALICYLIC ACID

phytomenadione

(vitamin K₁) is a natural form of VITAMIN K and is normally obtained from vegetables and dairy products. Phytomenadione can be used to treat vitamin K deficiency, but not a deficiency caused by malabsorption states (in such cases vitamin K₁ or MENADIOL SODIUM PHOSPHATE, the synthetic form of vitamin K₃, must be used). Administration is either oral in the form of tablets or by slow intravenous injection.

+▲ side-effects/warning: see VITAMIN K
✪ Related entry: Konakion

Picolax

(Nordic) is a proprietary, non-prescription preparation of the (*stimulant*) LAXATIVES sodium picosulphate and magnesium citrate. It can be used to evacuate the bowels before surgery, radiography, or endoscopy. It is available as a powder for making into an oral solution.

+▲ side-effects/warnings:
see SODIUM PICOSULPHATE;
see under MAGNESIUM SULPHATE

pilocarpine

is a PARASYMPATHOMIMETIC drug. It can be applied to the eye to treat glaucoma by improving drainage of aqueous fluid from the eye and to constrict the pupil of the eye after it has been dilated for ophthalmic examination. It is available as eye-drops.

+ side-effects: impaired focusing of the eye.
▲ warning: there can be systemic cholinergic actions if a sufficient amount is absorbed into the eye.
✪ Related entries: Isopto Carpine; Minims Pilocarpine Nitrate; Ocusert Pilo; Sno Pilo

pimozide

is an ANTIPSYCHOTIC drug, which is used to treat patients suffering from psychotic disorders such as schizophrenia, paranoia and mania. It can also be used to treat Gilles de la Tourette syndrome and in the short-term treatment of severe anxiety. Administration is oral in the form of tablets.

+▲ side-effects/warning: see under CHLORPROMAZINE HYDROCHLORIDE; but is less sedating. It is not to be given to patients who are breast-feeding, or with certain heart arrhythmias.
✪ Related entry: Orap

pindolol

is a BETA-BLOCKER that can be used as an ANTIHYPERTENSIVE treatment for raised blood pressure and as an ANTI-ANGINA treatment to relieve symptoms and improve exercise tolerance. Administration is oral in the form of tablets. It is also available, as an antihypertensive treatment, in the form of a COMPOUND PREPARATION with a DIURETIC.
+▲ side-effects/warnings: see under PROPRANOLOL HYDROCHLORIDE
✪ Related entries: Viskaldix; Visken

pipenzolate bromide

is an ANTICHOLINERGIC drug. It is used to assist in the treatment of gastrointestinal disorders that involve muscle spasm of the intestinal wall. Administration is oral in the form of tablets or a suspension.
+▲ side-effects/warning: see under ATROPINE SULPHATE
✪ Related entry: Piptalin

P

piperacillin

is a broad-spectrum ANTIBACTERIAL and
(PENICILLIN) ANTIBIOTIC drug. It is used to
treat many serious or compound forms of
bacterial infection, particularly those
caused by *Pseudomonas aeruginosa*.
Administration is by injection or infusion.
+▲ side-effects/warning: see under
BENZYLPENICILLIN
☉ Related entry: Tazocin

piperazine

is an ANTHELMINTIC drug (a
PHENOTHIAZINE DERIVATIVE), which is used
to treat infestation by roundworm or
threadworm. Administration is oral as
tablets, an oral powder, a syrup, or a
dilute elixir.
+ side-effects: there may be nausea and
vomiting with diarrhoea; there may also be
allergic reactions such as urticaria (itchy skin
rash). Rarely, there is dizziness, colic and lack
of muscular co-ordination ('worm wobble').
▲ warning: it should be administered with
caution to patients with certain kidney or liver
disorders, epilepsy, neurological disease, or
who are pregnant.
**☉ Related entries: De Witt's Worm
Syrup; Expelix; Pripsen Powder; Pripsen
Worm Elixir**

piperazine oestrone
sulphate

is a female SEX HORMONE, an OESTROGEN,
which is used in HRT (hormone
replacement therapy). Administration is
oral in the form of tablets.
+▲ side-effects/warning: see under
OESTROGEN
☉ Related entry: Harmogen

Piportil Depot

(Rhône-Poulenc Rorer) is a proprietary,
prescription-only preparation of the
ANTIPSYCHOTIC drug pipothiazine
palmitate. It can be used in maintenance
therapy of patients with psychotic
disorders such as chronic schizophrenia.
Administration is by a long-acting depot

deep intramuscular injection.
+▲ side-effects/warning: see PIPOTHIAZINE
PALMITATE

pipothiazine palmitate

(pipotiazine palmitate) is a
PHENOTHIAZINE DERIVATIVE, which is used
as an ANTIPSYCHOTIC in maintenance
therapy of patients with schizophrenia and
other psychoses. Administration is by
injection.
+▲ side-effects/warning: see under
CHLORPROMAZINE. It is not be administered to
patients with parkinsonism or confusional
states.
☉ Related entry: Piportil Depot

pipotiazine palmitate

See PIPOTHIAZINE PALMITATE

Pipril

(Lederle) is a proprietary, prescription-
only preparation of the broad-spectrum
ANTIBACTERIAL and (PENICILLIN)
ANTIBIOTIC drug PIPERACILLIN. It can be
used to treat many serious or compound
forms of bacterial infection, particularly
those caused by *Pseudomonas
aeruginosa*. It is available in a form for
injection and infusion.
+▲ side-effects/warning: see PIPERACILLIN

Piptalin

(Boehringer Mannheim) is a proprietary,
prescription-only COMPOUND PREPARATION
of the ANTICHOLINERGIC drug pipenzolate
bromide and the ANTIFOAMING AGENT
dimethicone. It can be used as an
ANTISPASMODIC for the symptomatic relief
of smooth muscle spasm in the
gastrointestinal tract. It is available as a
suspension.
+▲ side-effects/warning: see DIMETHICONE;
PIPENZOLATE BROMIDE

piracetam

is a recently introduced drug that is used
to treat cortical myoclonus (involuntary
spasmic contractions of muscles of the

body). Administration is oral as tablets or an oral solution.

✚▲ side-effects: diarrhoea, weight gain, sleepiness, insomnia, depression, rash and overactivity.

▲ warning: it should not be used in patients with severe liver or kidney impairment, or who are pregnant or breast-feeding. Withdrawal of treatment should be gradual.

○ **Related entry: Nootropll**

pirbuterol

is a SYMPATHOMIMETIC and BETA-RECEPTOR STIMULANT, which has beta$_2$-receptor selectivity. It is mainly used as a BRONCHODILATOR in reversible obstructive airways disease and as an ANTI-ASTHMATIC treatment in severe acute asthma. It can also be used for the alleviation of symptoms of chronic bronchitis and emphysema. Administration is by capsules or aerosol. (Patients should be cautioned not to exceed the stated dose and if a previously effective dose fails to relieve symptoms they should consult their doctor.)

✚▲ side-effects/warning: see under SALBUTAMOL

○ **Related entry: Exirel**

pirenzepine

is an ANTICHOLINERGIC drug with properties that are quite different from many other drugs in this class. It can reduce the production of gastric acids and digestive juices from the stomach, so reducing the acidity and without widespread side-effects. It can therefore be used as an ULCER-HEALING DRUG for gastric and duodenal ulcers. Administration is oral in the form of tablets.

✚ side-effects: rarely, there may be dry mouth and slight visual disturbance. Blood disorders have been reported.

▲ warning: do not administer to patients with an enlarged prostate gland, closed-angle glaucoma, paralytic ileus, pyloric stenosis, or who are pregnant. Use with care in those with

kidney impairment.

○ **Related entry: Gastrozepin**

piretanide

is a powerful (*loop*) DIURETIC drug, which can be used as an ANTIHYPERTENSIVE. Administration is oral in the form of capsules.

✚▲ side-effects/warning: see under FRUSEMIDE

○ **Related entry: Arelix**

Piriton

(Allen & Hanburys) is a proprietary, non-prescription preparation of the ANTIHISTAMINE drug chlorpheniramine maleate. It can be used to treat allergic conditions such as hay fever and urticaria. It is available as tablets and a syrup and is also available on a prescription-only basis in a form for injection.

✚▲ side-effects/warning: see CHLORPHENIRAMINE MALEATE

piroxicam

is a (NSAID) NON-NARCOTIC ANALGESIC and ANTIRHEUMATIC drug. It has a long duration of action and is used to treat pain and inflammation in rheumatic disease and other musculoskeletal disorders, including juvenile arthritis and acute gout. Administration can be oral in the form of capsules or soluble tablets, or as suppositories, or by injection, or as a gel for local application.

✚▲ side-effects/warning: see under NSAID. It may cause pain at the injection site; it may cause pancreatitis or gastrointestinal disturbances, especially in the elderly.

○ **Related entries: Feldene; Feldene Gel; Flamatrol; Larapam; Pirozip**

Pirozip

(Ashbourne) is a proprietary, prescription-only preparation of the (NSAID) NON-NARCOTIC ANALGESIC and ANTIRHEUMATIC drug piroxicam. It can be used to treat acute gout, arthritic and rheumatic pain and other musculoskeletal

P

disorders. It is available as capsules.
+▲ side-effects/warning: see PIROXICAM

Pitressin
(Parke-Davis) is a proprietary, prescription-only preparation of the HORMONE vasopressin. It can be administered either for diagnosis or as a DIABETES INSIPIDUS TREATMENT. Alternatively, it can be used to treat the bleeding of varices (varicose veins) in the oesophagus. It is available in a form for injection.
+▲ side-effects/warning: see VASOPRESSIN

pivampicillin
is a more readily absorbed form of the broad-spectrum ANTIBACTERIAL and (PENICILLIN) ANTIBIOTIC drug ampicillin. It is converted in the body to ampicillin after absorption and has similar actions and uses.
+▲ side-effects/warning: see under AMPICILLIN
❍ Related entry: Pondocillin

Piz Buin SPF 20 Sun Block Lotion
(Zyma Healthcare) is a proprietary, non-prescription SUNSCREEN lotion that protects the skin from UVA and UVB ultraviolet radiation (UVB-SPF 20). It is a cream-coloured skin lotion containing the pigment titanium dioxide along with butylmethoxydibenzoyl methane and octyl methoxy-cinnammimate. A patient whose skin condition requires this sort of protection may be prescribed it at the discretion of his or her doctor.
+▲ side-effects/warning: see TITANIUM DIOXIDE

pizotifen
is an ANTIHISTAMINE and SEROTONIN antagonist drug. It can be used as an ANTIMIGRAINE treatment, particularly for headaches in which blood pressure inside the blood vessels plays a part, such as migraine and cluster headache.

Administration is oral in the form of tablets or an elixir.
+ side-effects: anticholinergic effects, drowsiness, increased appetite and weight gain, occaisional nausea and dizziness.
▲ warning: administer with care to patients with urinary retention, kidney impairment, closed-angle glaucoma; or who are pregnant or breast-feeding. Drowsiness may impair the performance of skilled tasks such as driving.
❍ Related entry: Sanomigran

Plaquenil
(Sanofi Winthrop) is a proprietary, prescription-only preparation of hydroxychloroquine sulphate, which has ANTI-INFLAMMATORY and ANTIRHEUMATIC properties. It can be used to treat rheumatoid arthritis (including juvenile arthritis) and lupus erythematosus. It is available as tablets.
+▲ side-effects/warning: see HYDROXYCHLOROQUINE SULPHATE

Platet
(Nicholas) is a proprietary, non-prescription preparation of the (NSAID) NON-NARCOTIC ANALGESIC and ANTIRHEUMATIC drug aspirin, which can be used as an ANTIPLATELET aggregation (antithrombotic) drug. It can be used to reduce the formation of blood thrombi (clots) and is available as effervescent tablets.
+▲ side-effects/warning: see ASPIRIN

Plendil
(Schwarz) is a proprietary, prescription-only preparation of the CALCIUM-CHANNEL BLOCKER drug felodipine. It can be used as an ANTIHYPERTENSIVE treatment and is available as tablets.
+▲ side-effects/warning: see FELODIPINE

Plesmet
(Link) is a proprietary, non-prescription preparation of the drug ferrous glycine sulphate. It can be used as an IRON supplement in iron deficiency

ANAEMIA TREATMENT and is available as a syrup.

+▲ side-effects/warning: see FERROUS GLYCINE SULPHATE

plicamycin

(or mithramycin) is a CYTOTOXIC DRUG (of ANTIBIOTIC origin). It is used solely in the emergency control of calcium metabolism where there are excessive levels of calcium in the blood (hypercalaemia), which is caused by malignant disease. Administration is by injection.

+ side-effects: there may be nausea and vomiting, with hair loss. The blood-cell producing capacity of the bone marrow is reduced.

▲ warning: because the drug is toxic, the dose should be the minimum that is effective. Regular blood counts are essential during treatment. Administer with great caution to patients with kidney or liver disorders.

✪ Related entry: Mithracin

pneumococcal vaccine

is a VACCINE used for IMMUNIZATION against pneumonia. It is intended really only for those people at particular risk from infection and at risk from an identified pneumococcal strain prevalent within a community. The duration of protection is considered to be about five years. Administration is by subcutaneous or intramuscular injection.

+▲ side-effects/warning:
see under VACCINE

✪ Related entry: Pneumovax II

Pneumovax II

(Morson) is a proprietary, prescription-only VACCINE preparation of pneumococcal vaccine. It can be used for prevention of pneumococcal pneumonia in people for whom the risk of contracting the disease is unusually high. It is available in a form for injection.

+▲ side-effects/warning: see
PNEUMOCOCCAL VACCINE

podophyllum

is a KERATOLYTIC and caustic agent that can be used to treat and dissolve warts and also to reduce the production of new skin cells.

+▲ side-effects/warning: it may cause considerable irritation (particularly to eyes), avoid face, normal skin and open wounds. Do not use if pregnant or breast-feeding.

✪ Related entries: Condyline; Warticon; Warticon Fem

poldine methylsulphate

(poldine metilsulfate) is an ANTICHOLINERGIC drug. It can be used as an ANTISPASMODIC for the symptomatic relief of smooth muscle spasm in the gastrointestinal tract. Administration is oral in the form of tablets.

+▲ side-effects/warning: see under ATROPINE SULPHATE

✪ Related entry: Nacton

poldine metilsulfate

See POLDINE METHYLSULPHATE

Poliomyelitis Vaccine, Inactivated

(District Health Authorities)
(Pol/Vav – Inact) is a non-proprietary, prescription-only VACCINE preparation of poliomyelitis vaccine inactivated, (Salk). It can be used to provide immunity from infection by polio and is available in a form for injection.

+▲ side-effects/warning: see
POLIOMYELITIS VACCINE

Poliomyelitis Vaccine, Live (Oral)

(District Health Authorities)
(Pol/Vav – Oral) is a non-proprietary, prescription-only VACCINE preparation of poliomyelitis vaccine live, (oral) (Sabine), which contains 'live' but attenuated polio viruses. It can be used to confer immunity from infection and is available in a form for oral administration.

P

461

P

+▲ side-effects/warning: see POLIOMYELITIS VACCINE

poliomyelitis vaccine

is a VACCINE used for IMMUNIZATION that is available in two types. Poliomyelitis vaccine, inactivated (Salk) is a suspension of dead viruses injected into the body so that the body produces antibodies and becomes immune. Poliomyelitis vaccine live, (oral) (Sabine) is a suspension of live but attenuated polio viruses (of polio virus types 1, 2 and 3) for oral administration. In the UK, the live vaccine is more commonly used and the administration is generally simultaneous with diphtheria-pertussis-tetanus (triple) vaccine during the first year of life with a booster at school entry age. The inactivated vaccine remains available for those patients who, for some reason, cannot use the live vaccine.

+▲ side-effects/warning: see under VACCINE

Pollon-Eze

(Centra Healthcare) is a proprietary, non-prescription preparation of the ANTIHISTAMINE drug astemizole. It can be used to treat the symptoms of allergic disorders such as hay fever and urticaria and is available as tablets.

+▲ side-effects/warning: see ASTEMIZOLE

Pol/Vac (Inact)

is an abbreviation for POLIO MYELITIS VACCINE, INACTIVATED

Pol/Vac (Oral)

is an abbreviation for POLIO MYELITIS VACCINE, LIVE (ORAL)

polyestradiol phosphate

is a an analogue of OESTROGEN, a SEX HORMONE, that is used as an ANTICANCER treatment for cancer of the prostate gland. Administration is by intramuscular injection.

+▲ side-effects/warning: see under STILBOESTROL

◎ **Related entry: Estradurin**

Polyfax

(Cusi) is a proprietary, prescription-only COMPOUND PREPARATION of the ANTIBACTERIAL and ANTIBIOTIC drugs polymyxin B sulphate and bacitracin zinc. It can be used to treat infections of the skin and the eye and is available for topical application as a skin ointment, an eye ointment and as eye-drops.

+▲ side-effects/warning: see BACITRACIN ZINC; POLYMYXIN B SULPHATE

polymyxin

is the name of a group of ANTIBACTERIAL and ANTIBIOTIC drugs. They are active against Gram-negative bacteria, including *Pseudomonas aeruginosa* and are used to treat skin infections, burns and wounds. The antibiotics of this group can be administered by injection or topical application; though COLISTIN is not absorbed orally it can be used to sterilize the bowel. See also POLYMYXIN B SULPHATE.

polymyxin B sulphate

is an ANTIBACTERIAL and (POLYMYXIN) ANTIBIOTIC drug. It can be used to treat several forms of bacterial infection, particularly infections caused by Gram-negative bacteria such as *Pseudomonas aeruginosa*. Its use is restricted because it very toxic and because of this toxicity it is mainly administered topically as eye-drops, ear-drops, or ointments.

+▲ side-effects/warning: side-effects are minimal on topical application.

◎ **Related entries: Gregoderm; Maxitrol; Neosporin; Otosporin; Polyfax; Polytrim; Terra-Cortril; Tribiotic**

polynoxylin

is an ANTIFUNGAL and ANTIBACTERIAL drug. It can be used topically as a cream to treat minor skin infections.

◎ **Related entry: Anaflex**

polystyrene sulphonate resins

are used to treat excessively high levels of potassium in the blood, for example, in dialysis patients. Administration is either oral as a solution or by topical application in the form of a retention enema.

✛ side-effects: treatment by enemas may cause rectal ulcers.

▲ warning: some resins should not be given to patients with hyperparathyroidism, sarcoidosis, multiple myeloma, or metastatic cancer; avoid in those with congestive heart failure or impaired kidney function. An adequate fluid intake must be maintained.

○ Related entries: Calcium Resonium; Resonium A

Polytar Emollient

(Stiefel) is a proprietary, non-prescription preparation of coal tar. It can be used to treat psoriasis, eczema and dermatitis and is available as a liquid for adding to a bath.

✛▲ side-effects/warning: see COAL TAR

polythiazide

is one of the THIAZIDE class of DIURETICS. It can be used in ANTIHYPERTENSIVE treatment, either alone or in conjunction with other types of drugs and in the treatment of oedema (accumulation of fluid in the tissues) associated with congestive heart failure. Administration is oral in the form of tablets.

✛▲ side-effects/warning: see under BENDROFLUAZIDE

○ Related entry: Nephril

Polytrim

(Cusi) is a proprietary, prescription-only COMPOUND PREPARATION of the ANTIBACTERIAL and ANTIBIOTIC drugs trimethoprim and polymyxin B sulphate. It can be used to treat bacterial infections in the eye and is available as eye-drops and an eye ointment.

✛▲ side-effects/warning: see POLYMYXIN B SULPHATE; TRIMETHOPRIM

polyvinyl alcohol

is a constituent in several preparations that are used as artificial tears to treat dryness of the eye due to disease. Administration is by topical application as eye-drops.

○ Related entries: Hypotears; Liquifilm Tears; Sno Tears

Ponderax

(Servier) is a proprietary, prescription-only preparation of the APPETITE SUPPRESSANT drug fenfluramine hydrochloride. It can be used as a short-term, additional treatment in medical therapy for obesity. It is available as modified-release capsules (*Pacaps*).

✛▲ side-effects/warning: see FENFLURAMINE HYDROCHLORIDE

Pondocillin

(Leo) is a proprietary, prescription-only preparation of the broad-spectrum ANTIBACTERIAL and (PENICILLIN) ANTIBIOTIC drug pivampicillin. It can be used to treat systemic bacterial infections, infections of the upper respiratory tract, of the ear, nose and throat and of the urinogenital tracts. It is available as tablets.

✛▲ side-effects/warning: see PIVAMPICILLIN

Ponstan

(Parke-Davis) is a proprietary, prescription-only preparation of the (NSAID) NON-NARCOTIC ANALGESIC and ANTIRHEUMATIC drug mefenamic acid. It can be used to treat pain in rheumatoid arthritis, osteoarthritis and other musculoskeletal disorders and period pain. It is available as capsules, tablets (*Ponstan Forte*) and as a paediatric oral suspension.

✛▲ side-effects/warning: see MEFENAMIC ACID

Posalfilin

(Norgine) is a proprietary, non-prescription COMPOUND PREPARATION of

P

the KERATOLYTIC agents salicylic acid and podophyllum (resin). It can be used to treat and remove warts and verrucas (plantar warts) and is available as an ointment for topical application.
+▲ side-effects/warning: see PODOPHYLLUM; SALICYLIC ACID

Posiject

(Boehringer Ingelheim) is a proprietary, prescription-only preparation of the CARDIAC STIMULANT drug dobutamine hydrochloride, which has SYMPATHOMIMETIC and BETA-RECEPTOR STIMULANT properties. It can be used to treat serious heart disorders such as cardiogenic shock, septic shock, during heart surgery and in cardiac infarction. It works by increasing the heart's force of contraction and is available in a form for intravenous infusion.
+▲ side-effects/warning: see DOBUTAMINE HYDROCHLORIDE

Potaba

(Glenwood) is a proprietary, non-prescription preparation of potassium aminobenzoate. It can be used to treat scleroderma and Peyronie's disease and is available as capsules, tablets and as a powder in sachets (called envules).
+▲ side-effects/warning: see POTASSIUM AMINOBENZOATE

potassium aminobenzoate

is a drug that is used in the treatment of disorders associated with excess fibrous tissue, such as scleroderma and Peyronie's disease. There is uncertainty about how it works and how well. Administration is oral in the form of capsules, tablets, or a solution.
+ side-effects: there may be nausea; anorexia (if so discontinue treatment).
▲ warning: it should not be administered to patients who are taking sulphonamides and with caution to those with kidney disease.
464 **✪ Related entry: Potaba**

potassium canrenoate

is a mild DIURETIC drug of the *aldosterone-antagonist* type. It can be used to treat oedema (accumulation of fluid in the tissues) associated with aldosteronism (abnormal production of aldosterone by the adrenal gland), certain heart diseases and liver failure. Administration is by injection.
+▲ side-effects/warning: see under SPIRONOLACTONE. There may be nausea and vomiting and pain at the injection site.
✪ Related entry: Spiroctan-M

*potassium-channel activator

drugs work by opening pores in cell membranes that allow potassium ions to pass more readily, which has the effect of making them electrically less excitable. In blood vessels such drugs have VASODILATOR effects, which cause a reduction of the heart's workload and generally lowers blood pressure. The recently introduced drug of this type is NICORANDIL, which can be used to prevent and treat attacks of angina pectoris (ischaemic heart pain).

potassium chloride

is used primarily as a potassium supplement to correct potassium deficiency, especially due to or following severe loss of body fluids (eg. chronic diarrhoea) and treatment with drugs that deplete body reserves (eg. some DIURETICS). It may also be used as a substitute for natural salt (SODIUM CHLORIDE) in cases where sodium, for one reason or another, is inadvisable. Administration is either oral as tablets or by injection or intravenous infusion.
✪ Related entries:
Balanced Salt Solution; Burinex K; Diocalm Replenisher; Dioralyte; Diumide-K Continus; Glandosane; Lasikal; Lasix+K; Luborant; Neo-NaClex-K; Sando-K; Slow-K

potassium citrate

when administered orally has the effect of making the urine alkaline instead of acid. An action that is useful for relieving pain in some infections of the urinary tract or the bladder. Administration is oral in the form of tablets or a liquid solution.

✚ side-effects: there may be mild diuresis. Prolonged high dosage may lead to excessively high levels of potassium in the blood.

▲ warning: it should be administered with caution to patients with heart disease or impaired kidney function.

✪ Related entries: Balanced Salt Solution; Effercitrate

potassium hydroxyquinoline sulphate

is a drug that has both ANTIBACTERIAL and ANTIFUNGAL properties. It is used mostly as a constituent in anti-inflammatory and antibiotic creams and ointments, for example, in preparations used to treat acne.

✚ side-effects: rarely, it may cause sensitivity reactions.

✪ Related entries: Quinocort; Quinoderm Cream; Quinoderm Cream 5; Quinoderm Lotio-Gel 5%; Quinoped

potassium permanganate

is a general ANTISEPTIC agent. It can be used in solution for cleaning burns and abrasions and for maintaining asepsis in wounds that are suppurating or weeping.

✚▲ side-effects/warning: avoid contact with mucous membranes, to which it is an irritant. It stains skin and fabric.

✪ Related entry: Permitabs

povidone-iodine

is a complex of iodine on an organic carrier and is used as an ANTISEPTIC agent. It is topically applied to the skin, especially in sensitive areas (such as the vulva), acne of the scalp and is also used as a mouthwash. It works by slowly releasing the iodine it contains and is

available as a gel, an oral solution, or vaginal inserts (pessaries).

✚ side-effects: rarely, there may be sensitivity reactions.

▲ warning: these depend on the applications, but it should be used with care by patients with certain kidney diseases, who are pregnant or breast-feeding and on broken skin.

✪ Related entries: Betadine; Brush Off Cold Sore Lotion; Oilatum; Savlon Dry; Videne

Powerin Analgesic Tablets

(Whitehall Laboratories) is a proprietary, non-prescription COMPOUND PREPARATION of the (NSAID) NON-NARCOTIC ANALGESIC, ANTIRHEUMATIC and ANTIPYRETIC drug aspirin, the NON-NARCOTIC ANALGESIC drug paracetamol and the STIMULANT caffeine. It can be used to relieve mild to moderate pain, including headache, sore throat, toothache, muscle aches and pains, period pain and to relieve cold and flu symptoms. It is available as tablets and is not normally given to children under 12 years, except on medical advice.

✚▲ side-effects/warning: see ASPIRIN; CAFFEINE; PARACETAMOL

Pragmatar

(Bioglan) is a proprietary, non-prescription COMPOUND PREPARATION of coal tar (as cetyl alcohol-coal tar distillate), salicylic acid and sulphur. It can be used for psoriasis and eczema and is available as a cream.

✚▲ side-effects/warning: COAL TAR; SALICYLIC ACID; SULPHUR

pralidoxime mesylate

is an ANTIDOTE that is used to treat poisoning by organophosphorous compounds (eg. insecticides) in conjunction with an ANTICHOLINERGIC drug (usually ATROPINE SULPHATE). Administration is by injection.

✚ side-effects: drowsiness, dizziness, visual disturbances, muscular weakness, nausea,

P

headache, speeding of the heart and breathing, muscle weakness.

▲ warning: it should not be used to treat poisoning by carbamates or organophosphorous compounds without anticholinesterase activity. Use with caution in patients with myasthenia gravis or impaired kidney function.

pramoxine hydrochloride

is a LOCAL ANAESTHETIC drug, which is included in some proprietary preparations that are used for treating haemorrhoids. Administration is by topical application as a cream or suppositories.
○ Related entries: Anugesic-HC; Epifoam; Proctofoam HC

pravastatin

is used as a LIPID-LOWERING DRUG in hyperlipidaemia to reduce the levels, or change the proportions, of various lipids in the bloodstream. It is usually administered only to patients in whom a strict and regular dietary regime, alone, or some other therapy is not having the desired effect. Administration is oral in the form of tablets.
✛▲ side-effects/warning: see under SIMVASTATIN
○ Related entry: Lipostat

Praxilene

(Lipha) is a proprietary, non-prescription preparation of the VASODILATOR drug naftidrofuryl oxalate. It can be used to help improve blood circulation to the hands and feet when this is impaired, for example in peripheral vascular disease (Raynaud's phenomenon). It is available as tablets and in a form for injection.
✛▲ side-effects/warning: see NAFTIDROFURYL OXALATE

praziquantel

is an ANTHELMINTIC drug. It is the drug of choice (though not available in the UK) in treating infections caused by schistosomes, which are the worms that

can colonize the veins of a human host and cause bilharziasis and is also useful in the treatment of tapeworm infestation. It has a low toxicity and is administered orally.

prazosin hydrochloride

is an ALPHA-ADRENOCEPTOR BLOCKER drug. It is used as an ANTIHYPERTENSIVE treatment, often in conjunction with other classes of drug (such as BETA-BLOCKERS or DIURETICS), in congestive HEART FAILURE TREATMENT (because of its SMOOTH MUSCLE RELAXANT properties), in the treatment of urinary retention (eg. in benign prostatic hyperplasia) and in peripheral vascular disease (Raynaud's phenomenon). Administration is oral in the form of tablets.
✛ side-effects: postural hypotension (fall in blood pressure on standing), dizziness, headache, dry mouth and nasal congestion, failure to ejaculate, palpitations, frequent urination (and possibly incontinence). There may be weakness and drowsiness.
▲ warning: initially, it may cause marked postural hypotension, so the patient should lie down when given the drug or it should be taken on retiring to bed. It is not to be used in certain forms of congestive heart failure (eg. aortic stenosis). Administer with care to the elderly and to those with certain kidney disorders.
○ Related entries: Alphavase; Hypovase; Hypovase Benign Prostatic Hypertrophy

Precortisyl

(Roussel) is a proprietary, prescription-only preparation of the CORTICOSTEROID and ANTI-INFLAMMATORY drug prednisolone. It can be used in the treatment of allergic and rheumatic conditions, particularly those affecting the joints and soft tissues. It is available as tablets in several different forms and strengths (eg. *Precortisyl Forte*).
✛▲ side-effects/warning: see PREDNISOLONE

Predenema

(Pharmax) is a proprietary, prescription-only preparation of the CORTICOSTEROID drug prednisolone (as sodium metasulphobenzoate). It can be used as an ANTI-INFLAMMATORY treatment for rectal inflammation (eg. in ulcerative colitis and Crohn's disease). It is available as a retention enema.

✚▲ side-effects/warning: see PREDNISOLONE SODIUM PHOSPHATE

Predfoam

(Pharmax) is a proprietary, prescription-only preparation of the CORTICOSTEROID drug prednisolone (as sodium metasulphobenzoate). It can be used as an ANTI-INFLAMMATORY treatment for inflammation of the rectum (eg. in ulcerative colitis and Crohn's disease). It is available as a rectal foam enema.

✚▲ side-effects/warning: see PREDNISOLONE

Pred Forte

(Allergan) is a proprietary, prescription-only preparation of the CORTICOSTEROID and ANTI-INFLAMMATORY drug prednisolone (as acetate). It can be used to treat inflammatory conditions in and around the eye and is available as eye-drops.

✚▲ side-effects/warning: see PREDNISOLONE

Prednesol

(Glaxo) is a proprietary, prescription-only preparation of the CORTICOSTEROID and ANTI-INFLAMMATORY drug prednisolone. It can be used in the treatment of allergic and rheumatic conditions, particularly those affecting the joints and soft tissues. It is available as tablets.

✚▲ side-effects/warning: see PREDNISOLONE

prednisolone

is a synthetic, *glucocorticoid* CORTICOSTEROID with ANTI-INFLAMMATORY properties. It is used in the treatment of a number of rheumatic and allergic conditions (particularly those affecting the joints or the lungs) and collagen disorders. It is also an effective treatment for ulcerative colitis, inflammatory bowel disease, Crohn's disease, rectal or anal inflammation, haemorrhoids and as an IMMUNOSUPPRESSANT in the treatment of myasthenia gravis. It may also be used for systemic corticosteroid therapy. Administration (as prednisolone, prednisolone acetate, prednisolone, or sodium phosphate) can be oral in the form of tablets, or by topical application in the form of creams, lotions, ointments, suppositories, or a retention enema, or by injection.

✚▲ side-effects/warning: see under CORTICOSTEROIDS. The type and severity of any side-effects depends on the route of administration.

○ Related entries: Deltacortril Enteric; Deltastab; Minims Prednisolone; Precortisyl; Pred Forte; Predenema; Predfoam; Prednesol; Predsol; Predsol-N; Scheriproct

prednisone

is a CORTICOSTEROID that is converted in the body to the *glucocorticoid* corticosteroid PREDNISOLONE. It can be used as an ANTI-INFLAMMATORY drug for a variety of inflammatory and allergic disorders. Administration is oral in the form of tablets.

✚▲ side-effects/warning: see under CORTICOSTEROIDS

○ Related entry: Decortisyl

Predsol

(Evans) is a proprietary, prescription-only preparation of the CORTICOSTEROID drug prednisolone (as sodium phosphate). It can be used as an ANTI-INFLAMMATORY treatment for inflammation of the rectum (eg. in ulcerative colitis and Crohn's disease) and for non-infected, inflammatory ear and eye conditions. It is available as a retention enema, suppositories and as ear- or eye-drops.

✚▲ side-effects/warning: see PREDNISOLONE

P

Predsol-N

(Evans) is a proprietary, prescription-only COMPOUND PREPARATION of the CORTICOSTEROID drug prednisolone sodium phosphate and the ANTIBACTERIAL and (AMINOGLYCOSIDE) ANTIBIOTIC drug neomycin sulphate. It can be used to treat inflammatory ear and eye conditions and is available as ear- and eye-drops.
+▲ side-effects/warning: see NEOMYCIN SULPHATE; PREDNISOLONE SODIUM PHOSPHATE

Preferid

(Yamanouchi) is a proprietary, prescription-only preparation of the CORTICOSTEROID drug budesonide. It can be used to treat severe inflammatory skin disorders such as eczema and psoriasis and is available as a cream and an ointment.
+▲ side-effects/warning: see BUDESONIDE

Prefil

(Norgine) is a proprietary, non-prescription preparation of the (*bulking agent*) LAXATIVE sterculia. It can be used in the medical treatment of obesity, where it is intended to make a patient feel full. It is available as granules for solution.
+▲ side-effects/warning: see STERCULIA

Pregaday

(Evans) is a proprietary, non-prescription COMPOUND PREPARATION of ferrous fumarate and folic acid. It can be used as an IRON and folic acid supplement during pregnancy and is available as tablets.
+▲ side-effects/warning: see FERROUS FUMARATE; FOLIC ACID

Pregnyl

(Organon) is a proprietary, prescription-only preparation of the HORMONE human chorionic gonadotrophin (HCG). It can be used to treat undescended testicles and delayed puberty in boys and as an infertility treatment in women suffering from specific hormonal deficiency contributing to infertility. It is available in a form for injection.
+▲ side-effects/warning: see CHORIONIC GONADOTROPHIN

Premarin

(Wyeth) is a proprietary, prescription-only preparation of the OESTROGEN of conjugated oestrogens. It can be used in HRT and is available in the form of tablets in a calendar pack.
+▲ side-effects/warning: see CONJUGATED OESTROGENS

Prempak-C

(Wyeth) is a proprietary, prescription-only COMPOUND PREPARATION of the female SEX HORMONES the OESTROGEN conjugated oestrogens and the PROGESTOGEN norgestrel. It can be used in HRT and is available in the form of tablets in a calendar pack.
+▲ side-effects/warning: see CONJUGATED OESTROGENS; NORGESTREL

Prepadine

(Berk) is a proprietary, prescription-only preparation of the (TRICYCLIC) ANTIDEPRESSANT drug dothiepin hydrochloride. It can be used to treat depressive illness, especially in cases where some degree of sedation is deemed necessary. It is available as tablets and capsules.
+▲ side-effects/warning: see DOTHIEPIN HYDROCHLORIDE

Prepidil

(Upjohn) is a proprietary, prescription-only preparation of the PROSTAGLANDIN dinoprostone. It is used to induce labour and is administered as a cervical gel to the cervix.
+▲ side-effects/warning: see DINOPROSTONE

Prepulsid

(Janssen) is a proprietary, prescription-only preparation of the MOTILITY STIMULANT drug cisapride. It can be used to stimulate the stomach and intestine in a number of conditions and is available as tablets and a suspension.

✚▲ side-effects/warning: see CISAPRIDE

Prescal

(Ciba) is a proprietary, prescription-only preparation of the CALCIUM-CHANNEL BLOCKER drug isradipine. It can be used as an ANTIHYPERTENSIVE treatment and is available as tablets.

✚▲ side-effects/warning: see ISRADIPINE

Prestim

(Leo) is a proprietary, prescription-only COMPOUND PREPARATION of the BETA-BLOCKER drug timolol maleate and the (THIAZIDE) DIURETIC drug bendrofluazide. It can be used as an ANTIHYPERTENSIVE treatment for raised blood pressure and is available as tablets.

✚▲ side-effects/warning: see BENDROFLUAZIDE; TIMOLOL MALEATE

Prestim Forte

(Leo) is a proprietary, prescription-only COMPOUND PREPARATION of the BETA-BLOCKER drug timolol maleate and the (THIAZIDE) DIURETIC drug bendrofluazide. It can be used as an ANTIHYPERTENSIVE treatment for raised blood pressure and is available as tablets.

✚▲ side-effects/warning: see BENDROFLUAZIDE; TIMOLOL MALEATE

Priadel

(Delandale) is a proprietary, prescription-only preparation of the ANTIMANIA drug lithium (as lithium carbonate). It can be used to treat acute mania, manic-depressive bouts and recurrent depression. It is available as tablets (a liquid preparation of lithium citrate is also available).

✚▲ side-effects/warning: see LITHIUM

prilocaine hydrochloride

is a LOCAL ANAESTHETIC drug. It is used extensively for relatively minor surgical procedures, especially by injection in

dentistry and by surface anaesthesia and nerve block. Administration is by injection (in several forms) or by topical application as a cream.

✚▲ side-effects/warning: see under LIGNOCAINE HYDROCHLORIDE. It may cause methaemoglobinaemia (an abnormal form of haemoglobin that does not transport oxygen) that may require correction. Avoid its use in those who have anaemia or pre-existing methaemoglobinaemia.

○ Related entries: Citanest; Citanest with Octapressin; Emla

Primacor

(Sanofi Winthrop) is a proprietary, prescription-only preparation of the PHOSPHODIESTERASE INHIBITOR drug milrinone. It can be used, in the short term, in HEART FAILURE TREATMENT for acute heart failure, especially where other drugs have not been successful. It is available in a form for intravenous infusion or injection.

✚▲ side-effects/warning: see MILRINONE

Primalan

(Rhône-Poulenc Rorer) is a proprietary, prescription-only preparation of the ANTIHISTAMINE drug mequitazine. It can be used to treat the symptoms of allergic disorders such as hay fever and urticaria. and is available as tablets.

✚▲ side-effects/warning: see MEQUITAZINE

primaquine

is an ANTIMALARIAL drug. It is used to destroy parasitic forms in the liver that are not destroyed by chloroquine. Administration is oral in the form of tablets.

✚ side-effects: there may be nausea and vomiting, abdominal pain and blood disorders.

▲ warning: it should be administered with caution to patients who are pregnant or breast-feeding, or who have G6PD deficiency.

P

Primaxin

(Merck, Sharp & Dohme) is a proprietary, prescription-only COMPOUND PREPARATION of the ANTIBACTERIAL and (BETA-LACTAM) ANTIBIOTIC drug imipenem and the ENZYME INHIBITOR cilastatin, which is a combination known as imipenem with cilastatin. It can be used to treat infections such as those of the urethra and cervix and to prevent infection during operations. It is available in a form for injection or infusion.

✚▲ side-effects/warning: see IMIPENEM WITH CILASTATIN

primidone

is an ANTICONVULSANT and ANTI-EPILEPTIC drug, which is used in the treatment of all forms of epilepsy (except absence seizures) and of essential tremor. It is largely converted in the body to the BARBITURATE drug phenobarbitone and therefore has similar actions and effects. Administration is oral as tablets or an oral suspension.

✚▲ side-effects/warning: see under PHENOBARBITONE; but there may also be drowsiness, unsteady gait, nausea, rash and disturbances of vision.

❍ Related entry: Mysoline

Primolut N

(Schering Health) is a proprietary, prescription-only preparation of the PROGESTOGEN norethisterone. It can be used to treat uterine bleeding, abnormally heavy menstruation and other menstrual problems, endometriosis and for premenstrual tension syndrome. It is available in the form of tablets.

✚▲ side-effects/warning: see NORETHISTERONE

Primoteston Depot

(Schering Health) is a proprietary, prescription-only preparation of the male SEX HORMONE testosterone enanthate, which is an ANDROGEN. It can be used to treat hormonal deficiency in men and as an ANTICANCER treatment for hormone-related cancer in women. It is available in a form for long-acting (depot) injection.

✚▲ side-effects/warning: see TESTOSTERONE

Primperan

(Berk) is a proprietary, prescription-only preparation of the ANTI-EMETIC and ANTINAUSEANT drug metoclopramide hydrochloride. It can be used for the treatment of nausea and vomiting, particularly when associated with gastrointestinal disorders and after treatment with radiation or cytotoxic drugs. It also has gastric MOTILITY STIMULANT actions and can be used in the treatment of non-ulcer dyspepsia, gastric stasis and for prevention of reflux oesophagitis. It is available as tablets, an oral solution and in a form for injection.

✚▲ side-effects/warning: see METOCLOPRAMIDE HYDROCHLORIDE. Note the side-effects in young people in particular.

Prioderm

(Napp) is a proprietary, non-prescription preparation of the SCABICIDAL and PEDICULICIDAL drug malathion. It can be used to treat infestations of the scalp and pubic hair by lice (pediculosis), or of the skin by the itch-mite (scabies). It is available as a cream, a shampoo and a lotion. It is not normally used on children under six months, except on medical advice.

✚▲ side-effects/warning: see MALATHION

Pripsen Mebendazole

(Seton Healthcare) is a proprietary, non-prescription preparation of the ANTHELMINTIC drug mebendazole. It can be used to treat infections by threadworm and roundworm and is available as tablets. It is not normally given to children under two years, except on medical advice.

✚▲ side-effects/warning: see MEBENDAZOLE

Pripsen Powder

(Seton Healthcare) is a proprietary, non-prescription COMPOUND PREPARATION of the ANTHELMINTIC drug piperazine (as phosphate) and the *stimulant* LAXATIVE senna. It can be used to treat infections by threadworm and roundworm and is available as an oral powder. It is not normally given to children under one year, except on medical advice.

✚▲ side-effects/warning: see PIPERAZINE

Pripsen Worm Elixir

(Seton Healthcare) is a proprietary, non-prescription preparation of the ANTHELMINTIC drug piperazine (as citrate). It can be used to treat infections by threadworm and roundworm and is available as an oral powder. It is not normally given to children under one year, except on medical advice.

✚▲ side-effects/warning: see PIPERAZINE

Pro-Actidil

(Wellcome) is a proprietary, non-prescription preparation of the ANTIHISTAMINE drug triprolidine hydrochloride. It can be used to treat the symptoms of various allergic conditions, particularly hay fever and urticaria. It is available as tablets.

✚▲ side-effects/warning: see TRIPROLIDINE HYDROCHLORIDE

Pro-Banthine

(Baker Norton) is a proprietary, prescription-only preparation of the ANTICHOLINERGIC drug propantheline bromide. It can be used as an ANTISPASMODIC for gastrointestinal disorders involving spasm and in the treatment of adult enuresis (urinary incontinence). It is available as tablets.

✚▲ side-effects/warning: see PROPANTHELINE BROMIDE

probenecid

is a drug that alters the transport of chemicals by the kidneys and is used for two main purposes. First, by inhibiting the excretion from the body of certain ANTIBIOTICS (mainly the PENICILLINS and CEPHALOSPORINS), it increases their duration of action. Second, because it increases the excretion of uric acid from the blood, it can be used in the prevention of attacks of chronic gout, which involve high levels of uric acid (hyperuricaemia). Administration is oral in the form of tablets.

✚ side-effects: infrequently, there may be nausea and vomiting, but usually there is increased urination, headache and flushing, dizziness and rash; rarely, hypersensitivity, liver and kidney changes and blood disorders.

▲ warning: it is not to be used in patients with blood disorders, certain kidney disorders, porphyria, acute gout, or who are using aspirin or other salicylates. When first administering, certain concurrent treatments are required such as colchicine and a NSAID (not aspirin) and an adequate fluid intake must be maintained. Administer with caution to those with peptic ulcers, renal impairment, or G6PD deficiency.

○ Related entry: Benemid

probucol

is used as a LIPID-LOWERING DRUG in hyperlipidaemia to reduce the levels, or change the proportions, of various lipids in the bloodstream. Administration is oral in the form of tablets.

✚ side-effects: mild gastrointestinal upsets, nausea and vomiting; flatulence, diarrhoea, abdominal pain; rarely, irregular heartbeat and angio-oedema.

▲ warning: it should not be administered to patients who are pregnant or breast-feeding (avoid pregnancy for six months after stopping treatment).

○ Related entry: Lurselle

Procainamide Durules

(Astra) is a proprietary, prescription-only preparation of the ANTI-ARRHYTHMIC drug procainamide hydrochloride. It can be used to treat irregularities in the heart-beat, especially after a heart attack and is available as sustained-release tablets.

✚▲ side-effects/warning: see PROCAINAMIDE
HYDROCHLORIDE

procainamide hydrochloride

is a drug with LOCAL ANAESTHETIC
properties, which is used as an ANTI-
ARRHYTHMIC to treat heartbeat
irregularities, especially after a heart
attack. Administration can be oral as
tablets or modified-release tablets, or in a
form for injection.
✚ side-effects: there may be nausea,
diarrhoea, high temperature, depression, slow
heart rate and rashes. There may also be heart
failure and/or skin or blood disorders,
especially after prolonged treatment.
▲ warning: it should not be administered to
patients with heart failure, heart block, low
blood pressure, or who are breast-feeding;
administer with caution to those with asthma,
the neuromuscular disease myasthenia gravis,
lupus, impaired kidney function, or who are
pregnant.
❍ Related entries: Procainamide
Durules; Pronestyl

procaine

is a LOCAL ANAESTHETIC drug. Although
once popular, it is now seldom used
because it has been overtaken by
anaesthetics that are longer-lasting and
better absorbed through mucous
membranes. It cannot be used as a surface
anaesthetic because it is poorly absorbed.
However, it is still available and can be
used for regional anaesthesia or by
infiltration, usually in combination with
adrenaline. Administration (as procaine
hydrochloride) is by injection.
✚ side-effects: rarely, there are sensitivity
reactions.

procaine penicillin

is an ANTIBACTERIAL and PENICILLIN-type
ANTIBIOTIC drug, which is effectively a
rather insoluble salt of benzylpenicillin. It
is used mainly in long-lasting
intramuscular (depot) injections to treat

conditions such as syphilis and
gonorrhoea, but can also be used to treat
the equally serious condition gas gangrene
following amputation. Benzylpenicillin is
released slowly into the blood over a
period of days, therefore avoiding the
need for frequent injections.
Administration is by injection.
✚▲ side-effects/warning: see under
BENZYLPENICILLIN
❍ Related entry: Bicillin

procarbazine

is a CYTOTOXIC DRUG, which is used as an
ANTICANCER treatment for the lymphatic
cancer Hodgkin's disease. Administration
is oral in the form of capsules.
✚▲ side-effects/warning: see under
CYTOTOXIC DRUGS. Hypersensitivity rash.
❍ Related entry: Natulan

prochlorperazine

is a PHENOTHIAZINE DERIVATIVE drug. It is
used as an ANTIPSYCHOTIC in the treatment
of psychotic disorders such as
schizophrenia, as an ANXIOLYTIC in the
short-term treatment of anxiety and as an
ANTINAUSEANT in the prevention of nausea
caused by gastrointestinal disorder,
chemotherapy, radiotherapy, motion
sickness, or by the vertigo that results
from infection of the middle or inner ear.
Administration (as prochlorperazine
maleate or prochlorperazine mesylate)
can be oral as tablets, buccal tablets (left
to dissolve between the top lip and gum),
modified-release capsules, syrups or
effervescent granules, or topical as
suppositories, or by injection.
✚▲ side-effects/warning: see under
CHLORPROMAZINE HYDROCHLORIDE; but with
less sedation, muscle tremor and rigidity
disturbances.
❍ Related entries: Buccastem; Stemetil

Proctofibe

(Roussel) is a proprietary, non-
prescription preparation of the (*bulking
agent*) LAXATIVE bran with grain and citrus

fibre. It is avilable as tablets.
+▲ side-effects/warning: see BRAN

Proctofoam HC

(Stafford-Miller) is a proprietary,
prescription-only COMPOUND PREPARATION
of the CORTICOSTEROID and ANTI-
INFLAMMATORY drug hydrocortisone (as
acetate) and the LOCAL ANAESTHETIC drug
pramoxine hydrochloride. It can be used
to treat various painful conditions of the
anus and rectum and is available as a
foam in an aerosol.
+▲ side-effects/warning: see
HYDROCORTISONE; PRAMOXINE
HYDROCHLORIDE

Proctosedyl

(Roussel) is a proprietary, prescription-
only COMPOUND PREPARATION of the
CORTICOSTEROID and ANTI-INFLAMMATORY
drug hydrocortisone (as acetate) and the
LOCAL ANAESTHETIC drug cinchocaine
hydrochloride. It can be used to treat
various painful conditions of the anus and
rectum, including haemorrhoids. It is
available as an ointment and
suppositories.
+▲ side-effects/warning: see CINCHOCAINE;
HYDROCORTISONE

procyclidine hydrochloride

is an ANTICHOLINERGIC drug, which is used
in the treatment of some types of
parkinsonism (see ANTIPARKINSONISM). It
increases mobility and decreases rigidity
and tremor, but has only a limited effect
on bradykinesia. The tendency to produce
an excess of saliva is also reduced. It is
thought to work by correcting the over-
effectiveness of the NEUROTRANSMITTER
ACETYLCHOLINE (cholinergic excess),
which is caused by the dopamine
deficiency that occurs in parkinsonism.
Administration, which may be in
conjunction with other drugs used for the
relief of parkinsonism, is either oral as
tablets or a syrup, or by injection.
+▲ side-effects/warning: see under

BENZHEXOL HYDROCHLORIDE
۞ Related entries: Arpicolin; Kemadrin

Profasi

(Serono) is a proprietary, prescription-
only preparation of the HORMONE human
chorionic gonadotrophin (HCG). It can be
used to treat undescended testicles and
delayed puberty in boys and as an
infertility treatment for women suffering
from specific hormonal deficiency. It is
available in a form for injection.
+▲ side-effects/warning: see CHORIONIC
GONADOTROPHIN

Proflex Pain Relief

(Zyma Healthcare) is a proprietary,
non-prescription preparation of the
(NSAID) NON-NARCOTIC ANALGESIC and
ANTIRHEUMATIC drug ibuprofen. It can be
used for the symptomatic relief of
rheumatic and muscular pain, backache,
sprains, strains, lumbago and fibrositis. It
is available as a cream for massage into
the effected area.
+▲ side-effects/warning: see IBUPROFEN

Proflex Sustained Relief
Capsules

(Zyma Healthcare) is a proprietary, non-
prescription preparation of the (NSAID)
NON-NARCOTIC ANALGESIC and
ANTIRHEUMATIC drug ibuprofen. It can be
used for the relief of muscular pain,
rheumatic pain, lumbago and fibrositis. It
is available as tablets and is not normally
given to children under 12 years, except
on medical advice.
+▲ side-effects/warning: see IBUPROFEN

Proflex Tablets

(Zyma Healthcare) is a proprietary, non-
prescription preparation of the (NSAID)
NON-NARCOTIC ANALGESIC and
ANTIRHEUMATIC drug ibuprofen. It can be
used for the relief of sprains, strains,
rheumatic pain, lumbago, backache and
fibrositis. It is available as tablets and is
not normally given to children under 12

P years, except on medical advice.
✚▲ side-effects/warning: see IBUPROFEN

Progesic
(Lilly) is a proprietary, prescription-only preparation of the (NSAID) NON-NARCOTIC ANALGESIC and ANTIRHEUMATIC drug fenoprofen. It can be used to treat and relieve pain, particularly arthritic and rheumatic pain and other musculoskeletal disorders. It is available as tablets.
✚▲ side-effects/warning: see FENOPROFEN

progesterone
is a SEX HORMONE, a PROGESTOGEN, that is found predominantly in women, but also in men. In women, it is produced and secreted mainly by the ovaries (and also the placenta of pregnant women and the adrenal glands). It prepares the lining of the uterus (the endometrium) every menstrual cycle to receive a fertilized ovum. Most cycles do not result in fertilization (conception), but if a fertilized ovum does implant in the endometrium the resulting formation of a placenta ensures the continuation of the supply of progesterone and this prevents ovulation. In men, small quantities of progesterone are secreted by the testes and the adrenal glands. Therapeutically, progesterone is administered to women to treat various menstrual and gynaecological disorders. Administration is by topical application as anal or vaginal suppositories (pessaries), or by injection.
✚▲ side-effects/warning: see under PROGESTOGEN
○ Related entries: Cyclogest; Gestone

progestogen
is the name of the group of (STEROID) SEX HORMONES formed and released by the ovaries and placenta in women, the adrenal gland and in small amounts by the testes in men. Physiologically, progestogens prepare the lining of the uterus (endometrium) for pregnancy, maintain it throughout pregnancy and

prevent the further release of eggs (ovulation). They include the natural progestogen PROGESTERONE and those like it (DYDROGESTERONE, HYDROXYPROGESTERONE HEXANOATE and MEDROXYPROGESTERONE ACETATE) and the analogues of TESTOSTERONE (eg. NORGESTREL and NORETHISTERONE; and the recently introduced analogues DESOGESTREL, LEVONORGESTREL, NORGESTIMATE, GESTODENE. All are synthesized for therapeutic use and have many uses, including treatment of menstrual disorders (menorrhagia and severe dysmenorrhoea), endometriosis (inflammation of the tissues normally lining the uterus), in HRT (hormone replacement therapy), in recurrent (habitual) abortion, to relieve the symptoms of premenstrual syndrome and sometimes in the treatment of breast, endometrial and prostate cancers. The most common use is as constituents (with or without OESTROGENS) in ORAL CONTRACEPTIVES. Administration is oral.
✚ side-effects: depending on the dose, use and the particular progestogen administered; acne, skin rash, oedema (accumulation of fluid in the tissues), gastrointestinal disturbances, changes in libido, breast discomfort, premenstrual tension, irregular periods, sleep disturbances, or depression.
▲ warning: it should not be by patients with undiagnosed vaginal bleeding, certain cardiovascular disorders, porphyria, or certain cancers. Use with care in those with diabetes, heart, liver, or kidney disorders, or who are breast-feeding.

Prograf
(Fujisawa) is a proprietary, prescription-only preparation of the IMMUNOSUPPRESSANT drug tacrolimus. It can be used to prevent tissue rejection in transplant patients and is available as capsules and in a form for injection.
✚▲ side-effects/warning: see TACROLIMUS

proguanil hydrochloride

is an ANTIMALARIAL drug, which is used to prevent the contraction of malaria by visitors to tropical countries. Administration is oral as tablets.

✚ side-effects: there may be mild stomach disorders, diarrhoea, occasional skin reactions, mouth ulcers and hair loss.

▲ warning: it should be administered with caution to patients who suffer from severely impaired kidney function, or who are pregnant (folate supplements are required).

○ Related entry: Paludrine

Progynova

(Schering Health) is a proprietary, prescription-only preparation of the OESTROGEN oestradiol (as valerate). It can be used in HRT and is available as tablets.

✚▲ side-effects/warning: see OESTRADIOL

prolactin

is a HORMONE secreted into the bloodstream by the anterior pituitary gland in both men and women. Despite its name, it influences many aspects of body function, but its main role is indeed the control of lactation. Its release is influenced by the hypothalamus through a factor called prolactin-release inhibiting factor (PRIM), which is probably the NEUROTRANSMITTER mediator DOPAMINE. This fact is important, since it explains why the drug BROMOCRIPTINE, which stimulates dopamine RECEPTORS, can be used to suppress prolactin secretion and why a dopamine ANTAGONIST increases it. Bromocriptine, when clinically necessary, can therefore be used to prevent or suppress lactation after normal birth or in disease states where there is excessive secretion of prolactin with associated galactorrhea (excessive milk production). Overproduction of prolactin can also occur when there is a pituitary tumour or when patients are being treated with (dopamine antagonist) NEUROLEPTIC drugs, METOCLOPRAMIDE HYDROCHLORIDE, or METHYLDOPA.

Proleukin

(EuroCetus) is a proprietary, prescription-only preparation of the ANTICANCER drug aldesleukin (interleukin-2). It can be used mainly in the treatment of metastatic renal cell carcinoma. It is available in a form for injection.

✚▲ side-effects/warning: see ALDESLEUKIN

prolintane

is a STIMULANT drug, which is incorporated into some proprietary vitamin preparations and can be used to assist in the treatment of fatigue or lethargy.

▲ warning: it should not be taken by those with epilepsy or hyperthyroidism.

○ Related entry: Villescon

Proluton Depot

(Schering Health) is a proprietary, prescription-only preparation of the PROGESTOGEN (female SEX HORMONE) hydroxyprogesterone hexanoate. It can be used to treat recurrent (habitual) abortion and is available in a form for long-lasting (depot) injection.

✚▲ side-effects/warning: see HYDROXYPROGESTERONE HEXANOATE

promazine hydrochloride

is chemically one of the PHENOTHIAZINE DERIVATIVES. It is used as an ANTIPSYCHOTIC drug to tranquillize agitated and restless patients, especially the elderly. Administration is either oral as tablets or a suspension, or by injection.

✚▲ side-effects/warning: see under CHLORPROMAZINE HYDROCHLORIDE

○ Related entry: Sparine

promethazine hydrochloride

is an ANTIHISTAMINE drug, chemically a PHENOTHIAZINE DERIVATIVE, which also has HYPNOTIC and ANTUSSIVE properties. It is used to treat the symptoms of allergic conditions such as hay fever and urticaria (itchy skin rash) and can also be used in

P

the emergency treatment of anaphylactic shock. It has a SEDATIVE action and can be administered as a preoperative medication, to treat temporary sleep disorders and to sedate children. Administration is either oral as tablets or a dilute elixir, or by injection. See also PROMETHAZINE THEOCLATE.

+▲ side-effects/warning: see under CYCLIZINE; ANTIHISTAMINE. Intramuscular injections may be painful. Avoid its use in patients with porphyria. Because of its sedative side-effects, the performance of skilled tasks such as driving may be impaired.

○ Related entries:
Medised; Night Nurse Capsules; Night Nurse Liquid; Pamergan P100; Phenergan; Phensedyl Plus; Q-Mazine Syrup; Sominex

promethazine teoclate

See PROMETHAZINE THEOCLATE

promethazine theoclate

(promethazine teoclate) is chemically a PHENOTHIAZINE DERIVATIVE and is a form of the ANTIHISTAMINE drug promethazine hydrochloride, but with a slightly longer duration of action. It can be used as an ANTINAUSEANT to prevent nausea and vomiting caused by motion sickness or infection of the ear. Administration is oral in the form of tablets.

+▲ side-effects/warning: see under ANTIHISTAMINE. Because of its sedative property, the performance of skilled tasks such as driving may be impaired.

○ Related entry: Avomine

Prominal

(Sanofi Winthrop) is a proprietary, prescription-only preparation of the BARBITURATE drug methylphenobarbitone and is on the Controlled Drugs List. It can be used as an ANTICONVULSANT and ANTI-EPILEPTIC to treat most forms of epilepsy and is available as tablets.

+▲ side-effects/warning: see METHYLPHENOBARBITONE

Pronestyl

(Squibb) is a proprietary, prescription-only preparation of the ANTI-ARRHYTHMIC drug procainamide hydrochloride. It can be used to treat irregularities in the heartbeat, especially after a heart attack. It is available as tablets and in a form for injection.

+▲ side-effects/warning: see PROCAINAMIDE HYDROCHLORIDE

Propaderm

(Glaxo) is a proprietary, prescription-only preparation of the CORTICOSTEROID drug beclomethasone dipropionate. It can be used to treat severe, non-infective skin inflammation such as eczema. It is available as a cream and an ointment for topical application.

+▲ side-effects/warning: see BECLOMETHASONE DIPROPIONATE

propafenone hydrochloride

is an ANTI-ARRHYTHMIC drug, which is used to prevent and treat irregularities of the heartbeat. Administration is oral in the form of tablets.

+ side-effects: nausea, vomiting, diarrhoea or constipation; fatigue, headache, dizziness; rash, postural hypotension (especially in the elderly), dry mouth, blurred vision and occasionally heart and blood disorders.

▲ warning: it should be administered with care in the elderly, those who are pregnant, or with certain kidney or liver disorders. Avoid in patients with severe heart conditions, electrolyte imbalance and obstructive lung disease.

○ Related entry: Arythmol

Propain Tablets

(Panpharma) is a proprietary, non-prescription COMPOUND PREPARATION of the (OPIOID) NARCOTIC ANALGESIC drug codeine phosphate, the ANTIHISTAMINE drug diphenhydramine hydrochloride, the NON-NARCOTIC ANALGESIC and ANTIPYRETIC drug paracetamol and the STIMULANT caffeine. It can be used to relieve pain, including headache, migraine, muscular pain and period pain and to relieve cold and flu symptoms and fever. It is available as scored tablets and is not normally given to children under 12 years, except on medical advice.

✚▲ side-effects/warning: see CAFFEINE; CODEINE PHOSPHATE; DIPHENHYDRAMINE HYDROCHLORIDE; PARACETAMOL

propamidine isethionate

is an ANTIBACTERIAL drug, which is used specifically to treat infections of the eyelids or conjunctiva, including acanthamoeba keratitis (sometimes in conjunction with other drugs). Adminisration is by topical application in the form of eye-drops.

❂ Related entries: Brolene Eye Drops; Golden Eye Drops

Propanix

(Ashbourne) is a proprietary, prescription-only preparation of the BETA-BLOCKER drug propranolol hydrochloride. It can be used as an ANTIHYPERTENSIVE treatment for raised blood pressure, as an ANTI-ANGINA treatment to relieve symptoms and improve exercise tolerance and as an ANTI-ARRHYTHMIC to regularize heartbeat and to treat myocardial infarction. It can also be used as an ANTITHYROID drug for short-term treatment of thyrotoxicosis, as an ANTIMIGRAINE treatment to prevent attacks, as an ANXIOLYTIC treatment, particularly for symptomatic relief of tremor and palpitations and, with an ALPHA-ADRENOCEPTOR BLOCKER, in the acute treatment of phaeochromocytoma. It is available as modified-release capsules (*Propanix SR*).

✚▲ side-effects/warning: see PROPRANOLOL HYDROCHLORIDE

propantheline bromide

is an ANTICHOLINERGIC drug. It is used in the treatment of gastrointestinal disorders that involve muscle spasm of the intestinal wall, of urinary frequency and adult enuresis (urinary incontinence).

Administration is oral in the form of tablets.

✚▲ side-effects/warning: see under ATROPINE SULPHATE

❂ Related entry: Pro-Banthine

Propine

(Allergan) is a proprietary, prescription-only preparation of the SYMPATHOMIMETIC drug dipivefrine hydrochloride. It can be used as a GLAUCOMA TREATMENT to reduce intraocular pressure and is available as eye-drops.

✚▲ side-effects/warning: see DIPIVEFRINE HYDROCHLORIDE

propofol

is a GENERAL ANAESTHETIC drug. It is used in the induction and maintenance of anaesthesia and for the sedation of patients in intensive care on artificial ventilation. Recovery after treatment is rapid and without any hangover effect. Administration is by injection or infusion.

✚ side-effects: occasionally, there may be pain on intravenous injection. There may be slowing of the heart. Convulsions, anaphylaxis and delayed recovery have been reported.

▲ warning: the monitoring of certain body functions is advisable.

❂ Related entry: Diprivan

propranolol hydrochloride

is a BETA-BLOCKER that can be used as an ANTIHYPERTENSIVE treatment for raised blood pressure, as an ANTI-ANGINA treatment to relieve symptoms and improve exercise tolerance and as an ANTI-ARRHYTHMIC to regularize heartbeat and to treat and prevent myocardial infarction. It can also be used as an ANTITHYROID drug for short-term treatment of thyrotoxicosis, for the acute treatment of phaeochromocytoma, as an ANTIMIGRAINE treatment to prevent attacks and as an ANXIOLYTIC treatment, particularly for symptomatic relief of tremor and palpitations. Administration

P

can be oral as tablets, modified-release capsules or a syrup, or by injection. It is also available, as an antihypertensive treatment, in the form of COMPOUND PREPARATIONS with DIURETICS.

✚ side-effects: slowing of the heart rate, asthma-like symptoms and bronchospasm, gastrointestinal disturbances, poor circulation in the extremities, fatigue and sleep-disturbance; heart failure in susceptible patients. There are rare reports of rashes and dry eyes.

▲ warning: it should not be administered to patients with asthma or any disease of the airways, history of heart failure, cardiogenic shock, or certain abnormal heart rhythms. It should be administered with caution to those with certain liver or kidney disorders, in late pregnancy, who are breast-feeding, diabetics, or with myasthenia gravis.

○ Related entries: Angilol; Apsolol; Bedranol SR; Berkolol; Betadur CR; Beta-Prograne; Cardinol; Half-Betadur CR; Half-Beta-Prograne; Half-Inderal LA; Inderal; Inderal-LA; Inderetic; Inderex; Propanix; Sloprolol

propylthiouracil

is a drug that acts as an indirect HORMONE ANTAGONIST by inhibiting the thyroid gland's production of THYROID HORMONES, therefore treating an excess of thyroid hormones in the blood and the symptoms that it causes (thyrotoxicosis). Treatment can be on a maintenance basis over a long period (with dosage adjusted to optimum effect), or it can be used just before surgical removal of the thyroid gland. It is administered to patients who are sensitive to the antithyroid drug carbimazole. Administration is in the form of tablets.

✚▲ side-effects/warning: see under CARBIMAZOLE. Also, it may cause haemorrhage and precipitate lupus syndrome.

Prosaid

(BHR) is a proprietary, prescription-only preparation of the (NSAID) NON-NARCOTIC ANALGESIC and ANTIRHEUMATIC drug

naproxen. It can be used to relieve pain and inflammation, particularly rheumatic and arthritic pain and to treat other musculoskeletal disorders. It is available as tablets.

✚▲ side-effects/warning: see NAPROXEN

Proscar

(Merk Sharp & Dohme) is a proprietary, prescription-only preparation of the ANTI-ANDROGEN finasteride, which is an *indirect* SEX HORMONE ANTAGONIST. It can be used to treat benign prostatic hyperplasia in men and is available as tablets.

✚▲ side-effects/warning: see FINASTERIDE

prostacyclin

See EPOPROSTENOL

prostaglandin

is the name given to members of a family of LOCAL HORMONES (so-called because they exert their effects near to where they are formed), which are produced naturally by many organs and tissues in the body, both normally and in disease states. Naturally occurring members of the family include prostaglandin E_2 (DINOPROSTONE), prostaglandin $F_2\alpha$ (DINOPROST) and prostacyclin (EPOPROSTENOL). They are used therapeutically along with synthetic analogues (eg. MISOPROSTOL). The uses of the prostaglandins reflect their high potency in causing such bodily actions as contraction of the uterus, softening and dilation of the cervix and dilation of blood vessels. Similarly, the side-effects of these agents used as drugs reflect their other powerful actions; such as stimulating the intestine causing pain, diarrhoea, actions on the brain to cause fever and prolongation of bleeding.

Prostap SR

(Lederle) is a proprietary, prescription-only preparation of leuprorelin acetate, which is an analogue of the hypothalamic

HORMONE gonadorelin (gonadothrophin-releasing hormone; GnRH). It can be used as an ANTICANCER drug for cancer of the prostate gland and to treat endometriosis. It is available in a form for subcutaneous or intramuscular injection.
+▲ side-effects/warning: see LEUPRORELIN ACETATE

Prostigmin
(Roche) is a proprietary, prescription-only preparation of the ANTICHOLINESTERASE and PARASYMPATHOMIMETIC drug neostigmine. It can be used to stimulate bladder or intestinal activity and to treat myasthenia gravis. It is available in a form for injection (as neostigmine methylsulphate) and as tablets (as neostigmine bromide).
+▲ side-effects/warning: see NEOSTIGMINE

Prostin E2
(Upjohn) is a proprietary, prescription-only form of the PROSTAGLANDIN dinoprostone. It is used mainly to induce labour or to cause therapeutic abortion. It is available as tablets, as vaginal tablets (pessaries), a vaginal gel and in a form for injection.
+▲ side-effects/warning: see DINOPROSTONE

Prostin F2 alpha
(Upjohn) is a proprietary, prescription-only preparation of the PROSTAGLANDIN $F_2\alpha$ dinoprost. It is used mainly to induce therapeutic abortion because of its property of causing uterine contractions. It is available in a form for injection.
+▲ side-effects/warning: see DINOPROST

Prostin VR
(Upjohn) is a proprietary, prescription-only form of the PROSTAGLANDIN alprostadil (prostaglandin PGE_1). It is used to maintain newborn babies with heart defects (to maintain patent ductus arteriosus), while preparations are made for corrective surgery in intensive care. It is available in a form for infusion.

+▲ side-effects/warning: see ALPROSTADIL

Prosulf
(CP) is a proprietary, prescription-only preparation of protamine sulphate. It can be used to counteract heparin overdose and is available in a form for injection.
+▲ side-effects/warning: see PROTAMINE SULPHATE

protamine sulfate
See: PROTAMINE SULPHATE

protamine sulphate
(protamine sulfate) can be used to treat an overdose of heparin. Administration is by slow intravenous injection.
+▲ side-effects/warning: slowing of the heart rate, hypotension and flushing.
✪ Related entry: Prosulf

protamine zinc insulin
is a form of purified INSULIN, prepared as a sterile complex with protamine and zinc, used in DIABETIC TREATMENT to maintain diabetic patients. It is available in vials for injection and has a long duration of action.
+▲ side-effects/warning: see INSULIN
✪ Related entry:
Hypurin Protamine Zinc

Prothiaden
(Boots) is a proprietary, prescription-only preparation of the (TRICYCLIC) ANTIDEPRESSANT drug dothiepin hydrochloride. It can be used to treat depressive illness, especially in cases where some degree of sedation is deemed necessary. It is available as tablets and capsules.
+▲ side-effects/warning: see DOTHIEPIN HYDROCHLORIDE

protirelin
(thyrotrophin-releasing hormone; TRH), is a natural hypothalamic HORMONE produced and secreted by the hypothalamus. It in turn acts on the

P

anterior pituitary gland to produce and secrete thyrotrophin (thyroid-stimulating hormone; TRH), a hormone that then causes the production and secretion of yet other hormones in the body. Therapeutically, it is used primarily to assess thyroid function in patients who suffer from under-activity of the pituitary gland (hypopituitarism) or from over-activity of the thyroid gland (hyperthyroidism). Administration is either oral in the form of tablets or by injection.

✚ side-effects: there is commonly nausea. Treatment by injection may cause flushing, dizziness, faintness, raised blood pressure and pulse rate, a strange taste in the mouth and a desire to urinate. Occasionally, there may be bronchospasm.

▲ warning: administer with caution to patients with severe under-activity of the pituitary gland, myocardial ischaemia, asthma and obstructive airways disease, or who are pregnant.

⊙ Related entry: TRH-Cambridge

*proton-pump inhibitor

drugs are a recently introduced type of ULCER-HEALING DRUG. They work by inhibiting gastric and acid secretion in the parietal cells (acid-producing cells) of the stomach lining by interfering with the action of the ion pump that is responsible for the secretion of acid. They can be used to treat the symptoms of dyspepsia, which is caused by over-production of acid (hyperacidity), chronic problems associated with peptic ulcers (gastric or duodenal) and oesophagitis (inflammation of the oesophagus caused by regurgitation of acid and enzymes). They can also be used as an alternative to treatment with H2-ANTAGONISTS. Two notable examples of proton-pump inhibitor drugs are LANSOPRAZOLE and OMPERAZOLE.

protriptyline hydochloride

is an ANTIDEPRESSANT drug of the TRICYCLIC group. It is used particularly to

treat depressive illness in apathetic and withdrawn patients because it has a STIMULANT effect. Administration is oral in the form of tablets.

✚▲ side-effects/warning: see under AMITRIPTYLINE HYDROCHLORIDE; but is less sedating, so there may be anxiety, raised heart rate, lowered blood pressure; photosensitive rashes.

⊙ Related entry: Concordin

Provera

(Upjohn) is a proprietary, prescription-only preparation of the SEX HORMONE medroxyprogesterone acetate (a synthetic PROGESTOGEN). In women it can be used as an ANTICANCER drug for cancer of the breast or uterine endometrium and as a hormonal supplement for those whose progestogen level requires boosting (such as in endometriosis or dysfunctional uterine bleeding). It is available as tablets.

✚▲ side-effects/warning: see MEDROXYPROGESTERONE ACETATE

Pro-Viron

(Schering Health) is a proprietary, prescription-only preparation of mesterolone, which has ANDROGEN (male SEX HORMONE) activity. It can be used to make up hormonal deficiency and is available as tablets.

✚▲ side-effects/warning: see MESTEROLONE

proxymetacaine

is a LOCAL ANAESTHETIC drug. It can be used by topical application in ophthalmic treatments and is administered (as hydrochloride) in the form of eye-drops.

✚ side-effects: there may be slight stinging on initial application.

⊙ Related entry: Ophthaine

Prozac

(Dista) is a proprietary, prescription-only preparation of the (SSRI) ANTIDEPRESSANT drug fluoxetine hydrochloride, which has less SEDATIVE effects than some other antidepressants. It has recently been used to treat bulimia nervosa and is available as capsules and as a liquid.

+▲ side-effects/warning: see FLUOXETINE

pseudoephedrine hydrochloride

is a SYMPATHOMIMETIC drug with BRONCHODILATOR, VASOCONSTRICTOR and DECONGESTANT properties. It is sometimes used to treat obstructive airways disease, but is most commonly included in a number of proprietary preparations for treating cold symptoms. Its actions and effects are very similar to those of the closely related drug ephedrine hydrochloride.

+▲ side-effects/warning: see under EPHEDRINE HYDROCHLORIDE

✪ Related articles: Actifed Compound Linctus; Actifed Expectorant; Actifed Syrup; Actifed Tablets; Bronalin Dry Cough Elixir; Day Cold Comfort Capsules; Dimotane Expectorant; Dimotane with Codeine; Dimotane with Codeine Paediatric; Expulin Cough Linctus - Sugar Free; Galpseud; Galpseud Plus; Meltus Dry Cough Elixir, Adult; Meltus Junior Dry Cough Elixir; Night Cold Comfort Capsules; Phensedyl Plus; Robitussin Chesty Cough with Congestion; Sudafed Elixir; Sudafed Expectorant; Sudafed Linctus; Sudafed Tablets; Sudafed Co-Tablets; Tixylix Cough and Cold.

Psoradrate

(Procter & Gamble) is a proprietary, non-prescription COMPOUND PREPARATION of dithranol and urea. It can be used for subacute and chronic psoriasis and is available as a cream.

+▲ side-effects/warning: see DITHRANOL; UREA

Psoriderm

(Dermal) is a proprietary, non-prescription COMPOUND PREPARATION of coal tar (with lecithin). It can be used for psoriasis, eczema and dandruff. It is available as a cream, a scalp lotion and a bath emulsion.

+▲ side-effects/warning: see COAL TAR; LECITHIN

PsoriGel

(Novex) is a proprietary, non-prescription preparation of coal tar. It can be used to treat psoriasis and dermatitis and is available as a gel.

+▲ side-effects/warning: see COAL TAR

Psorin

(Thames) is a proprietary, non-prescription COMPOUND PREPARATION of dithranol, salicylic acid and coal tar. It can be used to treat psoriasis and dermatitis and is available as an ointment.

+▲ side-effects/warning: see COAL TAR; DITHRANOL; SALICYLIC ACID

Pulmadil

(3M Health Care) is a proprietary, prescription-only preparation of the BETA-RECEPTOR STIMULANT and SYMPATHOMIMETIC drug rimiterol hydrobromide. It can be used as a BRONCHODILATOR in reversible obstructive airways disease, as an ANTI-ASTHMATIC treatment in severe acute asthma and for the alleviation of symptoms of chronic bronchitis and emphysema. It is available as an aerosol inhalant.

+▲ side-effects/warning: see RIMITEROL HYDROBROMIDE

Pulmicort Inhaler

(Astra) is a proprietary, prescription-only preparation of the CORTICOSTEROID drug budesonide. It can be used to prevent asthma attacks and is available in inhalers; one preparation, *Pulmicort LS*, is used with the *Nebuhaler* or the *Spacer* inhaler devices.

+▲ side-effects/warning: see BUDESONIDE

Pulmicort Respules

(Astra) is a proprietary, prescription-only preparation of the CORTICOSTEROID drug

P

budesonide. It can be used to prevent asthma attacks and is available in *Respules* for inhalation.
+▲ side-effects/warning: see BUDESONID.

Pulmicort Turbohaler

(Astra) is a proprietary, prescription-only preparation of the CORTICOSTEROID drug budesonide. It can be used to prevent asthma attacks and is available as a dry-powder inhaler.
+▲ side-effects/warning: see BUDESONIDE

Pump-Hep

(Leo) is a proprietary, prescription-only preparation of the ANTICOAGULANT drug heparin (as heparin sodium). It can be used to treat various forms of thrombosis and is available in a form for injection.
+▲ side-effects/warning: see HEPARIN

purgatives

See LAXATIVE

Pur-In Isophane

(CP Pharmaceuticals) is a proprietary, non-prescription preparation of highly purified human ISOPHANE INSULIN. It is used as a DIABETIC TREATMENT to treat and maintain diabetic patients. It is available in vials and cartridges for the *Pur-In Pen* injection device and has an intermediate duration of action.
+▲ side-effects/warning: see INSULIN

Pur-In Mix 15/85

(CP Pharmaceuticals) is a proprietary, non-prescription preparation of human BIPHASIC ISOPHANE INSULIN (15% soluble/85% isophane). It is used as a DIABETIC TREATMENT to treat and maintain diabetic patients. It is available in vials and cartridges for the *Pur-In Pen* injection device and has an intermediate duration of action.
+▲ side-effects/warning: see INSULIN

Pur-In Mix 25/75

(CP Pharmaceuticals) is a proprietary,

non-prescription preparation of human BIPHASIC ISOPHANE INSULIN (25% soluble/75% isophane). It is used as a DIABETIC TREATMENT to treat and maintain diabetic patients. It is available in vials and cartridges for the *Pur-In Pen* injection device and has an intermediate duration of action.
+▲ side-effects/warning: see INSULIN

Pur-In Mix 50/50

(CP Pharmaceuticals) is a proprietary, non-prescription preparation of human BIPHASIC ISOPHANE INSULIN (50% soluble/50% isophane). It is used as a DIABETIC TREATMENT to treat and maintain diabetic patients. It is available in vials and cartridges for the *Pur-In Pen* injection device and has an intermediate duration of action.
+▲ side-effects/warning: see INSULIN

Puri-Nethol

(Wellcome) is a proprietary, prescription-only preparation of the (CYTOTOXIC) ANTICANCER drug mercaptopurine. It can be used in the treatment of acute leukaemias and is available as tablets.
+▲ side-effects/warning: see MERCAPTOPURINE

Pur-In Neutral

(CP Pharmaceuticals) is a proprietary, non-prescription preparation of highly purified human neutral SOLUBLE INSULIN. It is used as a DIABETIC TREATMENT to treat and maintain diabetic patients. It is available in vials and cartridges for the *Pur-In Pen* injection device and has a short duration of action.
+▲ side-effects/warning: see INSULIN

Pyopen

(Link) is a proprietary, prescription-only preparation of the ANTIBACTERIAL and (PENICILLIN) ANTIBIOTIC drug carbenicillin. It can be used to treat serious pseudomonal infections and is

available in a form for injection.
+▲ side-effects/warning: see CARBENICILLIN

Pyralvex

(Norgine) is a proprietary, non-prescription preparation of salicylic acid and rhubarb extract, which have a COUNTER-IRRITANT, or RUBEFACIENT, action. It can be applied to the mouth for symptomatic relief of pain from mouth ulcers and denture irritation. It is available as a cream and a gel and is not normally used for children, except on medical advice.
+▲ side-effects/warning: see SALICYLIC ACID

pyrantel

is an ANTHELMINTIC drug. It is used in the treatment of infections by roundworm, threadworm and hookworm. Administration is oral in the form of tablets.
+ side-effects: there may be diarrhoea, mild nausea and vomiting, anorexia, headache and sleep disturbances, dizziness and rash.
▲ warning: administer with care to patients with certain liver disorders, or who are pregnant.
◑ Related entry: Combantrin

pyrazinamide

is an ANTIBACTERIAL drug and is one of the major forms of ANTITUBERCULAR treatment. It is generally used in combination with other drugs, such as ISONIAZID and RIFAMPICIN, in order to cover resistance and for maximum effect. Because pyrazinamide is only active against dividing forms of *Mycobacterium tuberculosis*, it is most effective in the early stages of treatment (i.e. the first few months). Administration is oral in the form of tablets.
+ side-effects: there may be symptoms of liver malfunction, including high temperature, severe weight loss and jaundice. There may be nausea and vomiting, sensitivity reactions such as urticaria, joint pain and blood disorders.

▲ warning: it should not be administered to patients with liver damage or porphyria; it should be administered with caution to patients with impaired kidney function, diabetes, or gout.
◑ Related entry: Rifater

pyridostigmine

is an ANTICHOLINESTERASE drug that enhances the effects of the NEUROTRANSMITTER acetylcholine (and of certain cholinergic drugs). Because of this property, it has PARASYMPATHOMIMETIC actions and is sometimes used to stimulate the intestine. It is more commonly used to treat the neuromuscular transmission disorder myasthenia gravis. Administration can be oral as tablets or by injection.
+▲ side-effects/warning: see under NEOSTIGMINE but it has generally weaker parasympathomimetic actions.
◑ Related entry: Mestinon

pyrimethamine

is an ANTIMALARIAL drug, which is mainly used in combination with DAPSONE or SULFADOXINE to prevent or treat malaria. It can also be used, along with a sulphonamide, to treat the protozoal infection toxoplasmosis. Administration is oral in the form of tablets.
+ side-effects: there may be rashes, insomnia and blood disorders.
▲ warning: it should be administered with caution to patients with certain liver or kidney disorders, or who are taking folic acid supplements (eg. during pregnancy). A high dosage requires regular blood counts.
◑ Related entries: Daraprim; Maloprim

Pyrogastrone

(Sanofi Winthrop) is a proprietary, prescription-only COMPOUND PREPARATION of the CYTOPROTECTANT drug carbenoxolone sodium, the ANTACIDS aluminium hydroxide, magnesium trisilicate and sodium bicarbonate and the DEMULCENT alginic acid. It can be used as an ULCER-HEALING DRUG for benign gastric

Q

P ulceration and is available as tablets and an oral liquid.

✚▲ side-effects/warning: see ALGINIC ACID; ALUMINIUM HYDROXIDE; CARBENOXOLONE SODIUM; MAGNESIUM TRISILICATE; SODIUM BICARBONATE

Q-Mazine Syrup

(Seton Healthcare) is a proprietary, non-prescription preparation of the ANTIHISTAMINE drug promethazine hydochloride. It can be used as an ANTINAUSEANT for the treatment of motion sickness and also for allergic reactions such as urticaria. It is available as an oral liquid and is not normally given to children under one year, except on medical advice.

+▲ side-effects/warning: see PROMETHAZINE HYDOCHLORIDE

Quellada

(Stafford-Miller) is a proprietary, non-prescription preparation of the SCABICIDAL and PEDICULICIDAL drug lindane. It can be used to treat infestations of the pubic hair by lice (pediculosis) or of the skin by itch-mites (scabies). It is available as a lotion and is not normally used for children under six months, except on medical advice.

+▲ side-effects/warning: see LINDANE

Questran

(Bristol-Myers) is a proprietary, prescription-only preparation of the LIPID-LOWERING DRUG cholestyramine. It can be used in hyperlipidaemia to reduce the levels, or change the proportions, of lipids in the bloodstream. It has various other uses, including as an ANTIDIARRHOEAL and, in certain circumstances, in biliary disturbances (including pruritus in biliary obstruction, or biliary cirrhosis). It is available as a powder to be taken with liquids.

+▲ side-effects/warning: see CHOLESTYRAMINE

Questran A

(Bristol-Myers) is a proprietary, prescription-only preparation of the LIPID-LOWERING DRUG cholestyramine. It can be used in hyperlipidaemia to reduce the levels and change the proportions, of lipids in the bloodstream. It has various

other uses, including as an ANTIDIARRHOEAL and in biliary disturbances (including pruritus in biliary obstruction, or biliary cirrhosis). It is available as a powder (containing the sweetener aspartame) to be taken with liquids.

+▲ side-effects/warning: see CHOLESTYRAMINE

quinagolide

is a recently introduced drug with similar actions to BROMOCRIPTINE. It can be used to treat HORMONE disorders (hyperprolactinaemia disorders) such as prolactinoma. Administration is oral in the form of tablets.

+▲ side-effects/warning: see under BROMOCRIPTINE. There is also anorexia, abdominal pain, diarrhoea, insomnia, oedema (accumulation of fluid in the tissues), flushing and nasal congestion. It is not be given to patients who are pregnant.

✪ Related entry: Norprolac

quinalbarbitone sodium

is a BARBITURATE drug with a rapid onset of action. It is used as a HYPNOTIC to promote sleep in conditions of severe, intractable insomnia. Administration is oral in the form of capsules. Preparations containing quinalbarbitone sodium are on the Controlled Drugs List.

+▲ side-effects/warning: see under BARBITURATE

✪ Related entries: Seconal Sodium; Tuinal

quinapril

is an ACE INHIBITOR. It is a powerful VASODILATOR that can be used as an ANTIHYPERTENSIVE and in HEART FAILURE TREATMENT, often when other treatments are not appropriate. It is frequently used in conjunction with other classes of drug, particularly (THIAZIDE) DIURETICS. Administration is oral in the form of tablets.

Q

+▲ side-effects/warning: see under
CAPTOPRIL
**✪ Related entries: Accupro; Accuretic;
Acezide**

quinidine

is a CINCHONA ALKALOID and is chemically
related to QUININE. It is used as an ANTI-
ARRHYTHMIC drug to treat heartbeat
irregularities and is available as tablets.
+▲ side-effects/warning: see under
PROCAINAMIDE HYDROCHLORIDE. There may
also be other heart arrhythmias and a
number of blood disorders. It is not to be
given to patients with heart block.
✪ Related entry: Kinidin Durules

quinine

is a CINCHONA ALKALOID and was for a long
time the main treatment for malaria.
Today, it has been almost completely
replaced by synthetic and less toxic drugs
(eg. CHLOROQUINE). However, quinine is
still used (as quinine sulphate or quinine
hydrochloride) against falciparum malaria
in cases that prove to be resistant to the
newer drugs, or for emergency cases in
which large doses are necessary. It can
also be used to relieve nocturnal cramps.
Administration is either oral as tablets or
by infusion.
+ side-effects: toxic effects (especially in
overdose) – called *cinchonism* – include
nausea, headache, abdominal pain, visual
disturbances, tinnitus (ringing in the ears), a
rash and confusion. Some patients may
experience visual disturbances and temporary
blindness, sensitivity reactions and blood
disorders.
▲ warning: it should not be administered to
patients with certain optic nerve disorders or
haemoglobinurea. It should be administered
with caution to those who suffer from heart
block, atrial fibrillation, who have G6PD
deficiency, or who are pregnant.
✪ Related entry: Nicobrevin

Quinocort

(Quinoderm) is a proprietary,

prescription-only COMPOUND PREPARATION
of the ANTI-INFLAMMATORY and
CORTICOSTEROID drug hydrocortisone and
the ANTIFUNGAL and ANTIBACTERIAL drug
potassium hydroxyquinoline sulphate. It
can be used to treat inflammation,
particularly when associated with fungal
infections and is available as a cream for
topical application.
+▲ side-effects/warning: see
HYDROCORTISONE; POTASSIUM
HYDROXYQUINOLINE SULPHATE

Quinoderm Cream

(Quinoderm) is a proprietary, non-
prescription COMPOUND PREPARATION of
the KERATOLYTIC and ANTIMICROBIAL drug
benzoyl peroxide (10%) and the
ANTIFUNGAL and ANTIBACTERIAL drug
potassium hydroxyquinoline sulphate. It
can be used to treat acne and is available
as a cream for topical application.
+▲ side-effects/warning: see BENZOYL
PEROXIDE; POTASSIUM HYDROXYQUINOLINE
SULPHATE

Quinoderm Cream 5

(Quinoderm) is a proprietary, non-
prescription COMPOUND PREPARATION of
the KERATOLYTIC and ANTIMICROBIAL drug
benzoyl peroxide (5%) and the
ANTIFUNGAL and ANTIBACTERIAL drug
potassium hydroxyquinoline sulphate. It
can be used to treat acne and is available
as a cream for topical application.
+▲ side-effects/warning: see BENZOYL
PEROXIDE; POTASSIUM HYDROXYQUINOLINE
SULPHATE

Quinoderm Lotio-Gel 5%

(Quinoderm) is a proprietary, non-
prescription COMPOUND PREPARATION of
the KERATOLYTIC and ANTIMICROBIAL drug
benzoyl peroxide (5%) and the
ANTIFUNGAL and ANTIBACTERIAL drug
potassium hydroxyquinoline sulphate. It
can be used to treat acne and is available
as a cream for topical application.
+▲ side-effects/warning: see BENZOYL

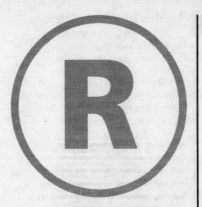

PEROXIDE; POTASSIUM HYDROXYQUINOLINE
SULPHATE

*quinolones

(4-quinolones) are ANTIBACTERIAL and
ANTIBIOTIC drugs, which are mainly used
to treat infections in patients who are
allergic to penicillin, or whose strain of
bacterium is resistant to standard
antibiotics. Although they are active
against a wide range of infective bacterial
organisms, they are usually more effective
against Gram-negative organisms and also
have useful activity against some Gram-
positive organisms (though not
anaerobes). They work by damaging the
internal structure of bacteria (i.e. they are
bactericidal). Chemically, they are related
to NALIDIXIC ACID and the names of more
recently introduced members end with -
oxacin. See ACROSOXACIN; CINOXACIN;
CIPROFLOXACIN; NORFLOXACIN; OFLOXACIN

Quinoped

(Quinoderm) is a proprietary, non-
prescription COMPOUND PREPARATION of
the ANTIFUNGAL drug potassium
hydroxyquinoline sulphate and the
KERATOLYTIC and ANTIMICROBIAL drug
benzoyl peroxide. It can be used to treat
fungal skin infections such as athlete's foot
and is available as a cream.
 side-effects/warning: see BENZOYL
PEROXIDE; POTASSIUM HYDROXYQUINOLINE
SULPHATE

R

Rabies Immunoglobulin

(Public Health Laboratory Service)
(Antirabies Immunoglobulin Injection) is
a non-proprietary, prescription-only
preparation of a SPECIFIC
IMMUNOGLOBULIN. It can be used in
IMMUNIZATION to give immediate immunity
against infection by rabies. It is available
in a form for intramuscular injection.

rabies immunoglobulin, human

is a SPECIFIC IMMUNOGLOBULIN that is used
in IMMUNIZATION to give immediate
passive immunity against infection by
rabies and can be used in conjunction
with RABIES VACCINE. Administration is by
intramuscular injection and injection at
the site of the bite.
○ Related entries: Rabies
Immunoglobulin

rabies vaccine

is a VACCINE used for the IMMUNIZATION to
prevent contracting rabies (but does not
treat people already infected with rabies).
It is administered to medical workers and
their relatives, who may come into contact
with rabid animals or with people who
have been bitten by an animal that might
be rabid. It can also be routinely
administered to people who work with
animals (eg. vets) to prevent contracting
rabies. The vaccine is of a type known as a
human diploid cell vaccine and is
administered by a course of injections.
○ Related entry: Rabies Vaccine BP
Pasteur Merieux

Rabies Vaccine BP Pasteur Merieux

(Merieux) is a proprietary, prescription-
only VACCINE preparation, which can be
used to prevent contracting rabies. It is
available in a form for injection.
✚▲ side-effects/warning: see RABIES VACCINE

Radian B Heat Spray

(Roche) is a proprietary, non-prescription
COMPOUND PREPARATION of camphor,
menthol, salicylic acid and ammonium
salicylate, which all have COUNTER-
IRRITANT, or RUBEFACIENT, actions. It can
be applied to the skin for symptomatic
relief of muscle and rheumatic pain,
sciatica, lumbago, fibrosis and muscle
stiffness. It is available as a spray and is
not normally used for children, except on
medical advice.
✚▲ side-effects/warning: see AMMONIUM
SALICYLATE; CAMPHOR; MENTHOL; SALICYLIC
ACID

Radian B Muscle Lotion

(Roche) is a proprietary, non-prescription
COMPOUND PREPARATION of camphor,
menthol, the (NSAID) NON-NARCOTIC
ANALGESIC and ANTIRHEUMATIC drug
ammonium salicylate and the KERATOLYTIC
agent salicylic acid. It is used as a
COUNTER-IRRITANT, or RUBEFACIENT, for the
symptomatic relief of muscle and
rheumatic pain, sciatica, lumbago, fibrosis
and muscle stiffness. It is available as a
spray for application to the skin and is not
normally used for children under six
years, except on medical advice.
✚▲ side-effects/warning: see AMMONIUM
SALICYLATE; CAMPHOR; MENTHOL; SALICYLIC
ACID

Radian B Muscle Rub

(Roche) is a proprietary, non-prescription
COMPOUND PREPARATION of camphor,
menthol, methyl salicylate and capsicum
oleoresin. It is used as a COUNTER-
IRRITANT, or RUBEFACIENT, for the
symptomatic relief of muscle and
rheumatic pain, sciatica, lumbago, fibrosis
and muscle stiffness. It is available as an
ointment for topical application to the skin
and is not normally used for children
under six years, except on medical advice.
✚▲ side-effects/warning: see CAMPHOR;
CAPSICUM OLEORESIN; MENTHOL; METHYL
SALICYLATE. It should not be used on
inflamed or broken skin, or on mucous
membranes.

Ralgex Cream

(SmithKline Beecham) is a proprietary, non-prescription COMPOUND PREPARATION of capsicum oleoresin, glycol salicylate and methyl nicotinate. It is used as a COUNTER-IRRITANT, or RUBEFACIENT, for the symptomatic relief of muscle pain and stiffness, sciatica, lumbago and fibrosis. It is available as a cream for topical application to the skin and is not normally used for children, except on medical advice.

✚▲ side-effects/warning: see CAPSICUM OLEORESIN; GLYCOL SALICYLATE; METHYL NICOTINATE

Ralgex Stick

(SmithKline Beecham) is a proprietary, non-prescription COMPOUND PREPARATION of menthol, methyl salicylate, glycol salicylate, ethyl salicylate and capsicum oleoresin. It can be used as a COUNTER-IRRITANT, or RUBEFACIENT, for the symptomatic relief of muscle pain and stiffness, sciatica, lumbago and fibrosis. It is available as an embrocation stick for topical application to the skin and is not normally used for children, except on medical advice.

✚▲ side-effects/warning: see CAPSICUM OLEORESIN; ETHYL SALICYLATE; GLYCOL SALICYLATE; MENTHOL; METHYL SALICYLATE

ramipril

is an ACE INHIBITOR and a powerful VASODILATOR. It can be used as an ANTIHYPERTENSIVE and in HEART FAILURE TREATMENT and sometimes following myocardial infarction (damage to heart muscle, usually after a heart attack). It is often used in conjunction with other classes of drug, particularly (THIAZIDE) DIURETICS. Administration is oral in the form of capsules.

✚▲ side-effects/warning: see under CAPTOPRIL

⊘ **Related entry: Tritace**

Ramysis

(ISIS) is a proprietary, prescription-only preparation of the ANTIBACTERIAL and (TETRACYCLINE) ANTIBIOTIC drug doxycycline. It can be used to treat infections of many kinds and is available as capsules.

✚▲ side-effects/warning: see DOXYCYCLINE

ranitidine

is an effective and extensively prescribed H_2-ANTAGONIST and ULCER-HEALING DRUG. It is used to assist in the treatment of benign peptic (gastric and duodenal) ulcers, to relieve heartburn in cases of reflux oesophagitis (caused by regurgitation of acid and enzymes into the oesophagus), Zollinger-Ellison syndrome and a variety of conditions where reduction of acidity is beneficial. It is now also available without prescription – in a limited amount and for short-term uses only – for the relief of heartburn, dyspepsia and hyperacidity. It works by reducing the secretion of gastric acid (by acting as a histamine receptor H_2-receptor antagonist), so reducing erosion and bleeding from peptic ulcers and allowing them a chance to heal. However, treatment with ranitidine should not start before a full diagnosis of gastric bleeding or serious pain has been made, because its action in restricting gastric secretions may possibly mask the presence of stomach cancer. It can also be used to treat ulceration induced by NSAID treatment. Administration can be oral in the form of tablets, effervescent tablets or a syrup, or by injection.

✚▲ side-effects/warning: see under CIMETIDINE; but it does not significantly inhibit microsomal drug-metabolizing enzymes.

⊘ **Related entries: Zantac; Zantac 75**

Rapifen

(Janssen) is a proprietary, prescription-only preparation of the (OPIOID) NARCOTIC ANALGESIC drug alfentanil (as hydrochloride) and is on the Controlled

Drugs List. It can be used in outpatient surgery, short operational procedures and for the enhancement of anaesthesia. It is available in a form for injection.

+▲ side-effects/warning: see ALFENTANIL

Rapitard MC

(Novo Nordisk) is a proprietary, non-prescription preparation of BIPHASIC INSULIN, highly purified bovine and porcine insulin and is used in DIABETIC TREATMENT to treat and maintain diabetic patients. It is available in vials for regular injection and has an intermediate duration of action.

+▲ side-effects/warning: see INSULIN

Rastinon

(Hoechst) is a proprietary, prescription-only preparation of the SULPHONYLUREA drug tolbutamide. It is used in DIABETIC TREATMENT for Type II diabetes (non-insulin-dependent diabetes mellitus; NIDDM; maturity-onset diabetes) and is available as tablets.

+▲ side-effects/warning: see TOLBUTAMIDE

razoxane

is a synthetic CYTOTOXIC DRUG, which is used to treat some forms of cancer, including leukaemia. Administration is oral in the form of tablets.

+▲ side-effects/warning: see under CYTOTOXIC DRUGS

☉ Related entry: Razoxin

Razoxin

(Zeneca) is a proprietary, prescription-only preparation of the (CYTOTOXIC) ANTICANCER drug razoxane. It can be used in the treatment of some cancers, for example, acute leukaemia and is available as tablets.

+▲ side-effects/warning: see RAZOXANE

*receptors

are proteins through which many drugs and natural mediators act to exert their effects. Receptors *recognize* and are

stimulated by, only their own mediators, including neurotransmitters, hormones and local hormones, or drugs that have been designed to mimic these mediators. They are usually situated on the surface membrane of cells and only require tiny amounts of a mediator or other chemical (called agonists) to trigger a reaction that can produce rapid and profound changes in that cell (for instance, biochemical changes of electrical effects). Another class of drug, the ANTAGONISTS, have a different type of action; they can *occupy* (in effect, physically block) the receptor without producing changes in the cell and prevent the agonist type of drug from acting. Examples of receptor types are alpha- and beta-adrenoceptors for ADRENALINE and NORADRENALINE; muscarinic and nicotinic cholinergic receptors for acetylcholine; H_1 and H_2 for histamine; and ANDROGEN OESTROGEN receptors for SEX HORMONE mediators. In all cases, synthetic drugs have been produced that act, either as agonists or antagonists, at these receptors.

Recormon

(Boehringer Mannheim) is a proprietary, prescription-only preparation of epoetin beta (synthesized human erythropoitetin beta). It can be used in ANAEMIA TREATMENT for conditions known to be associated with chronic renal failure in dialysis patients. It is available in a form for injection.

+▲ side-effects/warning: see EPOETIN

Redeptin

(SmithKline Beecham) is a proprietary, prescription-only preparation of the ANTIPSYCHOTIC drug fluspirilene. It can be used in the maintenance of schizophrenic patients and is available in a form for injection.

+▲ side-effects/warning: see FLUSPIRILENE

Redoxon

(Roche) is a proprietary, non-prescription

preparation of vitamin C (ascorbic acid). It can be used to treat the symptoms of vitamin C deficiency and is available as tablets and effervescent tablets.
+▲ side-effects/warning: see ASCORBIC ACID

Refolinon

(Pharmacia) is a proprietary, prescription-only preparation of folinic acid. It can be used to counteract the folate-antagonist activity and consequent toxic effects of certain ANTICANCER drugs, especially METHOTREXATE. It is available as tablets and in a form for injection.
+▲ side-effects/warning: see FOLINIC ACID

Regaine

(Upjohn) is a proprietary, prescription-only preparation of the VASODILATOR drug minoxidil. It can be used to treat male-pattern baldness (in men and women) and is available as a topical solution.
+▲ side-effects/warning: see MINOXIDIL

Regulan

(Procter & Gamble) is a proprietary, non-prescription preparation of the (*bulking agent*) LAXATIVE ispaghula husk. It can be used to treat a number of gastrointestinal disorders, including irritable bowel syndrome and diverticular disease. It is available as a powder for solution in water and is not normally given to children under six years, except on medical advice.
+▲ side-effects/warning: see ISPAGHULA HUSK

Reguletts

(Seton Healthcare) is a proprietary, non-prescription preparation of the (*stimulant*) LAXATIVE phenolphthalein. It can be used to relieve constipation and is available as pills. It is not normally given to children, except on medical advice.
+▲ side-effects/warning: see PHENOLPHTHALEIN

Regulose

(Intercare Products) is a proprietary, non-prescription preparation of the (*osmotic*) LAXATIVE lactulose. It can be used to relieve constipation and is available as an oral solution.
+▲ side-effects/warning: see LACTULOSE

Relaxit Micro-enema

(Pharmacia) is a proprietary, non-prescription preparation of sodium citrate (with sodium lauryl sulphate, sorbic acid, sorbitol and glycerol). It can be used as a LAXATIVE and is available as an enema.
+▲ side-effects/warning: SODIUM CITRATE

Relefact LH-RH

(Hoechst) is a proprietary, prescription-only preparation of gonadorelin (gonadotrophin-releasing hormone; GnRH). It can be used as a diagnostic aid in assessing the functioning of the pituitary gland and is available in a form for intravenous injection.
+▲ side-effects/warning: see GONADORELIN

Relefact LH-RH/TRH

(Hoechst) is a proprietary, prescription-only COMPOUND PREPARATION of gonadorelin (gonadotrophin-releasing hormone; GnRH) and protirelin (thyrotrophin-releasing hormone; TRH). It can be used as a diagnostic aid in assessing the functioning of the pituitary gland and is available in a form for intravenous injection.
+▲ side-effects/warning: see GONADORELIN; PROTIRELIN

Relifex

(Bencard) is a proprietary, prescription-only preparation of the (NSAID) NON-NARCOTIC ANALGESIC and ANTIRHEUMATIC drug nabumetone. It can be used to treat and relieve pain and inflammation, particularly arthritic and rheumatic pain and other musculoskeletal disorders. It is available as tablets and a sugar-free oral suspension.
+▲ side-effects/warning: see NABUMETONE

R

R

Remedeine
(Napp) is a proprietary, prescription-only COMPOUND ANALGESIC preparation of the NON-NARCOTIC ANALGESIC drug paracetamol and the (OPIOID) NARCOTIC ANALGESIC drug dihydrocodeine tartrate, in the ratio 500/20 mg. It can be used as a painkiller and is available as tablets (and also under the proprietary name *Forte Tablets* in a combination of 500/30 mg).
+▲ side-effects/warning: see DIHYDROCODEINE TARTRATE; PARACETAMOL

Remegel Original
(Warner-Wellcome) is a proprietary, non-prescription preparation of the ANTACID drug calcium carbonate. It can be used for the relief of heartburn, acid indigestion and upset stomach. It is available as chewable tablets and is not normally given to children, except on medical advice.
+▲ side-effects/warning: see CALCIUM CARBONATE

Remnos
(DDSA Pharmaceuticals) is a proprietary, prescription-only preparation of the BENZODIAZEPINE drug nitrazepam. It can be used as a relatively long-acting HYPNOTIC for the short-term treatment of insomnia, where a degree of sedation during the daytime is acceptable. It is available as tablets.
+▲ side-effects/warning: see NITRAZEPAM

Rennie Gold (Minty)
(Roche) is a proprietary, non-prescription preparation of the ANTACID calcium carbonate. It can be used for the relief of acid indigestion, heartburn, upset stomach, dyspepsia and biliousness. It is available as tablets and is not normally given to children, except on medical advice.
+▲ side-effects/warning: see CALCIUM CARBONATE

Rennie Rap-Eze
(Roche) is a proprietary, non-prescription preparation of the ANTACID calcium carbonate. It can be used for the relief of acid indigestion, heartburn, upset stomach, dyspepsia and biliousness. It is available as tablets and is not normally given to children, except on medical advice.
+▲ side-effects/warning: see CALCIUM CARBONATE

Rennie Tablets, Digestif
(Roche) is a proprietary, non-prescription COMPOUND PREPARATION of the ANTACIDS calcium carbonate and magnesium carbonate. It can be used for the relief of acid indigestion, heartburn, upset stomach, dyspepsia, biliousness and overindulgence. It is available as tablets and is not normally given to children under six years, except on medical advice.
+▲ side-effects/warning: see CALCIUM CARBONATE; MAGNESIUM CARBONATE

Replenine
(BPL) is a recently introduced proprietary, prescription-only (heat-treated) preparation of factor IX fraction, dried, which is prepared from human blood plasma. It can be used in treating patients with a deficiency in factor IX (haemophilia B) and is available in a form for infusion.
+▲ side-effects/warning: see FACTOR IX FRACTION, DRIED

reproterol hydrochloride
is a SYMPATHOMIMETIC and BETA-RECEPTOR STIMULANT with $beta_2$-receptor selectivity. It is mainly used as a BRONCHODILATOR in reversible obstructive airways disease and as an ANTI-ASTHMATIC in severe acute asthma. It can also be used for the alleviation of symptoms of chronic bronchitis and emphysema. Administration is by aerosol. (Patients should be cautioned not to exceed the stated dose and if a previously effective dose fails to relieve symptoms they should consult their doctor.)

+▲ side-effects/warning: see under
SALBUTAMOL
✪ Related entry: Bronchodil

Resiston One

(Fisons) is a proprietary, non-prescription
COMPOUND PREPARATION of the ANTI-
ALLERGIC drug sodium cromoglycate and
the SYMPATHOMIMETIC and DECONGESTANT
drug xylometazoline hydrochloride. It can
be used in the prevention of allergic
rhinitis and is available as a nasal aerosol.
+▲ side-effects/warning: see SODIUM
CROMOGLYCATE; XYLOMETAZOLINE
HYDROCHLORIDE

Resolve

(SmithKline Beecham) is a proprietary,
non-prescription preparation of the NON-
NARCOTIC ANALGESIC drug paracetamol,
vitamin C and various ANTACID salts. It can
be used to treat headache with stomach
upset or with nausea (eg. migraine). It is
available as effervescent granules for
dissolving and is not normally given to
children under 12 years, except on
medical advice.
+▲ side-effects/warning: see PARACETAMOL

Resonium A

(Sanofi Winthrop) is a proprietary, non-
prescription preparation of sodium
polystyrene sulphonate, which is a resin
that can be used to treat high blood
potassium levels, particularly in patients
who suffer from fluid retention or who
undergo kidney dialysis. It is available in
the form of a powdered resin for use as a
rectal enema or by mouth.
+▲ side-effects/warning: see under
POLYSTYRENE SULPHONATE RESINS

resorcinol

is a KERATOLYTIC agent, which, when
applied topically, causes skin to peel and
relieves itching. It is also used in
ointments and lotions for the treatment of
acne.
+ side-effects: there may be local irritation.

▲ warning: it is not to be used if there are
local infections; avoid the eyes, mouth and
mucous membranes.
✪ Related entry: Eskamel

Respacal

(UCB Pharma) is a proprietary,
prescription-only preparation of the BETA-
RECEPTOR STIMULANT tulobuterol
hydrochloride. It can be used as a
BRONCHODILATOR in reversible obstructive
airways disease, as an ANTI-ASTHMATIC in
severe acute asthma and for the alleviation
of symptoms of chronic bronchitis and
emphysema. It is available as tablets and a
syrup.
+▲ side-effects/warning: see TULOBUTEROL
HYDROCHLORIDE

Restandol

(Organon) is a proprietary, prescription-
only preparation of the ANDROGEN (male
SEX HORMONE) testosterone (as
undecanoate). It can be used to treat
deficiency in men and for breast cancer in
women. It is available as capsules.
+▲ side-effects/warning: see TESTOSTERONE

Retin-A

(Cilag) is a proprietary, prescription-only
preparation of the (retinoid) tretinoin. It
can be used to treat severe acne and is
available as a cream, a gel and a lotion.
+▲ side-effects/warning: see TRETINOIN

retinol

is the chemical term for vitamin A, which
is a fat-soluble vitamin that is found in
meats and milk products and is also
synthesized in the body from constituents
in green vegetables and carrots. Retinol is
essential for growth and the maintenance
of mucous surfaces. It is particularly
useful in supporting the part of the eye's
retina that allows vision in the dark and a
deficiency may cause night-blindness and
dry eyes. On the other hand, an excess
may cause hair loss, peeling of the skin,
joint pain and liver damage. It is

R

493

R

administered therapeutically to make up vitamin deficiency (which is rare in Western countries). Administration is mainly oral in the form of capsules or as an emulsion, but it can also be by injection. Derivatives of Vitamin A (retinoids) are used by topical application to treat acne.
○ Related entries: acitretin; isotretinoin.

Retrovir

(Wellcome) is a proprietary, prescription-only preparation of the ANTIVIRAL drug zidovudine (azidothymidine; AZT). It can be used in the treatment of AIDS and is available as capsules, a syrup and in a form for intravenous infusion.
+▲ side-effects/warning: see ZIDOVUDINE

Revanil

(Roche) is a proprietary, prescription-only preparation of the ANTIPARKINSONISM drug lysuride maleate and is available as tablets.
+▲ side-effects/warning: see LYSURIDE MALEATE

Rheumacin LA

(CP Pharmaceuticals) is a proprietary, prescription-only preparation of the (NSAID) NON-NARCOTIC ANALGESIC and ANTIRHEUMATIC drug indomethacin. It can be used to relieve pain and inflammation, particularly rheumatic and arthritic pain and to treat other musculoskeletal disorders (including acute gout and inflammation of joints and tendons). It is available as modified-release capsules.
+▲ side-effects/warning: see INDOMETHACIN

Rheumox

(Wyeth) is a proprietary, prescription-only preparation of the (NSAID) NON-NARCOTIC ANALGESIC and ANTIRHEUMATIC drug azapropazone. It can be used to relieve pain and inflammation only of severe rheumatoid arthritis, ankylosing spondylitis and acute gout. It is available as capsules and tablets.

+▲ side-effects/warning: see AZAPROPAZONE

Rhinocort

(Astra) is a proprietary, prescription-only preparation of the CORTICOSTEROID drug budesonide. It can be used to treat nasal rhinitis. It is available as a nasal aerosol, *Rhinocort Aqua nasal aerosol* and as a nasal spray, *Rhinocort Aqua nasal spray*.
+▲ side-effects/warning: see BUDESONIDE

Rhinolast

(ASTA Medica) is proprietary, prescription-only preparation of the ANTIHISTAMINE drug azelastine hydrochloride. It can be used for the symptomatic relief of allergic rhinitis and is available as a nasal spray.
+▲ side-effects/warning: see AZELASTINE HYDROCHLORIDE

Rhuaka Herbal Syrup

(Waterhouse) is a proprietary, non-prescription COMPOUND PREPARATION of the (*stimulant*) LAXATIVES senna, rhubarb and cascara liquid. It can be used to relieve constipation and is available as a syrup. It is not normally given to children under seven years, except on medical advice.
+▲ side-effects/warning: see RHUBARB; SENNA

rhubarb

in a powdered form is sometimes used as a *stimulant* LAXATIVE and is a constituent of some proprietary laxative preparations.
○ Related entries: Pyralvex; Rhuaka Herbal Syrup

Rhumalgan

(Lagap) is a proprietary, prescription-only preparation of the (NSAID) NON-NARCOTIC ANALGESIC and ANTIRHEUMATIC drug diclofenac sodium. It can be used to treat arthritic and rheumatic pain and other musculoskeletal disorders. It is available as tablets and modified-release tablets (*Rhumalgan SR*).

R

+▲ side-effects/warning: see DICLOFENAC
SODIUM

ribavirin
See TRIBAVIRIN

Ridaura
(Bencard) is a proprietary, prescription-
only preparation of the ANTIRHEUMATIC
drug auranofin. It can be used to treat
rheumatoid arthritis and is available as
tablets.
+▲ side-effects/warning: see AURANOFIN

Rideril
(DDSA Pharmaceuticals) is a proprietary,
prescription-only preparation of the
ANTIPSYCHOTIC drug thioridazine. It can be
used to treat and tranquillize psychotic
patients, particularly manic forms of
behavioural disturbance and in the short-
term treatment of anxiety. It is available as
tablets.
+▲ side-effects/warning: see THIORIDAZINE

rifabutin
is an ANTIBACTERIAL, ANTITUBERCULAR and
ANTIBIOTIC drug, which is a recently
introduced member of the rifamycin
family. It can be used for the prevention of
Mycobacterium avium infection in
immunocompromised patients and for the
treatment of pulmonary tuberculosis and
mycobacterial disease. Administration is
oral in the form of capsules.
+▲ side-effects/warning: see under
RIFAMPICIN; there may be blood and liver
disorders, nausea, vomiting and
hypersensitivity reactions. Urine, saliva and
other bodily secretions may turn orange-red.
○ **Related entry: Mycobutin**

Rifadin
(Merrell) is a proprietary, prescription-
only preparation of the ANTIBACTERIAL and
ANTIBIOTIC drug rifampicin. It can be used
as an ANTITUBERCULAR drug to treat
dapsone-resistant leprosy and other
serious infections. It is available as

capsules, as a syrup and in a form for
intravenous infusion.
+▲ side-effects/warning: see RIFAMPICIN

rifampicin
is an ANTIBACTERIAL, ANTITUBERCULAR and
ANTIBIOTIC drug. It is one of the principal
drugs used in the treatment of
tuberculosis, mainly in combination with
other antitubercular drugs, such as
isoniazid or pyrazinamide, in order to
cover resistance and for maximum effect.
It acts against Mycobacterium tuberculosis
and sensitive Gram-positive bacteria by
inhibiting the bacterial RNA polymerase
enzyme. It is also effective in the treatment
of leprosy, brucellosis, legionnaires'
disease and serious staphylococcal
infections. Additionally, it may be used to
prevent meningococcal meningitis and
Haemophilus influenzae (type b)
infection. Administration is either oral as
capsules, tablets or a syrup, or by
injection or infusion.
+ side-effects: there are many side-effects and
include: gastrointestinal problems involving
nausea, vomiting, diarrhoea and weight loss;
many patients also undergo the symptoms of
flu, breathlessness, collapse and shock. Rarely,
there is kidney failure, liver dysfunction,
jaundice, muscle weakness, alteration in the
composition of the blood and/or
discolouration of the urine, saliva and other
body secretions. Sensitivity reactions, such as
a rash or urticaria (itchy skin rash) and
menstrual disturbances.
▲ warning: it should not be administered to
patients with jaundice or porphyria; it should
be administered with caution to those with
impaired liver function, or who are pregnant
or breast-feeding. One other effect of the drug
is that soft contact lenses may become
discoloured. It may reduce the reliability of
the contraceptive pill.
○ **Related entries: Rifadin; Rifater;
Rifinah; Rimactane; Rimactazid**

Rifater
(Merrell) is a proprietary, prescription-

R

only COMPOUND PREPARATION of the ANTIBACTERIAL drugs rifampicin, isoniazid and pyrazinamide. It can be used in the ANTITUBERCULAR treatment of pulmonary tuberculosis in the initial, intensive phase. It is available as tablets.

✛▲ side-effects/warning: see ISONIAZID; PYRAZINAMIDE; RIFAMPICIN

Rifinah

(Merrell) is a proprietary, prescription-only COMPOUND PREPARATION of the ANTIBACTERIAL drugs rifampicin and isoniazid. It can be used in ANTITUBERCULAR treatment and is available as tablets in two strengths, *Rifinah 150* and *Rifinah 300*.

✛▲ side-effects/warning: see ISONIAZID; RIFAMPICIN

Rimacid

(Rima) is a proprietary, prescription-only preparation of the (NSAID) NON-NARCOTIC ANALGESIC and ANTIRHEUMATIC drug indomethacin. It can be used to treat the pain and inflammation of rheumatic disease and other musculoskeletal disorders. It is available as capsules.

✛▲ side-effects/warning: see INDOMETHACIN

Rimacillin

(Rima) is a proprietary, prescription-only preparation of the broad-spectrum ANTIBACTERIAL and (PENICILLIN) ANTIBIOTIC drug ampicillin. It can be used to treat systemic bacterial infections, infections of the upper respiratory tract, of the ear, nose and throat and the urinogenital tracts. It is available as capsules and an oral suspension.

✛▲ side-effects/warning: see AMPICILLIN

Rimactane

(Ciba) is a proprietary, prescription-only preparation of the ANTIBACTERIAL and ANTIBIOTIC drug rifampicin. It can be used as an ANTITUBERCULAR drug and may also be used to treat other serious infections. It is available as capsules, a

syrup and in a form for intravenous infusion.

✛▲ side-effects/warning: see RIFAMPICIN

Rimactazid

(Ciba) is a proprietary, prescription-only COMPOUND PREPARATION of the ANTIBACTERIAL drugs rifampicin and isoniazid. It can be used in ANTITUBERCULAR treatment and is available as tablets in two strengths, *Rimactazid 150* and *Rimactazid 300*.

✛▲ side-effects/warning: see ISONIAZID; RIFAMPICIN

Rimafen

(Norton; Rima) is a proprietary, prescription-only preparation of the (NSAID) NON-NARCOTIC ANALGESIC, ANTIRHEUMATIC and ANTIPYRETIC drug ibuprofen. It can be used to relieve pain, particularly the pain of rheumatic disease and other musculoskeletal disorders, period pain, pain following operations and fever. It is available as tablets.

✛▲ side-effects/warning: see IBUPROFEN

Rimapam

(Rima) is a proprietary, prescription-only preparation of the BENZODIAZEPINE drug diazepam. It can be used as an ANXIOLYTIC in the short-term treatment of anxiety, as a HYPNOTIC to relieve insomnia, as an ANTICONVULSANT and ANTI-EPILEPTIC for status epilepticus, as a SEDATIVE in preoperative medication, as a SKELETAL MUSCLE RELAXANT and to assist in the treatment of alcohol withdrawal symptoms. It is available as tablets.

✛▲ side-effects/warning: see under BENZODIAZEPINE

Rimapurinol

(Rima) is a proprietary, prescription-only preparation of the ENZYME INHIBITOR allopurinol, which is a XANTHINE OXIDASE INHIBITOR. It can be used to treat excess uric acid in the blood and so prevent renal stones and attacks of gout. It is

available as tablets.
+▲ side-effects/warning: see ALLOPURINOL

Rimifon

(Cambridge) is a proprietary,
prescription-only preparation of the
ANTIBACTERIAL drug isoniazid. It can be
used as an ANTITUBERCULAR drug and
usually in combination with other
antitubercular drugs. It is available in a
form for injection.
+▲ side-effects/warning: see ISONIAZID

rimiterol hydrobromide

is a SYMPATHOMIMETIC, a BETA-RECEPTOR
STIMULANT with beta$_2$-receptor selectivity.
It is mainly used as a BRONCHODILATOR in
reversible obstructive airways disease and
as an ANTI-ASTHMATIC treatment in severe
acute asthma. It can also be used for the
alleviation of symptoms of chronic
bronchitis and emphysema. Administration
is by aerosol. (Patients should be
cautioned not to exceed the stated dose
and if a previously effective dose fails to
relieve symptoms they should consult their
doctor.)
+▲ side-effects/warning: see under
SALBUTAMOL; but has a shorter duration of
action.
○ Related entry: Pulmadil

Rimoxallin

(Rima) is a proprietary, prescription-only
preparation of the broad-spectrum
ANTIBACTERIAL and (PENICILLIN)
ANTIBIOTIC drug amoxycillin. It can be
used to treat systemic bacterial infections,
infections of the upper respiratory tract, of
the ear, nose and throat and the
urinogenital tracts. It is available as
capsules and an oral suspension.
+▲ side-effects/warning: see AMOXYCILLIN

Rinatec

(Boehringer Ingelheim) is a proprietary,
prescription-only preparation of the
ANTICHOLINERGIC and BRONCHODILATOR
drug ipratropium bromide. It can be used

to treat watery rhinitis and is available as a
metered spray.
+▲ side-effects/warning: see IPRATROPIUM
BROMIDE. Avoid spraying near the eyes.

Risperdal

(Janssen; Organon) is a proprietary,
prescription-only preparation of the
recently introduced ANTIPSYCHOTIC drug
risperidone. It can be used to tranquillize
patients suffering from schizophrenia and
other psychotic disorders and is available
as tablets.
+▲ side-effects/warning: see RISPERIDONE

risperidone

is a recently introduced ANTIPSYCHOTIC
drug, which is used to tranquillize patients
suffering from schizophrenia and other
acute and chronic psychotic disorders.
Administration is oral in the form of
tablets.
+▲ side-effects/warning: see under
CHLORPROMAZINE HYDROCHLORIDE; but
agitation may occur more frequently and
there may be nausea, abdominal pain,
dyspepsia, anxiety, concentration difficulties,
headache, dizziness, fatigue and rhinitis.
○ Related entry: Risperdal

ritodrine hydrochloride

is a SYMPATHOMIMETIC and BETA-RECEPTOR
STIMULANT drug, which can be used in
obstetrics to prevent or delay premature
labour by relaxing the uterus.
Administration is either oral as tablets or
in form for intravenous injection.
+ side-effects: muscle tremor, nausea,
vomiting, sweating, palpitations and speeding
of the heart, hypotension (low blood
pressure), flushing and dilation of blood
vessels in the extremities. Infusion or high
doses can lead to a lowering of blood
potassium levels, increased uterine bleeding,
oedema of the lungs, chest pains, heart
arrhythmias, enlargement of the salivary
glands and changes in blood picture on
prolonged use.
▲ warning: administer with caution to

R

R patients with certain heart disorders, hypertension, disorders of the thyroid gland, diabetes and where there are low levels of blood potassium (hypokalaemia). Care must be taken with drug interactions. It should not be used in eclampsia and severe pre-eclampsia, heart disease, uterine infections, placenta praevia and other potential complications. Patient's should be monitored (pulse rate, pulmonary oedema and blood pressure).

◐ Related entry: Yutopar

Rivotril

(Roche) is a proprietary, prescription-only preparation of the BENZODIAZEPINE drug clonazepam. It can be used as a ANTICONVULSANT and ANTI-EPILEPTIC to treat all forms of epilepsy, especially myoclonus, status epilepticus. It is available as tablets and in a form for injection.

+▲ side-effects/warning: see CLONAZEPAM

Roaccutane

(Roche) is a proprietary, prescription-only preparation of isotretinoin. It can be used to treat severe acne that proves to be unresponsive to more common treatments. It is available as capsules.

+▲ side-effects/warning: see ISOTRETINOIN

Robaxin

(Shire) is a proprietary, prescription-only preparation of the SKELETAL MUSCLE RELAXANT drug methocarbamol. It can be used to relieve acute muscle spasm and is available as tablets and in a form for injection.

+▲ side-effects/warning: see METHOCARBAMOL

Robaxisal Forte

(Shire) is a proprietary, prescription-only COMPOUND PREPARATION of the SKELETAL MUSCLE RELAXANT drug methocarbamol and the (NSAID) NON-NARCOTIC ANALGESIC and ANTIRHEUMATIC drug aspirin. It can be used primarily in the short-term treatment of rheumatic pain and to relieve the symptoms of other musculoskeletal disorders. It is available as tablets.

+▲ side-effects/warning: see ASPIRIN; METHOCARBAMOL

Robinul

(Wyeth) is a proprietary, prescription-only preparation of the ANTICHOLINERGIC drug glycopyrronium bromide. It can be used before operations for drying up saliva and other secretions. It is available in a form for injection.

+▲ side-effects/warning: see GLYCOPYRRONIUM BROMIDE

Robinul-Neostigmine

(Wyeth) is a proprietary, prescription-only COMPOUND PREPARATION of the ANTICHOLINERGIC drug glycopyrronium bromide and the ANTICHOLINESTERASE drug neostigmine (as methylsulphate). It can be used at the end of operations to reverse the actions of competitive neuromuscular blocking agents. It is available in a form for injection.

+▲ side-effects/warning: see GLYCOPYRRONIUM BROMIDE; NEOSTIGMINE

Robitussin Chesty Cough with Congestion

(Whitehall Laboratories) is a proprietary, non-prescription preparation of the EXPECTORANT guaiphenesin and the SYMPATHOMIMETIC and DECONGESTANT drug pseudoephedrine hydrochloride. It can be used for the relief of chesty coughs and nasal congestion and is available as an oral liquid. It is not to be given to children under six years, except on medical advice.

+▲ side-effects/warning: GUAIPHENESIN; PSEUDOEPHEDRINE HYDROCHLORIDE

Robitussin Dry Cough

(Whitehall Laboratories) is a proprietary, non-prescription preparation of the (OPIOID) NARCOTIC ANALGESIC and ANTITUSSIVE drug dextromethorphan hydrobromide. It can be used for the

symptomatic relief of persistent dry, irritant cough and is available as an oral liquid. It is not to be given to children under six years, except on medical advice.
+▲ side-effects/warning: see DEXTROMETHORPHAN HYDROBROMIDE

Robitussin Junior Persistent Cough Medicine

(Whitchall Laboratories) is a proprietary, non-prescription preparation of the (OPIOID) NARCOTIC ANALGESIC and ANTITUSSIVE drug dextromethorphan hydrobromide. It can be used for the symptomatic relief of persistent dry, irritant cough in children and is available as an oral liquid. It is not to be given to children under one year, except on medical advice.
+▲ side-effects/warning: see DEXTROMETHORPHAN HYDROBROMIDE

RoC Total Sunblock Cream

(RoC) is a proprietary, non-prescription SUNSCREEN, which contains constituents that protect the skin from ultraviolet radiation. It contains several agents used to help protect the skin, including avobenzone and ethylhexyl-methoxycinnamate. A patient whose skin condition requires this sort of protection may be prescribed it at the discretion of his or her doctor.

Rocaltrol

(Roche) is a proprietary, prescription-only preparation of calcitriol, which is a VITAMIN D analogue. It can be used to treat vitamin D deficiency and is available as capsules.
+▲ side-effects/warning: see CALCITRIOL

Roccal

(Sanofi Winthrop) is a proprietary, non-prescription preparation of the ANTISEPTIC agent benzalkonium chloride. It can be used to cleanse wounds and the skin before operations and is available as a solution.
+▲ side-effects/warning: see BENZALKONIUM CHLORIDE

Roccal Concentrate 10X

(Sanofi Winthrop) is a proprietary, non-prescription preparation of the ANTISEPTIC agent benzalkonium chloride. It can be used to cleanse wounds and the skin before operations and is available as a solution.
+▲ side-effects/warning: see BENZALKONIUM CHLORIDE

Rocephin

(Roche) is a proprietary, prescription-only preparation of the ANTIBACTERIAL and (CEPHALOSPORIN) ANTIBIOTIC drug ceftriaxone. It can be used to treat bacterial infections and to prevent infection arising during and after surgery. It is available in a form for injection.
+▲ side-effects/warning: see CEFTRIAXONE

rocuronium bromide

is a *non-depolarizing* SKELETAL MUSCLE RELAXANT drug. It is used to induce muscle paralysis during surgery and is administered by injection.
+▲ side-effects/warning: see under TUBOCURARINE CHLORIDE; but with less cardiovascular side-effects; administer with care to patients with kidney and liver impairment.
✪ Related entry: Esmeron

Roferon-A

(Roche) is a proprietary, prescription-only preparation of interferon (in the form of alpha-2a, rbe). It can be used as an ANTICANCER drug in the treatment of hairy cell leukaemias, myelogenous leukaemia, certain renal cell carcinoma, cutaneous T-cell lymphoma, chronic active hepatitis B and AIDS-related Kaposi's sarcoma. It is available in a form for injection.
+▲ side-effects/warning: see INTERFERON

Rogitine

(Ciba) is a proprietary, prescription-only

R preparation of the ALPHA-ADRENOCEPTOR BLOCKER drug phentolamine mesylate. It can be used as an ANTIHYPERTENSIVE and in the diagnosis of phaeochromocytoma. It is available in a form for injection.
+▲ side-effects/warning: see PHENTOLAMINE MESYLATE

Rohypnol
(Roche) is a proprietary, prescription-only preparation of the BENZODIAZEPINE drug flunitrazepam. It can be used as a HYPNOTIC for the short-term treatment of insomnia and is available as tablets.
+▲ side-effects/warning: see FLUNITRAZEPAM

Rommix
(Ashbourne) is a proprietary, prescription-only preparation of the ANTIBACTERIAL and (MACROLIDE) ANTIBIOTIC drug erythromycin. It can be used to treat and prevent many forms of infection and is available as tablets and a liquid oral mixture.
+▲ side-effects/warning: see ERYTHROMYCIN

Ronicol
(Tillomed) is a proprietary, non-prescription preparation of the VASO-DILATOR drug nicotinyl alcohol. It can be used to help improve blood circulation to the hands and feet when this is impaired, for example in peripheral vascular disease (Raynaud's phenomenon). It is available as a suspension, tablets and as the stronger *Timespan* tablets.
+▲ side-effects/warning: see NICOTINYL ALCOHOL

rose bengal
is a dye that is used for ophthalmic diagnostic procedures in the eye. Administration is by topical application in the form of eye-drops.
◐ Related entry: Minims Rose Bengal

rosoxacin
See ACROSOXACIN

Rowachol
(Monmouth) is a proprietary, prescription-only preparation of plant oils, including terpenes (borneol, camphene, cineole, mendone, menthol and pipene in olive oil). It can be used to treat gallstones and bile and liver disorders in cases where surgery is not possible. It is available as capsules.
+▲ side-effects/warning: see TERPENES

Rowatinex
(Monmouth) is a proprietary, prescription-only preparation of plant oils, including terpenes. It can be used to help expulsion of urinary tract calculi (stones) and is available as capsules.
+▲ side-effects/warning: see TERPENES

Rubavax
(Merieux) is a proprietary, prescription-only preparation of a VACCINE that can be used for the prevention of rubella (German measles). It is available in a form for injection.
+▲ side-effects/warning: see RUBELLA VACCINE

*rubefacient
is another term for a COUNTER-IRRITANT. The name derives from the fact that these agents cause a reddening of the skin by causing the blood vessels of the skin to dilate, which gives a soothing feeling of warmth. The term *counter-irritant* refers to the idea that irritation of the sensory nerve endings alters or offsets pain in the underlying muscle or joints that are served by the same nerves.

Rubella Immunoglobulin
(SNBTS) (Antirubella Immunoglobulin Injection) is a non-proprietary, prescription-only preparation of a SPECIFIC IMMUNOGLOBULIN. It can be used in IMMUNIZATION to give immediate immunity against infection by rubella (German Measles). It is available in a form for intramuscular injection.

rubella immunoglobulin, human

is a SPECIFIC IMMUNOGLOBULIN that is used in IMMUNIZATION to give immediate *passive immunity* against infection by rubella (German measles), for example, in pregnancy. It is generally not required since most people have established immunity through vaccination with RUBELLA VACCINE at an early age. Administration is by intramuscular injection.
○ Related entry: Rubella Immunoglobulin

rubella vaccine

is a VACCINE used for IMMUNIZATION against rubella (German mealses). It is medically recommended for pre-pubertal girls between 10 and 14 years, for medical staff who as potential carriers of the virus might put pregnant women at risk from infection and also for women of child-bearing age, because German measles during pregnancy constitutes a serious risk to the foetus. As a precaution vaccination should not take place if the patient is pregnant or likely to become pregnant within the following three months. The vaccine is prepared as a freeze-dried suspension of live, but attenuated, viruses grown in cell cultures. Administration is by injection. The substitution of a universal vaccination programme in schools for boys and girls by the combined MR vaccine (against measles and rubella) and the MMR programme for infants has meant that the rubella vaccination treatment alone is likely to become obsolete.
○ Related entries: Almevax; Ervevax; Rubavax

Rub/Vac

is an abbreviation for RUBELLA VACCINE

Rusyde

(CP) is a proprietary, prescription-only preparation of the (*loop*) DIURETIC drug frusemide. It can be used to treat oedema, particularly pulmonary (lung) oedema in patients with chronic heart failure and low urine production due to kidney failure (oliguria). It is available as tablets.
✚▲ side-effects/warning: see FRUSEMIDE

rutosides

also known as oxerutins, are derivatives of rutin, which is a vegetable substance. They are thought to work by reducing the fragility and permeability of certain blood vessels and may therefore be effective in preventing small haemorrhages and swellings (though there are doubts as to their efficacy). In mixtures, called oxerutins, they are used to treat oedema (accumulation of fluid in the tissues) associated with chronic venous insufficiency.
✚ side-effects: flushing, rashes, headache and gastrointestinal disturbances.
○ Related entry: Paroven

Rynacrom

(Fisons) is a proprietary, non-prescription preparation of the ANTI-ALLERGIC drug sodium cromoglycate. It can be used in the prevention of allergic rhinitis (inflamed lining of the nose). It is available as a nasal spray and nose-drops.
✚▲ side-effects/warning: see SODIUM CROMOGLYCATE

Rynacrom Compound

(Fisons) is a proprietary, non-prescription COMPOUND PREPARATION of the ANTI-ALLERGIC drug sodium cromoglycate and the SYMPATHOMIMETIC and DECONGESTANT drug xylometazoline hydrochloride. It can be used in the prevention of allergic rhinitis and is available as a nasal spray and nasal-drops
✚▲ side-effects/warning: see SODIUM CROMOGLYCATE; XYLOMETAZOLINE HYDROCHLORIDE

Rythmodan

(Roussel) is a proprietary, prescription-

R

R only preparation of the ANTI-ARRHYTHMIC drug disopyramide (as disopyramide phosphate). It is available as capsules and in a form for injection.
✚▲ side-effects/warning: see DISOPYRAMIDE

Rythmodan Retard

(Roussel) is a proprietary, prescription-only preparation of the ANTI-ARRHYTHMIC drug disopyramide (as disopyramide phosphate). It is available as modified-release tablets.
✚▲ side-effects/warning: see DISOPYRAMIDE

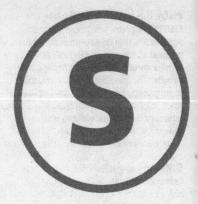

8SM

(BPL) is a proprietary, prescription-only preparation of dried human factor VIII fraction, which acts as a HAEMOSTATIC drug to reduce or stop bleeding in the treatment of disorders in which bleeding is prolonged and potentially dangerous (mainly haemophilia A). It is available in a form for intravenous infusion or injection
+▲ side-effects/warning. see FACTOR VIII FRACTION, DRIED

Sabril

(Merrell) is a proprietary, prescription-only preparation of the ANTICONVULSANT and ANTI-EPILEPTIC drug vigabatrin. It can be used to assist in the control of seizures that have not responded to other anti-epileptic drugs. It is available as tablets and a powder for oral administration.
+▲ side-effects/warning: see VIGABATRIN

Saizen

(Serono) is a proprietary, prescription-only preparation of somatropin, which is the biosynthetic form of the pituitary HORMONE human growth hormone. It can be used to treat hormonal deficiency and associated symptoms (in particular, short stature). It is available in a form for injection.
+▲ side-effects/warning: see SOMATROPIN

Salactol

(Dermal) is a proprietary, non-prescription preparation of the KERATOLYTIC agent salicylic acid (with lactic acid). It can be used to remove warts and hard skin and is available as a liquid paint.
+▲ side-effects/warning: see SALICYLIC ACID

Salamol

(Norton) is a proprietary, prescription-only preparation of the BETA-RECEPTOR STIMULANT salbutamol. It can be used as a BRONCHODILATOR in reversible obstructive airways disease, as an ANTI-ASTHMATIC treatment in severe acute asthma and for the alleviation of symptoms of chronic bronchitis and emphysema. It is available as a breath-actuated, metered aerosol inhalant.
+▲ side-effects/warning: see SALBUTAMOL

Salatac

(Dermal) is a proprietary, non-prescription preparation of the KERATOLYTIC agent salicylic acid (with lactic acid). It can be used to remove warts and hard skin and is available as a gel.
+▲ side-effects/warning: see SALICYLIC ACID

Salazopyrin

(Pharmacia) is a proprietary, prescription-only preparation of the AMINOSALICYLATE drug sulphasalazine. It can be used to treat active rheumatoid arthritis, ulcerative colitis and Crohn's disease. It is available as tablets, enteric-coated tablets, an oral suspension, suppositories and a retention enema.
+▲ side-effects/warning: see SULPHASALAZINE

Salazopyrin EN-Tabs

(Pharmacia) is a proprietary, prescription-only preparation of the AMINOSALICYLATE drug sulphasalazine. It can be used to treat active rheumatoid arthritis and ulcerative colitis and is available as enteric-coated tablets.
+▲ side-effects/warning: see SULPHASALAZINE

Salbulin

(3M Health Care) is a proprietary, prescription-only preparation of the BETA-RECEPTOR STIMULANT salbutamol (as salbutamol sulphate). It can be used as a BRONCHODILATOR in reversible obstructive airways disease, as an ANTI-ASTHMATIC treatment in severe acute asthma and for the alleviation of symptoms of chronic bronchitis and emphysema. It is available as a metered aerosol inhalant.
+▲ side-effects/warning: see SALBUTAMOL

S

salbutamol

is a SYMPATHOMIMETIC and BETA-RECEPTOR STIMULANT with good beta$_2$-receptor selectivity. It is mainly used as a BRONCHODILATOR in reversible obstructive airways disease and as an ANTI-ASTHMATIC treatment in severe acute asthma. It can also be used for the alleviation of symptoms of chronic bronchitis and emphysema and in obstetrics to prevent or delay premature labour by relaxing the uterus. It can be administered orally in the form of tablets, as modified-release tablets, as a sugar-free liquid, or as an inhalant from an aerosol, a nebulizer, an inhalation cartridge, a powder disc, or a ventilator. Alternatively, it can be administered by injection or infusion.

✚ side-effects: there may be a fine muscle tremor, particularly of the hands; headache and nervous tension, palpitations, dilation of blood vessels in the extremities, a speeding of the heart (normally minimal with aerosol administration) and very occasionally muscle cramps. Infusion or high doses can lead to a lowering of blood potassium levels. Some hypersensitivity reactions have been reported, including (paradoxical) bronchoconstriction, itchy rash (urticaria) and angio-oedema.

▲ warning: administer with caution to patients with certain disorders of the thyroid gland and heart, with hypertension, diabetes (in intravenous use) and who are breast-feeding, or pregnant (except when used to delay premature labour). Blood potassium levels should be monitored in severe asthma. There may be pain at the site of injection.

✚▲ side-effects/warning: for its use in labour, see under ritodrine hydrochloride.

✪ Related entries: Aerocrom; Aerolin Autohaler; Asmaven; Salamol; Salbulin; Salbutamol Cyclocaps; Steri-Neb Salamol; Ventide; Ventodisks; Ventolin; Volmax

Salbutamol Cyclocaps

(Du Pont) is a proprietary, prescription-only preparation of the BETA-RECEPTOR STIMULANT salbutamol (as salbutamol sulphate). It can be used as a BRONCHODILATOR in reversible obstructive airways disease, as an ANTI-ASTHMATIC treatment in severe acute asthma and for the alleviation of symptoms of chronic bronchitis and emphysema. It is available as capsules for use with the *Cyclohaler* device.

✚▲ side-effects/warning: see SALBUTAMOL

salcatonin

is a synthetic form of the THYROID HORMONE calcitonin (in the same form that is found in salmon). Its function is to lower the levels of calcium and phosphate in the blood and to regulate these levels with the correspondingly opposite action of a parathyroid hormone parathormone Therapeutically, it has the same effect and is used to lower blood levels of calcium when they are abnormally high (hypercalaemia) and to treat Paget's disease of the bone.

✚▲ side-effects/warning: see under CALCITONIN

✪ Related entries: Calsynar; Miacalcic

salicylate

is a termed used to describe a group of drugs that are chemically related to salicylic acid, which is a simple, single-ringed, organic molecule that occurs naturally as a component of salicin (a glycoside found in willow bark) and methyl salicylate (in oil of wintergreen). These natural products have been known for centuries to have antirheumatic actions, which derives from an inherent ANTI-INFLAMMATORY activity. Both the two natural medicines are irritant and poisonous if taken by mouth and the salt SODIUM SALICYLATE is rather irritant if administered orally. However, in 1899 the semi-synthetic drug the ester acetylsalicylic acid, was introduced under the name *Aspirin* as an ANALGESIC, ANTIPYRETIC and ANTIRHEUMATIC drug. Today, aspirin is still widely used as a generic drug and has been joined by a number of other salicylate drugs with similar actions and uses, for example, the aspirin-paracetamol ester BENORYLATE and the recently introduced drug DIFLUNISAL.

From the use of oil of wintergreen (containing methyl salicylate) as a topically applied treatment for muscle and joint aches and pains, several similar derivatives were developed with similar actions, for example, CHOLINE SALICYLATE, ETHYL SALICYLATE and GLYCOL SALICYLATE. Although it is not clear how these drugs act, it seems probable that they act as COUNTER-IRRITANTS, also known as RUBEFACIENTS.

Further uses of salicylates include the AMINOSALICYLATES (which contain a 5-aminosalicylic acid component), which are used to treat active Crohn's disease and to induce and maintain remission of the symptoms of ulcerative colitis and are also sometimes used to treat rheumatoid arthritis. Drugs in this group include MESALAZINE, OLSALAZINE SODIUM and SULPHASALAZINE, which combines within the one chemical both 5-aminosalicylic acid and the antibacterial SULPHONAMIDE.

In strong solution, salicylic acid is the standard, classic KERATOLYTIC agent, which can be used in the treatment of acne and to clear the skin of thickened, horny patches (hyperkeratoses) and scaly areas that occur in some forms of eczema, ichthyosis and psoriasis.

salicylic acid

is a KERATOLYTIC agent that also has some ANTIFUNGAL activity. It can be used to treat minor skin infections such as athlete's foot and psoriasis. It is also incorporated into some topical preparations that are rubbed into the skin as a COUNTER-IRRITANT, or RUBEFACIENT, treatment to relieve pain in soft tissues, including underlying muscle and joints. It is also used to remove warts and calluses. Administration is topical as a solution, a paint, or gel ointment; in combination with sulphur as an ointment,

a cream, or a shampoo; or with coal tar as an ointment.

✚ side-effects: there may be excessive drying, sensitivity and local irritation. After prolonged use there may be systemic effects.

▲ warning: avoid broken or inflamed skin. Certain preparations of this drug should not be used by diabetics or those with impaired blood circulation.

○ **Related entries:** Acnisal; Anthranol; Aserbine; Balneum with Tar; Baltar; benzoic acid ointment, compound, BP; Capasal; Clinitar; coal tar and salicylic acid ointment, BP; Cocois; Cuplex; Diprosalic; Dithrolan; Duofilm; Gelcosal; Gelcotar; Ionil T; Monphytol; Movelat Cream; Occlusal; Phytex; Posalfilin; Pragmatar; Psorin; Pyralvex; Radian B Heat Spray; Radian B Muscle Lotion; Salactol; Salatac; Verrugon; Warticon; Warticon Fem; zinc and salicylic acid paste, BP

Salivace

(Penn) is a proprietary, non-prescription COMPOUND PREPARATION of CARMELLOSE SODIUM and various other salts and constituents. It is used as a form of ARTIFICIAL SALIVA for application to the membranes of the mouth and throat in conditions that make the mouth abnormally dry (including after radiotherapy or in sicca syndrome). It is available as an aerosol.

Saliva Orthana

(Nycomed) is a proprietary, non-prescription preparation of gastric mucin (porcine). It can be used as a form of ARTIFICIAL SALIVA for application to the membranes of the mouth and throat in conditions that make the mouth abnormally dry. It is available as an aerosol and lozenges.

Salivix

(Thames) is a proprietary, non-prescription COMPOUND PREPARATION of acacia, malic acid and various other constituents. It is used as a form of ARTIFICIAL SALIVA for application to the membranes of the mouth and throat in conditions that make the mouth abnormally dry (including after radiotherapy or in sicca syndrome). It is available as pastilles.

salmeterol

is a recently introduced SYMPATHOMIMETIC and BETA-RECEPTOR STIMULANT with β_2-receptor selectivity. It is mainly used as a BRONCHODILATOR in reversible obstructive airways disease and as an ANTI-ASTHMATIC treatment in severe acute asthma. It can also be used for the alleviation of symptoms of chronic bronchitis and emphysema. It is similar to salbutamol but has a much longer duration of action. Therefore it may be used to prevent asthma attacks throughout the night after inhalation before going to bed and also for long-duration prevention of exercise-induced bronchospasm.
It is administered by inhalation as an aerosol or powder. It would normally be used in conjunction with long-term ANTI-INFLAMMATORY prophylactic (preventive) therapy (eg. with CORTICOSTEROIDS or SODIUM CROMOGLYCATE).

Patients should be cautioned that this drug should not be used for the relief of acute attacks and that corticosteroid treatment must be continued. Patients should also be cautioned not to exceed the stated dose and if a previously effective dose fails to relieve symptoms they should consult their doctor.
+▲ side-effects/warning: see under SALBUTAMOL; but the effects are more prolonged. There is a significant incidence of (paradoxical) bronchospasm.
✪ Related entry: Serevent

Salofalk

(Thames) is a proprietary, prescription-only preparation of the AMINOSALICYLATE drug mesalazine. It can be used to treat ulcerative colitis and is available as tablets.
+▲ side-effects/warning: see MESALAZINE

Saluric

(Merck, Sharp & Dohme) is a proprietary, prescription-only preparation of the (THIAZIDE) DIURETIC drug chlorothiazide. It can be used, either alone or in conjunction with other drugs, in the treatment of oedema and as an ANTIHYPERTENSIVE. It is available as tablets.
+▲ side-effects/warning: see CHLOROTHIAZIDE

Salzone

(Wallace Mfg.) is a proprietary, non-prescription preparation of the NON-NARCOTIC ANALGESIC and ANTIPYRETIC drug paracetamol. It can be used to releive mild to moderate pain and to reduce temperature in fever. It is available as a paediatric oral solution.
+▲ side-effects/warning: see PARACETAMOL

Sandimmun

(Sandoz) is a proprietary, prescription-only preparation of the IMMUNOSUPPRESSANT drug cyclosporin. It can be used to prevent tissue rejection in transplant patients, to treat severe, active rheumatoid arthritis and certain severe, resistant skin conditions (under specialist supervision). It is available as capsules, an oral solution and in a form for injection.
+▲ side-effects/warning: see CYCLOSPORIN

Sandocal

(Sandoz) is a proprietary, non-prescription preparation of calcium carbonate, calcium lactate gluconate, calcium carbonate and citric acid. It can be used as a MINERAL SUPPLEMENT in cases of calcium deficiency. It is available as effervescent tablets in two strengths, *Sandocal-400* and *Sandocal-1000*.
+▲ side-effects/warning: see CALCIUM CARBONATE

Sando-K

(Sandoz) is a proprietary, non-prescription MINERAL SUPPLEMENT that contains potassium chloride (with potassium bicarbonate). It is used to make up deficient blood levels of potassium and is available as effervescent tablets.

+▲ side-effects/warning: see POTASSIUM CHLORIDE

Sandostatin

(Sandoz) is a proprietary, prescription-only preparation of octreotide. It can be used as an ANTICANCER drug to treat the symptoms following the release of hormones from certain carcinoid tumours. It is available in a form for injection.

+▲ side-effects/warning: see OCTREOTIDE

Sanomigran

(Sandoz) is a proprietary, prescription-only preparation of the ANTIMIGRAINE drug pizotifen. It can be used to treat headache, particularly migraine and cluster headache and is available as tablets and an elixir.

+▲ side-effects/warning: see PIZOTIFEN

Saventrine

(Pharmax) is a proprietary, prescription-only preparation of the SYMPATHOMIMETIC isoprenaline (as isoprenaline hydrochloride). It can be used as a CARDIAC STIMULANT drug to treat a dangerously low heart rate or heart block. It is available as tablets and in a form for infusion (as *Saventrine IV*).

+▲ side-effects/warning: see ISOPRENALINE

Savlon Antiseptic Cream

(Zyma Healthcare) is a proprietary, non-prescription preparation of the ANTISEPTIC agents chlorhexidine (as gluconate) and cetrimide. It can be used to clean lesions, ranging from minor skin disorders or blisters to minor burns and small wounds and to prevent all types of infection from developing. It is available as a cream.

+▲ side-effects/warning: see CETRIMIDE; CHLORHEXIDINE

Savlon Bath Oil

(Zyma Healthcare) is a proprietary, non-prescription preparation of the EMOLLIENT liquid paraffin (and wool alcohols). It can be used for the symptomatic relief of contact dermatitis, atopic dermatitis (eczema), senile pruritus, ichthyosis and related dry skin disorders. It is available as a liquid to be added to a bath.

+▲ side-effects/warning: see LIQUID PARAFFIN

Savlon Dry

(Zyma Healthcare) is a proprietary, non-prescription preparation of the ANTISEPTIC agent povidone-iodine. It can be used for first aid treatment of cuts, grazes, minor burns and scalds. It is available as a spray.

+▲ side-effects/warning: SEE POVIDONE-IODINE

*scabicidal

drugs are used to kill the mites that cause scabies, which is an infestation by the itch-mite *Sarcoptes scabiei*. The female mite tunnels into the top surface of the skin in order to lay her eggs, causing severe irritation as she does so. Newly hatched mites, also causing irritation with their secretions, then pass easily from person to person on direct contact. Every member of an infected household should be treated and clothing and bedding should be disinfected. Treatment is usually with local application of a cream containing LINDANE, MALATHION, or PERMETHRIN, which kills the mites. BENZYL BENZOATE may also be used, but can be an irritant itself.

Schering PC4

(Schering Health) is a proprietary, prescription-only ORAL CONTRACEPTIVE that contains an OESTROGEN and a PROGESTOGEN, in this case ethinyloestradiol and levonorgestrel. It can

S be used after sexual intercourse has taken place (also known as the 'morning-after' pill).

+▲ side-effects/warning: see ETHINYLOESTRADIOL; LEVONORGESTREL

Scheriproct

(Schering Health) is a proprietary, prescription-only COMPOUND PREPARATION of the CORTICOSTEROID drug prednisolone hexanoate and the LOCAL ANAESTHETIC drug cinchocaine (as dibucaine hydrochloride). It can be used by topical application to treat haemorrhoids and is available as an ointment and suppositories.

+▲ side-effects/warning: see CINCHOCAINE; PREDNISOLONE HEXANOATE

Scholl Athlete's Foot Cream

(Scholl) is a proprietary, non-prescription preparation of the ANTIFUNGAL drug tolnaftate. It can be used to prevent and treat fungal infections responsible for athlete's foot and is available as a cream.

+▲ side-effects/warning: see TOLNAFTATE

Scholl Athlete's Foot Powder

(Scholl) is a proprietary, non-prescription preparation of the ANTIFUNGAL drug tolnaftate. It can be used to prevent and treat fungal infections responsible for athlete's foot and is available as a powder.

+▲ side-effects/warning: see TOLNAFTATE

Scholl Athlete's Foot Solution

(Scholl) is a proprietary, non-prescription preparation of the ANTIFUNGAL drug tolnaftate. It can be used to prevent and treat fungal infections responsible for athlete's foot and is available as a solution.

+▲ side-effects/warning: see TOLNAFTATE

Scholl Athlete's Foot Spray Liquid

(Scholl) is a proprietary, non-prescription

preparation of the ANTIFUNGAL drug tolnaftate. It can be used to prevent and treat athlete's foot and is available as an aerosol spray.

+▲ side-effects/warning: see TOLNAFTATE

Scoline

(Evans) is a proprietary, prescription-only preparation of the (*depolarizing*) SKELETAL MUSCLE RELAXANT drug suxamethonium chloride. It can be used to induce muscle paralysis during surgery and is available in a form for injection.

+▲ side-effects/warning: see SUXAMETHONIUM CHLORIDE

Scopoderm TTS

(Ciba) is a proprietary, prescription-only preparation of the ANTICHOLINERGIC drug hyoscine (as base). It can be used as an ANTINAUSEANT in the treatment of motion sickness. It is available as a self-adhesive patch that is placed on a hairless area of skin (usually behind an ear) and the drug is then released and absorbed through the skin.

+▲ side-effects/warning: see under HYOSCINE HYDROBROMIDE

scopolamine hydrobromide

is another name, which is standard in the USA, for hyoscine hydrobromide.

Sea-Legs

(Seton) is a proprietary, non-prescription preparation of the ANTIHISTAMINE and ANTINAUSEANT drug meclozine hydrochloride. It can be used to treat motion sickness and is available as tablets. It is not normally given to children under two years, except on medical advice.

+▲ side-effects/warning: see MECLOZINE HYDROCHLORIDE

Secaderm

(Fisons) is a proprietary, non-prescription COMPOUND PREPARATION of the ANTISEPTIC agent phenol, turpentine oil and terebene (with melaleuca oil). It can be used to

improve underlying blood circulation and is therefore used to treat such disorders as chilblains or varicose veins. It is available as an ointment (salve) for topical application.
+▲ side-effects/warning: see PHENOL; TURPENTINE OIL

Secadrex
(Rhône-Poulenc Rorer) is a proprietary, prescription-only COMPOUND PREPARATION of the BETA-BLOCKER drug acebutolol and the (THIAZIDE) DIURETIC drug hydrochlorothiazide. It can be used as an ANTIHYPERTENSIVE treatment for raised blood pressure and is available as tablets.
+▲ side-effects/warning: see ACEBUTOLOL; HYDROCHLOROTHIAZIDE

Seconal Sodium
(Lilly) is a proprietary, prescription-only preparation of the BARBITURATE drug quinalbarbitone sodium and is on the Controlled Drugs List. It can be used as a HYPNOTIC to treat persistent and intractable insomnia and is available as capsules.
+▲ side-effects/warning: see QUINALBARBITONE SODIUM

Sectral
(Rhône-Poulenc Rorer) is a proprietary, prescription-only preparation of the BETA-BLOCKER drug acebutolol. It can be used as an ANTIHYPERTENSIVE treatment for raised blood pressure, as an ANTI-ANGINA treatment to relieve symptoms and improve exercise tolerance and as an ANTI-ARRHYTHMIC to regularize heartbeat and to treat myocardial infarction. It is available as capsules and tablets.
+▲ side-effects/warning: see ACEBUTOLOL

Securon
(Knoll) is a proprietary, prescription-only preparation of the CALCIUM-CHANNEL BLOCKER drug verapamil hydrochloride. It can be used as an ANTIHYPERTENSIVE, as an ANTI-ANGINA drug in the prevention of

attacks and as an ANTI-ARRHYTHMIC to correct certain heart irregularities. It is available as tablets and in a form for injection.
+▲ side-effects/warning: see VERAPAMIL HYDROCHLORIDE

Securon SR
(Knoll) is a proprietary, prescription-only preparation of the CALCIUM-CHANNEL BLOCKER drug verapamil hydrochloride. It can be used as an ANTIHYPERTENSIVE and as an ANTI-ANGINA drug in the prevention of attacks. It is available as modified-release tablets.
+▲ side-effects/warning: see VERAPAMIL HYDROCHLORIDE

Securopen
(Bayer) is a proprietary, prescription-only preparation of the ANTIBACTERIAL and (PENICILLIN) ANTIBIOTIC drug azlocillin. It is mainly used to treat pseudomonal infections of the urinary tract, upper respiratory tract and septicaemia. It is available in a form for infusion or injection.
+▲ side-effects/warning: see AZLOCILLIN

*sedative
drugs calm and soothe, relieving anxiety and nervous tension and disposing a patient towards drowsiness. They are used particularly as a premedication prior to surgery. Many sedatives are HYPNOTIC drugs (such as the BARBITURATES), but are administered in doses lower than those used to induce sleep. The terms *minor tranquillizer* or ANXIOLYTIC are commonly used to describe benzodiazepine sedatives that relieve anxiety without causing excessive sleepiness.

Seldane
(Marrion Merrell Dow) is a proprietary, non-prescription preparation of the ANTIHISTAMINE drug terfenadine. It can be used to treat the symptoms of allergic disorders such as hay fever and allergic

S

skin conditions. It is available as tablets and is not normally given to children, except on medical advice.

✚▲ side-effects/warning: see TERFENADINE

Select-A-Jet Dopamine

(IMS) is a proprietary, prescription-only preparation of the SYMPATHOMIMETIC and CARDIAC STIMULANT drug dopamine (as dopamine hydrochloride). It can be used to treat cardiogenic shock following a heart attack or during heart surgery. It is available as a liquid in vials for dilution and infusion.

✚▲ side-effects/warning: see DOPAMINE

selegiline

is an ENZYME INHIBITOR, which is used in ANTIPARKINSONISM treatment because it inhibits the enzyme that breaks down the neurotransmitter DOPAMINE in the brain. It is thought that dopamine deficiency in the brain causes Parkinson's disease. It is often used in combination with LEVODOPA (which is converted to dopamine in the brain) to treat the symptoms of parkinsonism. Its enzyme-inhibiting property in effect supplements and extends the action of levodopa and (in many but not all patients) it also minimizes some side-effects. Administration is oral in the form of tablets.

✚ side-effects: hypotension, nausea and vomiting, confusion and agitation.

▲ warning: in some patients, side-effects are aggravated by the combination of selegiline and levodopa and the dose of levodopa may have to be reduced.

⊙ Related entry: Eldepryl

selenium sulphide

is a substance that is used as an anti-dandruff agent in some shampoos.

⊙ Related entries: Lenium; Selsun

Selsun

(Abbott) is a proprietary, non-prescription

shampoo that contains SELENIUM SULPHIDE, which is used as an anti-dandruff agent.

Semi-Daonil

(Hoechst) is a proprietary, prescription-only preparation of the SULPHONYLUREA drug glibenclamide. It is used in DIABETIC TREATMENT for Type II diabetes (non-insulin-dependent diabetes mellitus; NIDDM; maturity-onset diabetes) and is available as tablets (at half the strength of DAONIL tablets).

✚▲ side-effects/warning: see GLIBENCLAMIDE

Semitard MC

(Novo Nordisk) is a proprietary, non-prescription preparation of highly purified porcine INSULIN ZINC SUSPENSION (AMORPHOUS). It is used in DIABETIC TREATMENT to treat and maintain diabetic patients. It is available in vials for injection and has an intermediate duration of action.

✚▲ side-effects/warning: see under INSULIN

Semprex

(Wellcome) is a proprietary, prescription-only preparation of the ANTIHISTAMINE drug acrivastine. It can be used to treat the symptoms of allergic disorders such as hay fever and urticaria. It is available as capsules.

✚▲ side-effects/warning: see ACRIVASTINE

Senlax

(Intercare Products) is a proprietary, non-prescription preparation of the (*stimulant*) LAXATIVE senna. It can be used to relieve constipation and is available as a chocolate bar. It is not normally given to children under six years, except on medical advice.

✚▲ side-effects/warning: see SENNA

senna

is a traditional, powerful *stimulant* LAXATIVE, which is still in fairly widespread use. It works by increasing the muscular activity of the intestinal walls and may take from 8 to 12 hours to have any relieving effect on constipation. Senna preparations can also be administered to evacuate the bowels before an abdominal X-ray or prior to endoscopy or surgery.

✚ side-effects: it may cause griping, abdominal cramp and discoloured urine.

▲ warning: it should not be administered to patients who suffer from intestinal blockage.

✪ Related entries: Calfig California Syrup of Figs; Manevac; Nylax Tablets; Pripsen Powder; Rhuaka Herbal Syrup; Senlax; Senokot Granules; Senokot Syrup; Senokot Tablets

Senokot Granules

(Reckitt & Coleman) is a proprietary, non-prescription preparation of the (*stimulant*) LAXATIVE senna. It can be used to relieve constipation and is available as granules. It is not normally given to children under six years, except on medical advice.

✚▲ side-effects/warning: see SENNA

Senokot Syrup

(Reckitt & Coleman) is a proprietary, non-prescription preparation of the (*stimulant*) LAXATIVE senna. It can be used to relieve constipation and is available as a syrup. It is not normally given to children under six years, except on medical advice.

✚▲ side-effects/warning: see SENNA

Senokot Tablets

(Reckitt & Coleman) is a proprietary, non-prescription preparation of the (*stimulant*) LAXATIVE senna. It can be used to relieve constipation and is available as tablets. It is not normally given to children, except on medical advice.

✚▲ side-effects/warning: see SENNA

Septrin

(Wellcome) is a proprietary, prescription-only COMPOUND PREPARATION of the (SULPHONAMIDE) ANTIBACTERIAL drug sulphamethoxazole and the antibacterial drug trimethoprim, which is a combination called co-trimoxazole. It can be used to treat bacterial infections, especially infections of the urinary tract, prostatitis and bronchitis. It is available as tablets, as soluble tablets, as a suspension (in adult and paediatric strengths) and in a form for intravenous infusion.

✚▲ side-effects/warning: see CO-TRIMOXAZOLE

Serc

(Duphar) is a proprietary, prescription-only preparation of the drug betahistine hydrochloride, which has ANTINAUSEANT properties. It can be used to treat nausea associated with vertigo, tinnitus and hearing loss in Ménière's disease. It is available as tablets.

✚▲ side-effects/warning: see BETAHISTINE HYDROCHLORIDE

Serenace

(Baker Norton) is a proprietary, prescription-only preparation of the ANTIPSYCHOTIC drug haloperidol. It can be used to treat psychotic disorders, especially schizophrenia and the hyperactive, euphoric condition mania and to tranquillize patients undergoing behavioural disturbance. It can also be used in the short-term treatment of severe anxiety, for some involuntary motor disturbances and for intractable hiccup. It is available as a liquid, tablets, capsules and in a form for injection.

✚▲ side-effects/warning: see HALOPERIDOL

Serevent

(Allen & Hanbury) is a proprietary, prescription-only preparation of the BETA-RECEPTOR STIMULANT drug salmeterol (as xinafoate; hydroxynaphthoate). It can be used as a BRONCHODILATOR in reversible obstructive airways disease and as an ANTI-ASTHMATIC treatment. It is a recently introduced drug with unusual properties, in that it has a very prolonged duration of action. Therefore it is not to be used for the relief of acute attacks, but instead is largely used to give overnight protection (though it should be taken in conjunction with corticosteroids or similar drugs). It is available as an aerosol and as a powder for inhalation using the *Diskhaler* device. (Patients should be cautioned that this drug should not be used for the relief of acute attacks and that corticosteroid treatment must be continued. Patients should also be cautioned not to exceed the stated dose and if a previously effective dose fails to relieve symptoms they should consult their doctor.)

✚▲ side-effects/warning: see SALMETEROL

sermorelin

is an analogue of growth hormone releasing-hormone (somatorelin; GHRH). It is used therapeutically in a newly introduced test primarily to assess secretion of growth hormone. Administration is by injection.

✚ side-effects: it may cause flushing of the face and pain at injection site.

▲ warning: administer with care to patients with epilepsy, hypothyroidism, or who are being treated with antithyroid drugs. Do not use in pregnancy or breast-feeding. Caution must be taken when prescribing to those who are obese, hyperglycaemic, or have increased fatty acids in their blood.

✪ Related entry: Geref 50

Serophene

(Serono) is a proprietary, prescription-only preparation of the HORMONE ANTAGONIST and ANTI-OESTROGEN clomiphene citrate. It can be used as an infertility treatment and is available as tablets.

✚▲ side-effects/warning: see CLOMIPHENE CITRATE

serotonin

(5-HT) is a natural mediator in the body with NEUROTRANSMITTER and LOCAL HORMONE roles. As a neurotransmitter in

the brain, it mediates chemical messages on its release to excite or inhibit other nerves. It also interacts with a range of RECEPTORS (specific types of recognition sites on cells). A number of important drug classes have been developed that work by mimicking, modifying, or antagonizing serotonin's actions, including drugs that selectively modify its effect at receptors.

Serotonin levels in the brain are thought to be an important determinant of mood and ANTIDEPRESSANT drugs modify levels of serotonin (and other monoamines such as NORADRENALINE). The most recently developed class of antidepressant, the SSRI class (eg. FLUOXETINE), is named after the drugs' mechanisms of action – selective serotonin re-uptake inhibitors. The recently introduced ANXIOLYTIC drug BUSPIRONE HYDROCHLORIDE is thought to work by stimulating a certain type of serotonin receptor in the brain and can be used for the short-term relief of anxiety. Serotonin is also involved in the process of perception and its function is thought to be disrupted in psychotic illness (eg. schizophrenia); part of the evidence for this is that drugs such as LSD both induce mental states with psychotic features and are able to interact with some types of serontin receptors.

Serotonin and its receptors also have other important roles. For example, a newly developed class of ANTINAUSEANT and ANTI-EMETIC drugs are 5-HT_3-receptor antagonists (eg. GRANISETRON, ONDANSETRON and TROPISETRON) and are of particular value in treating vomiting caused by radiotherapy and chemotherapy by, in part, blocking the local hormone actions of serotonin in the intestine. SUMATRIPTAN, another recently developed drug, can be injected to treat acute migraine attacks and works by producing a rapid constriction of blood vessels surrounding the brain through stimulating serotonin 5-HT_1 receptors.

Seroxat

(SmithKline Beecham) is a proprietary, prescription-only preparation of the (SSRI) ANTIDEPRESSANT drug paroxetine, which has less SEDATIVE effects than some other antidepressants. It is available as tablets.

+▲ side-effects/warning: see PAROXETINE

sertraline

is an ANTIDEPRESSANT drug of the recently developed SSRI group. It is used to treat depressive illness and has the advantage over some other antidepressant drugs because it has relatively less SEDATIVE and ANTICHOLINERGIC side-effects. It is available as tablets.

+▲ side-effects/warning: see under FLUOXETINE

○ Related entry: Lustral

Setlers Tablets Peppermint Flavour

(SmithKline Beecham) is a proprietary, non-prescription preparation of the ANTACID calcium carbonate. It can be used for the relief of heartburn, indigestion, dyspepsia, nausea and flatulence. It is available as tablets and is not normally given to children under 12 years, except on medical advice.

+▲ side-effects/warning: see CALCIUM CARBONATE

Setlers Tums-Assorted Fruit Flavour

(SmithKline Beecham) is a proprietary, non-prescription preparation of the ANTACID calcium carbonate. It can be used for the relief of heartburn, indigestion, dyspepsia, nausea and flatulence. It is available as tablets and is not normally given to children, except on medical advice.

+▲ side-effects/warning: see CALCIUM CARBONATE

Sevredol

(Napp) is a proprietary, prescription-only preparation of the (OPIOID) NARCOTIC ANALGESIC drug morphine sulphate and is on the Controlled Drugs List. It can be used primarily to relieve pain following surgery, or the pain experienced during the final stages of terminal malignant disease. It is available as tablets.

+▲ side-effects/warning: see under OPIOID

*sex hormones

are endocrine (blood-borne) HORMONES that largely determine the development of the internal and external genitalia and secondary sexual characteristics (growth of hair, breasts and depth of voice). For convenience they are divided into male and female hormones, but both groups are produced to some extent by both sexes. They are all STEROIDS and chemically very similar. The main *male sex hormones* are called ANDROGENS, of which TESTOSTERONE is the principal member. In men, androgens are produced primarily by the testes; in both men and women, they are also produced by the adrenal glands; and in women, small quantities are secreted by the ovaries. In medicine, there are a number of synthetic androgens that are used to make up hormonal deficiency and which can also be used in ANTICANCER treatment.

Female sex hormones are called OESTROGENS and PROGESTERONE. They are produced and secreted mainly by the ovary and the placenta during pregnancy; and to a lesser extent, in men and women, by the adrenal cortex and, in men, by the the testes.

Natural and synthetic oestrogens are used therapeutically, sometimes in combination with PROGESTOGENS, to treat menstrual, menopausal or other gynaecological problems, as ORAL CONTRACEPTIVES (and as parenteral contraceptives by injection or implantation) and for HRT (hormone replacement therapy). See also: ANTI-OESTROGEN; ANTI-ANDROGEN; CONTRACEPTIVE.

S

S | ## silver sulphadiazine

is a compound ANTIBACTERIAL preparation
of silver and the SULPHONAMIDE drug
sulphadiazine. It has a broad spectrum of
antibacterial activity, as well as the
astringent and antiseptic properties of the
silver and is used primarily to inhibit
infection of burns and bedsores. It is
available as a cream for topical
application.
✚ side-effects: side-effects are rare, but there
may be sensitivity reactions including rashes.
▲ warning: it should not be administered to
patients who are allergic to sulphonamides; it
should be administered with caution to those
with impaired function of the liver or kidneys.
⊕ Related entry: Flamazine

simethicone

is a name for activated DIMETHICONE.

simple eye ointment

is a non-proprietary, bland, sterile
preparation of liquid paraffin and wool fat
in yellow soft paraffin. It is used as an eye
treatment both as a night-time eye
lubricant (in conditions that cause dry
eyes) and to soften the crusts caused by
infections of the eyelids (blepharitis).
✚▲ side-effects/warning: see LIQUID
PARAFFIN; WOOL FAT; YELLOW SOFT PARAFFIN

Simplene

(Smith & Nephew) is a proprietary,
prescription-only preparation of the
SYMPATHOMIMETIC hormone adrenaline. It
can be used in the treatment of glaucoma,
but not closed-angle glaucoma and is
available as eye-drops.
✚▲ side-effects/warning: see ADRENALINE

simvastatin

is used as a LIPID-LOWERING DRUG in
hyperlipidaemia to reduce the levels, or
change the proportions, of various lipids
in the bloodstream. It is usually
administered only to patients in whom a
strict and regular dietary regime, alone, is
not having the desired effect.

Administration is oral in the form of
tablets.
✚ side-effects: constipation or diarrhoea;
nausea and headache; flatulence with
abdominal discomfort, rash; insomnia; rarely,
liver and other complaints.
▲ warning: it should not be administered to
patients who are pregnant or breast-feeding
(and avoid pregnancy for at least one month
after stopping treatment). Patients should be
checked for normal liver function before and
during treatment; avoid high alcohol
consumption and report any muscle pain.
⊕ Related entry: Zocor

Sinemet

(Du Pont) is a proprietary, prescription-
only COMPOUND PREPARATION of the drugs
levodopa and carbidopa, which is a
combination called co-careldopa. It can
be used to treat parkinsonism, but not the
parkinsonian symptoms induced by drugs
(see ANTIPARKINSONISM). It is available as
tablets with a levodopa/carbidopa ratio of
1:10.
✚▲ side-effects/warning: see LEVODOPA

Sinemet CR

(Du Pont) is a proprietary, prescription-
only COMPOUND PREPARATION of the drugs
levodopa and carbidopa, which is a
combination called co-careldopa. It can
be used to treat parkinsonism, but not the
parkinsonian symptoms induced by drugs
(see ANTIPARKINSONISM). It is available as
modified-release tablets with a
carbidopa/levodopa ratio of 1:4.
✚▲ side-effects/warning: see LEVODOPA

Sinemet LS

(Du Pont) is a proprietary,
prescription-only COMPOUND PREPARATION
of the drugs levodopa and carbidopa,
which is a combination called
co-careldopa. It can be used to treat
parkinsonism, but not the parkinsonian
symptoms induced by drugs
(see ANTIPARKINSONISM). It is available
as tablets with a carbidopa/levodopa

ratio of 1:4.

✚▲ side-effects/warning: see LEVODOPA

Sinemet-Plus

(Du Pont) is a proprietary, prescription-only COMPOUND PREPARATION of the drugs levodopa and carbidopa, which is a combination called co-careldopa. It can be used to treat parkinsonism, but not the parkinsonian symptoms induced by drugs (see ANTIPARKINSONISM). It is available as tablets with a levodopa/carbidopa ratio of 25:100.

✚▲ side-effects/warning: see LEVODOPA

Sinequan

(Pfizer) is a proprietary, prescription-only preparation of the (TRICYCLIC) ANTIDEPRESSANT drug doxepin. It can be used to treat depressive illness, especially in cases where sedation is required. It is available as capsules.

✚▲ side-effects/warning: see DOXEPIN

Sinthrome

(Geigy) is a proprietary, prescription-only preparation of the synthetic ANTICOAGULANT drug nicoumalone. It can be used to prevent the formation of clots in heart disease, after heart surgery (especially following implantation of prosthetic heart valves) and to prevent venous thrombosis and pulmonary embolism. It is available as tablets.

✚▲ side-effects/warning: see NICOUMALONE

Siopel

(Zeneca) is a proprietary, non-prescription preparation of the ANTISEPTIC agent cetrimide and the ANTIFOAMING AGENT dimethicone. It can be used as a BARRIER CREAM to treat and dress itching or infected skin, nappy rash and bedsores and also to protect and sanitize a stoma (an outlet on the skin surface following the surgical curtailment of the intestines). It is available as a cream.

✚▲ side-effects/warning: see CETRIMIDE; DIMETHICONE

*skeletal muscle relaxants

act to reduce tone or spasm in the voluntary (skeletal) muscles of the body. They include those drugs – called *neuromuscular blocking drugs* – that are used in surgical operations to paralyse skeletal muscles that are normally under voluntary nerve control (but because the muscles involved in respiration are also paralysed, the patient usually needs to be artificially ventilated). The use of these drugs means that lighter levels of anaesthesia are required. Drugs of this sort work by acting at *nicotinic* RECEPTORS on the muscle that recognize ACETYLCHOLINE, the NEUROTRANSMITTER released from nerves to contract the muscle. There are two sorts of drug that achieve this effect, the *non-depolarizing* skeletal muscle relaxants (eg. GALLAMINE TRIETHIODIDE, TUBOCURARINE CHLORIDE and VECURONIUM BROMIDE) and the *depolarizing* skeletal muscle relaxants (eg. SUXAMETHONIUM CHLORIDE). The action of the non-depolarizing blocking agents may be reversed at the end of the operation, so that normal respiration may return, by administering an ANTICHOLINESTERASE drug (eg. NEOSTIGMINE). DANTROLENE SODIUM acts directly on skeletal muscle and can be used to relieve muscle spasm.

There are some quite different drugs (eg. BACLOFEN and DIAZEPAM) that effect muscle tone but do not work in the same way as the skeletal muscle relaxants discussed above, instead they act at some site in the central nervous system to reduce nervous activity and indirectly lower muscle tone. These drugs are used when some defect or disease causes spasm in muscle. All the drugs discussed in this entry are quite distinct from SMOOTH MUSCLE RELAXANTS.

Skinoren

(Schering Health) is a proprietary, prescription-only preparation of azelaic acid, which has mild ANTIBACTERIAL and

S KERATOLYTIC properties. It can be used to treat skin conditions such as acne and is available as a cream.
+▲ side-effects/warning: see AZELAIC ACID

Slo-Indo

(Generics) is a proprietary, prescription-only preparation of the (NSAID) NON-NARCOTIC ANALGESIC and ANTIRHEUMATIC drug indomethacin. It can be used to relieve the pain and inflammation of rheumatic disease, acute gout and other inflammatory musculoskeletal disorders and also period pain. It is available as modified-release capsules.
+▲ side-effects/warning: see INDOMETHACIN

Slo-Phyllin

(Lipha) is a proprietary, non-prescription preparation of the BRONCHODILATOR drug theophylline. It can be used as an ANTI-ASTHMATIC and chronic bronchitis treatment. It is available as modified-release capsules for prolonged effect.
+▲ side-effects/warning: see THEOPHYLLINE

Sloprolol

(CP) is a proprietary, prescription-only preparation of the BETA-BLOCKER drug propranolol hydrochloride. It can be used as an ANTIHYPERTENSIVE treatment for raised blood pressure, as an ANTI-ANGINA treatment to relieve symptoms and improve exercise tolerance and as an ANTI-ARRHYTHMIC to regularize heartbeat and to treat myocardial infarction. It can also be used as an ANTITHYROID drug for short-term treatment of thyrotoxicosis, as an ANTIMIGRAINE treatment to prevent attacks, as an ANXIOLYTIC treatment, particularly for symptomatic relief of tremor and palpitations, and, with an ALPHA-ADRENOCEPTOR BLOCKER, in the acute treatment of phaeochromocytoma. It is available as modified-release capsules.
+▲ side-effects/warning: see PROPRANOLOL HYDROCHLORIDE

Slow-Fe

(Ciba) is a proprietary, non-prescription preparation of the drug ferrous sulphate. It can be used as an IRON supplement in iron deficiency ANAEMIA TREATMENT and is available as modified-release tablets.
+▲ side-effects/warning: see FERROUS SULPHATE

Slow-Fe Folic

(Ciba) is a proprietary, non-prescription COMPOUND PREPARATION of ferrous fumarate and folic acid. It can be used as an IRON and folic acid supplement during pregnancy and is available as tablets.
+▲ side-effects/warning: see FERROUS SULPHATE; FOLIC ACID

Slow-K

(Ciba) is a proprietary, non-prescription preparation of potassium chloride. It can be used as a potassium supplement to make up a blood deficiency of potassium and is available as modified-release tablets.

Slow-Trasicor

(Ciba) is a proprietary, prescription-only preparation of the BETA-BLOCKER drug oxprenolol hydrochloride. It can be used as an ANTIHYPERTENSIVE treatment for raised blood pressure, as an ANTI-ANGINA treatment to relieve symptoms and improve exercise tolerance and as an ANTI-ARRHYTHMIC to regularize heartbeat and to treat myocardial infarction. It can also be used as an ANXIOLYTIC treatment, particularly for symptomatic relief of tremor and palpitations. It is available as modified-release tablets.
+▲ side-effects/warning: see OXPRENOLOL HYDROCHLORIDE

Slozem

(Lipha) is a proprietary, prescription-only preparation of the CALCIUM-CHANNEL BLOCKER diltiazem hydrochloride. It can be used as an ANTIHYPERTENSIVE and ANTI-ANGINA drug and is available in the form of

modified-release capsules.
+▲ side-effects/warning: see DILTIAZEM
HYDROCHLORIDE

smallpox vaccine

(Var/Vac) consists of a suspension of live
(but attenuated) viruses and was used in
IMMUNIZATION to prevent infection with
smallpox. However, it is no longer
required anywhere in the world because
global eradication of smallpox has now
been achieved. The smallpox vaccine also
works against other poxes (such as
vaccinia) and is still used for specialist
centres where researchers work with
dangerous viruses. Technically, therefore,
smallpox vaccine is still available on
prescription.
+▲ side-effects/warning: see under VACCINE

*smooth muscle relaxants

act on smooth (involuntary) muscles
(such as the intestines and blood vessels)
throughout the body to reduce spasm
(ANTISPASMODIC), cause relaxation and to
decrease motility. They can work by a
variety of mechanisms, though the term is
often reserved for those drugs that act
directly on smooth muscle, rather than
those that work indirectly through
blocking or modifying the action of
vasoconstrictor HORMONES or
NEUROTRANSMITTERS (eg. ACE INHIBITORS,
ALPHA-ADRENOCEPTOR BLOCKERS and BETA-
BLOCKERS). Smooth muscle relaxants may
be used for a number of purposes: drugs
that dilate blood vessels may be used in
ANTIHYPERTENSIVE treatment to lower
blood pressure (eg. CALCIUM-CHANNEL
BLOCKERS and HYDRALAZINE for long-term
treatment and SODIUM NITROPRUSSIDE for a
hypertensive crisis); in ANTI-ANGINA
treatment to treat angina pectoris (eg.
calcium-channel blockers for long-term
prevention and GLYCERYL TRINITRATE for
acute attacks); to improve circulation in
the extremities in the treatment of
peripheral vascular disease (eg. INOSITOL
NICOTINATE and OXPENTIFYLLINE); in ANTI-

ASTHMATIC treatment as BRONCHODILATORS
(eg. BETA-RECEPTOR STIMULANTS and
THEOPHYLLINE); to reduce spasm or colic
of the intestine (eg. MEBEVERINE); to relax
the uterus in premature labour (beta-
receptor stimulants). Drugs of the smooth
muscle relaxant class are quite distinct
from SKELETAL MUSCLE RELAXANTS.

Sno Phenicol

(Smith & Nephew) is a proprietary,
prescription-only preparation of the
ANTIBACTERIAL and ANTIBIOTIC drug
chloramphenicol. It can be used to treat
bacterial infections in the eye and is
available as eye-drops.
+▲ side-effects/warning: see
CHLORAMPHENICOL

Sno Pilo

(Smith & Nephew) is a proprietary,
prescription-only preparation of the
PARASYMPATHOMIMETIC drug pilocarpine.
It can be used in GLAUCOMA TREATMENT
and to facilitate inspection of the eye. It is
available as eye-drops.
+▲ side-effects/warning: see PILOCARPINE

Sno Tears

(Smith & Nephew) is a proprietary, non-
prescription preparation of polyvinyl
alcohol. It can be used as artificial tears
where there is dryness of the eye due to
disease and is available as eye-drops.
+▲ side-effects/warning: see POLYVINYL
ALCOHOL
arning: see AMYLOBARBITONE

sodium acid phosphate

is a mineral salt which mainly uses has in
combination either with other phosphorus
salts as a phosphorus supplement or a
proprietary enema and or to treat
infections of the urinary tract. Available in
proprietary LAXATIVE preparations in forms
for enema, suppository and as oral tablets.
**✪ Related entries: Carbalax; Fleet
Ready-to-use Enema; Fletchers'
Phosphate Enema; Phosphate-Sandoz**

S **Sodium Amytal**
(Lilly) is a proprietary, prescription-only
preparation of the BARBITURATE drug
amylobarbitone (as sodium) and is on the
Controlled Drugs List. It can be used as a
HYPNOTIC to treat persistent and
intractable insomnia and is available as
capsules and in a form for injection.
✚▲ side-effects/warning: see
AMYLOBARBITONE

sodium aurothiomalate

is a form in which gold can be used as an
ANTI-INFLAMMATORY and ANTIRHEUMATIC
drug in the treatment of severe conditions
of active rheumatoid arthritis and juvenile
arthritis. It works extremely slowly and
takes several months to have any
beneficial effect. Administration is by
injection.
✚ side-effects: severe reactions in a few
patients and blood disorders; skin reactions,
mouth ulcers; rarely, peripheral nerve
disorders, fibrosis, liver toxicity and jaundice,
hair loss and colitis.
▲ warning: it should not be administered to
patients with blood disorders or bone marrow
disease, severe kidney or liver disease; certain
skin disorders, lupus erythematosus, fibrosis;
or who are pregnant or breast-feeding.
Regular blood counts and monitoring of a
wide range of body functions during
treatment is necessary.
○ Related entry: Myocrisin

sodium bicarbonate

is an ANTACID that is used for the rapid
relief of indigestion. It is a constituent of
many proprietary preparations that are
used to relieve hyperacidity, dyspepsia and
for the symptomatic relief of heartburn
and a peptic ulcer. It is also sometimes
used in infusion media to replace lost
electrolytes, or to relieve conditions of
severe metabolic acidosis – when the
acidity of body fluids is badly out of
balance with the alkalinity – which may
occur in kidney failure or diabetic coma.
Administration is oral as tablets, capsules,

a liquid, or a powder.
✚ side-effects: belching, when used as an
antacid.
▲ warning: it should not be taken by patients
with impaired kidney function, or who are on
a low-sodium diet.
○ Related entries: Actron; Alka-Seltzer
Original; Andrews Answer; Bismag
Tablets; Bisodol Antacid Powder;
Bisodol Antacid Tablets; Bisodol Extra
Tablets; Bisodol Heartburn; Caved-S;
Eno; Gastrocote; Gastron; Gaviscon
250; Gaviscon Liquid; Japps Health
Salts; Magnatol; Min-I-Jet Sodium
Bicarbonate; Original Andrews Salts;
Phosphate-Sandoz; Pyrogatrone

sodium bicarbonate, BP

is an non-proprietary liquid formulation of
sodium bicarbonate and can be used as an
ANTACID. It is rapidly acting and, as with
other antacids containing carbonate,
causes belching and alkalosis if taken in
excessive doses. It is available as a
solution.
✚▲ side-effects/warning: see SODIUM
BICARBONATE

sodium calciumedetate

is a CHELATING AGENT, which is used as an
ANTIDOTE to poisoning by heavy metals,
especially lead. It works by forming a
chemical complex that is inactive and is
excreted safely from the body.
Administration is by injection.
✚ side-effects: nausea, cramp and kidney
damage in overdosage.
▲ warning: administer with caution to
patients with impaired kidney function.
○ Related entry: Ledclair

sodium carboxymethyl cellulose

See CARMELLOSE SODIUM

sodium cellulose phosphate

is used to reduce high calcium levels in
the bloodstream by inhibiting calcium

absorption from food. It is available as sachets of powder for solution in water.

✚ side-effects: it may cause diarrhoea and occasionally produces magnesium deficiency.

▲ warnings: do not use in patients with congestive heart failure or certain other heart conditions, or where dietary sodium is restricted. Administer with care to patients who are breast-feeding, pregnant, who have certain kidney disorders and in growing children.

❂ Related entry: Calcisorb

sodium chlodronate

is a drug that affects calcium metabolism and is used to treat high calcium levels associated with malignant tumours and bone lesions. Administration is oral in the form of tablets or slow intravenous infusion. Dietary counselling of patients is advised, particularly with regard to avoiding food containing calcium during oral treatment.

✚ side-effects: there may be nausea and diarrhoea and skin reactions. There may be lowered calcium levels (hypocalcaemia).

▲ warning: it should not be administered to patients with certain kidney disorders, or who are pregnant or breast-feeding. Kidney and liver function and white cell count should be monitored; an adequate fluid intake should be maintained.

❂ Related entries: Bonefos; Loron

sodium chloride

is an essential constituent of the human body for both blood and tissues. It is the major form in which the mineral element sodium appears. Sodium is involved in the balance of body fluids, in the nervous system and is essential for the functioning of the muscles. Sodium chloride, or salt, is contained in many foods, but too much salt can lead to oedema (the accumulation of fluids in the tissues), dehydration, and/or hypertension (high blood pressure). Therapeutically, sodium chloride is widely used as saline solution (0.9%) or dextrose saline (to treat

dehydration and shock), as a medium with which to effect bladder irrigation, as a sodium supplement in patients with low sodium levels, as an eye-wash, nose-drops, a mouthwash and by topical application in solution as a cleansing lotion.

✚ side-effects: overdosage can lead to hypertension, dehydration, or oedema.

▲ warning: it should be administered with caution to patients with heart failure, hypertension, fluid retention, or impaired kidney function.

❂ Related entries: Balanced Salt Solution; Diocalm Replenisher; Dioralyte; Glandosane; Luborant; Minims Sodium Chloride

sodium citrate

is an alkaline compound, which is used to treat mild infections of the urinary tract (especially cystitis) in which the urine is acid. It is available in several proprietary compound LAXATIVE preparations and is administered orally.

✚ side-effects: there may be dry mouth and mild diuresis.

▲ warning: it should be administered with caution to patients with impaired kidney function or heart disease, or who are pregnant.

❂ Related entries: Balanced Salt Solution; Diocalm Replenisher; KLN Suspension; Lemsip; Lemsip, Junior; Micolette Micro-enema; Picolax; Relaxit Micro-enema; Vicks Original Formula Cough Syrup

sodium cromoglicate
See SODIUM CROMOGLYCATE

sodium cromoglycate

(sodium cromoglicate) is an ANTI-ALLERGIC drug. It is used to prevent recurrent asthma attacks (but not to treat acute attacks) and allergic symptoms in the eye (eg. allergic conjunctivitis), intestine (eg. food allergy) and elsewhere. It is not clear how it works, but its ANTI-

S INFLAMMATORY activity appears to involve a reduction in the release of inflammatory mediators. Administration is usually by inhalation from an aerosol or nebulizer, or from an applicator that squirts dry powder, eye-drops, eye ointment, nasal drops, or a nasal spray.

✚ side-effects: depending on the route of administration, there may be coughing or transient bronchospasm. Inhalation of the dry powder preparation may cause irritation of the throat. Local irritation in the nose. Nausea, vomiting, or joint pain.

❍ Related entries: Aerochrom; Brol-eze Eye Drops; Hay-Crom; Intal; Nalcrom; Opticrom; Opticrom Allergy Eye Drops; Optrex Hayfever Allergy Eye Drops; Resiston One; Rynacrom; Rynacrom Compound; Vividrin

sodium fusidate
See FUSIDIC ACID

sodium fusidate gauze dressing, BP
See FUCIDIN INTERTULLE

sodium hyaluronate
is a visco-elastic polymer that is normally present in the aqueous and vitreous humour of the eye. It can be used during surgical procedures on the eye and is administered by injection.

✚ side-effects: occasional hypersensitivity reactions, short-lived rise in intraocular pressure (pressure in the eyeball).

❍ Related entry: Healonid

sodium hypochlorite
is a powerful oxidizing agent, which can be used in solution as an ANTISEPTIC for cleansing abrasions, burns and ulcers. It is not commonly used today because it can be an irritant to some people. There are a number of non-proprietary solutions available in various concentrations.

✚▲ side-effects/warning: it can have an irritant effect and can bleach fabrics.

❍ Related entry: Chlorasol

sodium nitrite
is a compound that is used in the emergency treatment of cyanide poisoning and often in combination with sodium thiosulphate. Administration is by injection. See ANTIDOTE.

✚ side-effects: flushing and headache.

sodium nitroprusside
is a VASODILATOR drug that is used acutely as an ANTIHYPERTENSIVE to control severe hypertensive crises, as a HEART FAILURE TREATMENT and as a HYPOTENSIVE for controlled low blood pressure in surgery. Administration is by infusion.

✚ side-effects: headache, dizziness, sweating, nausea and retching, palpitations; there may also be abdominal pain, anxiety and blood disorders.

▲ warning: it should not be administered to patients with severe impaired liver function or vitamin B_{12} deficiency; it should be administered with caution to those with impaired kidney function, impaired brain blood circulation, hypothyroidism, who are elderly, pregnant, or breast-feeding; or have ischaemic heart disease.

❍ Related entry: Nipride

sodium perborate
is an ANTISEPTIC agent and is used in solution as a mouthwash.

▲ warning: it should not be used continuously or borate poisoning may occur; use with care in those with renal impairment.

❍ Related entry: Bocasan

sodium picosulfate
See SODIUM PICOSULPHATE

sodium picosulphate
(sodium picosulfate) is a *stimulant* LAXATIVE. It works by stimulating motility of the intestine and can be used to relieve constipation and to prepare patients for X-ray, endoscopy, or surgery. Administration is oral in the form of an elixir or as a powder for solution.

✚ side-effects: abdominal cramps.

▲ warning: it should not be administered to patients who suffer from intestinal blockage.
✪ **Related entries: Laxoberal; Picolax**

sodium salicylate

is a soluble (NSAID) NON-NARCOTIC ANALGESIC and ANTIRHEUMATIC drug. It can be used to treat rheumatic disease and other musculoskeletal disorders. Administration is oral in the form of a mixture or as tablets. See also SALICYLATES and SALICYLIC ACID.
✚▲ side-effects/warning: see NSAID.
✪ **Related entries: Doan's Backache Pills; Jackson's Febrifuge**

sodium stibogluconate

is an ANTIPROTOZOAL drug. It can be used to treat various forms of the tropical disease leishmaniasis, or kala-azar, which is caused by parasitic protozoa transmitted in sandfly bites and which leaves extensive, unsightly lesions on the skin. Administration is by slow intravenous or intramuscular injection.
✚ side-effects: there may be vomiting, coughing and chest pain, or anorexia. The injection may be painful.
▲ warning: it should not be administered to patients with pneumonia, certain heart, liver, or kidney disorders.
✪ **Related entry: Pentostam**

sodium tetradecyl sulphate

is a drug used in sclerotherapy, which is a technique to treat varicose veins by the injection of an irritant solution. Administration is by injection.
✚▲ side-effects/warning: see under ETHANOLAMINE OLEATE
✪ **Related entry: STD**

sodium thiosulphate

is a compound that is used in the emergency treatment of cyanide poisoning and often in combination with sodium nitrite. Administration is by injection. See ANTIDOTE.

sodium valproate

is an ANTICONVULSANT and ANTI-EPILEPTIC drug. It is a valuable drug for treating all forms of epilepsy, particularly tonic-clonic seizures (grand mal) in primary generalized epilepsy. Administration is either oral as tablets, a liquid or capsules, or by injection.
✚ side effects: nausea and gastric irritation, unsteady gait and muscle tremor, increased appetite and weight gain, temporary hair loss, oedema (accumulation of fluid in the tissues), blood changes, impaired liver function, effects on blood and liver, menstrual disorders, rashes, growth of breasts in men.
▲ warning: it should not be administered to patients with liver disease or a family history of liver dysfunction. Administer with caution to patients who are pregnant or breast-feeding, or who have porphyria or lupus erythematosus.
✪ **Related entries: Convulex; Epilim; Epilim Chrono; Epilim Intravenous; Orlept**

Sofradex

(Roussel) is a proprietary, prescription-only COMPOUND PREPARATION of the broad-spectrum ANTIBACTERIAL and (AMINOGLYCOSIDE) ANTIBIOTIC drug framycetin sulphate and the ANTI-INFLAMMATORY and CORTICOSTEROID drug dexamethasone. It can be used to treat inflammation and infection in the eye or outer ear and is available as drops and an ointment.
✚▲ side-effects/warning: see DEXAMETHASONE; FRAMYCETIN SULPHATE

Soframycin

(Roussel) is a proprietary, prescription-only preparation of the broad-spectrum, ANTIBACTERIAL and (AMINOGLYCOSIDE) ANTIBIOTIC drug framycetin sulphate. It can be used to treat infection of the skin, an open wound, or of the eye and is available as eye-drops and an eye ointment for topical application.

S ✚▲ side-effects/warning: see FRAMYCETIN SULPHATE

Solarcaine

(Schering-Plough) is a proprietary, non-prescription COMPOUND PREPARATION of the LOCAL ANAESTHETIC drug benzocaine and the ANTISEPTIC agent triclosan. It can be used to treat local pain and skin irritation. It is available as a cream, a lotion and a spray for topical application.
✚▲ side-effects/warning: see BENZOCAINE; TRICLOSAN

Solpadeine Capsules

(Sterling Research) is a proprietary, non-prescription COMPOUND PREPARATION of the NON-NARCOTIC ANALGESIC drug paracetamol, the (OPIOID) NARCOTIC ANALGESIC drug codeine phosphate (a combination known as co-codamol) and the STIMULANT caffeine. It can be used to relieve headache, period pain and rheumatic and musculoskeletal pain. It is available as capsules and is not to be given to children under 12 years, except on medical advice.
✚▲ side-effects/warning: see CAFFEINE; CODEINE PHOSPHATE; PARACETAMOL

Solpadeine Soluble Tablets

(Sterling Research) is a proprietary, non-prescription COMPOUND PREPARATION of the NON-NARCOTIC ANALGESIC drug paracetamol, the (OPIOID) NARCOTIC ANALGESIC drug codeine phosphate (a combination known as co-codamol) and the STIMULANT caffeine. It can be used to relieve headache, period pain and rheumatic and musculoskeletal pain. It is available as soluble tablets and is not to be given to children under seven years, except on medical advice.
✚▲ side-effects/warning: see CAFFEINE; CODEINE PHOSPHATE; PARACETAMOL

Solpadeine Tablets

(Sterling Research) is a proprietary, non-prescription COMPOUND PREPARATION of the NON-NARCOTIC ANALGESIC drug paracetamol, the (OPIOID) NARCOTIC ANALGESIC drug codeine phosphate (a combination known as co-codamol) and the STIMULANT caffeine. It can be used to relieve headache, period pain and rheumatic and musculoskeletal pain. It is available as tablets and is not to be given to children under 12 years, except on medical advice.
✚▲ side-effects/warning: see CAFFEINE; CODEINE PHOSPHATE; PARACETAMOL

Solpadol

(Sterling-Winthrop) is a proprietary, prescription-only COMPOUND ANALGESIC preparation of the (OPIOID) NARCOTIC ANALGESIC and ANTITUSSIVE drug codeine phosphate and the NON-NARCOTIC ANALGESIC drug paracetamol (a combination known as co-codamol). It can be used as a painkiller and is available as tablets (*Caplets*).
✚▲ side-effects/warning: see CODEINE PHOSPHATE; PARACETAMOL

soluble insulin

(neutral insulin; insulin injection) is a form of animal (porcine or bovine) or human insulin prepared as a sterile solution and used in DIABETIC TREATMENT to treat and maintain diabetic patients. It is available in vials for injection and has a short duration of action. It is the form of insulin that is used in diabetic emergencies.
✚▲ side-effects/warning: see INSULIN
✪ Related entries: Human Actrapid; Human Velosulin; Humulin S; Hypurin Neutral; Pur-In Neutral; Velosulin

Solu-Cortef

(Upjohn) is a proprietary, prescription-only preparation of the CORTICOSTEROID and ANTI-INFLAMMATORY drug hydrocortisone (as sodium succinate). It can be used to treat inflammation, allergic symptoms and shock. It is available in a form for injection.

+▲ side-effects/warning: see
HYDROCORTISONE

Solu-Medrone
(Upjohn) is a proprietary, prescription-only preparation of the CORTICOSTEROID and ANTI-INFLAMMATORY drug methylprednisolone (as acetate). It can be used in the treatment of allergic disorders, shock and cerebral oedema. It is available in a form for injection.
+▲ side-effects/warning: see
METHYLPREDNISOLONE

somatotropin
is a name for the pituitary HORMONE human growth hormone (HGH). It was isolated from the pituitary glands of cadavers, which when used to treat short stature (dwarfism) brought with it the risk of acquiring Creutzfeldt-Jakob disease due to contamination. It has now been replaced in the UK by SOMATROPIN, which is a biosynthetic form of human growth hormone and so has no risk of contamination.

somatropin
(biosynthetic human growth hormone) is the name given to the synthetic form of the pituitary HORMONE human growth hormone. The name is used to distinguish it from the natural human product somatotropin (HGH) that it replaced in the UK. Somatropin was isolated from the pituitary glands of cadavers and consequently brought with it the risk of acquiring Creutzfeldt-Jakob disease due to contamination. Somatropin is used to treat short stature (dwarfism) when the condition is due to growth hormone deficiency (eg. in Turner syndrome). It is only used when the bones are still forming and is administered by injection.
+ side-effects: there may be reactions at injection sites and swelling due to accumulation of lymph in tissues (in Turner syndrome).
▲ warnings: it should not be used by pregnant women and given with caution to those with diabetes, other pituitary hormone deficiencies, or open bone epiphyses.
✪ Related entries: Genotropin; Humatrope; Norditropin; Saizen

Sominex
(SmithKline Beecham) is a proprietary, non-prescription preparation of the ANTIHISTAMINE drug promethazine hydrochloride, which is a PHENOTHIAZINE DERIVATIVE with marked SEDATIVE properties. It can be used to help induce sleep in the treatment of temporary sleep disturbances and is available as tablets. It is not normally given to children under 16 years, except on medical advice.
+▲ side-effects/warning: see PROMETHAZINE HYDROCHLORIDE

Somnite
(Norgine) is a proprietary, prescription-only preparation of the BENZODIAZEPINE drug nitrazepam. It can be used as a relatively long-acting HYPNOTIC for the short-term treatment of insomnia, where a degree of sedation during the daytime is acceptable. It is available as an oral suspension.
+▲ side-effects/warning: see NITRAZEPAM

Soneryl
(Rhône-Poulenc Rorer) is a proprietary, prescription-only preparation of the BARBITURATE drug butobarbitone and is on the Controlled Drugs List. It can be used as a HYPNOTIC to treat persistent and intractable insomnia and is available as tablets.
+▲ side-effects/warning: see
BUTOBARBITONE

Soni-Slo
(Lipha) is a proprietary, non-prescription preparation of the VASODILATOR and ANTI-ANGINA drug isosorbide dinitrate. It can be used in HEART FAILURE TREATMENT and to treat and prevent angina pectoris. It is available as modified-release capsules.

+▲ side-effects/warning: see ISOSORBIDE DINITRATE

Sootheye

(Rhône-Poulenc Rorer is a proprietary, non-prescription preparation of the ASTRINGENT agent zinc sulphate. It can be used for the symptomatic relief of minor eye irritation and is available as eye-drops for topical application.
+▲ side-effects/warning: see ZINC SULPHATE

Sorbichew

(Stuart) is a proprietary, non-prescription preparation of the VASODILATOR and ANTI-ANGINA drug isosorbide dinitrate. It can be used in HEART FAILURE TREATMENT and to treat and, in particular, prevent angina pectoris. It is available as chewable tablets.
+▲ side-effects/warning: see ISOSORBIDE DINITRATE

Sorbid SA

(Stuart) is a proprietary, non-prescription preparation of the VASODILATOR and ANTI-ANGINA drug isosorbide dinitrate. It can be used to treat and, in particular, prevent angina pectoris. It is available as modified-release sublingual tablets in two strengths, *Sorbid-20 SA* and *Sorbid-20 SA*.
+▲ side-effects/warning: see ISOSORBIDE DINITRATE

sorbitol

is a sweet-tasting carbohydrate, which is used as a sugar-substitute (particularly by diabetics) and as the carbohydrate component in some nutritional supplements that are administered by injection or infusion. It is also used as a constituent of ARTIFICIAL SALIVA.
✪ Related entries: Glandosane; Luborant

Sorbitrate

(Stuart) is a proprietary, non-prescription preparation of the VASODILATOR and ANTI-ANGINA drug isosorbide dinitrate. It can be

used in HEART FAILURE TREATMENT and to treat and, in particular, prevent angina pectoris. It is available as tablets.
+▲ side-effects/warning: see ISOSORBIDE DINITRATE

Sotacor

(Bristol-Myers) is a proprietary, prescription-only preparation of the BETA-BLOCKER drug sotalol hydrochloride. It is used as an ANTIHYPERTENSIVE treatment for raised blood pressure, as an ANTI-ANGINA treatment to relieve symptoms and improve exercise tolerance and as an ANTI-ARRHYTHMIC to regularize heartbeat and to treat myocardial infarction. It can also be used as an ANTITHYROID drug for short-term treatment of thyrotoxicosis. It is available as tablets or in a form for injection.
+▲ side-effects/warning: see SOTALOL HYDROCHLORIDE

sotalol hydrochloride

is a BETA-BLOCKER that can be used as an ANTIHYPERTENSIVE treatment for raised blood pressure, as an ANTI-ANGINA treatment to relieve symptoms and improve exercise tolerance and as an ANTI-ARRHYTHMIC to regularize heartbeat and to treat and prevent myocardial infarction. It can also be used as an ANTITHYROID drug for short-term treatment of thyrotoxicosis. Administration can be oral as tablets or by injection. It is also available, as an antihypertensive treatment, in the form of a COMPOUND PREPARATION with a DIURETIC.
+▲ side-effects/warnings: see under PROPRANOLOL HYDROCHLORIDE. It may cause abnormal heart rhythms and care must be taken to avoid low blood potassium when used with diuretics.
✪ Related entries: Beta-Cardone; Sotacor; Sotazide; Tolerzide

Sotazide

(Bristol-Myers) is a proprietary, prescription-only COMPOUND PREPARATION of the BETA-BLOCKER drug sotalol hydrochloride and the (THIAZIDE) DIURETIC drug hydrochlorothiazide. It can be used as an ANTIHYPERTENSIVE treatment for raised blood pressure and is available as tablets.

+▲ side-effects/warning: see HYDROCHLOROTHIAZIDE; SOTALOL HYDROCHLORIDE

Sparine

(Wyeth) is a proprietary, prescription-only preparation of the ANTIPSYCHOTIC drug promazine hydrochloride. It can be used to soothe agitated and restless patients, particularly elderly patients. It is available as tablets, a suspension and in a form for injection

+▲ side-effects/warning: see PROMAZINE HYDROCHLORIDE

spasmolytic

See ANTISPASMODIC

Spasmonal

(Norgine) is a proprietary, non-prescription preparation of the ANTISPASMODIC drug alverine citrate. It can be used to treat muscle spasm of the gastrointestinal tract and is available as capsules.

+▲ side-effects/warning: see ALVERINE CITRATE

specific immunoglobulin

is used to give immediate *passive immunity*. Protection is achieved by administering a blood component prepared in much the same way as NORMAL IMMUNOGLOBULIN (HNIG), except that the blood plasma pooled is from donors with high levels of the particular antibody that is required (eg. for hepatitis B, rabies, rubella, tetanus, or varicella-zoster). Administration is by injection.

✪ Related entries: anti-D (Rh₀) immunoglobulin; hepatitis B immuno-globulin (HBIG); rabies immuno-globulin; rubella immunoglobulin; tetanus immunoglobulin; varicella-zoster immunoglobulin (VZIG)

spectinomycin

is an ANTIBACTERIAL and ANTIBIOTIC drug. It is used almost exclusively to treat gonorrhoea caused by Gram-negative organisms resistant to penicillin, or in patients who are allergic to penicillin. It is an AMINOGLYCOSIDE-like antibiotic, in that it is related both in structure and by the way it works to that group of drugs. Administration is by deep intramuscular injection.

+ side-effects: there may be nausea and vomiting; high temperature and dizziness; urticaria (itchy skin rash); fever.

▲ warning: it is essential that both sexual partners undergo treatment even if only one shows symptoms. Administer with caution to patients who are pregnant or breast-feeding.

✪ Related entry: Trobicin

Spectraban Lotion

(Stiefel) is a proprietary, non-prescription SUNSCREEN lotion. It contains constituents that protect the skin from ultraviolet radiation, including padimate-O and aminobezoic acid, with UVB protection (SPF25). A patient whose skin condition requires this sort of protection may be prescribed it at the discretion of his or her doctor.

+▲ side-effects/warning: see AMINOBENZOIC ACID

Spectraban Ultra

(Stiefel) is a proprietary, non-prescription SUNSCREEN lotion. It conatins constituents that protect the skin from ultraviolet radiation, including padimate-O, aminobenzoic acid, oxybenzone and butylmethoxydibenzoyl, with both UVB (SPF28) and UVA protection (SPF 6). A patient whose skin condition requires this sort of protection may be prescribed it at

S the discretion of his or her doctor.

✚▲ side-effects/warning: see
AMINOBENZOIC ACID

*spermicidal contraceptive

drugs kill sperm and are intended to be used as an adjunct to barrier methods of contraceptive method is being used such as the condom (sheath) or diaphragm (Dutch cap), but should never be regarded as a sole means of contraception. Most spermicidal preparations consist of a spermicide, which is usually chemically an alcohol ester (eg. nonoxinol, octoxinol; p-di-isobutylphenoxypolyethoxyethanol), within a jelly liquid or cream base. Administration is topical in the form of vaginal inserts (pessaries), creams, gels, pastes, foams in aerosols and soluble films.

○ Related entries: C-Film; Delfen; Double Check; Duracreme; Duragel; Gynol II; Ortho-Creme; Ortho-Gynol; Orthoforms; Staycept

Spiro-Co

(Baker Norton) is a proprietary, prescription-only COMPOUND PREPARATION of the (aldosterone-antagonist and potassium-sparing) DIURETIC drug spironolactone and the (potassium-depleting, THIAZIDE) diuretic hydroflumethiazide (a combination called co-flumactone 25/25). It can be used in congestive HEART FAILURE TREATMENT and is available as tablets.

✚▲ side-effects/warning: see
HYDROFLUMETHIAZIDE; SPIRONOLACTONE

Spiro-Co 50

(Baker Norton) is a proprietary, prescription-only COMPOUND PREPARATION of the (aldosterone-antagonist and potassium-sparing) DIURETIC drug spironolactone and the (potassium-depleting, THIAZIDE) diuretic hydroflumethiazide

(a combination called co-flumactone 50/50). It can be used in congestive HEART FAILURE TREATMENT and is available as tablets.

✚▲ side-effects/warning: see
HYDROFLUMETHIAZIDE; SPIRONOLACTONE

Spiroctan

(Boehringer Mannheim) is a proprietary, prescription-only preparation of the (potassium-sparing and aldosterone-antagonist) DIURETIC drug spironolactone, which is often used in conjunction with other types of diuretics, such as the THIAZIDES. It can be used to treat oedema associated with aldosteronism, in congestive heart failure, kidney disease and fluid retention and ascites caused by cirrhosis of the liver. It is available as tablets and capsules.

✚▲ side-effects/warning: see
SPIRONOLACTONE

Spiroctan-M

(Boehringer Mannheim) is a proprietary, prescription-only preparation of the (aldosterone-antagonist) DIURETIC drug potassium canrenoate. It can be used to treat oedema associated with aldosteronism, heart disease and liver failure. It is available in a form for injection.

✚▲ side-effects/warning: POTASSIUM CANRENOATE

Spirolone

(Berk) is a proprietary, prescription-only preparation of the (aldosterone-antagonist and potassium-sparing) DIURETIC drug spironolactone, which is often used in conjunction with other types of diuretics, such as the THIAZIDES. It can be used to treat oedema associated with aldosteronism, congestive heart failure, kidney disease and fluid retention and ascites caused by cirrhosis of the liver. It is available as tablets.

✚▲ side-effects/warning: see
SPIRONOLACTONE

spironolactone

is a DIURETIC drug of the *aldosterone-antagonist* type. It is also *potassium-sparing* and so can be used in conjunction with other types of diuretic, such as the THIAZIDES, which cause loss of potassium, to obtain a more beneficial action. It can be used to treat oedema (accumulation of fluid in the tissues) associated with aldosteronism (abnormal production of aldosterone by the adrenal gland), in congestive HEART FAILURE TREATMENT, kidney disease and fluid retention and ascites caused by cirrhosis of the liver. Administration is oral in the form of tablets, capsules, or an oral suspension.
✚ side-effects: gastrointestinal disturbances, impotence and gynaecomastia (enlargements of breasts) in men; irregular periods in women; skin rashes, lethargy, raised blood potassium and lowered blood sodium levels; disturbances of liver, blood and bone function.
▲ warning: it should not be administered to patients with severe kidney failure; raised potassium or lowered sodium levels in the blood; who are pregnant or breast-feeding; or who have Addison's disease. Administer with caution to those with certain liver or kidney disorders (blood electrolytes should be monitored).
❍ Related entries: Aldactide 25; Aldactide 50; Aldactone; Laractone; Lasilactone; Spiro-Co; Spiro-Co 50; Spiroctan; Spirolone; Spirospare

Spirospare

(Ashbourne) is a proprietary, prescription-only preparation of the (*aldosterone-antagonist* and *potassium-sparing*) DIURETIC drug spironolactone, which is often used in conjunction with other types of diuretic, such as the THIAZIDES, that cause loss of potassium. It can be used in congestive HEART FAILURE TREATMENT, to treat oedema associated with aldosteronism, kidney disease and fluid retention and ascites caused by cirrhosis of the liver. It is available as tablets.
✚▲ side-effects/warning: see SPIRONOLACTONE

Sporanox

(Janssen) is a proprietary, prescription-only preparation of the ANTIFUNGAL drug itraconazole. It can be used to treat candidiasis infections of the vagina, vulva and oropharynx and ringworm infections of the skin. It is available as capsules.
✚▲ side-effects/warning: see ITRACONAZOLE

Sprilon

(Perstorp) is a proprietary, non-prescription COMPOUND PREPARATION of zinc oxide, the ANTIFOAMING AGENT dimethicone, wool fat, wool alcohol and paraffins. It can be used as a BARRIER CREAM to treat leg ulcers, bedsores, or applied to areas of the skin that require protection from urine or faeces (as in nappy rash or around a stoma – an outlet on the skin surface following the surgical curtailment of the intestines). It is available as an aerosol.
✚▲ side-effects/warning: DIMETHICONE; LIQUID PARAFFIN; WOOL ALCOHOL; WOOL FAT; ZINC OXIDE

squill linctus, opiate

is a non-prescription preparation that combines several soothing liquids, including tolu syrup, the (OPIOID) ANTITUSSIVE camphorated tincture of opium and anhydrous morphine, into a cough linctus (also known as *Gee's Linctus*).
✚▲ side-effect/warning: see under OPIOID

*SSRI

drugs are ANTIDEPRESSANT drugs that are used to relieve the symptoms of depressive illness (eg. FLUOXETINE and PAROXETINE). Like the MONOAMINE-OXIDASE INHIBITORS (MAOIs) and TRICYCLIC antidepressant drugs, the SSRI class is thought to work by modifying the actions of mood-modifying amine NEUROTRANSMITTERS in the brain. The abbreviation SSRI stands for *Selective*

S

Serotonin Re-uptake Inhibitor, because the mechanism of action is thought to be principally through inhibiting the amine-pump responsible for the re-uptake of the neurotransmitter 5-hydroxytryptamine (5-HT, SEROTONIN) into nerve endings within the brain. This recently developed class of drug seems to be effective in at least some patients and has the advantage of being less SEDATIVE than the tricyclics and with less ANTICHOLINERGIC side-effects such as effects on the heart. Treatment often takes some weeks before beneficial effects are achieved. Treatment should not begin immediately before or after other types of antidepressant have been taken. Withdrawal of treatment must be gradual. See under FLUOXETINE for principal actions and side-effects, though VENLAFAXINE also inhibits re-uptake of both serotonin and NORADRENALINE. See also FLUVOXAMINE MALEATE and SERTRALINE.

Stafoxil

(Yamanouchi) is a proprietary, prescription-only preparation of the ANTIBACTERIAL and (PENICILLIN) ANTIBIOTIC drug flucloxacillin. It can be used to treat bacterial infections, especially staphylococcal infections that prove to be resistant to penicillin. It is available as capsules.

✚▲ side-effects/warning: see FLUCLOXACILLIN

stanozolol

is an *anabolic* STEROID. It can be used to assist the metabolic synthesis of protein in the body and to treat hereditary angio-oedema. Administration is oral in the form of tablets.

✚▲ side-effects/warning: see under NANDROLONE; with headache, euphoria, dyspepsia, depression and cramp; there have been reports of hair loss and jaundice.

❂ Related entry: Stromba

Staril

(Squibb) is a proprietary, prescription-

only preparation of the ACE INHIBITOR fosinopril. It can be used as an ANTIHYPERTENSIVE treatment and is available as tablets.

✚▲ side-effects/warning: see FOSINOPRIL

Staycept

(Syntex) is a proprietary, non-prescription SPERMICIDAL CONTRACEPTIVE for use in combination with barrier methods of contraception (such as a condom). It is available as pessaries, which contain nonoxinol, or as a jelly containing octoxinol.

✚▲ side-effects/warning: see NONOXINOL; OCTOXINOL

STD

(STD Pharmaceutical) is a proprietary, prescription-only preparation of the drug sodium tetradecyl sulphate. It is used in scleropathy, which is a technique to treat varicose veins by the injection of an irritant solution. It is available in a form for injection.

✚▲ side-effects/warning: see SODIUM TETRADECYL SULPHATE

Stelazine

(SmithKline Beecham) is a proprietary, prescription-only preparation of the (PHENOTHIAZINE) ANTIPSYCHOTIC drug trifluoperazine. It can be used to treat and tranquillize psychotic patients (such as schizophrenics), particularly those experiencing behavioural disturbances. The drug can also be used in the short-term treatment of severe anxiety and as an ANTI-EMETIC and ANTINAUSEANT for nausea and vomiting caused by an underlying disease or by drug therapies. It is available as tablets, capsules (*Spansules*), a liquid and in a form for injection.

✚▲ side-effects/warning: see TRIFLUOPERAZINE

Stemetil

(Rhône-Poulenc Rorer) is a proprietary, prescription-only preparation of the

PHENOTHIAZINE DERIVATIVE drug prochlorperazine (as maleate or mesylate), which has many applications. In this preparation it is used as an ANTINAUSEANT to relieve the symptoms of nausea caused by cytotoxic drugs in the treatment of cancer and by the vertigo and loss of balance experienced due to infections of the inner and middle ear. It can also be used as an ANTIPSYCHOTIC for schizophrenia and other psychoses and for the short-term treatment of severe anxiety. It is available as tablets, effervescent granules, a syrup, suppositories and in a form for injection.

+▲ side-effects/warning: see PROCHLORPERAZINE.

sterculia

is a vegetable gum that can absorb large amounts of water and is used as a *bulking agent* LAXATIVE. It works by increasing the overall mass of faeces and so stimulating bowel movement, though the full effect may not be achieved for several hours. It is a useful alternative for patients who cannot tolerate bran in treating a range of bowel conditions, including diverticular disease and irritable bowel syndrome. More controversially, sterculia is also used to treat serious obesity with the intention that small amounts of food ingested may be bulked up internally, so making the patient feel full. Administration is oral in the form of granules to be taken with water.

+▲ side-effects/warning: see under ISPAGHULA HUSK

✪ Related entries: Alvercol; Normacol; Normacol Plus; Prefil

Steri-Neb Ipratropium

(Baker Norton) is a proprietary, prescription-only preparation of the ANTICHOLINERGIC and BRONCHODILATOR drug ipratropium bromide. It can be used to treat the symptoms of chronic bronchitis and is available as a nebulizer solution unit.

+▲ side-effects/warning: see IPRATROPIUM BROMIDE

Steri-Neb Salamol

(Baker Norton) is a proprietary, prescription-only preparation of the BETA-RECEPTOR STIMULANT salbutamol (as salbutamol sulphate). It can be used as a BRONCHODILATOR in reversible obstructive airways disease, as an ANTI-ASTHMATIC treatment in severe acute asthma and for the alleviation of symptoms of chronic bronchitis and emphysema. It is available as a nebulizer solution unit.

+▲ side-effects/warning: see SALBUTAMOL

Steripod Chlorhexidine

(Seton Healthcare) is a proprietary, non-prescription preparation of the ANTISEPTIC agent chlorhexidine (as gluconate). It can be used for swabbing and cleaning wounds and burns and is available as a solution.

+▲ side-effects/warning: see CHLORHEXIDINE

*steroids

are a class of naturally occurring and synthetic agents whose structure is based chemically on a steroid nucleus (a rather complex structure that consists of three, six-member rings and one, five-member ring). There are a number of important groups of chemicals in the body that are steroids, including all the CORTICOSTEROID HORMONES of the adrenal cortex (glucocorticoid or mineralocorticoids), all the SEX HORMONES (i.e. ANDROGENS, PROGESTOGENS and anabolic steroids), all VITAMINS of the VITAMIN D group (CALCIFEROL and analogues) and the bile acids (i.e. CHENODEOXYCHOLIC ACID and analogues). Synthetic chemical analogues of the majority of these have an important part in medicine.

Ster-Zac Bath Concentrate

(Hough) is a non-prescription preparation of the ANTISEPTIC agent

S

triclosan. It can be used for staphylococcal skin infections and is available as concentrates for adding to a bath.

+▲ side-effects/warning: see TRICLOSAN

Stesolid

(Dumex) is a proprietary, prescription-only preparation of the BENZODIAZEPINE drug diazepam. It can be used as an ANXIOLYTIC for the sort-term treatment of anxiety, as a HYPNOTIC to relieve insomnia, as an ANTICONVULSANT and ANTI-EPILEPTIC for status epilepticus, as a SEDATIVE in preoperative medication, as a SKELETAL MUSCLE RELAXANT and to assist in the treatment of alcohol withdrawal symptoms. It is available as a rectal solution.

+▲ side-effects/warning: see DIAZEPAM

Stiedex

(Stiefel) is a proprietary, prescription-only preparation of the CORTICOSTEROID and ANTI-INFLAMMATORY drug desoxymethasone. It can be used in the treatment of severe, acute inflammation and chronic skin disorders, including psoriasis. It is available as a cream and a lotion for topical application.

+▲ side-effects/warning: see DESOXYMETHASONE

Stiemycin

(Stiefel) is a proprietary, prescription-only preparation of the ANTIBACTERIAL and (MACROLIDE) ANTIBIOTIC drug erythromycin. It can be used to treat acne and is available as a solution for topical application.

+▲ side-effects/warning: see ERYTHROMYCIN

stilboestrol

(diethylstilbestrol) is a synthetic SEX HORMONE with OESTROGEN activity. It is useful in HRT (hormone replacement therapy) in women following the menopause. It is sometimes used in low dosage as an ANTICANCER treatment for cancer of the prostate gland in men and in post-menopausal women for breast cancer and vaginal atrophy. Administration can be oral in the form of tablets or as vaginal inserts (pessaries).

+ side-effects: nausea, thrombosis, fluid retention. In men, breast growth and impotence; in women, bleeding on withdrawal. There may be high blood calcium levels and bone pain when used for breast cancer.

▲ warning: it should not be administered to patients with certain cardiovascular or liver disorders.

✪ Related entries: Apstil; Tampovagan

Stilnoct

(Lorex) is a proprietary, non-prescription preparation of the recently introduced HYPNOTIC drug zolpidem tartrate. It can be used for the short-term treatment of insomnia and is available as tablets.

+▲ side-effects/warning: see ZOLPIDEM TARTRATE

*stimulant

drugs activate body systems or functions. In general, the term is used to describe drugs that stimulate the central nervous system. Therapeutically, they can be used to treat patients suffering from narcolepsy (extreme tendency to fall asleep when engaged in monotonous activities or when in quiet surroundings). There is a tendency for those who use stimulant drugs on a regular basis to become drug dependant and show a withdrawal syndrome when they stop taking the drug. Preparations of one of the most powerful and best-known stimulants DEXAMPHETAMINE SULPHATE are on the Controlled Drugs List. CAFFEINE and related compounds are mild stimulants and for medical purposes caffeine is incorporated into several proprietary COMPOUND ANALGESIC preparations that are used as cold remedies.

S

Streptase

(Hoechst) is a proprietary, prescription-only preparation of the FIBRINOLYTIC drug streptokinase. It can be used to treat thrombosis and embolism and is available in a form for injection.
+▲ side-effects/warning: see STREPTOKINASE

streptokinase

is an enzyme that is used therapeutically as an FIBRINOLYTIC drug, because it has the property of breaking up blood clots. It is used rapidly in serious conditions such as venous thrombi, pulmonary embolism and myocardial infarction. Administration is by injection or infusion.
+ side-effects: nausea, vomiting and bleeding. There may be allergic reaction such as a rash and a high temperature and also back pain.
▲ warning: it should not be administered to patients with disorders of coagulation; who are liable to bleed (vaginal bleeding, peptic ulceration, recent trauma, or surgery); acute pancreatitis, or oesophageal varices. Administer with care in those who are pregnant.
۞ Related entries: Kabikinase; Streptase

streptomycin

is an ANTIBACTERIAL and ANTIBIOTIC drug, which is an original member of the AMINOGLYCOSIDE family. In the UK today, it is used almost exclusively for the treatment of tuberculosis, in combination with other antibiotics. Treatment takes between 6 and 18 months. Administration is normally by injection.
+▲ side-effects/warning: see under GENTAMICIN; there may also be hypersensitivity reactions and loss of sensation in the mouth.

Stromba

(Sanofi Winthrop) is a proprietary, prescription-only preparation of the *anabolic* STEROID stanozolol. It can be used to treat angio-oedema and is available as tablets.
+▲ side-effects/warning: see STANOZOLOL

Stugeron

(Janssen) is a proprietary, non-prescription preparation of the ANTIHISTAMINE drug cinnarizine. It can be used as an ANTINAUSEANT to treat nausea and vomiting caused by the vertigo and loss of balance that is experienced in vestibular disease. It can also be used as a VASODILATOR to treat peripheral vascular disease (Raynaud's phenomenon). It is available as tablets.
+▲ side-effects/warning: see CINNARIZINE

Stugeron Forte

(Janssen) is a proprietary, non-prescription preparation of the ANTIHISTAMINE drug cinnarizine and can be used as an ANTINAUSEANT. It also has VASODILATOR properties that affect the blood vessels of the hands and feet and so may be used to improve the circulation in peripheral vascular disease (Raynaud's phenomenon). It is available as tablets.
+▲ side-effects/warning: see CINNARIZINE

Sublimaze

(Janssen) is a proprietary, prescription-only preparation of the (OPIOID) NARCOTIC ANALGESIC drug fentanyl (as hydrochloride) and is on the Controlled Drugs List. It can be used to treat moderate to severe pain, mainly during operations and to enhance the effect of a BARBITURATE general anaesthetic. It is available in a form for injection.
+▲ side-effects/warning: see FENTANYL

sucralfate

is a drug that is a complex of aluminium hydroxide and sulphated sucrose. It can be used as a long-term treatment of gastric and duodenal ulcers It has very little ANTACID action, but is thought to work as a CYTOPROTECTANT by forming a barrier over an ulcer, so protecting it from acid and the

S enzyme pepsin and allowing it to heal. Administration is oral in the form of tablets.

✚ side-effects: constipation, diarrhoea, nausea, indigestion, gastric discomfort, dry mouth, skin rash and itching, insomnia, dizziness, vertigo and drowsiness.

▲ warning: it should be administered with caution to patients with kidney disease, or who are pregnant or breast-feeding.

○ Related entry: Antepsin

Sudafed Elixir

(Wellcome) is a proprietary, non-prescription preparation of the SYMPATHOMIMETIC and DECONGESTANT drug pseudoephedrine hydrochloride. It can be used for the symptomatic relief of allergic and vasomotor rhinitis and colds and flu. It is available as a liquid and is not normally given to children under two years, except on medical advice.

✚▲ side-effects/warning: see PSEUDOEPHEDRINE HYDROCHLORIDE

Sudafed Expectorant

(Wellcome) is a proprietary non-prescription COMPOUND PREPARATION of the SYMPATHOMIMETIC and DECONGESTANT drug pseudoephedrine hydrochloride and the EXPECTORANT guaiphenesin. It can be used for the symptomatic relief of upper respiratory tract disorders accompanied by productive cough. It is available as a liquid and is not normally given to children under two years, except on medical advice.

✚▲ side-effects/warning: see GUAIPHENESIN; PSEUDOEPHEDRINE HYDROCHLORIDE

Sudafed Linctus

(Wellcome) is a proprietary, non-prescription COMPOUND PREPARATION of the SYMPATHOMIMETIC and DECONGESTANT drug pseudoephedrine hydrochloride and the (OPIOID) ANTITUSSIVE and NARCOTIC ANALGESIC drug dextromethorphan hydrobromide. It can be used for the symptomatic relief of dry coughs accompanied by congestion of the upper airways. It is available as a liquid and is not normally given to children under two years, except on medical advice.

✚▲ side-effects/warning: see DEXTROMETHORPHAN HYDROBROMIDE; PSEUDOEPHEDRINE HYDROCHLORIDE

Sudafed-Co Tablets

(Wellcome) is a proprietary, non-prescription COMPOUND PREPARATION of the SYMPATHOMIMETIC and DECONGESTANT drug pseudoephedrine hydrochloride and the NON-NARCOTIC ANALGESIC drug paracetamol. It can be used for the symptomatic relief of conditions where upper respiratory congestion is associated with raised body temperature or pain, including colds and flu. It is available as tablets and is not normally given to children under six years, except on medical advice.

✚▲ side-effects/warning: see PARACETAMOL; PSEUDOEPHEDRINE HYDROCHLORIDE

Sudafed Nasal Spray

(Wellcome) is a proprietary, non-prescription preparation of the SYMPATHOMIMETIC and VASOCONSTRICTOR drug oxymetazoline hydrochloride. It can be used as a NASAL DECONGESTANT for symptomatic relief of nasal congestion associated with a wide variety of upper respiratory tract disorders. It is available as a nasal spray and is not normally given to children under six years, except on medical advice.

✚▲ side-effects/warning: see OXYMETAZOLINE HYDROCHLORIDE

Sudafed Tablets

(Wellcome) is a proprietary, non-prescription preparation of the SYMPATHOMIMETIC and DECONGESTANT drug pseudoephedrine hydrochloride. It can be used for the symptomatic relief of allergic rhinitis, colds and flu. It is available as tablets and is not normally given to children under 12 years, except on

medical advice.
+▲ side-effects/warning: see
PSEUDOEPHEDRINE HYDROCHLORIDE

Sudocrem Antiseptic Cream

(Pharmax) is a proprietary, non-prescription COMPOUND PREPARATION of zinc oxide, benzyl alcohol, benzyl benzoate, hypoallergenic lanolin and various other minor constituents. It can be used as an EMOLLIENT and a BARRIER CREAM for nappy rash and incontinence dermatitis.
+▲ side-effects/warning: BENZYL BENZOATE; LANOLIN; ZINC OXIDE

sulconazole nitrate

is an (AZOLE) ANTIFUNGAL drug. It is used to treat skin infections, particularly those caused by tinea. Administration is by topical application in the form of a cream.
+▲ side-effects/warning: see under CLOTRIMAZOLE. Avoid contact with the eyes.
❂ Related entry: Exelderm

Suleo-C

(Napp) is a proprietary, non-prescription preparation of the PEDICULICIDAL drug carbaryl. It can be used to treat infestations of the scalp and pubic hair by lice (pediculosis). It is available as a lotion and a shampoo and is not normally used for children under six months, except on medical advice.
+▲ side-effects/warning: see CARBARYL

Suleo-M

(Napp) is a proprietary, non-prescription preparation of the SCABICIDAL and PEDICULICIDAL drug malathion. It can be used to treat infestations of the scalp and pubic hair by lice (pediculosis) and of the skin by itch-mites (scabies). It is available as a lotion and is not normally used for children under six months, except on medical advice.
+▲ side-effects/warning: see
MALATHION

sulfadiazine

See SULPHADIAZINE

sulfadoxine

is a long-acting (SULPHONAMIDE) ANTIBACTERIAL drug. It is used solely in combination with the ANTIMALARIAL drug PYRIMETHAMINE to prevent or treat malaria.
+▲ side-effects/warning: there may be serious side-effects; administer with caution to patients who are pregnant or breast-feeding.
❂ Related entry: Fansidar

sulfametopyrazine

is a long-acting (SULPHONAMIDE) ANTIBACTERIAL drug. It is used primarily in the treatment of chronic bronchitis and infections of the urinary tract. Administration is oral in the form of tablets.
+▲ side-effects/warning: see under CO-TRIMOXAZOLE
❂ Related entry: Kelfizine W

sulfasalazine

See SULPHASALAZINE

sulfinpyrazone

See SULPHINPYRAZONE

sulindac

is a (NSAID) NON-NARCOTIC ANALGESIC and ANTIRHEUMATIC drug. It is used to treat pain and inflammation in rheumatic disease and other musculoskeletal disorders. Administration is oral in the form of tablets.
+▲ side-effect/warning: see under NSAID. Administer with care to patients who have had kidney stones. An adequate fluid intake must be maintained.
❂ Related entry: Clinoril

sulphabenzamide

is a (SULPHONAMIDE) ANTIBACTERIAL drug. It is combined with two similar drugs, sulphacetamide and sulphathiazole, in a proprietary preparation that can be used

S

to treat bacterial infections of the vagina and the cervix and to prevent infection following gynaecological surgery. Administration is by topical application as vaginal tablets (pessaries) or a cream.
✚ side-effects: there may be sensitivity reactions.
▲ warning: it should not be used by patients with severe kidney damage, or who are pregnant.
◯ Related entry: Sultrin

sulphacetamide
is a (SULPHONAMIDE) ANTIBACTERIAL drug. It is combined with two similar drugs, sulphabenzamide and sulphathiazole, in a proprietary preparation that can be used to treat bacterial infections of the vagina and the cervix and to prevent infection following gynaecological surgery. Administration is by topical application as vaginal tablets (pessaries) or a cream.
✚ side-effects: there may be sensitivity reactions.
▲ warning: it should not be used by patients with severe kidney damage, or who are pregnant.
◯ Related entry: Sultrin

sulphadiazine
(sulfadiazine) is a (SULPHONAMIDE) ANTIBACTERIAL drug. It can be used to treat serious bacterial infections, particularly meningococcal meningitis and to prevent recurrence of rheumatic fever. Administration is either oral as tablets or by injection or infusion.
✚▲ side-effects/warning: see CO-TRIMOXAZOLE. It should not be administered to patients with severe kidney damage.

sulphadimethoxine
is a (SULPHONAMIDE) ANTIBACTERIAL drug. It can be used to treat the eye disorder trachoma, which is common in underdeveloped countries. Administration is oral in the form of tablets. It is not available in the UK.

sulphadimidine
is a (SULPHONAMIDE) ANTIBACTERIAL drug. It can be used to treat serious bacterial infections, particularly infections of the urinary tract and meningococcal meningitis. Administration is oral in the form of tablets.
✚▲ side-effects/warning: see under CO-TRIMOXAZOLE

sulpha drugs
See SULPHONAMIDES

sulphamethoxazole
is a (SULPHONAMIDE) ANTIBACTERIAL drug. It can be used, in combination with another antibacterial drug trimethoprim (a combination called co-trimoxazole), to treat a wide range of serious infections, especially of the urinary tract, the upper respiratory tract and prostate.
✚▲ side-effects/warning: see under CO-TRIMOXAZOLE
◯ Related entries: Bactrim; Chemotrim; Comixco; Comox; Fectrim; Laratrim; Septrin

sulphasalazine
(sulfasalazine) is an AMINOSALICYLATE drug, which combines within the one chemical a SULPHONAMIDE constituent (with ANTIBACTERIAL properties) and an aminosalicylate (5-aminosalicylic acid) component. It can be used to treat active Crohn's disease and to induce and maintain remission of the symptoms of ulcerative colitis. It is also sometimes used to treat rheumatoid arthritis. Administration can be oral as a suspension or tablets, or as suppositories or a retention enema.
✚ side-effects: nausea, vomiting and discomfort in the upper abdomen; rash, headache; rarely, fever, blood disorders and a number of other complaints.
▲ warning: it should not be administered to patients known to be sensitive to salicylates (aspirin-type drugs) or to sulphonamides; it should be administered with caution to those

with liver or kidney disease, G6PD deficient, or who are pregnant or breast-feeding.
○ Related entries: Salazopyrin; Salazopyrin EN-Tabs

sulphathiazole

is a (SULPHONAMIDE) ANTIBACTERIAL drug. It is combined with two similar drugs, sulphacetamide and sulphabenzamide, in a proprietary preparation that can be used to treat bacterial infections of the vagina and the cervix and to prevent infection following gynaecological surgery. Administration is by topical application as vaginal tablets (pessaries) or a cream.
✚ side-effects: there may be sensitivity reactions.
▲ warning: it should not be used by patients with severe kidney damage, or who are pregnant.
○ Related entry: Sultrin

sulphinpyrazone

(sulfinpyrazone) is a drug that is used to treat and prevent gout and renal hyperurea. It works by promoting the excretion of uric acid in the urine. Administration is oral in the form of tablets.
✚ side-effects: gastrointestinal disturbances, allergic skin reactions, salt and water retention, rarely blood disorders, ulceration and bleeding in the gastrointestinal tract, kidney failure and changes in liver function.
▲ warning: see under probenecid. Regular blood counts are advisable and avoid using in patients with NSAID hypersensitivity or heart disease.
○ Related entry: Anturan

*sulphonamides

(sulpha or sulfa drugs) are derivatives of a red dye called sulphanilamide and have the property of preventing the growth of bacteria. They were the first group of drugs suitable for ANTIMICROBIAL use as relatively safe ANTIBACTERIAL agents. Today, they, along with other similar synthetic classes of chemotherapeutic drugs, are commonly referred to as ANTIBIOTICS, although, strictly speaking, they are not *antibiotics* (in the literal sense of agents produced by, or obtained from, microorganisms, that inhibit the growth of, or destroy, other micro-organisms). Their antibacterial action stems from their chemical similarity to a compound required by bacteria to generate the essential growth factor, folic acid. This similarity inhibits the production of folic acid by bacteria (and therefore growth), while the human host is able to utilize folic acid in the diet. Most sulponamides are administered orally and are rapidly absorbed into the blood. They are short-acting and may have to be taken several times a day. Their quick progress through the body and excretion in the urine makes them particularly suited for the treatment of urinary infections. One or two sulphonamides are long-acting (and may be used to treat diseases such as malaria or leprosy) and another one or two are poorly absorbed (consequently, they were, until recently, used to treat intestinal infections). The best-known and most-used sulphonamides include SULPHADIAZINE, SULPHADIMIDINE and SULFAMETOPYRAZINE. Sulphonamides tend to cause side-effects, particularly nausea, vomiting, diarrhoea and headache, some of which (especially sensitivity reactions) may become serious. For instance, bone-marrow damage may result from prolonged treatment. Such serious hypersensitivity reactions are more of a risk with the longer-acting sulphonamides, which can accumulate in the body. As a general rule, patients being treated with sulphonamides should try to avoid sunlight. The sulphonamides are largely being replaced by newer antibacterials with greater activity, fewer problems with bacterial resistance and less risk of side-effects. See CO-TRIMOXAZOLE; SILVER SULPHADIAZINE; SULFADOXINE; SULPHADIMETHOXINE; SULPHAMETHOXAZOLE; SULPHONE.

S

sulphone

drugs are closely related to the SULPHONAMIDES. They have similar therapeutic action and are therefore used for similar purposes. They are particularly successful in preventing the growth of the bacteria responsible for leprosy, malaria and tuberculosis. The only member of this group that is still commonly used is the valuable drug DAPSONE.

sulphonylurea

drugs are derived from a sulphonamide and have the effect of reducing blood levels of glucose, so they can be used in DIABETIC TREATMENT. They work by promoting the secretion of INSULIN from the pancreas and are thus useful in treating the form of hyperglycaemia that occurs in Type II diabetes (non-insulin-dependent diabetes mellitus; NIDDM; maturity-onset diabetes) where there is still some insulin production. They should be used in conjunction with a modified diet.
See: CHLORPROPAMIDE; GLIBENCLAMIDE; GLICLAZIDE; GLIPIZIDE; GLIQUIDONE; TOLAZAMIDE; TOLBUTAMIDE.

sulphur

is a non-metallic element, which was thought to be active against external parasites and fungal infections of the skin, but this would now appear to have little scientific basis. Consequently, sulphur now has a less common use in creams, ointments and lotions for treating skin disorders such as acne, dermatitis and psoriasis.
○ **Related entries: Cocois; Eskamel; Pragnatar**

sulpiride

is an ANTIPSYCHOTIC drug, which is used to treat the symptoms of schizophrenia (to increase an apathetic and withdrawn patient's awareness) and, quite separately from its antipsychotic uses, disorders that may cause tremor, tics, involuntary

movements, or involuntary utterances (such as Gilles de la Tourette syndrome). Administration is oral in the form of tablets.
✚▲ side-effects/warning: see under CHLORPROMAZINE HYDROCHLORIDE; but is less sedating and does not cause jaundice or skin reactions. Administer with care to patients with porphyria and avoid its use in those who are breast-feeding.
○ **Related entries: Dolmatil; Sulpitil**

Sulpitil

(Pharmacia) is a proprietary, prescription-only preparation of the ANTIPSYCHOTIC drug sulpiride. It can be used, at a low dose, to treat the symptoms of schizophrenia (to increase an apathetic and withdrawn patient's awareness) and at a higher dose and quite separately from its antipsychotic uses, to treat other conditions that may cause tremor, tics, involuntary movements, or involuntary utterances (such as Gilles de la Tourette syndrome). It is available as tablets.
✚▲ side-effects/warning: see SULPIRIDE

Sultrin

(Cilag) is a proprietary, prescription-only COMPOUND PREPARATION of the (SULPHONAMIDE) ANTIBACTERIAL drugs sulphacetamide, sulphabenzamide and sulphathiazole. It can be used to treat bacterial infections of the vagina and the cervix and to prevent infection following gynaecological surgery. It is available as vaginal tablets (pessaries) and a cream.
✚▲ side-effects/warning: see SULPHACETAMIDE; SULPHABENZAMIDE; SULPHATHIAZOLE

sumatriptan

is a recently introduced ANTIMIGRAINE drug, which is used to treat acute migraine attacks (but not to prevent attacks) and cluster headache. It works by producing a rapid constriction of blood vessels surrounding the brain (by stimulating SEROTONIN receptors). Administration is

either oral as tablets or by self-injection.
✛ side-effects: chest pain and tightness in the chest (sometimes intense, angina-like pain), sensation of tingling, heaviness, pressure, heat, flushing, dizziness, a feeling of weakness, loss of sensation in the extremities, drowsiness and fatigue, changes in liver function, reports of nausea and vomiting, also transient pain at the injection site.
▲ warning: it should not be given to the elderly or children, or to patients with ischaemic heart disease or a history of heart attack, coronary vasospasm, certain types of angina, or uncontrolled hypertension. Administer with care to patients with conditions predisposing to coronary heart disease, liver or kidney impairment, or who are pregnant or breast-feeding. Drowsiness may impair the performance of skilled tasks such as driving.
❍ Related entry: Imigran

Sun E45

(Crookes Healthcare) is the name of a range of proprietary, non-prescription SUNSCREEN lotions. They contain titanium dioxide, aminobenzoic acid, padimate-O, oxybenzone and butylmethoxydibenzoyl, which provide protection from ultraviolet radiation (factors 15-25; but with both UVA and UVB protection). *Sun E45* is available as *Sunblock Cream (SPF25)* and *Ultra Protection Lotion (SPF15)* and both are water resistant. A patient whose skin condition requires this sort of preparation may be prescribed it at the discretion of his or her doctor.
✛▲ side-effect/warning: see AMINOBENZOIC ACID; TITANIUM DIOXIDE

*sunscreen

preparations are creams and lotions that contain chemical agents which partly block the passage of ultraviolet radiation from the sun and in certain radiation therapies to the skin. Ultraviolet radiation harms the skin and exacerbates many skin conditions. It can be divided into two wavelength bands: UVB causes sunburn and contributes to skin cancer and aging; UVA causes problems by sensitizing the skin to certain drugs and, in the long term, may contribute to skin cancers. A number of substances offer protection against UVB, but are less effective against UVA. Some preparations also contain substances, such as TITANIUM DIOXIDE, which are reflective and provide some protection against UVA. The sun protection factor, or SPF, of a preparation indicates the degree of protection against burning by UVB. For example, an SPF of 4 allows a person to stay in the sun four-times longer than an unprotected person without burning. A star-rating system is used by some sunscreens to indicate the degree of protection against UVA relative to UVB. For example, a rating of 4 stars means equal protection against UVA and UVB; lower ratings mean greater protection against UVB than UVA. Sunscreens with an SPF greater than 15 may be prescribed for patients whose skin condition require this sort of preparation (eg. those abnormally sensitive to UV radiation due to genetic disorders, or to radiotherapy, or those with recurrent or chronic herpes simplex labialis).
❍ Related entries: Coppertone Ultrashade 23; Piz Buin SPF 20 Sun Block Lotion; RoC Total Sunblock Cream; Spectraban Lotion; Spectraban Ultra; Sun E45; Uvistat

Suprane

(Pharmacia) is a proprietary, prescription-only preparation of the inhalant GENERAL ANAESTHETIC drug desflurane. It can be used for the induction and maintenance of anaesthesia and is available in a form for inhalation.
✛▲ side-effects/warning: see DESFLURANE

Suprax

(Lederle) is a proprietary, prescription-only preparation of the ANTIBACTERIAL and (CEPHALOSPORIN) ANTIBIOTIC drug cefixime. It can be used to treat acute

S

bacterial infections by Gram-positive and Gram-negative organisms, particularly infections of the urinary tract. It is available as capsules, tablets and a paediatric oral suspension.
✚▲ side-effects/warning: see CEFIXIME

Suprecur

(Hoechst) is a proprietary, prescription-only preparation of the HORMONE buserelin, which is a form of gonadotrophin-releasing hormone. It can be used in women to treat endometriosis and in men as an ANTICANCER treatment for cancer of the prostate gland. It is available as a nasal spray.
✚▲ side-effects/warning: see BUSERELIN

Suprefact

(Hoechst) is a proprietary, prescription-only preparation of the HORMONE buserelin, which is a form of gonadotrophin-releasing hormone. It can be used in men as an ANTICANCER treatment for cancer of the prostate gland and in women for endometriosis. It is available as a nasal spray and in a form for injection.
✚▲ side-effects/warning: see BUSERELIN

Surgam

(Roussel) is a proprietary, prescription-only preparation of the (NSAID) NON-NARCOTIC ANALGESIC and ANTIRHEUMATIC drug tiaprofenic acid. It can be used to treat the pain of rheumatic disease and other musculoskeletal disorders. It is available as tablets and modified-release capsules (*Surgam SA*).
✚▲ side-effects/warning: see TIAPROFENIC ACID

Surmontil

(Rhône-Poulenc Rorer) is a proprietary, prescription-only preparation of the (TRICYCLIC) ANTIDEPRESSANT drug trimipramine. It can be used to treat depressive illness, especially in cases where there is a need for sedation. It is

available as tablets and as capsules (in the form of trimipramine maleate).
✚▲ side-effects/warning: see TRIMIPRAMINE

Suscard

(Pharmax) is a proprietary, non-prescription preparation of the VASODILATOR and ANTI-ANGINA drug glyceryl trinitrate. It can be used in HEART FAILURE TREATMENT and to treat and prevent angina pectoris. It is available as modified-release buccal tablets (which dissolve between the upper lip and gums).
✚▲ side-effects/warning: see GLYCERYL TRINITRATE

Sustac

(Pharmax) is a proprietary, non-prescription preparation of the VASODILATOR and ANTI-ANGINA drug glyceryl trinitrate. It can be used to treat and prevent angina pectoris and is available as modified-release tablets.
✚▲ side-effects/warning: see GLYCERYL TRINITRATE

Sustamycin

(Boehringer Mannheim) is a proprietary, prescription-only preparation of the ANTIBACTERIAL and (TETRACYCLINE) ANTIBIOTIC drug tetracycline. It can be used to treat infections of many kinds and is available as modified-release capsules.
✚▲ side-effects/warning: see TETRACYCLINE

Sustenon 100

(Organon) is a proprietary, prescription-only preparation of the ANDROGEN (male SEX HORMONE) testosterone (as propionate, isocaproate and phenylpropionate). It can be used to treat testosterone deficiency in men and is available in a form for long-lasting depot injection.
✚▲ side-effects/warning: see TESTOSTERONE

Sustenon 250

(Organon) is a proprietary, prescription-only preparation of the ANDROGEN (male

SEX HORMONE) testosterone (as propionate and phenylpropionate). It can be used to treat testosterone deficiency in men and is available in a form for depot (long-lasting) injection.

+▲ side-effects/warning: see TESTOSTERONE

suxamethonium chloride

is a *depolarizing* SKELETAL MUSCLE RELAXANT drug. It is used to induce muscle paralysis during surgery and is administered by injection.

+ side-effects: there may be muscle pain afterwards and repeated doses may cause prolonged muscle paralysis.

▲ warning: it should not be administered to patients with severe liver disease or severe burns. Prolonged paralysis occurs infrequently where there is abnormal plasma cholinesterases and under certain other circumstances.

۞ Related entries: Anectine; Scoline

Symmetrel

(Geigy) is a proprietary, prescription-only preparation of the ANTIPARKINSONISM drug amantadine hydrochloride, which also has some ANTIVIRAL activity. It is used to treat parkinsonism, but not the parkinsonian symptoms induced by drugs. It can also be used to prevent certain types of influenza and to treat herpes zoster (shingles). It is available as capsules and as a syrup.

+▲ side-effects/warning: see AMANTADINE HYDROCHLORIDE

*sympathomimetics

are drugs that have effects that mimic those of the sympathetic nervous system. There are two main types (though several sympathomimetics belong to both types): the alpha-adrenoceptor stimulants (eg. PHENYLEPHRINE HYDROCHLORIDE and OXYMETAZOLINE HYDROCHLORIDE) are VASOCONSTRICTORS and are used particularly in NASAL DECONGESTANTS and preparations for relieving cold symtpoms; the other type is the BETA-RECEPTOR STIMULANTS (eg. salbutamol,

ORCIPRENALINE SULPHATE and TERBUTALINE SULPHATE) which are widely used as BRONCHODILATORS, particularly in ANTI-ASTHMATIC treatment and also as CARDIAC STIMULANTS (eg. ISOPRENALINE. A distinction may be made between the *direct sympathomimetics* such as those examples given above, which achieve selectivity of action within the body by only acting at one receptor (recognition site for HORMONES or NEUROTRANSMITTERS) type, as compared to the *indirect sympathomimetics* (eg. EPHEDRINE HYDROCHLORIDE and PSEUDOEPHEDRINE HYDROCHLORIDE) that work by releasing noradrenaline and adrenaline from nerves of the sympathetic nervous system and adrenal medulla and consequently show no selectivity of action, which therapeutically is a disadvantage.

See: ADRENALINE; DOBUTAMINE HYDROCHLORIDE; DOPAMINE; FENOTEROL HYDROCHLORIDE; METARAMINOL; METHOXAMINE HYDROCHLORIDE; NORADRENALINE; PIRBUTEROL; REPROTEROL HYDROCHLORIDE; RIMITEROL HYDROCHLORIDE; SALBUTAMOL

Synacthen

(Ciba) is a proprietary, prescription-only preparation of tetracosactrin, which is an analogue of the pituitary HORMONE CORTICOTROPHIN (ACTH) that stimulates the adrenal gland to produce corticosteroid hormones. It may be therapeutically useful to stimulate the adrenal gland when it is suppressed by chronic corticosteroid administration, however, the primary use of this drug is to test adrenal gland function. It is available in a form for injection.

+▲ side-effects/warning: see TETRACOSACTRIN

Synacthen Depot

(Ciba) is a proprietary, prescription-only preparation of tetracosactrin (and a zinc complex), which is an analogue of the pituitary HORMONE CORTICOTROPHIN

(ACTH) that stimulates the adrenal gland to produce corticosteroid hormones. It may be therapeutically useful to stimulate the adrenal gland when it is suppressed by chronic corticosteroid administration, however, the primary use of this drug is to test adrenal gland function. It is available in a form for injection.

+▲ side-effects/warning: see TETRACOSACTRIN

Synalar

(Zeneca) is a proprietary, prescription-only preparation of the CORTICOSTEROID and ANTI-INFLAMMATORY drug fluocinolone acetonide. It can be used to treat severe, acute inflammatory skin disorders such as eczema and psoriasis. It is available as a cream, gel, or ointment in three strengths, *Synalar*, *Synalar 1 in 4 Dilution* and *Synalar 1 in 10 Dilution*.

+▲ side-effects/warning: see FLUOCINOLONE ACETONIDE

Synalar C

(Zeneca) is a proprietary, prescription-only COMPOUND PREPARATION of the CORTICOSTEROID and ANTI-INFLAMMATORY drug fluocinolone acetonide and the ANTIMICROBIAL drug clioquinol. It can be used to treat skin infections with inflammation and is available as an ointment and a cream for topical application.

+▲ side-effects/warning: see CLIOQUINOL; FLUOCINOLONE ACETONIDE

Synalar N

(Zeneca) is a proprietary, prescription-only COMPOUND PREPARATION of the CORTICOSTEROID and ANTI-INFLAMMATORY drug fluocinolone acetonide and the ANTIBACTERIAL and (AMINOGLYCOSIDE) ANTIBIOTIC drug neomycin sulphate. It can be used to treat skin infections with inflammation and is available as an ointment and a cream for topical application.

+▲ side-effects/warning: see FLUOCINOLONE ACETONIDE; NEOMYCIN SULPHATE

Synarel

(Syntex) is a proprietary, prescription-only preparation of nafarelin, which is an analogue of the hypothalamic HORMONE GONADORELIN (gonadothrophin-releasing hormone; GnRH). It can be used to treat endometriosis and is available as a nasal spray.

+▲ side-effects/warning: see NAFARELIN

Syndol

(Marion Merrell Dow) is a proprietary, non-prescription COMPOUND PREPARATION of the NON-NARCOTIC ANALGESIC drug paracetamol, the (OPIOID) NARCOTIC ANALGESIC drug codeine phosphate, the ANTIHISTAMINE drug doxylamine succinate and the STIMULANT caffeine. It can be used to treat mild to moderate pain, including tension headache, toothache, period pain, muscle pain, neuralgia and pain following surgery. It is available as tablets and is not normally given to children, except on medical advice.

+▲ side-effects/warning: see CAFFEINE; CODEINE PHOSPHATE; DOXYLAMINE SUCCINATE; PARACETAMOL

Synflex

(Syntex) is a proprietary, prescription-only preparation of the (NSAID) NON-NARCOTIC ANALGESIC and ANTIRHEUMATIC drug naproxen (as sodium). It can be used to relieve pain and inflammation, particularly rheumatic and arthritic pain and also of acute gout, other musculoskeletal disorders and period pain. It is available as tablets.

+▲ side-effects/warning: see NAPROXEN

Synkavit

(Cambridge) is a proprietary, non-prescription preparation of menadiol sodium phosphate (VITAMIN K_3). It can be used to treat certain types of vitamin K deficiency and is available as tablets.

+▲ warning/side-effects: see MENADIOL SODIUM PHOSPHATE

Synphase

(Syntex) is a proprietary, prescription-only COMPOUND PREPARATION that can be used as a (*triphasic*) ORAL CONTRACEPTIVE (and also for certain menstrual problems) of the type that combines an OESTROGEN and a PROGESTOGEN, in this case ethinyloestradiol and norethisterone. It is available in the form of tablets in a calendar pack.
+▲ side-effects/warning: see ETHINYLOESTRADIOL; NORETHISTERONE

Syntaris

(Syntex) is a proprietary, prescription-only preparation of the CORTICOSTEROID drug flunisolide. It can be used to treat nasal allergy (such as hay fever) and is available as a nasal spray.
+▲ side-effects/warning: see FLUNISOLIDE

Syntex Menophase

(Syntex) is a proprietary, prescription-only COMPOUND PREPARATION of the female SEX HORMONES mestranol (an OESTROGEN) and norethisterone (a PROGESTOGEN). It can be used in HRT and is available in the form of tablets in a calendar pack.
+▲ side-effects/warning: see MESTRANOL; NORETHISTERONE

Syntocinon

(Sandoz) is a proprietary, prescription-only preparation of the natural PITUITARY HORMONE oxytocin, which causes increased contraction of the uterus during labour and stimulates lactation. It can be administered therapeutically to induce or assist labour and, in conjunction with ergometrine maleate (*Syntometrine*), to control bleeding following incomplete abortion and to aid delivery of the placenta under medical supervision. It is available in a form for injection or infusion.
+▲ side-effects/warning: see OXYTOCIN

Syntometrine

(Sandoz) is a proprietary, prescription-only COMPOUND PREPARATION of the ALKALOID ergometrine maleate and the natural HORMONE oxytocin. It can be usd to assist the third and final stage of labour (delivery of the placenta) and to control postnatal bleeding following incomplete abortion. It is available in a form for injection.
+▲ side-effects/warning: see ERGOMETRINE MALEATE; OXYTOCIN

Syntopressin

(Sandoz) is a proprietary, prescription-only preparation of lypressin, which is an analogue of the pituitary HORMONE vasopressin (antidiuretic hormone, ADH). It may be used as a pituitary-originated DIABETES INSIPIDUS TREATMENT and is available as a nasal spray.
+▲ side-effects/warning: see LYPRESSIN

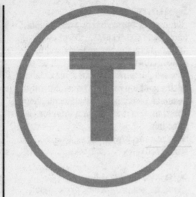

T

T/Gel

(Neutrogena) is a proprietary, non-prescription preparation of coal tar. It can be used to treat skin conditions such as dandruff and psoriasis of the scalp and is available as a shampoo.

✚▲ side-effects/warning: see COAL TAR

tacrolimus

is an IMMUNOSUPPRESSANT drug (a MACROLIDE ANTIBIOTIC) that is used paticularly to limit tissue rejection during and following organ transplant surgery (particularly of liver or kidney). Administration is either oral or by intravenous infusion.

✚▲ side-effects/warning: see under CYCLOSPORIN: do not use if sensitive to macrolide antibiotics, or pregnant or breast-feeding. Monitor body function.

✺ **Related entry: Prograf**

Tagamet

(SmithKline Beecham) is a proprietary preparation of the H$_2$-ANTAGONIST and ULCER-HEALING DRUG cimetidine. It is available on prescription or without a prescription in a limited amount and for short-term uses only. It can be used to treat benign peptic ulcers (in the stomach or duodenum), gastro-oesophageal reflux, dyspepsia and associated conditions. It is available as tablets, effervescent tablets, a syrup and in a form for injection or infusion.

✚▲ side-effects/warning: see CIMETIDINE

Tambocor

(3M Health Care) is a proprietary, prescription-only preparation of the ANTI-ARRHYTHMIC drug flecainide acetate. It can be used to treat heartbeat irregularities and is available as tablets and in a form for injection.

✚▲ side-effects/warning: see FLECAINIDE ACETATE

Tamofen

(Pharmacia) is a proprietary,

prescription-only preparation of the sex HORMONE ANTAGONIST drug tamoxifen. It inhibits the effect of OESTROGENS and because of this is used primarily as an ANTICANCER drug for cancers that depend on the presence of oestrogen in women, particularly breast cancer. It may also be used to treat certain conditions of infertility. It is available as tablets.

+▲ side-effects/warning: see TAMOXIFEN

tamoxifen

is a sex HORMONE ANTAGONIST, an ANTI-OESTROGEN. It antagonizes the natural oestrogen present in the body and can be useful in treating infertility in women whose condition is linked to the persistent presence of oestrogens and a consequent failure to ovulate. A second and major use, is as an ANTICANCER drug in the treatment of existing oestrogen-dependent breast cancer (both in pre- and post-menopausal women). A related, but still experimental, use is as a prophylactic (preventive) treatment in women considered to be at risk of developing breast cancer. Administration is oral in the form of tablets.

+ side-effects: hot flushes, vaginal bleeding or discharge, suppression of menstruation, itching vulva, gastrointestinal upsets, oedema, hair loss, blood disturbances (fall in platelet count and porphyria), visual disturbances and liver dysfunction. Some patients with breast cancer may experience pain.

▲ warning: it should not be administered to patients who are pregnant or breast-feeding. There may be swelling within the ovaries, raised blood calcium (associated with bone cancer), or adverse changes in the endometrial lining of the uterus.

✪ Related entries: Emblon; Noltam; Nolvadex; Oestrifen; Tamofen

Tampovagan

(Norgine) is a proprietary, prescription-only preparation of a form of stilboestrol, which is a SEX HORMONE analogue with OESTROGEN activity. It can be used to treat conditions of the vagina caused by hormonal deficiency (generally atrophic vaginitis in the menopause). It is available as vaginal inserts (pessaries).

+▲ side-effects/warning: see STILBOESTROL

Tancolin

(Roche) is a proprietary, non-prescription preparation of the (OPIOID) ANTITUSSIVE and NARCOTIC ANALGESIC drug dextromethorphan hydrobromide and vitamin C. It can be used for the symptomatic relief of coughs, particularly those associated with infection in the upper respiratory tract. It is available as a liquid and is not to be given to children under six months.

+▲ side-effects/warning: see DEXTROMETHORPHAN HYDROBROMIDE

Tarcortin

(Stafford-Miller) is a proprietary, prescription-only COMPOUND PREPARATION of the CORTICOSTEROID drug hydrocortisone and coal tar. It can be used to treat eczema and psoriasis and is available as a cream for topical application.

+▲ side-effects/warning: see COAL TAR; HYDROCORTISONE

Targocid

(Merrell) is a proprietary, prescription-only preparation of the ANTIBACTERIAL and ANTIBIOTIC drug teicoplanin. It can be used for serious infections such as endocarditis, dialysis-associated peritonitis and infections due to *Staphylococcus aureus*. It is available in a form for injection.

+▲ side-effects/warning: see TEICOPLANIN

Tarivid

(Hoechst, Roussel) is a proprietary, prescription-only preparation of the ANTIBACTERIAL and (QUINOLONE) ANTIBIOTIC drug ofloxacin. It can be used to treat infections, particularly complicated infections of the urinary tract,

T cervical infections, septicaemia and gonorrhoea. It is available as tablets and in a form for intravenous infusion.
+▲ side-effects/warning: see OFLOXACIN

Tavegil

(Sandoz) is a proprietary, non-prescription preparation of the ANTIHISTAMINE drug clemastine (as hydrogen fumarate). It can be used to treat the symptoms of allergic disorders such as hay fever and urticaria. It is available as tablets and a liquid.
+▲ side-effects/warning: see CLEMASTINE

Taxol

(Bristol-Myers; Squibb) is a proprietary, prescription-only preparation of the (CYTOTOXIC) ANTICANCER drug paclitaxel. It can be used to treat ovarian cancer and is available in a form for intravenous infusion.
+▲ side-effects/warning: see PACLITAXEL

Tazocin

(Lederle) is a proprietary, prescription-only COMPOUND PREPARATION of the broad-spectrum ANTIBACTERIAL and (PENICILLIN) ANTIBIOTIC drug piperacillin and the ENZYME INHIBITOR tazobactam, which, by preventing degradation by bacterium-derived beta-lactamase, confers *penicillinase-resistance* to the antibiotic. It can be used to treat many serious or compound forms of bacterial infection including skin infections, septicaemia and of the respiratory and urinary tracts, particularly infections caused by *Pseudomonas aeruginosa*. It is available in a form for injection or infusion.
+▲ side-effects/warning: see PIPERACILLIN

TCP Antiseptic Throat Pastilles (Blackcurrant Flavour)

(Charwell) is a proprietary, non-prescription preparation of TCP liquid antiseptic, which contains the ANTISEPTIC agent phenol (with halogenated phenols).

It can be used for the relief of minor sore throats.
+▲ side-effects/warning: see PHENOL

TCP Liquid Antiseptic

(Charwell) is a proprietary, non-prescription preparation of the ANTISEPTIC agent phenol (with halogenated phenols). It can be used for the symptomatic relief of sore throat including those associated with colds and flu. It is available as a solution for use as a gargle.
+▲ side-effects/warning: see PHENOL

Tears Naturale

(Alcon) is a proprietary, non-prescription preparation of hypromellose (with dextran '70'). It can be used as artificial tears for tear deficiency and is available as eye-drops.
+▲ side-effects/warning: see HYPROMELLOSE

Teejel Gel

(Seton Healthcare) is a proprietary, non-prescription COMPOUND PREPARATION of the ANTISEPTIC agent cetalkonium chloride and choline salicylate, which is a COUNTER-IRRITANT, or RUBEFACIENT. It can be applied to the mouth for the symptomatic relief of pain from mouth ulcers, cold sores, denture irritation, inflammation of the tongue and teething in infants. It is not normally given to children under four months, except on medical advice.
+▲ side-effects/warning: see CHOLINE SALICYLATE

Tegretol

(Geigy) is a proprietary, prescription-only preparation of the ANTICONVULSANT and ANTI-EPILEPTIC drug carbamazepine. It can be used in the preventive treatment of most forms of epilepsy (except absence seizures), for trigeminal neuralgia, in the treatment of diabetes insipidus and in the management of manic-depressive illness. It is available as tablets, chewable tablets,

a liquid, suppositories and as modified-release tablets called *Tegretol Retard*.
+▲ side-effects/warning: see
CARBAMAZEPINE

teicoplanin

is an ANTIBACTERIAL and ANTIBIOTIC drug, which is one of the glycopeptide family and is similar to VANCOMYCIN, but with a longer duration of action so it can be taken only once a day. It has activity primarily against Gram-positive bacteria and works by inhibiting the synthesis of components of the bacterial cell wall. It can be used in the treatment of serious infections, including endocarditis, dialysis-associated peritonitis, severe burns and for infections caused by *Staphylococcus aureus*. Administration is by injection or infusion.
+ side-effects: there may be diarrhoea, nausea and vomiting, headache; severe allergic reactions, bronchospasm, fever and rash; blood disorders; ringing in the ears and mild loss of hearing; local reactions at the injection site; loss of balance has been reported.
▲ warning: tests on liver and kidney function are required, also blood counts and hearing tests. Administer with caution to patients who are elderly, pregnant, or breast-feeding. Its use may have deleterious effects on the organs of the ear, on the kidney and liver; blood concentrations of the drug in the blood, along with liver and kidney function, should be monitored during treatment.
✪ Related entry: Targocid

temazepam

is a BENZODIAZEPINE drug, which is used as a relatively short-acting HYPNOTIC for the short-term treatment of insomnia and as a preoperative medication.
Administration is oral as gel-filled capsules (which come in several forms, eg. *Temazepam Gelthix*), an oral solution, or as tablets.
+▲ side-effects/warning: see under
BENZODIAZEPINE

Temgesic

(Reckitt & Colman) is a proprietary, prescription-only preparation of the (OPIOID) NARCOTIC ANALGESIC drug buprenorphine (as hydrochloride) and is on the Controlled Drugs List. It can be used to treat all forms of pain and is available as sublingual tablets (to be retained under the tongue) and in a form for injection.
+▲ side-effects/warning: see
BUPRENORPHINE

temocillin

is a new ANTIBACTERIAL and (PENICILLIN) ANTIBIOTIC drug. It is used primarily to treat forms of infection that other penicillins are incapable of countering, due to the production of the enzyme penicillinase by the bacteria concerned. However, temocillin is not inactivated by the penicillinase enzymes produced, for example, by certain Gram-negative bacteria (but not *Pseudomonas aeruginosa*), however, it is not active against Gram-positive bacteria, such as in infections of the urinary tract. It is therefore classed as a *penicillinase-resistant* penicillin. Administration is either oral in the form of capsules or by injection.
+▲ side-effects/warning: see under
BENZYLPENICILLIN
✪ Related entry: Temopen

Temopen

(Bencard) is a proprietary, prescription-only preparation of the ANTIBACTERIAL and (PENICILLIN) ANTIBIOTIC drug temocillin. It can be used to treat bacterial infections, especially certain Gram-negative bacterial infections that prove to be resistant to penicillin, but is not active against Gram-positive bacteria. It is available in a form for injection.
+▲ side-effects/warning: see TEMOCILLIN

Tenchlor

(Berk) is a proprietary, prescription-only

T

T

COMPOUND PREPARATION of the BETA-BLOCKER drug atenolol and the DIURETIC drug chlorthalidone (a combination called co-tenidone). It can be used as an ANTIHYPERTENSIVE treatment for raised blood pressure and is available as tablets.
+▲ side-effects/warning: see ATENOLOL; CHLORTHALIDONE

Tenif

(Stuart) is a proprietary, prescription-only COMPOUND PREPARATION of the BETA-BLOCKER drug atenolol and the CALCIUM-CHANNEL BLOCKER nifedipine. It can be used as an ANTIHYPERTENSIVE treatment for raised blood pressure and is available as capsules.
+▲ side-effects/warning: see ATENOLOL; NIFEDIPINE

Tenoret 50

(Stuart) is a proprietary, prescription-only COMPOUND PREPARATION of the BETA-BLOCKER drug atenolol and the DIURETIC drug chlorthalidone. It can be used as an ANTIHYPERTENSIVE treatment for raised blood pressure and is available as tablets.
+▲ side-effects/warning: see ATENOLOL; CHLORTHALIDONE

Tenoretic

(Stuart) is a proprietary, prescription-only COMPOUND PREPARATION of the BETA-BLOCKER drug atenolol and the DIURETIC drug chlorthalidone. It can be used as an ANTIHYPERTENSIVE treatment for raised blood pressure and is available as tablets.
+▲ side-effects/warning: see ATENOLOL CHLORTHALIDONE

Tenormin

(Stuart) is a proprietary, prescription-only preparation of the BETA-BLOCKER drug atenolol. It can be used as an ANTIHYPERTENSIVE treatment for raised blood pressure, as an ANTI-ANGINA treatment to relieve symptoms and improve exercise tolerance and as an ANTI-ARRHYTHMIC to regularize heartbeat

and to treat myocardial infarction. It is available as tablets, a syrup and in a form for injection.
+▲ side-effects/warning: see ATENOLOL

tenoxicam

is a (NSAID) NON-NARCOTIC ANALGESIC and ANTIRHEUMATIC drug. It has a long duration of action and is used to treat pain and inflammation in rheumatic disease and other musculoskeletal disorders. Administration is either oral in the form of tablets or by intramuscular or intravenous injection.
+▲ side-effect/warning: see under NSAID.
✪ Related entry: Clinoril

Tensium

(DDSA Pharmaceuticals) is a proprietary, prescription-only preparation of the BENZODIAZEPINE drug diazepam. It can be used as an ANXIOLYTIC for the short-term treatment of anxiety, as a HYPNOTIC to relieve insomnia, as an ANTICONVULSANT and ANTI-EPILEPTIC for status epilepticus, as a SEDATIVE in preoperative medication, as a SKELETAL MUSCLE RELAXANT and to assist in the treatment of alcohol withdrawal symptoms. It is available as tablets.
+▲ side-effects/warning: see under BENZODIAZEPINE

Tenuate Dospan

(Merrell) is a proprietary, prescription-only preparation of the APPETITE SUPPRESSANT diethylpropion hydrochloride and is on the Controlled Drugs List. It can be used in the medical treatment of obesity, but only in the short term and under strict medical supervision. It is available as modified-release tablets.
+▲ side-effects/warning: see DIETHYLPROPION HYDROCHLORIDE

Teoptic

(CIBA Vision) is a proprietary, prescription-only preparation of the BETA-BLOCKER drug carteolol hydrochloride. It

can be used for GLAUCOMA TREATMENT and is available as eye-drops.
✚▲ side-effects/warning: see CARTEOLOL HYDROCHLORIDE

terazosin
is an ALPHA-ADRENOCEPTOR BLOCKER drug. It is used as an ANTIHYPERTENSIVE treatment and also, because of its SMOOTH MUSCLE RELAXANT properties, in the treatment of urinary retention (eg. in benign prostatic hyperplasia). Administration is oral in the form of tablets.
✚ side-effects: there may be lack of energy, urinary frequency, dizziness, swelling and peripheral oedema (accumulation of fluid in the tissues).
warning: the first dose may cause collapse (due to hypotension), so it should be taken on retiring to bed or when lying down.
◎ Related entries: Hytrin; Hytrin BPH

terbinafine
is an ANTIFUNGAL drug, which is used to treat ringworm infections of the skin and fungal infections of the nails. Unlike most other antifungals it can be taken by mouth and so is available as tablets as well as a cream.
✚ side-effects: there may be loss of appetite, abdominal discomfort, nausea and diarrhoea, headache, muscle and joint ache and urticaria (itchy skin rash), unusual skin disturbances, light sensitivity, taste disturbances and liver disorders.
▲ warning: it should be used with care where there is abnormal liver or kidney function, in pregnancy and breast-feeding. Avoid contact of the cream with the eyes.
◎ Related entry: Lamisil

terbutaline sulphate
is a SYMPATHOMIMETIC and a BETA-RECEPTOR STIMULANT with good beta$_2$-receptor selectivity. It is mainly used as a BRONCHODILATOR in reversible obstructive airways disease, as an ANTI-ASTHMATIC treatment in severe acute asthma and for

the alleviation of symptoms of chronic bronchitis and emphysema. It can also be used in obstetrics to prevent or delay premature labour by relaxing the uterus. It is administered by injection, tablets, modified-release tablets, a sugar-free liquid, or in an inhalant form
✚▲ side-effects/warning: see under SALBUTAMOL (and RITODRINE HYDROCHLORIDE for use in labour).
◎ Related entries: Bricanyl; Monovent

terfenadine
is a recently developed ANTIHISTAMINE drug with less sedative side-effects than some older members of its class. It can be used for the symptomatic relief of allergic symptoms such as hay fever and urticaria (itchy skin rash). Administration is oral in the form of tablets or as a suspension.
✚▲ side-effects/warning: see under ANTIHISTAMINE. Although the incidence of sedative and anticholinergic effects is low, there may still be drowsiness which may impair the performance of skilled tasks such as driving. Certain serious disturbances of heart rhythm have been observed after excessive dose and when used in combination with certain other drugs (including a number of antibiotics, antidepressants, antipsychotics and anti-arrhythmics). Hair loss has been reported.
◎ Related entries: One-A-Day Antihistamine Tablets; Seldane; Triludan

terlipressin
is a form of the pituitary HORMONE antidiuretic hormone (ADH) or vasopressin. It can be used as a VASOCONSTRICTOR to treat bleeding from varices (varicose veins) in the oesophagus. Administration is by injection.
✚▲ side-effects/warning: see under VASOPRESSIN; but side-effects are usually milder.
◎ Related entry: Glypressin

T

terpenes

are chemically unsaturated hydrocarbons that are found in terpene plant oils and resins. Examples include CINEOLE, MENTHOL, pinene and squalene. Examples that are chemically larger include the caratenoids and VITAMIN A. Mixtures of some terpenes are used to treat gallstone disorders. Menthol, which is the most widely used of all the terpenes, is included in inhalant preparations intended to clear nasal or catarrhal congestion in conditions such as colds, rhinitis (inflammation of the nasal mucous membrane), or sinusitis. It is also included in some COUNTER-IRRITANT, or RUBEFACIENT, preparations that are rubbed into the skin to relieve muscle or joint pain.

✚▲ side-effects/warning: there seem to be only a few adverse reactions with topical application, even though their action would appear to involve irritation of sensory nerve endings. Some interact with contraceptives or coagulants that are administered orally.

Terra-Cortril

(Pfizer) is a proprietary, prescription-only COMPOUND PREPARATION of the ANTI-INFLAMMATORY and CORTICOSTEROID drug hydrocortisone (as acetate) and the ANTIBACTERIAL and (TETRACYCLINE) ANTIBIOTIC drug oxytetracycline. It can be used for local or topical application to treat skin disorders in which bacterial or other infection is also implicated. It is available as a topical ointment and as a suspension. *Terra-Cortril Ear Suspension* also contains the (POLYMYXIN) antibiotic drug polymyxin B sulphate.

✚▲ side-effects/warning: see HYDROCORTISONE; OXYTETRACYCLINE; POLYMYXIN B SULPHATE

Terra-Cortril Nystatin

(Pfizer) is a proprietary, prescription-only COMPOUND PREPARATION of the ANTI-INFLAMMATORY and CORTICOSTEROID drug

hydrocortisone (as acetate), the ANTIFUNGAL and ANTIBIOTIC drug nystatin and the ANTIBACTERIAL and (TETRACYCLINE) antibiotic drug oxytetracycline. It can be used to treat skin disorders caused by fungal or bacterial infection. It is available as a cream.

✚▲ side-effects/warning: see HYDROCORTISONE; NYSTATIN; OXYTETRACYCLINE

Terramycin

(Pfizer) is a proprietary, prescription-only preparation of the ANTIBACTERIAL and (TETRACYCLINE) ANTIBIOTIC drug oxytetracycline. It can be used to treat a wide range of infections and is available as tablets and capsules.

✚▲ side-effects/warning: see OXYTETRACYCLINE

Tertroxin

(Link) is a proprietary, prescription-only preparation of liothyronine sodium, which is a form of the THYROID HORMONE triiodothyronine. It can be used to make up hormonal deficiency (hypothyroidism) and therefore to treat the associated symptoms. It is available as tablets.

✚▲ side-effects/warning: see LIOTHYRONINE SODIUM

Testosterone

(Organon) is a proprietary, prescription-only preparation of the ANDROGEN (male SEX HORMONE) testosterone (as propionate and phenylpropionate). It can be used to treat testosterone deficiency in men and women (as part of HRT). It is available as an implant.

✚▲ side-effects/warning: see TESTOSTERONE

testosterone

is an ANDROGEN and the principal male SEX HORMONE. It is produced (in men) mainly in the testes with other androgens that promote the development and maintenance of the male sex organs and in the development of the secondary male sexual characteristics. It is also made in small amounts in women. Therapeutically, it can be administered to treat hormonal deficiency, for instance for delayed puberty, certain cancers (eg. breast cancer in women) and in HRT (hormone replacement therapy) in menopausal women. Administration is either oral in the form of capsules, or by injection or depot injection.

+▲ side-effects/warning: see under ANDROGEN

✪ Related entries: Primoteston Depot; Restandol; Sustenon 100; Sustenon 250; Testosterone; Virormone

Tet/Vac/Ads

is an abbreviation for ADSORBED TETANUS VACCINE.

Tet/Vac/FT

is an abbreviation for TETANUS VACCINE, which is prepared from tetanus formol toxoid, the plain vaccine and is not adsorbed onto a carrier.

Tetabulin

(Immuno) (Tetanus Immunoglobulin Injection) is a proprietary, prescription-only preparation of tetanus immunoglobulin, human (HTIG), which is a SPECIFIC IMMUNOGLOBULIN. It can be used in IMMUNIZATION to give immediate *passive immunity* against infection by the tetanus organism. Administration is by intramuscular injection.

Tetanus Immunoglobulin

(BLS; SNBTS) (Antitetanus Immunoglobulin Injection) is a non-proprietary, prescription-only preparation of tetanus immunoglobulin, human (HTIG), which is a SPECIFIC IMMUNOGLOBULIN that can be used in IMMNNUNIZATION to give immediate *passive immunity* against infection by the tetanus organism. Administration is by intramuscular injection.

Tetanus Immunoglobulin for Intravenous Use

(SNBTS) is a non-proprietary, prescription-only preparation of tetanus immunoglobulin, human (HTIG), which is a SPECIFIC IMMUNOGLOBULIN that can be used in IMMUNIZATION to give immediate passive immunity against infection by the tetanus organism. Administration is by intravenous injection.

tetanus immunoglobulin, human

(HTIG) is a SPECIFIC IMMUNOGLOBULIN, which is a form of immunoglobulin used for IMMUNIZATION to give immediate *passive immunity* against infection by tetanus. It is mostly used as an added precaution in treating patients with contaminated wounds. It can be considered just a precautionary measure because today almost everybody has established immunity through a VACCINE administered at an early age and vaccination is in any case readily available for those at risk. Administration is by intramuscular injection.

✪ Related entries: Tetabulin; Tetanus Immunoglobulin; Tetanus Immunoglobulin for Intravenous Use

Tetanus Immunoglobulin Injection

See TETABULIN

tetanus toxoid

See TETANUS VACCINE

Tetanus Vaccine

(Evans) (Tet/Vac/FT) is a non-proprietary, prescription-only VACCINE preparation of a the *toxoid-type* TETANUS VACCINE. It can be used for provide active immunization against tetanus and is available in a form for injection.

tetanus vaccine

(tetanus toxoid) is used in IMMUNIZATION to provide protection against infection by

T

the tetanus organism. It is a *toxoid-type* VACCINE, which is a vaccine made from a toxin produced by bacteria, in this case tetanus bacteria, that is modified to make it non-infective and which then stimulates the body to form the appropriate antitoxin (antibody). In tetanus vaccine, the bacterial toxoid is adsorbed onto a mineral carrier and is usually given as one constituent of the *triple vaccine* ADSORBED DIPHTHERIA, TETANUS and PERTUSSIS VACCINE (DTPer/Vac/Ads) or the *double vaccine* ADSORBED DIPHTHERIA AND TETANUS VACCINE (DT/Vac/Ads), which are administered during early life. However, tetanus vaccine can be administered by itself at any age for those who are at special risk from being infected. Administration is by intramuscular or subcutaneous injection and a 'booster' injection is given after ten years.

○ Related entries: Adsorbed Diphtheria and Tetanus Vaccine for Adults and Adolescents; Adsorbed Tetanus Vaccine; Clostet; Tetanus Vaccine; Trivac-AD

tetrabenazine

is a drug that is used to assist a patient to regain voluntary control of movement, or at least to lessen the extent of involuntary movements, in Huntingdon's chorea and related disorders. It is thought to work by reducing the amount of DOPAMINE in the nerves in the brain. Administration is oral in the form of tablets.

✚ side-effects: drowsiness, gastrointestinal disturbance, depression, hypotension, extrapyramidal symptoms (muscle tremor and rigidity).

▲ warning: administer with caution to patients who are pregnant and avoid its use in those who are breast-feeding. Because of its drowsiness effect, the performance of skilled tasks such as driving may be impaired.

○ Related entry: Nitoman

Tetrabid-Organon

(Organon) is a proprietary, prescription-

only preparation of the ANTIBACTERIAL and (TETRACYCLINE) ANTIBIOTIC drug tetracycline. It can be used to treat infections of many kinds (including acne) and is available as modified-release capsules.

✚▲ side-effects/warning: see TETRACYCLINE

Tetrachel

(Berk) is a proprietary, prescription-only preparation of the ANTIBACTERIAL and (TETRACYCLINE) ANTIBIOTIC drug tetracycline. It can be used to treat infections of many kinds and is available as capsules and tablets.

✚▲ side-effects/warning: see TETRACYCLINE

tetracosactide

See TETRACOSACTRIN

tetracosactrin

(tetracosactide) is a synthetic HORMONE, an analogue of the pituitary hormone corticotrophin (ACTH), which acts on the adrenal glands to release corticosteroids, especially HYDROCORTISONE. It is used to test adrenal function and is administered by intramuscular or intravenous injection.

✚▲ side-effects/warning: see under CORTICOSTEROIDS. There is a risk of anaphylaxis.

○ Related entries: Synacthen; Synacthen Depot

tetracycline

is a broad-spectrum ANTIBACTERIAL and ANTIBIOTIC drug. It is one of the TETRACYCLINES and gave its name to this family of similar antibiotics. It can be used to treat many forms of infection, for example infections of the urinary and respiratory tracts, of the genital organs, ears, eyes, mouth ulcers and skin (acne). Administration can be oral as capsules, tablets or liquids, or by infusion.

✚ side-effects: there may be nausea and vomiting with diarrhoea; headache and visual disturbances. Occasionally, there is sensitivity to light or other sensitivity reactions such as rashes (if so, discontinue treatment). Rarely, pancreatitis and colitis.

▲ warning: it should not be administered to patients who are aged under 12 years, because of tooth colouration, or who are pregnant or breast-feeding. Administer with caution to those with impaired liver or kidney function.

○ Related entries: Achromycin; Deteclo; Mysteclin; Sustamycin; Tetrabid-Organon; Tetrachel; Topicycline

tetracyclines

are a group of very broad-spectrum ANTIBACTERIAL and ANTIBIOTIC drugs. Apart from being effective against bacteria, they also inhibit the growth of chlamydia (a virus-like bacterium that causes genitourinary tract infections, eye infections and psittacosis *Chlamydia psittaci*), rickettsia (a virus-like bacterium that causes, for example, Q fever and typhus *Rickettsia typhi*) and mycoplasma (a minute nonmotile organism that causes, for example, mycoplasmal pneumonia *Mycoplasma pneumoniae*). The tetracyclines act by inhibiting protein biosynthesis in sensitive micro-organisms and penetrate human macrophages and are therefore useful in combating micro-organisms such as mycoplasma that can survive and multiply within macrophages. Although they have been used to treat a very wide range of infections, the development of bacterial resistance has meant that their uses have become more specific. Treatment of atypical pneumonia due to chlamydia, rickettsia, or mycoplasma is a notable indication for tetracyclines, while treatment of chlamydial urethritis and pelvic inflammatory disease is another. They are also used to treat brucellosis and Lyme disease and are effective in treating exacerbations of chronic bronchitis and acne. Most tetracyclines are more difficult to absorb in a stomach that contains milk, antacids (calcium salts or magnesium salts), or iron salts (eg. in anaemia treatment); and most (except doxycycline

and minicycline) may exacerbate kidney failure, so should be avoided when treating patients with kidney disease. They may be deposited in growing bone and teeth (causing staining and potential deformity), so they should not be administered to children under 12 years or to pregnant women. The best-known and most-used tetracyclines include TETRACYCLINE (which they were all named after), DOXYCYCLINE and OXYTETRACYCLINE. The members of the tetracycline family have generic names ending -*cycline*. Administration is oral in the form of capsules, tablets, or liquids. See CHLORTETRACYCLINE; DEMECLOCYCLINE HYDROCHLORIDE; LYMECYCLINE; MINOCYCLINE.

Tetralysal 300

(Pharmacia) is a proprietary, prescription-only preparation of the ANTIBACTERIAL and (TETRACYCLINE) ANTIBIOTIC drug lymecycline. It can be used to treat infections of many kinds and is available as capsules.
+▲ side-effects/warning: see LYMECYCLINE

Theo-Dur

(Astra) is a proprietary, non-prescription preparation of the BRONCHODILATOR drug theophylline. It can be used as an ANTI-ASTHMATIC and for the treatment of chronic bronchitis. It is available as modified-release tablets.
+▲ side-effects/warning: see THEOPHYLLINE

theophylline

is a BRONCHODILATOR drug that is mainly used as an ANTI-ASTHMATIC and for the treatment of bronchitis. Chemically, it is classed as a xanthine. Administration is oral in the form of tablets and capsules (mainly modified-release forms capable of maintaining actions for up to 12 hours), as a liquid and in a form for injection. It is also available in the form of chemical derivatives, eg. AMINOPHYLLINE.
+ side-effects: there may be nausea and

gastrointestinal disturbances, headache, an increase or irregularity in the heartbeat, and/or insomnia; convulsions may occur when given intravenously.

▲ warning: safety depends very much on the concentration in the blood, but this depends on many factors including whether the patient smokes or drinks, their age and concurrent drug therapy. For this reason treatment should initially be gradual and progressively increased until control of bronchospasm is achieved. Administer with caution to patients who suffer from certain heart or liver disorders, who are pregnant or breast-feeding and where there is a risk of low blood potassium (hypokalaemia). It should not be used in patients with porphyria.

○ Related entries: Anestan Bronchial Tablets; Do-Do Tablets; Franol; Franol Plus; Franolyn For Chesty Coughs; Labophylline; Lasma; Nuelin; Nuelin SA; Slo-Phyllin; Theo-Dur; Uniphyllin Continus

Thephorin

(Sinclair) is a proprietary, non-prescription preparation of the ANTIHISTAMINE drug phenindamine tartrate. It can be used to treat the symptoms of allergic disorders such as hay fever and urticaria. It is available as tablets.

✚▲ side-effects/warning: see PHENINDAMINE TARTRATE

thiabendazole

(tiabendazole) is an AZOLE drug. It is used in the treatment of infestations by worm parasites, particularly those of the *Strongyloides* species that reside in the intestines but may migrate into the tissues. It is also used to treat other worm infestations resistant to common drugs. The usual course of treatment is intensive.

✚ side-effects: there may be nausea, vomiting, diarrhoea and anorexia; dizziness and drowsiness; and headache and itching. Possible hypersensitivity reactions include fever with chills, rashes and other skin disorders and occasionally tinnitus (ringing in the ears) or liver damage.

▲ warning: it should be administered with caution to patients with impaired kidney or liver function. Treatment should be withdrawn if hypersensitivity reactions occur. It is not to be administered to pregnant women. It may impair performance of skilled tasks such as driving.

○ Related entry: Mintezol

*thiazides

have a DIURETIC action: they inhibit sodium reabsorption at the beginning of the distal convoluted tubule of the kidney and may be used for prolonged periods. Their uses include ANTIHYPERTENSIVE treatment (either alone or in conjunction with other types of diuretic or other drugs) and the treatment of oedema (accumulation of fluid in the tissues) associated with congestive heart failure. There may be some depletion of potassium, but this can be treated with potassium supplements or the co-administering of *potassium-sparing* diuretics. Administration is oral in the form of tablets. See: BENDROFLUAZIDE; BENZTHIAZIDE; CHLOROTHIAZIDE; CHLORTHALIDONE; CLOPAMIDE; CYCLOPENTHIAZIDE; HYDROCHLOROTHIAZIDE; HYDROFLUMETHIAZIDE; INDAPAMIDE; MEFRUSIDE; METOLAZONE; POLYTHIAZIDE; XIPAMIDE.

thioguanine

is a CYTOTOXIC DRUG, which is used as an ANTICANCER drug in the treatment of acute leukaemias. Administration is oral in the form of tablets.

✚▲ side-effects/warning: see under CYTOTOXIC DRUGS

○ Related entry: Lanvis

thiopental sodium

See THIOPENTONE SODIUM

Thiopentone Sodium

(IMS) is a proprietary, prescription-only preparation of the GENERAL ANAESTHETIC drug thiopentone sodium. It can be used for the induction of anaesthesia and is available in a form for injection.
+▲ side-effects/warning: see THIOPENTONE SODIUM

thiopentone sodium

(thiopental sodium) is a BARBITURATE drug. It can be used as a GENERAL ANAESTHETIC for induction and maintenance of anaesthesia during very short operations. Administration is by injection.
+▲ side-effects/warning: see under BARBITURATE. It is not to be given to patients with porphyria.
✪ Related entries: Intraval Sodium; Thiopentone Sodium

thioridazine

is a recently introduced ANTIPSYCHOTIC drug, which is used to treat and tranquillize psychotic patients (such as schizophrenics), particularly those experiencing behavioural disturbances. The drug may also be used for the short-term treatment of anxiety and to calm agitated, elderly patients. Administration is oral in the form of tablets, a suspension, or a syrup.
+▲ side-effects/warning: see under CHLORPROMAZINE HYDROCHLORIDE; but has less sedative, hypothermia and extrapyramidal (muscle tremor and rigidity) symptoms; but is more likely to cause hypotension and there may be eye disorders and sexual dysfunction. Avoid its use in patients with porphyria.
✪ Related entries: Melleril; Rideril

Thiotepa

(Lederle) is a proprietary, prescription-only preparation of the (CYTOTOXIC) ANTICANCER drug thiotepa. It can be used in the treatment of tumours in the bladder or other body cavities. Administration is by instillation in the body cavity.
+▲ side-effects/warning: see THIOTEPA

thiotepa

is a CYTOTOXIC DRUG, which is used as an ANTICANCER drug in the treatment of tumours in the bladder and sometimes for breast cancer. It works by interfering with the DNA of new-forming cells, so preventing cell replication. Administration is by instillation in the body cavity.
+▲ side-effects/warning: see under CYTOTOXIC DRUGS
✪ Related entry: Thiotepa

thrombolytic drugs

break up or dissolve thrombi (blood clots). See FIBRINOLYTIC.

thymol

is obtained from the essential oil of the plant thyme. It can be used as a weak ANTISEPTIC, particularly in mouthwash preparations for oral or dental hygiene and also in DECONGESTANT preparations for inhalation. It is sometimes used in combination with the essential oils of other plants.
✪ Related entries: compound thymol glycerin, BP; Karvol Decongestant Capsules

thymoxamine

(moxisylyte) is an ALPHA-ADRENOCEPTOR BLOCKER drug. It can be used, because of its VASODILATOR properties, in the treatment of peripheral vascular disease (Raynaud's phenomenon). Administration is oral in the form of tablets.
+ side-effects: dizziness and headache, diarrhoea, liver toxicity and flushing.
▲ warning: it should not be administered to patients with certain liver disorders. Administer with caution to patients with diabetes.
✪ Related entry: Opilon

thyroid hormones

are secreted by the thyroid gland at the

T base of the neck. There are two major forms, both containing iodine: THYROXINE (L-thyroxine; T_4(80%) and TRIIODOTHYRONINE (L-tri-iodothronine; T_3(20%). They are transported in the bloodstream to control function throughout the body. Both these hormones, in the form of their sodium salts, are used therapeutically to make up a hormonal deficiency on a regular maintenance basis and to treat associated symptoms. They may also be used in the treatment of goitre, thyroid cancer, myxoedema and cretinism. A third hormone, CALCITONIN, is secreted by a different cell type in the thyroid gland and has a different physiological role. It is concerned with lowering calcium levels in the blood (an action which is used therapeutically).

✚▲ side-effects/warning: see under LIOTHYRONINE SODIUM; THYROXINE SODIUM

thyroid-stimulating hormone
See THYROTROPHIN

thyrotrophin
(thyroid-stimulating hormone; TSH) is an anterior pituitary HORMONE. It controls the release of THYROID HORMONES from the thyroid gland and is itself controlled by the hypothalamic hormone TRH (thyrotrophin-releasing hormone) and by high levels of thyroid hormone in the blood. In the case of clinical defects at some stage in this system of control, diagnostic tests are necessarily a matter for specialist clinics. Nowadays, it is considered less helpful to make direct diagnosis using thyrotrophin itself in stimulation tests, because it is easier to chemically measure the concentration of thyrotrophin and thyroid hormones (T_3 and T_4) in the blood.

thyrotrophin-releasing hormone
See PROTIRELIN

thyroxine
is one of the natural blood-borne (endocrine) HORMONES released by the thyroid gland. The other major THYROID HORMONE is TRIIODOTHYRONINE. In turn, the release of these hormones is regulated by the endocrine hormone THYROTROPHIN (thyroid-stimulating hormone; TSH), which is secreted by the pituitary gland. Therapeutically, thyroxine is used in the form of THYROXINE SODIUM (sodium L-throxine; T_4).

thyroxine sodium
(sodium L-thyroxine; T_4) is a preparation of THYROXINE, which is one of the two main natural THYROID HORMONES. It is used therapeutically to make up a hormonal deficiency on a regular maintenance basis and to treat associated symptoms. It may also be used in the treatment of goitre and thyroid cancer. Administration is oral in the form of tablets.

✚ side-effects: there may be heartbeat irregularities and increased heart rate, angina pain; headache, muscle cramp, flushing and sweating, diarrhoea, restlessness and weight loss.

▲ warning: administer with caution to patients with certain cardiovascular disorders, impaired adrenal glands, or prolonged myxoedema.

✪ Related entry: Eltroxin

thiabendazole
See TIABENDAZOLE

tiaprofenic acid
is a (NSAID) NON-NARCOTIC ANALGESIC and ANTIRHEUMATIC drug. It is used to treat pain and inflammation in rheumatic disease and other musculoskeletal disorders. Administration is oral in the form of tablets or capsules.

✚▲ side-effects/warning: see under NSAID. It may cause cystitis and bladder irritation and so should not be used where there is a history of urinary tract disorders and treatment must

be stopped if adverse effects occur (such as increased frequency of urination, pain, or blood in the urine).
○ Related entry: Surgam

tibolone

(Organon) is a drug that has both OESTROGEN and PROGESTOGEN activity. It can be used to treat menopausal problems in HRT (hormone replacement therapy). Administration is oral in the form of tablets.
+▲ side-effects/warning: see under OESTROGEN; PROGESTOGEN
○ Related entry: Livial

Ticar

(Link) is a proprietary, prescription-only preparation of the ANTIBACTERIAL and (PENICILLIN) ANTIBIOTIC drug ticarcillin. It can be used to treat serious infections such as septicaemia and peritonitis and also infections of the respiratory and urinary tracts. It is available in a form for injection or infusion.
+▲ side-effects/warning: see TICARCILLIN

ticarcillin

is an ANTIBACTERIAL and (PENICILLIN) ANTIBIOTIC drug. It has improved activity against a number of important Gram-negative bacteria, including *Pseudomonas aeruginosa*. It can be used to treat serious infections such as septicaemia and peritonitis and also infections of the respiratory and urinary tracts. One of its proprietary forms also contains CLAVULANIC ACID. Administration is by injection or infusion.
+▲ side-effects/warning: see under BENZYLPENICILLIN
○ Related entries: Ticar; Timentin

Tilade

(Fisons) is a proprietary, prescription-only preparation of the ANTI-ASTHMA drug nedocromil sodium. It can be used to prevent recurrent attacks of asthma and is available in a form for inhalation.
+▲ side-effects/warning: see NEDOCROMIL SODIUM

Tildiem

(Lorex) is a proprietary, prescription-only preparation of the CALCIUM-CHANNEL BLOCKER drug diltiazem hydrochloride. It can be used as as an ANTIHYPERTENSIVE and as an ANTI-ANGINA drug in the prevention of attacks. It is available as tablets.
+▲ side-effects/warning: see DILTIAZEM HYDROCHLORIDE

Tildiem LA

(Lorex) is a proprietary, prescription-only preparation of the CALCIUM-CHANNEL BLOCKER drug diltiazem hydrochloride. It can be used as as an ANTIHYPERTENSIVE and as an ANTI-ANGINA drug in the prevention of attacks. It is available as modified-release capsules (which should be taken with food).
+▲ side-effects/warning: see DILTIAZEM HYDROCHLORIDE

Tildiem Retard

(Lorex) is a proprietary, prescription-only preparation of the CALCIUM-CHANNEL BLOCKER drug diltiazem hydrochloride. It can be used as as an ANTIHYPERTENSIVE and as an ANTI-ANGINA drug in the prevention of attacks. It is available as modified-release tablets.
+▲ side-effects/warning: see DILTIAZEM HYDROCHLORIDE

Timecef

(Roussel) is a proprietary, prescription-only preparation of the ANTIBACTERIAL and (CEPHALOSPORIN) ANTIBIOTIC drug cefodizime. It can be used to treat infections of the lower respiratory tract, such as pneumonia and bronchopneumonia and of the urinary tract, including cystitis and pyelonephritis. It is available in a form for injection.
+▲ side-effects/warning: see CEFODIZIME

T

Timentin

(Beecham) is a proprietary, prescription-only COMPOUND PREPARATION of the ANTIBACTERIAL and (PENICILLIN) ANTIBIOTIC drug ticarcillin and the ENZYME INHIBITOR clavulanic acid, which inhibits enzymes produced by some bacteria and thereby imparting *penicillinase-resistance* on ticarcillin. This combination can be used to treat serious infections that occur in patients whose immune systems are undermined by disease or drugs and where the responsible micro-organism is resistant to ticarcillin alone. (Patients with such conditions are generally in hospital.) It is available in a form for injection or infusion.

+▲ side-effects/warning: see CLAVULANIC ACID; TICARCILLIN

Timodine

(Reckitt & Colman) is a proprietary, prescription-only COMPOUND PREPARATION of the CORTICOSTEROID drug hydrocortisone, the ANTIFUNGAL and ANTIBIOTIC drug nystatin and the ANTISEPTIC agent benzylalkonium chloride. It can be used to treat fungal infections and mild skin inflammation. It is available as a cream for topical application.

+▲ side-effects/warning: see BENZYLALKONIUM CHLORIDE; HYDROCORTISONE; NYSTATIN

timolol maleate

is a BETA-BLOCKER that can be used as an ANTIHYPERTENSIVE treatment for raised blood pressure, as an ANTI-ANGINA treatment to relieve symptoms and improve exercise tolerance and as an ANTI-ARRHYTHMIC to regularize heartbeat and to treat and prevent myocardial infarction. It can also be used as an ANTIMIGRAINE treatment to prevent attacks. Administration is oral in the form of tablets. Additionally, it can be used as a GLAUCOMA TREATMENT when it is given as eye-drops. It is also available, as an antihypertensive treatment, in the form of

a COMPOUND PREPARATION with a DIURETIC.

+▲ side-effects/warnings: see under PROPRANOLOL HYDROCHLORIDE

○ Related entries: Betim; Blocadren; Glaucol; Moducren; Prestim; Prestim Forte; Timoptol

Timoptol

(Merck, Sharp & Dohme) is a proprietary, prescription-only preparation of the BETA-BLOCKER drug timolol maleate. It can be used for GLAUCOMA TREATMENT and is available as eye-drops (in *Ocumeter* units).

+▲ side-effects/warning: see CARTEOLOL HYDROCHLORIDE

Timpron

(Berk) is a proprietary, prescription-only preparation of the (NSAID) NON-NARCOTIC ANALGESIC and ANTIRHEUMATIC drug naproxen. It can be used to relieve pain of musculoskeletal disorders, particularly rheumatic and arthritic pain and acute gout. It is available as tablets.

+▲ side-effects/warning: see NAPROXEN

Tinaderm Cream

(Schering-Plough) is a proprietary, non-prescription preparation of the ANTIFUNGAL drug tolnaftate. It can be used to treat athlete's foot and is available as a cream.

+▲ side-effects/warning: see TOLNAFTATE

Tinaderm-M

(Schering-Plough) is a proprietary, prescription-only COMPOUND PREPARATION of the ANTIFUNGAL and ANTIBIOTIC drug nystatin and the antifungal drug tolnaftate. It can be used to treat *Candida* fungal infections of the skin and nails and is available as a cream.

+▲ side-effects/warning: see NYSTATIN; TOLNAFTATE

Tinaderm Plus Powder

(Schering-Plough) is a proprietary, non-prescription preparation of the

ANTIFUNGAL drug tolnaftate. It can be used to treat athlete's foot and is available as a powder.

+▲ side-effects/warning: see TOLNAFTATE

Tinaderm Plus Powder Aerosol

(Schering-Plough) is a proprietary, non-prescription preparation of the ANTIFUNGAL drug tolnaftate. It can be used to treat athlete's foot and is available as a powder spray.

+▲ side-effects/warning: see TOLNAFTATE

tinidazole

is an (AZOLE) ANTIMICROBIAL drug with ANTIBACTERIAL and ANTIPROTOZOAL properties. It can be used to treat anaerobic infections such as bacterial vaginitis and protozoal infections such as giardiasis, trichomoniasis and amoebiasis. It can also be used to treat acute ulcerative gingivitis and to prevent infection following abdominal surgery. Administration is oral in the form of tablets.

+▲ side-effects/warning: see under METRONIDAZOLE

✪ Related entry: Fasigyn

Tinset

(Janssen) is a proprietary, non-prescription preparation of the ANTIHISTAMINE drug oxatomide. It can be used to treat allergic conditions such as hay fever and urticaria and is available as tablets.

+▲ side-effects/warning: see OXATOMIDE

tinzaparin

is a low molecular weight version of heparin. It has some advantages as an ANTICOAGULANT when used for long-term prevention of venous thrombo-embolism, particularly in orthopaedic use. Administration is by injection.

+▲ side-effects/warning: see under HEPARIN

✪ Related entry: Innohep

tioconazole

is an (AZOLE) ANTIFUNGAL drug, which is used to treat fungal infections of the nails. It is available as a lotion and a cream which are applied to the nails and surrounding area.

+ side-effects: there may be local irritation.

✪ Related entry: Trosyl

Tisept

(Seton Healthcare) is a proprietary, non-prescription COMPOUND PREPARATION of the ANTISEPTIC agents chlorhexidine (as gluconate) and cetrimide. It can be used as a general skin disinfectant and as an antiseptic for cleaning wounds. It is available as a solution.

+▲ side-effects/warning: see CETRIMIDE; CHLORHEXIDINE

titanium dioxide

is a white pigment incorporated into several SUNSCREEN preparations. It provides some degree of protection from ultraviolet UVA and UVB radiation.

✪ Related entries: Piz Buin SPF 20 Sun Block Lotion; Sun E45.

Tixylix Cough and Cold

(Intercare Products) is a proprietary, non-prescription COMPOUND PREPARATION of the (OPIOID) ANTITUSSIVE drug pholcodine, the ANTIHISTAMINE chlorpheniramine maleate and the SYMPATHOMIMETIC and DECONGESTANT drug pseudoephedrine hydrochloride. It can be used for the relief of dry, tickly coughs, runny nose and congestion. It is available as a syrup and is not normally given to children under one year, except on medical advice.

+▲ side-effects/warning: see CHLORPHENIRAMINE MALEATE; PHOLCODINE; PSEUDOEPHEDRINE HYDROCHLORIDE

Tixylix Inhalant

(Intercare Products) is a proprietary, non-prescription COMPOUND PREPARATION of aromatic oils (turpentine oils, eucalyptus

T

oil, camphor and menthol). It can be used for the symptomatic relief of colds, catarrh, flu and hay fever. It is available as capsules that are sprinkled over bed linen or nightwear, or inhaled after being mixed with hot water. It is not normally given to children under three months, except on medical advice.

Tobralex

(Alcon) is a proprietary, prescription-only preparation of the ANTIBACTERIAL and (AMINOGLYCOSIDE) ANTIBIOTIC drug tobramycin. It can be used to treat bacterial infections of the eye and is available as eye-drops.

✚▲ side-effects/warning: see TOBRAMYCIN

tobramycin

is an ANTIBACTERIAL and ANTIBIOTIC drug, which is a member of the AMINOGLYCOSIDE group. It is effective against some Gram-positive and Gram-negative bacteria and is used primarily for the treatment of serious Gram-negative infections caused by *Pseudomonas aeruginosa*, because it is significantly more active against this organism than gentamicin (the most commonly used of this class of antibiotic). Like other aminoglycosides, it is not absorbed from the intestine (except in the case of local infection or liver failure) and so is administered by injection when treating systemic disease. It is also available as eye-drops to treat bacterial infections of the eye.

✚▲ side-effects/warning: see under GENTAMICIN

⊙ Related entries: Nebcin; Tobralex

tocainide hydrochloride

is an ANTI-ARRHYTHMIC drug that is an analogue of the LOCAL ANAESTHETIC drug LIGNOCAINE HYDROCHLORIDE. It can be used to treat heartbeat irregularities, but, because of its high incidence of blood toxicity, generally only when more common drugs have

been found to be ineffective.
Administration is oral in the form of tablets.

✚ side-effects: there may be nausea, vomiting and gastrointestinal disturbance; a number of blood disturbances, tremor and liver impairment; visual hallucinations and confusion; dizziness and loss of sensation are not uncommon and may lead to convulsions.

▲ warning: it should not be used in patients with heart block; and administered with extreme caution to those with severely impaired liver or kidney function, heart failure, or who are elderly or pregnant. Regular and frequent blood counts are essential.

⊙ Related entry: Tonocard

tocopherol

(vitamin E) is a general name that is used to describe a group of substances known collectively as vitamin E. Good food sources include eggs, vegetable oils, wheat germ and green vegetables. Although deficiency is rare, it can be caused by malabsorption in conditions such as cystic fibrosis, abetalipoproteinaemia and chronic cholestasis. The form of tocopherol most used in therapy to make up vitamin deficiency is ALPHA TOCOPHERYL ACETATE. Administration is oral in the form of tablets or capsules.

✚▲ side-effects/warning: see under ALPHA TOCOPHERYL ACETATE

⊙ Related entry: Vitamin E Suspension

tocopheryl acetate

See ALPHA TOCOPHERYL ACETATE

Tofranil

(Geigy) is a proprietary, prescription-only preparation of the (TRICYCLIC) ANTIDEPRESSANT drug imipramine hydrochloride. It can be used to treat depressive illness, particularly in patients who are withdrawn and apathetic and may also be used to treat bed-wetting at night by children. It is available as tablets and a syrup.

✚▲ side-effects/warning: see IMIPRAMINE HYDROCHLORIDE

Tolanase
(Upjohn) is a proprietary, prescription-only preparation of the SULPHONYLUREA drug tolazamide. It is used in DIABETIC TREATMENT for Type II diabetes (non-insulin-dependent diabetes mellitus; NIDDM; maturity-onset diabetes) and is available as tablets.
✚▲ side-effects/warning: see TOLAZAMIDE

tolazamide
is as SULPHONYLUREA drug. It is used in DIABETIC TREATMENT for Type II diabetes (non-insulin-dependent diabetes mellitus; NIDDM; maturity-onset diabetes) and is administered orally as tablets.
✚▲ side-effects/warning: see under GLIBENCLAMIDE
✪ Related entry: Tolanase

tolbutamide
is a SULPHONYLUREA drug. It is used in DIABETIC TREATMENT for Type II diabetes (non-insulin-dependent diabetes mellitus; NIDDM; maturity-onset diabetes) and is administered orally as tablets.
✚▲ side-effects/warning: see under GLIBENCLAMIDE; but it may be used in renal impairment and the elderly.
✪ Related entry: Rastinon

Tolectin
(Cilag) is a proprietary, prescription-only preparation of the (NSAID) NON-NARCOTIC ANALGESIC and ANTIRHEUMATIC drug tolmetin. It can be used to treat the pain and inflammation of rheumatic disease and other musculoskeletal disorders. It is available as capsules.
✚▲ side-effects/warning: see TOLMETIN

Tolerzide
(Bristol-Myers) is a proprietary, prescription-only COMPOUND PREPARATION of the BETA-BLOCKER drug sotalol hydrochloride and the DIURETIC drug hydrochlorothiazide. It can be used as an ANTIHYPERTENSIVE treatment for raised blood pressure and is available as tablets.
✚▲ side-effects/warning: see HYDROCHLOROTHIAZIDE; SOTALOL HYDROCHLORIDE.

tolmetin
is a (NSAID) NON-NARCOTIC ANALGESIC and ANTIRHEUMATIC drug. It is used to treat the pain of rheumatic disease and other musculoskeletal disorders in juvenile arthritis. Administration is oral in the form of capsules.
✚▲ side-effects/warning: see under NSAID.
✪ Related entry: Tolectin

tolnaftate
is a mild ANTIFUNGAL drug, which is used primarily in the topical treatment of infections caused by the tinea species (eg. athlete's foot). Administration is in the form of a cream, a powder, or a solution.
✚▲ side-effects/warning: rarely, sensitivity reactions.
✪ Related entries: Mycil Athlete's Foot Ointment; Mycil Athlete's Foot Spray; Mycil Powder; Scholl Athlete's Foot Cream; Scholl Athlete's Foot Powder; Scholl Athlete's Foot Solution; Scholl Athlete's Foot Spray Liquid; Tinaderm Cream; Tinaderm Plus Powder; Tinaderm Plus Powder Aerosol; Tinaderm-M

Tonocard
(Astra) is a proprietary, prescription-only preparation of the ANTI-ARRHYTHMIC drug tocainide hydrochloride. It can be used to correct heart irregularities and is available as tablets.
✚▲ side-effects/warning: see TOCAINIDE HYDROCHLORIDE

Topal
(Novex) is a proprietary, non-prescription COMPOUND PREPARATION of the ANTACIDS aluminium hydroxide and magnesium carbonate and the DEMULCENT agent

T

alginic acid. It can be used to treat heartburn, severe indigestion and the symptoms of hiatus hernia. It is available as chewable tablets.

+▲ side-effects/warning: see ALGINIC ACID; ALUMINIUM HYDROXIDE; MAGNESIUM CARBONATE

Topicycline

(Monmouth) is a proprietary, prescription-only preparation of the ANTIBACTERIAL and (TETRACYCLINE) ANTIBIOTIC drug tetracycline (as hydrochloride). It can be used to treat acne and is available as a solution for topical application.

+▲ side-effects/warning: see TETRACYCLINE

Topilar

(Bioglan) is a proprietary, prescription-only preparation of the CORTICOSTEROID and ANTI-INFLAMMATORY drug fluclorolone acetonide. It can be used to treat severe, acute inflammatory skin disorders, such as eczema and psoriasis, that are unresponsive to less potent corticosteroids. It is available as a cream or ointment for topical application.

+▲ side-effects/warning: see FLUCLOROLONE ACETONIDE

Toradol

(Syntex) is a proprietary, prescription-only preparation of the (NSAID) NON-NARCOTIC ANALGESIC drug ketorolac trometamol. It can be used in the short-term management of moderate to severe acute postoperative pain. It is available as tablets and in a form for injection.

+▲ side-effect/warning: see KETOROLAC TROMETAMOL

torasemide

is a powerful DIURETIC drug of the *loop diuretic* type. It can be used to treat oedema (accumulation of fluid in the tissues), particularly pulmonary (lung) oedema in patients with chronic heart failure, low urine production due to

kidney failure (oliguria) and as an ANTIHYPERTENSIVE. Administration can be oral in the form of tablets or by injection or infusion.

+▲ side-effects/warning: see under FRUSEMIDE. It should not be used by patients who are pregnant or breast-feeding.

◯ Related entry: Torem

Torem

(Boehringer Mannheim) is a proprietary, prescription-only preparation of the (*loop*) DIURETIC drug torasemide. It can be used to treat oedema, particularly pulmonary (lung) oedema in patients with chronic heart failure and low urine production due to kidney failure (oliguria). It is available as tablets and in a form for injection or infusion.

+▲ side-effects/warning: see TORASEMIDE

Totamol

(CP) is a proprietary, prescription-only preparation of the BETA-BLOCKER drug atenolol. It can be used as an ANTIHYPERTENSIVE treatment for raised blood pressure, as an ANTI-ANGINA treatment to relieve symptoms and improve exercise tolerance and as an ANTI-ARRHYTHMIC to regularize heartbeat and to treat myocardial infarction. It is available as tablets.

+▲ side-effects/warning: see ATENOLOL

Tracrium

(Wellcome) is a proprietary, prescription-only preparation of the (*non-depolarizing*) SKELETAL MUSCLE RELAXANT drug atracurium besylate. It can be used to induce muscle paralysis during surgery and is available in a form for injection.

+▲ side-effects/warning: see ATRACURIUM BESYLATE

tramadol hydrochloride

is a recently introduced NARCOTIC ANALGESIC drug, which is similar to morphine in relieving pain, but probably with fewer side-effects. However, there

T

seem to be some differences in the mechanism by which it produces analgesia and it may not represent a typical OPIOID. Administration is either oral in the form of capsules or by intramuscular or intravenous injection.
+▲ side-effects/warning: see under OPIOID. Hypotension, hypertension and anaphylactic reactions have been reported. Administer with care to epileptics since convulsions have been reported. It should not be given to those who are pregnant or breast-feeding.
✪ Related entry: Zydol

tramazoline hydrochloride

is a SYMPATHOMIMETIC and VASOCONSTRICTOR drug, which can be used as a NASAL DECONGESTANT to treat allergic rhinitis (inflammation of the nasal mucous membrane). Administration is topical as an aerosol.
+▲ side-effects/warning: see under EPHEDRINE HYDROCHLORIDE
✪ Related entry: Dexa-Rhinaspray

Tramil 500 Analgesic Capsules

(Whitehall Laboratories) is a proprietary, non-prescription preparation of the NON-NARCOTIC ANALGESIC and ANTIPYRETIC drug paracetamol. It can be used to treat many forms of pain, including headache, migraine, muscular pain and period pain and also to relieve the symptoms of feverish colds and flu. It is available as tablets and is not normally given to children under 12 years, except on medical advice.
+▲ side-effects/warning: see PARACETAMOL

Trancopal

(Sanofi Winthrop) is a proprietary, prescription-only preparation of the ANXIOLYTIC drug chlormezanone. It is used principally in the short-term treatment of anxiety and insomnia and is available as tablets.
+▲ side-effects/warning: see CHLORMEZANONE

Trandate

(DF) is a proprietary, prescription-only preparation of the mixed BETA-BLOCKER and ALPHA-ADRENOCEPTOR BLOCKER drug labetalol hydrochloride. It can be used as an ANTIHYPERTENSIVE to reduce blood pressure, including in pregnancy, after myocardial infarction, in angina and during surgery. It is available as tablets or in a form for injection.
+▲ side-effects/warning: see LABETALOL HYDROCHLORIDE

trandolapril

is an ACE INHIBITOR and a powerful VASODILATOR. It can be used in ANTIHYPERTENSIVE treatment and often in conjunction with other classes of drug, particularly (THIAZIDE) DIURETICS. Administration is oral in the form of capsules
+▲ side-effects/warning: see under CAPTOPRIL
✪ Related entries: Gopten; Odrik

tranexamic acid

is an antifibrinolytic drug. It is used to stem bleeding in circumstances such as dental extraction in a haemophiliac patient or menorrhagia (excessive period bleeding). It works by inhibiting plasminogen, which is one of the blood's natural anticoagulant factors. Administration can be oral in the form of tablets or a syrup, or by injection.
+ side-effects there may be nausea and vomiting with diarrhoea; an injection may cause temporary giddiness.
▲ warning: it should be administered with caution to those with impaired kidney function. Prolonged treatment requires regular eye checks and liver function tests.
✪ Related entry: Cyklokapron

*tranquillizer

drugs calm, soothe and relieve anxiety and many also cause some degree of sedation. Although somewhat misleading, they are often classified in two groups *major*

T *tranquillizers* and *minor tranquillizers*. The major tranquillizers, which are also called NEUROLEPTICS or ANTIPSYCHOTIC drugs, are used primarily to treat severe mental disorders such as psychoses (including schizophrenia and mania). They are extremely effective in restoring a patient to a calmer, less-disturbed state of mind. The hallucinations, both auditory and visual, the gross disturbance of logical thinking and to some extent the delusions typical of psychotic states are generally well controlled by these drugs. Violent, aggressive behaviour that presents a danger to the patients themselves and to those that look after them, is also effectively treated by major tranquillizers. For this reason they are often used in the *management* of difficult, aggressive, antisocial individuals. Major tranquillizers that are commonly administered include the PHENOTHIAZINE DERIVATIVES (eg. CHLORPROMAZINE HYDROCHLORIDE, PROCHLORPERAZINE and THIORIDAZINE) and such drugs as FLUPENTHIXOL, FLUSPIRILENE and HALOPERIDOL. Minor tranquillizers are also *calming drugs*, but they are ineffective in the treatment of psychotic states. Their principal applications are as ANXIOLYTIC, HYPNOTIC and SEDATIVE drugs. The best-known and most-used minor tranquillizers are undoubtedly the BENZODIAZEPINES (eg. DIAZEPAM and CHLORDIAZEPOXIDE). However, prolonged treatment with minor tranquillizers can lead to dependence (addiction).

Transiderm-Nitro

(Geigy) is a proprietary, non-prescription preparation of the VASODILATOR and ANTI-ANGINA drug glyceryl trinitrate. It can be used to treat and prevent angina pectoris and to prevent phlebitis (inflammation in the veins). It is avialable as a self-adhesive dressing (patch), which, when placed on the chest wall, is then absorbed through the skin to give lasting relief.

✚▲ side-effects/warning: see GLYCERYL TRINITRATE

Transvasin Heat Rub

(Seton Healthcare) is a proprietary, non-prescription COMPOUND PREPARATION of the COUNTER-IRRITANT, or RUBEFACIENT, agents terahydrofurfuryl salicylate, hexyl nicotinate and ethyl salicylate. It can be used for the symptomatic relief of muscular aches and pains and is available as a cream for topical application to the skin.

✚▲ side-effects/warning: ETHYL SALICYLATE

Tranxene

(Boehringer Ingelheim) is a proprietary, prescription-only preparation of the ANXIOLYTIC drug clorazepate dipotassium. It can be used principally for the short-term treatment of anxiety and is available as capsules.

✚▲ side-effects/warning: see CLORAZEPATE DIPOTASSIUM

tranylcypromine

is an ANTIDEPRESSANT drug of the MONOAMINE-OXIDASE INHIBITOR (MAOI) class. It also has some STIMULANT effect which means that it is not as frequently used as other antidepressants. Administration is oral in the form of tablets.

✚▲ side-effects/warning: see under PHENELZINE; but do not use in patients with overactive thyroid secretion. It can cause hypertensive crisis, throbbing headache and insomnia (if taken in the evenings), but is less likely to cause liver damage.

❍ Related entry: Parnate

Trasicor

(Ciba) is a proprietary, prescription-only preparation of the BETA-BLOCKER drug oxprenolol hydrochloride. It can be used as an ANTIHYPERTENSIVE treatment for raised blood pressure, as an ANTI-ANGINA treatment to relieve symptoms and improve exercise tolerance and as an ANTI-ARRHYTHMIC to regularize heartbeat and to treat myocardial infarction. It can also be used as an ANXIOLYTIC treatment, particularly for symptomatic relief of tremor and palpitations. It is available as tablets.

+▲ side-effects/warning: see OXPRENOLOL HYDROCHLORIDE

Trasidrex

(Ciba) is a proprietary, prescription-only COMPOUND PREPARATION of the BETA-BLOCKER drug oxprenolol hydrochloride and the (THIAZIDE) DIURETIC drug cyclopenthiazide. It can be used as an ANTIHYPERTENSIVE treatment for raised blood pressure and is available as tablets.

+▲ side-effects/warning: see CYCLOPENTHIAZIDE; OXPRENOLOL HYDROCHLORIDE

Trasylol

(Bayer) is a proprietary, prescription-only preparation of aprotinin, which is a drug used to prevent life-threatening clot-formation, for instance in open-heart surgery, removal of tumours and in surgical procedures in patients with certain blood disorders (hyperplasminaemias). It is available in a from for injection.

+▲ side-effects/warning: see APROTININ

Travasept 100

(Baxter) is a proprietary, non-prescription COMPOUND PREPARATION of the ANTISEPTIC agents cetrimide and chlorhexidine (as acetate). It can be used for cleaning wounds and burns and is available as a solution.

+▲ side-effects/warning: see CETRIMIDE; CHLORHEXIDINE

Travogyn

(Schering Health) is a proprietary, prescription-only preparation of the ANTIFUNGAL drug isoconazole (as nitrate). It can be used in the treatment of fungal infections of the vagina and is available as vaginal tablets (pessaries).

+▲ side-effects/warning: see ISOCONAZOLE

Traxam

(Lederle) is a proprietary, prescription-only preparation of the drug felbinac (an active metabolite of fenbufen), which has (NSAID) NON-NARCOTIC ANALGESIC and COUNTER-IRRITANT, or RUBEFACIENT, actions. It can be used for the symptomatic relief of underlying muscle or joint pain and is available as a foam or gel for topical application to the skin. It is not normally used for children, except on medical advice.

+▲ side-effects/warning: see under FENBUFEN; but adverse effects on topical application are limited.

trazodone hydrochloride

is a TRICYCLIC-related ANTIDEPRESSANT drug. It is used to treat depressive illness, particularly in cases where some degree of SEDATION is required. Administration is oral in the form of capsules, tablets, or a liquid.

+▲ side-effects/warning: see under AMITRIPTYLINE HYDROCHLORIDE; but it has less ANTICHOLINERGIC actions. Occasionally, it may cause prolonged penile erection (priapism).

✪ Related entry: Molipaxin

Trental

(Hoechst) is a proprietary, non-prescription preparation of the VASODILATOR drug oxpentifylline. It can be used to help improve blood circulation to the hands and feet when this is impaired, for example in peripheral vascular disease (Raynaud's phenomenon). It is available as tablets.

+▲ side-effects/warning: see OXPENTIFYLLINE

Treosulfan

(Medac) is a proprietary, prescription-only preparation of the (CYTOTOXIC) ANTICANCER drug treosulfan. It can be used in the treatment of ovarian cancer and is available as capsules

T

and in a form for injection.
✚▲ side-effects/warning: see TREOSULFAN

treosulfan

is a CYTOTOXIC DRUG, which is used as an
ANTICANCER drug specifically in the
treatment of ovarian cancer. It works by
interfering with the DNA of new-forming
cells, so preventing cell replication.
Administration is either oral in the form of
capsules or by injection.
✚▲ side-effects/warning: see under
CYTOTOXIC DRUGS
✪ Related entry: Treosulfan

tretinoin

is chemically a retinoid (a derivative of
RETINOL, or vitamin A) and can be used to
treat acne. Administration is topical as a
cream, gel, or lotion applied to the skin.
✚ side-effects: there may be irritation or skin
peeling, redness, changes in skin
pigmentation and sensitivity to light.
▲ warning: it should not be applied to
broken skin. It should be kept away from the
eyes, mouth and mucous membranes. It is
not to be used in combination with other
keratolytics, or with sun-ray lamps. Do not
use if pregnant, or where there is eczema or
sunburned skin.
✪ Related entry: Retin-A

TRH

See PROTIRELIN

TRH-Cambridge

(Roche) is a proprietary,
prescription-only preparation of the
natural pituitary HORMONE
thyrotrophin-releasing hormone
(TRH or protirelin). It can be used
primarily in diagnosing thryoid
function in patients who suffer from
over-activity of the thyroid gland
(hyperthyroidism), or under-activity
of the pituitary gland (hypopituitarism).
It is available in a form for injection.
✚▲ side-effects/warning: see
PROTIRELIN

Tri-Adcortyl

(Squibb) is a proprietary, prescription-
only COMPOUND PREPARATION of the
ANTI-INFLAMMATORY and CORTICOSTEROID
drug triamcinolone acetonide, the
ANTIBACTERIAL and ANTIBIOTIC drugs
gramicidin and neomycin sulphate and the
ANTIFUNGAL and antibiotic drug nystatin. It
can be used for the treatment of severe
infective skin inflammation, such as
eczema and psoriasis, especially in cases
that have not responded to less-powerful
therapies. It is available as a cream and an
ointment for topical application.
✚▲ side-effects/warning: see GRAMICIDIN;
NEOMYCIN SULPHATE; NYSTATIN;
TRIAMCINOLONE ACETONIDE

Tri-Adcortyl Otic

(Squibb) is a proprietary, prescription-
only COMPOUND PREPARATION of the
ANTI-INFLAMMATORY and CORTICOSTEROID
drug triamcinolone acetonide, the
ANTIBACTERIAL and ANTIBIOTIC drugs
gramicidin and neomycin sulphate and the
ANTIFUNGAL and antibiotic drug nystatin. It
can be used for the treatment of severe
infective inflammation of the outer ear and
is available as an eye ointment.
✚▲ side-effects/warning: see GRAMICIDIN;
NEOMYCIN SULPHATE; NYSTATIN;
TRIAMCINOLONE ACETONIDE

Triadene

(Schering Health) is a proprietary,
prescription-only COMPOUND PREPARATION
that can be used as a (*triphasic*) ORAL
CONTRACEPTIVE (and also for certain
menstrual problems) of the type that
combines an OESTROGEN and a
PROGESTOGEN, in this case
ethinyloestradiol and gestodene. It is
available in the form of tablets in a
calendar pack.
✚▲ side-effects/warning: see
ETHINYLOESTRADIOL; GESTODENE

triamcinolone

is a synthetic CORTICOSTEROID with ANTI-

INFLAMMATORY and ANTI-ALLERGIC properties. It is used to suppress the symptoms of inflammation, especially when it is caused by allergic disorders. Administration is either oral as tablets or, for conditions such as hay fever and asthma, by injection.

+▲ side-effects/warning: see under CORTICOSTEROIDS

☉ Related entry: Ledercort

triamcinolone acetonide

is a synthetic CORTICOSTEROID with ANTI-INFLAMMATORY and ANTI-ALLERGIC properties. It is used to suppress the symptoms of inflammation, especially when it is caused by allergic disorders. It is sometimes administered as a systemic medication (in the form of an injection) to relieve conditions such as hay fever and asthma, but it is usually given by local injection to treat skin inflammation due to rheumatoid arthritis and bursitis. There are several proprietary cream preparations available that are mainly used to treat severe, non-infective skin inflammation such as eczema, but one or two are used for treating inflammation in the mouth.

+▲ side-effects/warning: see under CORTICOSTEROIDS. The type and severity of any side-effects depends on the route of administration.

☉ Related entries: Adcortyl; Adcortyl in Orabase; Adcortyl Intra-articular/Intradermal; Adcortyl with Graneodin; Audicort; Aureocort; Kenalog; Kenalog Intra-articular/Intramuscular; Nystadermal; Tri-Adcortyl; Tri-Adcortyl Otic

triamcinolone hexacetonide

is a CORTICOSTEROID with ANTI-INFLAMMATORY and ANTI-ALLERGIC properties. It is used to suppress the symptoms of inflammation in soft tissues. Administration is by injection.

+▲ side-effects/warning: see under CORTICOSTEROIDS

☉ Related entry: Lederspan

Triam-Co

(Baker Norton) is a proprietary, prescription-only COMPOUND PREPARATION of the (THIAZIDE) DIURETIC drug hydrochlorothiazide and the (*potassium-sparing*) diuretic triamterine (a combination called co-triamterzide 50/25). It can be used in the treatment of oedema and as an ANTIHYPERTENSIVE. It is available as tablets.

+▲ side-effects/warning: see HYDROCHLOROTHIAZIDE; TRIAMTERINE

triamterene

is a mild DIURETIC drug of the *potassium-sparing* type, which causes the retention of potassium. It is therefore used as an alternative to or, more commonly, in combination with other diuretics that normally cause a loss of potassium from the body (such as the THIAZIDES and *loop diuretics*). It can be used to treat oedema (accumulation of fluid in the tissues), as an ANTIHYPERTENSIVE (in combination with other drugs) and in congestive HEART FAILURE TREATMENT.

+ side-effects: gastrointestinal upsets, skin rashes, dry mouth, fall in blood pressure on standing; and raised blood potassium. There are also reports of blood disorders and light-sensitivity.

▲ warning: see under AMILORIDE HYDROCHLORIDE. Blood tests for potassium and urea are required, particularly in the elderly or in patients with impaired kidney function. The urine may be coloured blue.

☉ Related entries: Dyazide; Dytac; Dytide; Frusene; Kalspare

triazole

drugs are members of a chemical family that include the ANTIFUNGAL drugs FLUCYTOSINE and ITRACONAZOLE. They work by damaging the fungal cell membrane by inhibiting an enzyme called demethylase.

T

tribavirin

(ribavirin) is an ANTIVIRAL drug that inhibits a wide range of DNA and RNA viruses. It can be used to treat severe bronchiolitis caused by the syncytial virus in infants and certain other serious diseases (including lassa fever). It is administered by either nebulization or aerosol inhalation.

✚ side-effects: reticulocytosis and effects on the respiratory system.

▲ warning: it should not be used during pregnancy.

❂ Related entry: Virazid

Tribiotic

(3M Health Care) is a proprietary, prescription-only COMPOUND PREPARATION of the ANTIBACTERIAL and ANTIBIOTIC drug neomycin sulphate, polymyxin B sulphate and bacitracin zinc. It can be used to treat infections of the skin and is available as a spray.

✚▲ side-effects/warning: see BACITRACIN ZINC; NEOMYCIN SULPHATE; POLYMYXIN B SULPHATE

triclofos elixir

See TRICLOFOS ORAL SOLUTION, BP

triclofos oral solution, BP

(triclofos elixir) is a non-proprietary, prescription-only preparation of the HYPNOTIC drug triclofos sodium. It is used to treat insomnia in children and the elderly and is available as an elixir.

✚▲ side-effects/warning: see TRICLOFOS SODIUM

triclofos sodium

is a drug that is used as a HYPNOTIC to treat insomnia. Administration is oral in the form of an oral solution.

✚▲ side-effects/warning: see under CHLORAL HYDRATE; but with less stomach irritation.

triclosan

is an ANTISEPTIC agent, which is used to prevent the spread of an infection on the skin. It is available as a hand rub and a powder to be added to a bath.

✚▲ side-effects/warning: avoid contact with the eyes.

❂ Related entries: Solarcaine; Ster-Zac Bath Concentrate

*tricyclic

drugs are one of the three main classes of ANTIDEPRESSANT drugs that are used to relieve the symptoms of depressive illness. They are well established class of drugs, having been used for many years, but they do have SEDATIVE actions and many other side-effects. Since depression is commonly associated with loss of appetite and sleep disorders, an early benefit of tricyclic treatment may be an improvement of these symptoms. Some are also useful in the management of panic attacks and bed-wetting in children. Chemically, they are mainly dibenzazepine or dibenzcycloheptene derivatives and notable examples include AMITRIPTYLINE HYDROCHLORIDE, IMIPRAMINE HYDROCHLORIDE, DOXEPIN and DOTHIEPIN HYDROCHLORIDE. Some examples are chemically not tricyclics because they do not have the characteristic three-ringed structure, but are pharmacologically similar so are often classed under this heading (eg. MIANSERIN HYDROCHLORIDE). Treatment often takes some weeks to show maximal beneficial effects. Anxious or agitated patients respond better to those tricyclics which have more pronounced sedative properties (eg. amitriptyline and doxepin), whereas withdrawn patients are prescribed less-sedative tricyclics (eg. imipramine). See under amitriptyline hydrochloride for principal uses and side-effects.

Tridil

(Du Pont) is a proprietary, prescription-only preparation of the VASODILATOR and ANTI-ANGINA drug glyceryl trinitrate. It can be used in HEART FAILURE TREATMENT and to treat and prevent angina pectoris. It is

available in a form for injection.
+▲ side-effects/warning: see GLYCERYL
TRINITRATE

trientine dihydrochloride

is a CHELATING AGENT that is used to reduce
the abnormally high levels of copper in the
body that occur in Wilson's disease. It is
given to patients who cannot tolerate the
more commonly used drug PENICILLAMINE.
Administration is oral in the form of
capsules.
+ side-effects: nausea.
▲ warning: administer with care to patients
who are pregnant.
**✪ Related entry: Trientine
Dihydrochloride Capsules**

Trientine Dihydrochloride Capsules

(K & K-Greeff) is a proprietary,
prescription-only preparation of the
CHELATING AGENT trientine
dihydrochloride. It can be used to reduce
the abnormally high levels of copper in the
body that occur in Wilson's disease. It is
given to patients who cannot tolerate the
more commonly used drug PENICILLAMINE.
It is available as capsules.
+▲ side-effects/warning: see TRIENTINE
DIHYDROCHLORIDE

trifluoperazine

is chemically a PHENOTHIAZINE DERIVATIVE.
It is used as a powerful ANTIPSYCHOTIC
drug to treat and tranquillize psychotic
patients (such as schizophrenics),
particularly those experiencing some form
of behavioural disturbance. It can also be
used for the short-term treatment of
severe anxiety and as an ANTI-EMETIC and
ANTINAUSEANT for severe nausea and
vomiting caused by underlying disease or
drug therapies. Administration is either
oral as tablets, capsules (*Spansules*) or a
liquid, or by injection.
+▲ side-effects/warning: see under
CHLORPROMAZINE HYDROCHLORIDE; but with
less sedation, hypotension, hypothermia and

anticholinergic effects; though there is a
greater frequency of various movement
disturbances, including extrapyramidal
symptoms (muscle tremor and rigidity).
✪ Related entry: Stelazine

trifluperidol

is a powerful ANTIPSYCHOTIC drug, which
is used to treat and tranquillize psychotic
patients (such as schizophrenics),
particularly those experiencing manic,
behavioural disturbances. Administration
is oral in the form of tablets.
+▲ side-effects/warning: see under
HALOPERIDOL
✪ Related entry: Triperidol

Trifyba

(Sanofi Winthrop) is a proprietary, non-
prescription preparation of the natural
(*bulking agent*) LAXATIVE bran (wheat
fibre) and is available as a powder.
+▲ side-effects/warning: see BRAN

trihexyphenidyl hydrochloride

See BENZHEXOL HYDROCHLORIDE

Triiodothyronine

(Link) is a proprietary,
prescription-only preparation of
liothyronine sodium, which is a
form of the THYROID HORMONE
triiodothyronine. It can be used to
make up hormonal deficiency
(hypothyroidism) and to treat the
associated symptoms. It is available
in a form for injection.
+▲ side-effects/warning: see
LIOTHYRONINE SODIUM

triiodothyronine

(L-tri-iodothyronine; T_3) is the natural
form of one of the two main THYROID
HORMONES. Therapeutically, as
liothyronine sodium, it is used to make up
hormonal deficiency (hypothyroidism)
and to treat associated symptoms
(myxoedema). It may also be used in the

treatment of goitre and thyroid cancer.
+▲ side-effects/warning: see under
LIOTHYRONINE SODIUM

trilostane

is an ENZYME INHIBITOR. It inhibits the
production of both *glucocorticoid* and
mineralocorticoid CORTICOSTEROIDS by
the adrenal glands. It can therefore be
used to treat conditions that result from
the excessive secretion of corticosteroids
into the bloodstream (such as Cushing's
syndrome). It can also be used to treat
postmenopausal breast cancer.
Administration is oral in the form of
capsules.
+ side-effects: flushing, swelling and tingling
of the mouth, congested nose, nausea,
vomiting, diarrhoea; rarely, rashes and blood
changes.
▲ warning: it is not to be given to patients
who are pregnant, breast-feeding, or children;
administer with caution to those with breast
cancer (concurrent corticosteroids are
required), or impaired liver or kidney
function.
◎ Related entry: Modrenal

Triludan

(Merrell) is a proprietary, non-
prescription preparation of the
ANTIHISTAMINE drug terfenadine. It can be
used to treat the symptoms of allergic
disorders such as hay fever and urticaria.
It is available as tablets in two strengths
(the stronger preparation is called
Triludan Forte) and as a suspension for
dilution. (It may be purchased without a
prescription only in a limited quantity and
for children over six years).
+▲ side-effects/warning: see TERFENADINE

TrimaxCo

(Ashbourne) is a proprietary prescription-
only COMPOUND PREPARATION of the
(*potassium-sparing*) DIURETIC drug
triamterine and the (THIAZIDE) diuretic
drug hydrochlorothiazide (a combination
also called co-triamterzide 50/25). It can

be used in the treatment of oedema and as
an ANTIHYPERTENSIVE. It is available as
tablets.
+▲ side-effects/warning: see
HYDROCHLOROTHIAZIDE; TRIAMTERINE

trimeprazine tartrate

(alimemazine tartrate) is an
ANTIHISTAMINE drug that is chemically a
PHENOTHIAZINE DERIVATIVE. It can be used
to treat the symptoms of allergic
disorders, particularly urticaria (itchy skin
rash) and pruritis (itching). It also has
SEDATIVE and ANTINAUSEANT properties and
is used as a premedication prior to
surgery. Administration is oral in the form
of tablets and a syrup.
+▲ side-effects/warning: see under
ANTIHISTAMINE. Because of its sedative
property, the performance of skilled tasks such
as driving may be impaired.
◎ Related entry: Vallergan

trimetaphan camsilate

See TRIMETAPHAN CAMSYLATE

trimetaphan camsylate

(trimetaphan camsilate) is a GANGLION
BLOCKER drug. It lowers blood pressure by
reducing vascular tone normally induced
by the sympathetic nervous system. It is
short-acting and can be used as a
HYPOTENSIVE for controlled blood
pressure during surgery. Administration is
by injection or intravenous infusion.
+ side-effects: there may be an increase in
the heart rate and depression of respiration,
increased intraocular pressure, dilated pupils
and constipation.
▲ warning: it should be administered with
caution to patients with certain heart or
kidney disorders, diabetes, Addison's disease,
degenerative disease of the brain and in the
elderly. It is not to be given to patients who are
pregnant or with severe arteriosclerosis.
◎ Related entry: Arfonad

trimethoprim

is an ANTIBACTERIAL drug, which is similar

to the SULPHONAMIDES. It is used to treat and prevent the spread of many forms of bacterial infection, but particularly infections of the urinary and respiratory tracts. It has been used in combination with the sulphonamide drug SULPHAMETHOXAZOLE, because the combined effect is considered to be greater than twice the individual effect of either drug. This is the basis of the medicinal compound CO-TRIMOXAZOLE. More recently there has been a move away from the compound preparation to the use of trimethoprim alone. It is effective in many situations and lacks the side-effects of sulphamethoxazole. Administration is either oral as tablets or a suspension, or by injection.

✚ side-effects: there may be nausea, vomiting and gastrointestinal disturbances; rashes may break out with pruritus (itching) and there msy be effects on blood constituents.

▲ warning: it should not be administered to newborn babies; to patients who are pregnant; who have severely impaired kidney function, or porphyria. Dosage should be reduced for patients with poor kidney function, or who are breast-feeding. Prolonged treatment requires frequent blood counts.

❍ Related entries: Bactrim; Chemotrim; Comixco; Comox; Fectrim; Ipral; Laratrim; Monotrim; Polytrim; Septrin; Trimogal; Trimopan; Triprimix

Tri-Minulet

(Wyeth) is a proprietary, prescription-only COMPOUND PREPARATION that can be used as a (*triphasic*) ORAL CONTRACEPTIVE (and for also certain menstrual problems) of the type that combines an OESTROGEN and a PROGESTOGEN, in this case ethinyloestradiol and gestodene. It is available in the form of tablets in a calendar pack.

✚▲ side-effects/warning: see ETHINYLOESTRADIOL; GESTODENE

trimipramine

is an ANTIDEPRESSANT drug of the TRICYCLIC class. It is used to treat depressive illness, especially in cases where SEDATION is required. Administration is oral in the form of capsules or tablets.

✚▲ side-effects/warning: see under AMITRIPTYLINE HYDROCHLORIDE

❍ Related entry: Surmontil

Trimogal

(Lagap) is a proprietary, prescription-only preparation of the ANTIBACTERIAL drug trimethoprim. It can be used to treat infections of the upper respiratory tract (particularly bronchitis) and the urinary tract. It is available as tablets.

✚▲ side-effects/warning: see TRIMETHOPRIM

Trimopan

(Berk) is a proprietary, prescription-only preparation of the ANTIBACTERIAL drug trimethoprim. It can be used to treat infections of the upper respiratory tract (particularly bronchitis) and the urinary tract. It is available as a sugar-free suspension.

✚▲ side-effects/warning: see TRIMETHOPRIM

Trimovate

(Glaxo) is a proprietary, prescription-only COMPOUND PREPARATION of the CORTICOSTEROID drug clobetasone butyrate, the ANTIBACTERIAL and (TETRACYCLINE) ANTIBIOTIC drug oxytetracycline and the ANTIFUNGAL and antibiotic drug nystatin. It can be used to treat skin infections and is available as a cream for topical application.

✚▲ side-effects/warning: see CLOBETASONE BUTYRATE; NYSTATIN; OXYTETRACYCLINE

Trinordiol

(Wyeth) is a proprietary, prescription-only COMPOUND PREPARATION that can be used as a (*triphasic*) ORAL CONTRACEPTIVE (and for certain menstrual problems) of the type that combines an OESTROGEN and a PROGESTOGEN, in this case ethinyloestradiol and levonorgestrel. It is

T

available in the form of tablets in a
calendar pack.
✚▲ side-effects/warning: see
ETHINYLOESTRADIOL; LEVONORGESTREL

TriNovum

(Ortho) is a proprietary, prescription-only
COMPOUND PREPARATION that can be used
as a (*triphasic*) ORAL CONTRACEPTIVE (and
also for certain menstrual problems) of
the type that combines an OESTROGEN and
a PROGESTOGEN, in this case
ethinyloestradiol and norethisterone. It is
available in the form of tablets in a
calendar pack.
✚▲ side-effects/warning: see
ETHINYLOESTRADIOL; NORETHISTERONE

TriNovum ED

(Ortho) is a proprietary, prescription-only
COMPOUND PREPARATION that can be used
as a (*triphasic*) ORAL CONTRACEPTIVE (and
also for certain menstrual problems) of
the type that combines an OESTROGEN and
a PROGESTOGEN, in this case
ethinyloestradiol and norethisterone. It is
available in the form of tablets in a
calendar pack.
✚▲ side-effects/warning: see
ETHINYLOESTRADIOL; NORETHISTERONE

Triogesic Tablets

(Intercare Products) is a proprietary, non-
prescription COMPOUND PREPARATION of
the NON-NARCOTIC ANALGESIC drug
paracetamol and the SYMPATHOMIMETIC
and DECONGESTANT drug
phenylpropanolamine hydrochloride. It
can be used to treat nasal and sinus
congestion and associated pain. Unlike
many decongestants it is available as
tablets and is not normally given to
children under six years, except on
medical advice.
✚▲ side-effects/warning: see PARACETAMOL;
PHENYLPROPANOLAMINE HYDROCHLORIDE

Triominic

(Intercare Products) is a proprietary, non-

prescription COMPOUND PREPARATION of
the SYMPATHOMIMETIC and
VASOCONSTRICTOR drug
phenylpropanolamine hydrochloride and
the ANTIHISTAMINE pheniramine maleate. It
can be used as a NASAL DECONGESTANT for
the relief of nasal congestion and allergic
rhinitis. It is available as tablets and is not
normally given to children under six years,
except on medical advice.
✚▲ side-effects/warning: see
PHENIRAMINE MALEATE;
PHENYLPROPANOLAMINE HYDROCHLORIDE

Triperidol

(Lagap) is a proprietary, prescription-only
preparation of the ANTIPSYCHOTIC drug
trifluperidol. It can be used to treat
psychotic patients (including
schizophrenics), particularly those
experiencing manic, behavioural
disturbances. It is available as tablets.
✚▲ side-effects/warning: see
TRIFLUPERIDOL

tripotassium dicitratobismuthate

(bismuth chelate) is a CYTOPROTECTANT
drug. It coats the mucosa of the stomach
and can be used as an ULCER-HEALING
DRUG for benign peptic ulcers in the
stomach and duodenum. It may have a
specific action on the bacterial organism
Helicobacter pylori, which is associated
with peptic ulcers. Administration is oral
in the form of tablets or as a suspension.
✚ side-effects: the compound may darken the
tongue and the faeces and cause nausea and
vomiting.
▲ warning: it should not be given to patients
with kidney impairment or who are pregnant.
✪ Related entries: De-Nol; De-Noltab

Triprimix

(Ashbourne) is a proprietary,
prescription-only preparation of the
ANTIBACTERIAL drug trimethoprim. It can
be used to treat infections of the upper
respiratory tract (particularly bronchitis)

and the urinary tract. It is available as tablets.

✚▲ side-effects/warning: see TRIMETHOPRIM

triprolidine hydrochloride

is an ANTIHISTAMINE drug. It can be used for the symptomatic relief of allergic symptoms such as hay fever and urticaria (itchy skin rash). It is also used in some cough and decongestant preparations. Administration is oral in the form of tablets.

✚▲ side-effects/warning: see under ANTIHISTAMINE. Because of its sedative property, the performance of skilled tasks such as driving may be impaired.

❍ Related entries: Actifed Compound Linctus; Actifed Expectorant; Actifed Junior Cough Relief; Actifed Syrup; Actifed Tablets; Pro-Actidil

Triptafen

(Forley) is a proprietary, prescription-only COMPOUND PREPARATION of the ANITDEPRESSANT drug amitriptyline hydrochloride and the ANTIPSYCHOTIC drug perphenazine, in the ratio of 12.5:1. It can be used to treat depressive illness, particularly in association with anxiety and is available as tablets. *Triptafen-M* is a similar preparation but with a lower proportion of amitriptyline hydrochloride (5:1).

✚▲ side-effects/warning: see AMITRIPTYLINE HYDROCHLORIDE; PERPHENAZINE

Trisequens

(Novo Nordisk) is a proprietary, prescription-only COMPOUND PREPARATION of the female SEX HORMONES oestradiol and oestriol (both OESTROGENs) and norethisterone (as acetate; a PROGESTOGEN). It can be used to treat menopausal problems, including in HRT. It is available as tablets in the form of a calendar pack and also in a higher strength form, *Trisequens Forte*.

✚▲ side-effects/warning: see NORETHISTERONE; OESTRADIOL; OESTRIOL

trisodium edetate

is a CHELATING AGENT that binds to calcium and forms an inactive complex. It can therefore be used as an ANTIDOTE to treat conditions in which there is excessive calcium in the bloodstream (hypercalcaemia) and can also be used in the form of a solution to treat calcification of the cornea, or lime burns, of the eye. Administration for treating hypercalcaemia is by intravenous infusion and for the eye it is by topical application of a solution.

✚ side-effects: nausea, diarrhoea and cramps; pain in the limb where it is injected. An overdose may lead to kidney damage.

▲ warning: do not give to patients with impaired kidney function.

❍ Related entry: Limclair

Tritace

(Hoechst) is a proprietary, prescription-only preparation of the ACE INHIBITOR ramipril. It can be used as an ANTIHYPERTENSIVE and in HEART FAILURE TREATMENT, often in conjunction with other classes of drug. It is available as capsules.

✚▲ side-effects/warning: see RAMIPRIL

Trivax-AD

(Evans) is a proprietary, prescription-only version of the VACCINE preparation known as ADSORBED DIPHTHERIA, TETANUS and PERTUSSIS VACCINE (DTPer/Vac/Ads), when supplied direct by District Health Authorities and which is commonly referred to as *triple vaccine* because it combines the (toxoid) vaccines for diphtheria and pertussis (whooping cough) with the TETANUS VACCINE adsorbed onto a mineral carrier. It is available in a form for injection.

✚▲ side-effects/warning: see DIPHTHERIA VACCINES; PERTUSSIS VACCINE; TETANUS VACCINE

Trobicin

(Upjohn) is a proprietary, prescription-only preparation of the ANTIBACTERIAL and

T

(AMINOGLYCOSIDE) ANTIBIOTIC drug
spectinomycin. It is used specifically in the
treatment of gonorrhoea in patients who
are allergic to penicillins, or in cases
resistant to penicillins. It is available in a
form for injection.
✚▲ side-effects/warning: see
SPECTINOMYCIN

tropicamide

is a short-acting ANTICHOLINERGIC drug,
which can be used to dilate the pupil and
paralyse the focusing of the eye for
ophthalmic examination. Administration is
topical in the form of eye-drops.
✚▲ side-effects/warning: see under ATROPINE
SULPHATE; but there should be few side-effects
with topical administration, apart from
blurred vision. It should not be used in
patients with raised intraocular pressure
(pressure in the eyeball) .
❍ Related entries: Minims Tropicamide;
Mydriacyl; NODS Tropicamide.

tropisetron

is a recently introduced ANTI-EMETIC and
ANTINAUSEANT drug. It gives relief from
nausea and vomiting, especially in patients
receiving radiotherapy or chemotherapy
and where other drugs have been
ineffective. It acts by blocking the action of
the naturally occurring mediator
SEROTONIN. Administration is either oral as
capsules or by injection
✚ side-effects: constipation, diarrhoea,
abdominal pain, headache, fatigue and
dizziness (which may impair the performance
of skilled tasks such as driving).
▲ warning: administer with care to patients
with hypertension, or who are pregnant or
breast-feeding.
❍ Related entry: Navoban

Tropium

(DDSA Pharmaceuticals) is a proprietary,
prescription-only preparation of the
BENZODIAZEPINE drug chlordiazepoxide. It
can be used as an ANXIOLYTIC for the
short-term treatment of anxiety and to
alleviate acute alcohol withdrawal
symptoms. It is available as capsules.
✚▲ side-effects/warning: see
CHLORDIAZEPOXIDE

Trosyl

(Pfizer) is a proprietary, prescription-only
preparation of the ANTIFUNGAL drug
tioconazole. It can be used to treat fungal
infections of the nails and is available as a
cream and a nail solution.
✚▲ side-effects/warning: see TIOCONAZOLE

Tryptizol

(Morson) is a proprietary, prescription-
only preparation of the (TRICYCLIC)
ANTIDEPRESSANT drug amitriptyline
hydrochloride. It can be used in the
treatment of depressive illness, especially
in cases where sedation is required and
also to prevent bed-wetting at night by
children. It is available as tablets,
capsules, as a sugar-free liquid for dilution
and in a form for injection.
✚▲ side-effects/warning: see AMITRIPTYLINE
HYDROCHLORIDE

tryptophan

is an amino acid present in an ordinary,
well-balanced diet and from which the
natural body substance serotonin (5-
hydroxytryptamine; 5-HT) is derived.
Dysfunction of serotonin, in its
NEUROTRANSMITTER role in nerve-tracts in
the brain, is thought to contribute to
depression. Therapeutic administration of
tryptophan has been used in
ANTIDEPRESSANT treatment, but was
withdrawn from use because of an
association with a dangerous side-effect
called eosinophilia-myalgia syndrome. It
has been reintroduced for use in patients
only where no alternative treatment is
suitable and with registration and constant
blood-monitoring. Administration is oral
in the form of tablets.
✚ side-effects: light-headedness, drowsiness,
headache, nausea, eosinophilia-myalgia
syndrome.

▲ warning: it should not be administered to patients known to have defective metabolism of tryptophan in the diet, or who have a history of eosinophilia-myalgia syndrome. Administer with caution to those who are pregnant or breast-feeding.
○ Related entry. Optimax

TSH
See THYROTROPHIN

Tub/Vac/BCG (Dried)
is an abbreviation for the freeze-dried version of BCG VACCINE (against tuberculosis), which is administered by intradermal injection. See also Tub/Vac/BCG (Perc).

Tub/Vac/BCG (Perc)
is an abbreviation for the live version of BCG VACCINE (against tuberculosis) for *percutaneous* administration by multiple puncture of the skin. See also; TUB/VAC/BCG (DRIED).

tubocurarine chloride
is a *non-depolarizing* SKELETAL MUSCLE RELAXANT drug. It is used to induce muscle paralysis during surgery and is administered by injection.
✚ side-effects: histamine may be released, causing rash on the chest and neck; there may be a fall in blood pressure.
○ Related entry: Jexin

Tuinal
(Lilly) is a proprietary, prescription-only COMPOUND PREPARATION of the BARBITURATE drugs amylobarbitone (as sodium) and quinalbarbitone sodium and is on the Controlled Drugs List. It can be used as a HYPNOTIC to treat persistent and intractable insomnia and is available as tablets.
✚▲ side-effects/warning: see AMYLOBARBITONE; QUINALBARBITONE SODIUM

tulobuterol hydrochloride
is a SYMPATHOMIMETIC and BETA-RECEPTOR STIMULANT drug. It is mainly used as a BRONCHODILATOR in reversible obstructive airways disease and as an ANTI-ASTHMATIC treatment in severe acute asthma. It can also be used for the alleviation of symptoms of chronic bronchitis and emphysema. Administration is oral as tablets or a syrup.
✚▲ side-effects/warning: see under SALBUTAMOL. Avoid in pregnancy and certain kidney or liver disorders.
○ Related entries: Brelomax; Respacal

turpentine oil
is a COUNTER IRRITANT, or RUBEFACIENT, agent. It is included in certain COMPOUND PREPARATIONS that are used for the symptomatic relief of pain associated with rheumatism, neuralgia, fibrosis and sprains and stiffness of the joints. It is also used, along with other constituents, as an inhalant in DECONGESTANT preparations for the relief of cold symptoms.
○ Related entries: BN Liniment; Ellimans Universal Embrocation; Goddard's Embrocation; Mentholatum Deep Heat Rub; Secaderm; Tixylix Inhalant

Tylex
(Cilag) is a proprietary, prescription-only COMPOUND ANALGESIC preparation of the (OPIOID) NARCOTIC ANALGESIC and ANTITUSSIVE drug codeine phosphate and the NON-NARCOTIC ANALGESIC drug paracetamol (a combination known as co-codamol 30/500). It can be used as a painkiller and is available as capsules.
✚▲ side-effects/warning: see CODEINE PHOSPHATE; PARACETAMOL

Typhim VI
(Merieux) is a proprietary, prescription-only VACCINE preparation of the typhoid vaccine and is available in a form for injection.
✚▲ side-effects/warning: see TYPHOID VACCINE

T

Typhoid Vaccine

(Department of Health) is a non-proprietary, prescription-only VACCINE preparation of the typhoid vaccine and is available in a form for injection.

+▲ side-effects/warning: see
TYPHOID VACCINE

typhoid vaccine

is a suspension of dead typhoid bacteria. However, full protection is not guaranteed and travellers at risk are advised not to eat uncooked food or to drink untreated water. It is administered either orally or by deep subcutaneous or intramuscular injection.

Tyrocane Junior Antiseptic Lozenges

(Seton Healthcare) is a proprietary, non-prescription preparation of the ANTISEPTIC agent cetylpyridinium chloride. It can be used for the relief of minor throat infections. It is not normally given to children under six years, except on medical advice.

▲ warning: see CETYLPYRIDINIUM CHLORIDE

Tyrocane Throat Lozenges

(Seton Healthcare) is a proprietary, non-prescription COMPOUND PREPARATION of the ANTISEPTIC agents cetylpyridinium chloride and tyrothricin and the LOCAL ANAESTHETIC drug benzocaine. It can be used for the relief of pain and minor infections in the mouth and throat. It is not normally given to children under 12 years, except on medical advice.

+▲ side-effects/warning: see
BENZOCAINE; CETYLPYRIDINIUM CHLORIDE;
TYROTHRICIN

tyrothricin

is a weak ANTISEPTIC agent that is incorporated in some lozenges for sore throats.

✪ Related entries: Merocaine Lozenges;
Tyrocane Throat Lozenges; Tyrozets

Tyrozets

(Centra Healthcare) is a proprietary, non-prescription COMPOUND PREPARATION of the ANTISEPTIC agent tyrothricin and the LOCAL ANAESTHETIC drug benzocaine. It can be used to relieve minor mouth and throat irritations and is available as lozenges. It is not normally given to children under three years, except on medical advice.

+▲ side-effects/warning: see BENZOCAINE;
TYROTHRICIN

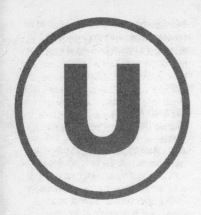

Ubretid
(Rhône-Poulenc Rorer) is a proprietary, prescription-only preparation of the ANTICHOLINESTERASE and PARASYMPATHOMIMETIC drug distigmine bromide. It can be used to stimulate bladder and intestinal activity and to treat myasthenia gravis. It is available as tablets or in form for injection.

+▲ side-effects/warning: see DISTIGMINE BROMIDE

Ucerax
(UCB Pharma) is a proprietary, prescription-only preparation of the ANTIHISTAMINE drug hydroxyzine hydrochloride, which has some additional ANXIOLYTIC properties. It can be used for the relief of allergic symptoms such as itching and mild rashes and also for short-term treatment of anxiety. It is available as tablets and as a syrup.

+▲ side-effects/warning: see HYDROXYZINE HYDROCHLORIDE

Ukidan
(Serono) is a proprietary, prescription-only preparation of the FIBRINOLYTIC drug urokinase. It can be used to treat serious conditions such as venous thrombi, pulmonary embolism, peripheral vascular occlusion, clots in the eye and myocardial infarction. It is available in a form for injection.

+▲ side-effects/warning: see UROKINASE

*ulcer-healing drugs
are used to promote healing of ulceration of the gastric (stomach) and duodenal (first part of small intestine) linings and so are used in the treatment of peptic ulcers. A number of classes of drugs may be used, including H₂-ANTAGONISTS (eg. CIMETIDINE and RANITIDINE), PROTON-PUMP INHIBITORS (eg. OMEPRAZOLE), selective ANTICHOLINERGIC drugs (eg. PIRENZEPINE), PROSTAGLANDIN analogues (eg. MISOPROSTOL), BISMUTH CHELATE COMPOUNDS (eg. TRIPOTASSIUM

U

U DICITATROBISMUTHATE) and certain other drugs with poorly understood modes of action, including LIQUORICE derivatives (eg. CARBENOXOLONE SODIUM). The first three classes act principally by reducing the secretion of peptic acid by the stomach's mucosal lining. The other drugs have complex actions that include a beneficial increase in blood flow to the mucosa, alterations in protective secretions, or antimicrobial actions against an infection by the bacterial organism *Helicobacter pylori*, which is associated with peptic ulcers. Other types of drug may reduce the discomfort of peptic ulcers without necessarily being ulcer-healing drugs (eg. ANTACIDS and non-specific antocholinergics).

Ultec

(Berk) is a proprietary preparation of the H₂-ANTAGONIST and ULCER-HEALING DRUG cimetidine. It is available on prescription or without a prescription in a limited amount and for short-term uses only. It can be used to treat benign peptic ulcers (in the stomach or duodenum), gastro-oesophageal reflux, dyspepsia and associated conditions. It is available as tablets.

+▲ side-effects/warning: see CIMETIDINE

Ultra Clearasil Maximum Strength

(Procter & Gamble) is a proprietary, non-prescription preparation of the KERATOLYTIC and ANTIMICROBIAL drug benzoyl peroxide (10%). It can be used to treat acne, spots and pimples and is available as a cream for topical application.

+▲ side-effects/warning: see BENZOYL PEROXIDE

Ultra Clearasil Regular Strength

(Procter & Gamble) is a proprietary, non-prescription preparation of the KERATOLYTIC and ANTIMICROBIAL drug benzoyl peroxide (5%). It can be used to treat acne, spots and pimples and is available as a cream for topical application.

+▲ side-effects/warning: see BENZOYL PEROXIDE

Ultradil Plain

(Schering Health) is a proprietary, prescription-only preparation of the CORTICOSTEROID and ANTI-INFLAMMATORY drug fluocortolone (as fluocortolone hexanoate and fluocortolone pivalate). It can be used to treat severe, inflammatory skin disorders such as eczema and psoriasis and is available as a cream and an ointment for topical application.

+▲ side-effects/warning: see FLUOCORTOLONE

Ultralanum Plain

(Schering Health) is a proprietary, prescription-only preparation of the CORTICOSTEROID and ANTI-INFLAMMATORY drug fluocortolone (as fluocortolone hexanoate and fluocortolone pivalate). It can be used to treat severe, inflammatory skin disorders such as eczema and psoriasis and is available as a cream and an ointment for topical application.

+▲ side-effects/warning: see FLUOCORTOLONE

Ultraproct

(Schering Health) is a proprietary, prescription-only COMPOUND PREPARATION of the CORTICOSTEROID and ANTI-INFLAMMATORY drug fluocortolone (as hexanoate) and the LOCAL ANAESTHETIC cinchocaine (as dibucaine hydrochloride). It can be used to treat haemorrhoids and is available as an ointment and suppositories for topical application.

+▲ side-effects/warning: see CINCHOCAINE; FLUOCORTOLONE

undecenoate

See UNDECENOIC ACID

undecenoic acid
and its salts (eg. zinc undecenoate) have ANTIFUNGAL activity and are incorporated into a number of topical preparations for the treatment of fungal infections of the skin, particularly athlete's foot. Administration is by ointments, creams, dusting powders, or shampoos.
○ **Related entries: Ceanel Concentrate; Mycota Cream; Mycota Powder; Mycota Spray**

Unguentum Merck
(Merck) is a proprietary, non-prescription COMPOUND PREPARATION of liquid paraffin, white soft paraffin and several other constituents. It can be used as an EMOLLIENT for dry skin and related disorders and is available as a cream.
+▲ side-effects/warning: see LIQUID PARAFFIN; WHITE SOFT PARAFFIN

Unihep
(Leo) is a proprietary, prescription-only preparation of the ANTICOAGULANT drug heparin (as heparin sodium). It can be used to treat various forms of thrombosis and is available in a form for injection.
+▲ side-effects/warning: see HEPARIN

Uniparin
(CP) is a proprietary, prescription-only preparation of the ANTICOAGULANT drug heparin (as heparin sodium). It can be used to treat various forms of thrombosis and is available in a form for injection.
+▲ side-effects/warning: see HEPARIN

Uniparin Calcium
(CP) is a proprietary, prescription-only preparation of the ANTICOAGULANT drug heparin (as heparin calcium). It can be used to treat various forms of thrombosis and is available in a form for injection.
+▲ side-effects/warning: see HEPARIN

Uniphyllin Continus
(Napp) is a proprietary, non-prescription preparation of the BRONCHODILATOR drug theophylline. It can be used as an ANTI-ASTHMATIC and to treat bronchitis. It is available as modified-release tablets for prolonged effect and a lower dose tablet for children.
+▲ side-effects/warning: see THEOPHYLLINE

Uniroid-HC
(Unigreg) is a proprietary, prescription-only COMPOUND PREPARATION of the CORTICOSTEROID hydrocortisone and the LOCAL ANAESTHETIC drug cinchocaine. It can be used by topical application to treat haemorrhoids and is available as an ointment and as suppositories.
+▲ side-effects/warning: see CINCHOCAINE; HYDROCORTISONE

Unisept
(Seton Healthcare) is a proprietary, non-prescription preparation of the ANTISEPTIC agent chlorhexidine (as gluconate). It can be used to clean wounds and is available in sachets for making up into a solution.
+▲ side-effects/warning: see CHLORHEXIDINE

Unisomnia
(Unigreg) is a proprietary, prescription-only preparation of the BENZODIAZEPINE drug nitrazepam. It can be used as a relatively long-acting HYPNOTIC for the short-term treatment of insomnia, where a degree of sedation during the daytime is acceptable. It is available as tablets.
+▲ side-effects/warning: see NITRAZEPAM

Univer
(Rhône-Poulenc Rorer) is a proprietary, prescription-only preparation of the CALCIUM-CHANNEL BLOCKER drug verapamil hydrochloride. It can be used as as an ANTIHYPERTENSIVE and an ANTI-ANGINA drug in the prevention of attacks. It is available as modified-release capsules.
+▲ side-effects/warning: see VERAPAMIL HYDROCHLORIDE

U

urea

is a chemical incorporated as a HYDRATING AGENT into a number of skin preparations, for example, creams that are used to treat eczema and psoriasis. It is also included in ear-drop preparations used for dissolving and washing out earwax.
○ Related entries: Alphaderm; Aquadrate; Calmurid; Calmurid HC; Exterol; Nutraplus; Otex; Psoradrate

Uriben

(RP Drugs) is a proprietary, prescription-only preparation of the ANTIBACTERIAL and (QUINOLONE) ANTIBIOTIC drug nalidixic acid. It can be used to treat infections, particularly those of the urinary tract and is available as an oral suspension.
+▲ side-effects/warning: see NALIDIXIC ACID

Urispas

(Syntex) is a proprietary, prescription-only preparation of the ANTICHOLINERGIC drug flavoxate hydrochloride. It can be used as an ANTISPASMODIC in the treatment of urinary frequency and incontinence and is available as tablets.
+▲ side-effects/warning: see FLAVOXATE HYDROCHLORIDE

urofollitrophin

is a form of the pituitary HORMONE follicle-stimulating hormone (FSH), which is also found in and can be prepared from, urine from menopausal women. Urofollitrophin is used as an infertility treatment in women whose infertility is due to abnormal pituitary gland function, or who do not respond to the commonly used fertility drug clomiphene citrate. It is also used in superovulation treatment for assisted conception, such as in *in vitro* fertilization.
+▲ side-effects/warning: see under HUMAN MENOPAUSAL GONADOTROPHINS
○ Related entries: Metrodin High Purity; Orgafol

Urokinase

(Leo) is a proprietary, prescription-only preparation of the FIBRINOLYTIC drug urokinase. It can be used to treat serious conditions such as venous thrombi, pulmonary embolism, peripheral vascular occlusion, clots in the eye and myocardial infarction. It is available in a form for injection.
+▲ side-effects/warning: see UROKINASE

urokinase

is an enzyme that is used therapeutically as a FIBRINOLYTIC drug, because it has the property of breaking up blood clots by activating plasmin formation, which then digests the fibrin that forms the clot. It can be used rapidly in serious conditions such as venous thrombi, pulmonary embolism, peripheral vascular occlusion and clots in the eye. Administration is by injection.
+ side-effects: nausea, vomiting and bleeding.
▲ warning: it should not be administered to patients with disorders of coagulation; who are liable to bleed (vaginal bleeding, peptic ulceration, recent trauma or surgery); acute pancreatitis, oesophageal varices, or who are pregnant.
○ Related entries: Ukidan; Urokinase

Uromitexan

(ASTA Medica) is a proprietary, prescription-only preparation of of the drug MESNA. It is used to combat the haemorrhagic cystitis, which is a serious complication caused by certain CYTOTOXIC DRUGS. It is available in a form for injection.
+▲ side-effects/warning: see MESNA

ursodeoxycholic acid

is a drug that can dissolve some gallstones *in situ*. Administration is oral in the form of capsules or tablets.
+▲ side-effects/warning: see under CHENODEOXYCHOLIC ACID; though liver

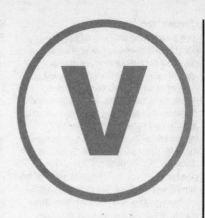

changes have not been reported and diarrhoea is rare.
○ Related entries: Combidol; Destolit; Ursofalk

Ursofalk
(Thames) is a proprietary, prescription-only preparation of ursodeoxycholic acid. It can be used to dissolve gallstones and is available as capsules.
+▲ side-effects/warning: see URSODEOXYCHOLIC ACID

Utinor
(Merck, Sharp & Dohme) is a proprietary, prescription-only preparation of the ANTIBACTERIAL and (QUINOLONE) ANTIBIOTIC drug norfloxacin. It can be used to treat infections, particularly of the urinary tract and is available as tablets.
+▲ side-effects/warning: see NORFLOXACIN

Utovlan
(Syntex) is a proprietary, prescription-only preparation of the PROGESTOGEN norethisterone. It can be used to treat uterine bleeding, abnormally heavy menstruation, endometriosis, premenstrual tension syndrome and other menstrual problems. In the form of tablets.
+▲ side-effects/warning: see NORETHISTERONE

Uvistat
(Windsor Healthcare) is the name of a range of proprietary, non-prescription SUNSCREEN preparations. The preparations contain titanium dioxide, ethylhexyl-methoxycinnaminate and avobenzone, which protect the skin from UVA and UVB ultraviolet radiation. They are available as skin creams (SPF30), a water-resistant cream (SPF20), babysun cream (SPF22) and as a lipscreen (SPF15). A patient whose skin condition requires one of these preparations may be prescribed it at the discretion of his or her doctor.

V

*vaccine

is a preparation that is used for IMMUNIZATION and to confer what is known as *active immunity* against specific diseases: that is, they cause a patient's own body to create a defence, in the form of antibodies, against the disease. Vaccines can be one of three types. The first type of vaccines are those administered in the form of a suspension of *dead* viruses (eg. INFLUENZA VACCINE) or bacteria (eg. TYPHOID VACCINE). The second type may be *live* but weakened, or attentuated, viruses (eg. RUBELLA VACCINE) or bacteria (eg. BCG VACCINE). The third and final type of vaccines are *toxoids*, which are suspensions containing extracts of the toxins released by the invading organism which then stimulate the formation of antibodies against the toxin of the disease, rather than the organism itself. Vaccines that incorporate dead micro-organisms or toxoids generally require a series of administrations (most often three) to build up a sufficient supply of antibodies in the body. 'Booster' shots may thereafter be necessary at regular intervals to reinforce immunity, for example, after ten years in the case of the tetanus vaccine. Vaccines that incorporate live micro-organisms may confer immunity with a single dose, because the organisms multiply within the body, although some live vaccines still require three administrations, for example, oral poliomyelitis vaccine.

✚ side-effects: side-effects range from little or no reactions to severe discomfort, high temperature and pain; a mild form of the disease (eg. measles) and rarely, anaphylactic shock.

▲ warning: vaccination should not be administered to patients who have a febrile (feverish) illness or any form of infection. Vaccines containing live material should not be administered routinely to patients who are pregnant, or who are known to have an immunodeficiency disorder.

580 ✪ Related entries: adsorbed diphtheria

and tetanus vaccine; adsorbed diphtheria, anthrax vaccine; cholera vaccine; diphtheria vaccines; hepatitis B vaccine; measles vaccine; meningococcal polysaccharide vaccine; MMR vaccine; MR vaccine; pertussis vaccine; pneumococcal vaccine; poliomyelitis vaccine; rabies vaccine; smallpox vaccine; tetanus and pertussis vaccine; tetanus vaccine; yellow fever vaccine

Vagifem

(Novo Nordisk) is a proprietary, prescription-only preparation of the female SEX HORMONE oestradiol (an OESTROGEN). It can be used to treat conditions of the vagina caused by hormonal deficiency (generally, atrophic vaginitis in the menopause). It is available as vaginal tablets (pessaries) that come with disposable applicators.

✚▲ side-effects/warning: see OESTRADIOL

Vaginyl

(DDSA Pharmaceuticals) is a proprietary, prescription-only preparation of the ANTIMICROBIAL drug metronidazole, which has both ANTIPROTOZOAL and ANTIBACTERIAL properties. It can be used to treat a range of infections, including those that may occur following surgery, vaginosis and dental infections and ulcers. The antiprotozoal activity is effective against the organisms that cause amoebic dysentery, giardiasis and trichomoniasis. It is available as tablets.

✚▲ side-effects/warning: see METRONIDAZOLE

Valclair

(Sinclair) is a proprietary, prescription-only preparation of the BENZODIAZEPINE drug diazepam. It can be used as an ANXIOLYTIC for the short-term treatment of anxiety, as a HYPNOTIC to relieve insomnia, as an ANTICONVULSANT and ANTI-EPILEPTIC for status epilepticus, as a SEDATIVE in preoperative medication, as a SKELETAL

MUSCLE RELAXANT and to help alleviate alcohol withdrawal symptoms. It is available as suppositories.

✚▲ side-effects/warning: see DIAZEPAM

Valenac

(Shire) is a proprietary, prescription-only preparation of the (NSAID) NON-NARCOTIC ANALGESIC and ANTIRHEUMATIC drug diclofenac sodium. It can be used to treat arthritic and rheumatic pain and other musculoskeletal disorders. It is available as tablets.

✚▲ side-effects/warning: see DICLOFENAC SODIUM

Valium

(Roche) is a proprietary, prescription-only preparation of the BENZODIAZEPINE drug diazepam. It can be used as an ANXIOLYTIC for the short-term treatment of anxiety, as a HYPNOTIC to relieve insomnia, as an ANTICONVULSANT and ANTI-EPILEPTIC for status epilepticus, as a SEDATIVE in preoperative medication, as a SKELETAL MUSCLE RELAXANT and to help alleviate alcohol withdrawal symptoms. It is available as tablets, an oral solution and a form for injection.

✚▲ side-effects/warning: see DIAZEPAM

Vallergan

(Rhône-Poulenc Rorer) is a proprietary, prescription-only preparation of the ANTIHISTAMINE drug trimeprazine tartrate. It can be used to treat the symptoms of allergic disorders, particularly urticaria and pruritis. It also has SEDATIVE and ANTINAUSEANT properties and can be used for premedication prior to surgery. It is available as tablets and a syrup.

✚▲ side-effects/warning: SEE TRIMEPRAZINE TARTRATE

Valoid

(Wellcome) is a proprietary, preparation of the ANTIHISTAMINE and ANTINAUSEANT drug cyclizine (as lactate). It can be used to treat nausea, vomiting, vertigo, motion sickness and disorders of the balance function of the inner ear. It is available without prescription as tablets and in a form for injection only on prescription.

✚▲ side-effects/warning: see ANTIHISTAMINE; CYCLIZINE

valproic acid

See under SODIUM VALPROATE

Valrox

(Shire) is a proprietary, prescription-only preparation of the (NSAID) NON-NARCOTIC ANALGESIC and ANTIRHEUMATIC drug naproxen. It can be used to relieve the pain of musculoskeletal disorders, particularly rheumatic and arthritic pain and acute gout. It is available as tablets.

✚▲ side-effects/warning: see NAPROXEN

Vancocin

(Lilly) is a proprietary, prescription-only preparation of the ANTIBACTERIAL and ANTIBIOTIC drug vancomycin (as hydrochloride). It can be used to treat certain infections such as pseudomembranous colitis and certain types of endocarditis. It is available as capsules (*Matrigel*) and in a form for injection.

✚▲ side-effects/warning: see VANCOMYCIN

vancomycin

is an ANTIBACTERIAL and ANTIBIOTIC drug. It is primarily active against Gram-positive bacteria and works by inhibiting the synthesis of components of the bacterial cell wall. It is only used in special situations, for example in the treatment of pseudomembranous colitis (a superinfection of the gastrointestinal tract), which can occur after treatment with broad-spectrum antibiotics. Another use is in the treatment of multiple-drug-resistant staphylococcal infections, particularly endocarditis. Administration is oral as capsules to treat colitis and by infusion for systemic infections.

✚ side-effects: these include kidney damage

V

and tinnitus (ringing in the ears). There may be blood disorders, chills, fever, rashes and other complications.

▲ warning: it should not be administered to patients with impaired kidney function, or who are deaf. Administer with caution to patients who are pregnant or breast-feeding. Blood counts, kidney function tests and hearing tests are required.

○ Related entry: Vancocin

Varicella-Zoster Immunoglobulin (VZIG)

(Public Health Laboratory Service) (Antivaricella-Zoster Immunoglobulin) is a non-proprietary, prescription-only preparation of a SPECIFIC IMMUNOGLOBULIN and is used to give immediate immunity against infection by varicella-zoster (chickenpox) virus. Administration is by intramuscular injection.

varicella-zoster immunoglobulin (VZiG)

is a SPECIFIC IMMUNOGLOBULIN, which is a form of immunoglobulin that is used in IMMUNIZATION to give immediate *passive immunity* against infection by the varicella-zoster virus (chickenpox), but is used only in IMMUNOSUPPRESSED patients at risk, including infants and pregnant women. (Varicella VACCINE is also available, but only on a named-patient basis). Administration is by intramuscular injection.

○ Related entry: Varicella-Zoster Immunoglobulin (VZIG)

Varidase Topical

(Lederle) is a proprietary, prescription-only preparation of the powdered enzymes streptokinase and streptodornase. It can be used, with a desloughing agent, to cleanse and soothe skin ulcers. It can also be administered through a catheter to dissolve clots in the urinary bladder. It is available as a powder.

➕▲ side-effects/warning: see STREPTOKINASE

Var/Vac

is an abbreviation for variola vaccine (in fact made from vaccinia virus). See SMALLPOX VACCINE

Vascace

(Roche) is a proprietary, prescription-only preparation of the ACE INHIBITOR cilazapril. It can be used as an ANTIHYPERTENSIVE in conjunction with other classes of drug, particularly (THIAZIDE) DIURETICS. It is available as tablets.

➕▲ side-effects/warning: see CILAZAPRIL

Vaseline Dermacare

(Elida Gibbs) is a proprietary, non-prescription COMPOUND PREPARATION of white soft paraffin and dimethicone. It can be used as an EMOLLIENT for dry skin, eczema, scaly or itchy skin and related disorders. It is available as a cream and a lotion.

➕▲ side-effects/warning: DIMETHICONE; WHITE SOFT PARAFFIN

*vasoconstrictor

drugs cause a narrowing (constricting) of the blood vessels and therefore a reduction in blood flow and an increase in blood pressure. They are used to increase blood pressure in circulatory disorders, in cases of shock, or in cases where pressure has fallen during lengthy or complex surgery. Different vasoconstrictors work in different ways, but many are SYMPATHOMIMETICS with alpha-adrenoceptor stimulant properties. Most vasoconstrictors have an effect on mucous membranes and therefore may be used to relieve nasal congestion (eg. OXYMETAZOLINE HYDROCHLORIDE and XYLOMETAZOLINE HYDROCHLORIDE). Some are used to prolong the effects of local anaesthetics (eg. ADRENALINE). Vasoconstrictors used in circulatory shock include NORADRENALINE, METHOXAMINE HYDROCHLORIDE and PHENYLEPHRINE HYDROCHLORIDE.

*vasodilator

drugs dilate blood vessels and thereby increase blood flow. Theoretically, they would be expected to be HYPOTENSIVE and therefore could be used to lower blood pressure. However, in practice, there may be compensatory mechanisms that maintain blood pressure by redistributing blood within the body, or by changing heart function. Drugs of this class work in a number of different ways: some are SMOOTH MUSCLE RELAXANTS that act directly on the blood vessels (eg. nitrite and nitrate compounds and CALCIUM-CHANNEL BLOCKERS); whereas others act indirectly by blocking or modifying the action of HORMONES or NEUROTRANSMITTERS (eg. ALPHA-ADRENOCEPTOR BLOCKERS and ACE INHIBITORS). Vasodilator drugs are used for a number of purposes, including as ANTI-ANGINA drugs (eg. GLYCERYL TRINITRATE), in acute hypertensive crisis (eg. SODIUM NITROPRUSSIDE), as ANTIHYPERTENSIVES to treat chronic raised blood pressure (eg. HYDRALAZINE HYDROCHLORIDE and NIFEDIPINE) and to treat poor circulation in the extremities (peripheral vascular disease, or Raynaud's Phenomenon: eg. INOSITOL NICOTINATE).

Vasogen Cream

(Pharmax) is a proprietary, non-prescription COMPOUND PREPARATION of zinc oxide, dimethicone and calamine. It can be used for nappy rash, bedsores and the skin around a stoma (an outlet on the skin surface following surgical curtailment of the intestines). It is available as a cream.

+▲ side-effects/warning: see CALAMINE; DIMETHICONE; ZINC OXIDE

vasopressin

is one of the pituitary HORMONES secreted by the posterior lobe of the pituitary gland. It is also known as *antidiuretic hormone*, or ADH. Therapeutically, it is used mainly to treat pituitary-originated diabetes insipidus, but it is a powerful

VASOCONSTRICTOR and can also be used to treat bleeding from varices (varicose veins) of the oesophagus. There are several forms of vasopressin (DESMOPRESSIN, LYPRESSIN and TERLIPRESSIN), which all differ in their duration of action and uses. Preparations include nose-drops, nasal spray, injections and solutions for infusion.

+ side-effects: peripheral vasoconstriction with pallor of skin; nausea, belching, abdominal cramps and an urge to defecate; hypersensitivity reactions, constriction of coronary arteries (possibly leading to angina and heart pain),

▲ warning: doses should be adjusted to individual response in order to balance water levels in the body. Great care is necessary in patients with asthma, epilepsy, certain kidney disorders, migraine, heart failure, who are pregnant, or have certain vascular disorders. Treatment must not be prolonged and should be carefully and regularly monitored; intermittent treatment is needed to avoid water overloading.

⊙ Related entry: Pitressin

Vasoxine

(Wellcome) is a proprietary, prescription-only preparation of the SYMPATHOMIMETIC and VASOCONSTRICTOR drug methoxamine hydrochloride. It can be used to treat cases of acute hypotension, particularly where blood pressure has dropped because of induction of general anaesthesia. It is available in a form for injection or infusion.

+▲ side-effects/warning: see METHOXAMINE HYDROCHLORIDE

vecuronium bromide

is a (*non-depolarizing*) SKELETAL MUSCLE RELAXANT drug. It is used to induce muscle paralysis during surgery and is administered by injection.

+▲ side-effects/warning: see under TUBOCURARINE CHLORIDE; but it does not generally cause the release of histamine.

⊙ Related entry: Norcuron

V

Veganin Tablets

(Warner Wellcome) is a proprietary, non-prescription COMPOUND ANALGESIC preparation of the NON-NARCOTIC ANALGESIC and ANTIRHEUMATIC drug aspirin, the non-narcotic and ANTIPYRETIC drug paracetamol and the (OPIOID) NARCOTIC ANALGESIC and ANTITUSSIVE drug codeine phosphate. It can be used to treat the symptoms of flu, headache, rheumatism, toothache and period pain. It is available as tablets and is not to be given to children under 12 years, except on medical advice.

✚▲ side-effects/warning: see ASPIRIN; CODEINE PHOSPHATE; PARACETAMOL

Veil

(Blake) is a proprietary, non-prescription preparation that is used to mask scars and other skin disfigurements. It is available as a cream and a powder and may be obtained on prescription under certain circumstances.

Velbe

(Lilly) is a proprietary, prescription-only preparation of the (CYTOTOXIC) ANTICANCER drug vinblastine sulphate. It can be used in the treatment of cancers, particularly lymphomas, acute leukaemias and some solid tumours. It is available in a form for injection.

✚▲ side-effects/warning: see VINBLASTINE SULPHATE

Velosef

(Squibb) is a proprietary, prescription-only preparation of the ANTIBACTERIAL and (CEPHALOSPORIN) ANTIBIOTIC drug cephradine. It can be used to treat a wide range of bacterial infections, particularly streptococcal infections of the skin and soft tissues, the urinary and upper respiratory tracts and middle ear; and also to prevent infection during surgery. It is available as capsules, a syrup and in a form for injection.

✚▲ side-effects/warning: see CEPHRADINE

Velosulin

(Novo Nordisk, Wellcome) is a proprietary form of highly purified porcine SOLUBLE INSULIN. It is used in DIABETIC TREATMENT for treating and maintaining diabetic patients. It is available in the form of vials for injection and has a short duration of action.

✚▲ side-effects/warning: see under INSULIN

venlafaxine

is an ANTIDEPRESSANT drug of the SSRI group. It can be used to treat depressive illness and has the advantage over some other antidepressant drugs in that it works by inhibiting uptake of the NEUROTRANSMITTERS SEROTONIN and NORADRENALINE and so has less sedative and ANTICHOLINERGIC side-effects. Administration is oral as tablets.

✚▲ side-effects/warning: see under FLUOXETINE. There may also be changes in liver enzymes.

○ Related entry: Efexor

Veno's Cough Mixture

(SmithKline Beecham) is a proprietary, non-prescription preparation of a syrup containing glucose and treacle. It is not normally given to children under three years, except on medical advice.

Veno's Expectorant

(SmithKline Beecham) is a proprietary, non-prescription preparation of the EXPECTORANT guaiphenesin with glucose and treacle. It is not normally given to children under three years, except on medical advice.

✚▲ side-effects/warning: see GUAIPHENESIN

Veno's Honey and Lemon

(SmithKline Beecham) is a proprietary, non-prescription preparation of a syrup containing lemon juice, honey and glucose. It is not normally given to children under one year, except on medical advice.

Ventide

(Allen & Hanburys) is a proprietary, prescription-only COMPOUND PREPARATION of the CORTICOSTEROID beclomethasone dipropionate and the SYMPATHOMIMETIC, BRONCHODILATOR and BETA-RECEPTOR STIMULANT drug salbutamol. It can be used as a treatment for the symptomatic relief of obstructive airways disease, as an ANTI-ASTHMATIC and to treat chronic bronchitis. It is available as an aerosol inhalant.

✚▲ side-effects/warning: see BECLOMETHASONE DIPROPIONATE; SALBUTAMOL

Ventodisks

(Allen & Hanburys) is a proprietary, prescription-only preparation of the BETA-RECEPTOR STIMULANT drug salbutamol (as salbutamol sulphate). It can be used as a BRONCHODILATOR in reversible obstructive airways disease, as an ANTI-ASTHMATIC treatment in severe acute asthma and for the alleviation of the symptoms of chronic bronchitis and emphysema. It is available in the form of disks for use with the *Diskhaler* device.

✚▲ side-effects/warning: see SALBUTAMOL

Ventolin

(Allen & Hanburys) is a proprietary, prescription-only preparation of the BETA-RECEPTOR STIMULANT drug salbutamol (as salbutamol sulphate). It can be used as a BRONCHODILATOR in reversible obstructive airways disease, as an ANTI-ASTHMATIC treatment in severe acute asthma and for the alleviation of the symptoms of chronic bronchitis and emphysema. It is available in many forms: as tablets, a sugar-free syrup, ampoules for injection, an infusion fluid, an aerosol-metered inhalant, as ampoules for nebulization spray (under the name *Nebules*), as a respirator solution and as a powder for inhalation (under the name *Rotacaps*).

✚▲ side-effects/warning: see SALBUTAMOL

Vepesid

(Bristol-Myers) is a proprietary, prescription-only preparation of the (CYTOTOXIC) ANTICANCER drug etoposide. It can be used in the treatment of cancers, particularly lymphoma or small cell carcinoma of the bronchus or testicle. It is available as capsules and in a form for injection.

✚▲ side-effects/warning: see ETOPOSIDE

Veracur

(Typharm) is a proprietary, non-prescription preparation of the KERATOLYTIC agent formaldehyde. It can be used to treat warts, especially verrucas (plantar warts) and is available as a gel.

✚▲ side-effects/warning: see FORMALDEHYDE

verapamil hydrochloride

is a CALCIUM-CHANNEL BLOCKER. It is used as an ANTI-ANGINA drug in the prevention and treatment of attacks, as an ANTI-ARRHYTHMIC to correct heart irregularities and as an ANTIHYPERTENSIVE treatment. Administration can be oral as tablets, capsules, or an oral liquid, or by injection or infusion.

✚ side-effects: there may be constipation, nausea and vomiting; headache, dizziness, flushing, fatigue; swollen ankles; rarely, there may be impairment of liver function; allergic skin reactions; gynaecomastia (enlargement of breasts in males); abnormal growth of the gums on prolonged treatment. After intravenous injection there may be a fall in blood pressure, a slowing of the heart, heart block, or heart irregularities.

▲ warning: it should not be taken by patients with certain heart disorders or porphyria. Administer with caution in patients with certain liver disorders and who are pregnant or breast-feeding.

✪ Related entries: Berkatens; Cordilox; Geangin; Half Securon SR; Securon; Securon SR; Univer

Veripaque

(Sanofi Winthrop) is a proprietary, non-

V

V prescription preparation of the (*stimulant*) LAXATIVE oxyphenisatin. It can be used to promote bowel movement (for instance, before colonic surgery or a barium enema) and is available as an enema.

✚▲ side-effects/warning: see OXYPHENISATIN

Vermox

(Janssen) is a proprietary, prescription-only preparation of the ANTHELMINTIC drug mebendazole. It can be used to treat infections by roundworm, threadworm, whipworm and hookworm and similar intestinal parasites. It is available as chewable tablets and a liquid oral suspension.

✚▲ side-effects/warning: see MEBENDAZOLE

Verrugon

(Pickles) is a proprietary, non-prescription preparation of the KERATOLYTIC agent salicylic acid. It can be used to used to remove warts and hard skin and is available as an ointment.

✚▲ side-effects/warning: see SALICYLIC ACID

Verucasep

(Galen) is a proprietary, non-prescription preparation of the KERATOLYTIC agent glutaraldehyde. It can be used to treat warts and to remove hard, dead skin. It is available as a gel for topical application to the skin.

✚▲ side-effects/warning: see GLUTARALDEHYDE

Vibramycin

(Invicta) is a proprietary, prescription-only preparation of the ANTIBACTERIAL and (TETRACYCLINE) ANTIBIOTIC drug doxycycline. It can be used to treat a wide range of infections and is available as capsules.

✚▲ side-effects/warning: see DOXYCYCLINE

Vibramycin D

(Invicta) is a proprietary, prescription-only preparation of the ANTIBACTERIAL and

(TETRACYCLINE) ANTIBIOTIC doxycycline. It can be used to treat a wide range of infections and is available as soluble tablets.

✚▲ side-effects/warning: see DOXYCYCLINE

Vicks Children's Vaposyrup

(Procter & Gamble) is a proprietary, non-prescription preparation of the (OPIOID) ANTITUSSIVE and NARCOTIC ANALGESIC drug dextromethorphan hydrobromide. It can be used for relieving and calming coughs and is available as a syrup. It is not normally given to children under three years, except on medical advice.

✚▲ side-effects/warning: see DEXTROMETHORPHAN HYDROBROMIDE

Vicks Coldcare Capsules

(Procter & Gamble) is a proprietary, non-prescription COMPOUND PREPARATION of the NON-NARCOTIC ANALGESIC and ANTIPYRETIC drug paracetamol, the ANTITUSSIVE and (OPIOID) NARCOTIC ANALGESIC drug dextromethorphan hydrobromide and the SYMPATHOMIMETIC and DECONGESTANT drug phenylpropanolamine hydrochloride. It can be used for the symptomatic relief of colds and flu and is available as capsules. It is not normally given to children under six years, except on medical advice.

✚▲ side-effects/warning: see DEXTROMETHORPHAN HYDROBROMIDE; PARACETAMOL; PHENYLPROPANOLAMINE HYDROCHLORIDE

Vicks Original Formula Cough Syrup

(Procter & Gamble) is a proprietary, non-prescription COMPOUND PREPARATION of the EXPECTORANT guaiphenesin, the ANTISEPTIC agent cetylpyridinium chloride and sodium citrate. It can be used for relieving a productive cough and is available as a syrup. It is not normally given to children under six years, except on medical advice.

+▲ side-effects/warning: see
CETYLPYRIDINIUM CHLORIDE;
GUAIPHENESIN

Vicks Sinex Decongestant Nasal Spray

(Procter & Gamble) is a proprietary, non-prescription preparation of the
SYMPATHOMIMETIC and VASOCONSTRICTOR drug oxymetazoline hydrochloride, along with menthol and cineole. It can be used as a NASAL DECONGESTANT for the symptomatic relief of nasal congestion associated with a wide variety of upper respiratory tract disorders, such as hay fever and colds. It is available as a nasal spray and is not normally given to children under six years, except on medical advice.
+▲ side-effects/warning: see
OXYMETAZOLINE HYDROCHLORIDE

Vicks Vaposyrup for Chesty Coughs

(Procter & Gamble) is a proprietary, non-prescription preparation of the EXPECTORANT guaiphenesin. It can be used for relieving coughs and to loosen the throat and is available as a syrup. It is not normally given to children under two years, except on medical advice.
+▲ side-effects/warning: see
GUAIPHENESIN

Vicks Vaposyrup for Chesty Coughs and Nasal Congestion

(Procter & Gamble) is a proprietary, non-prescription COMPOUND PREPARATION of the SYMPATHOMIMETIC and DECONGESTANT drug phenylpropanolamine hydrochloride and the EXPECTORANT guaiphenesin. It can be used for the short-term, symptomatic relief of nasal congestion and upper airways infections. It is available as a syrup and is not normally given to children under six years, except on medical advice.
+▲ side-effects/warning: see
GUAIPHENESIN; PHENYLPROPANOLAMINE HYDROCHLORIDE

Vicks Vaposyrup for Dry Coughs and Nasal Congestion

(Procter & Gamble) is a proprietary, non-prescription preparation of the (OPIOID) ANTITUSSIVE and NARCOTIC ANALGESIC drug dextromethorphan hydrobromide and the SYMPATHOMIMETIC and DECONGESTANT drug phenylpropanolamine hydrochloride. It can be used for the symptomatic relief of short-term upper airways infections. It is available as a syrup and is not normally given to children under six years, except on medical advice.
+▲ side-effects/warning: see
DEXTROMETHORPHAN HYDROBROMIDE;
PHENYLPROPANOLAMINE HYDROCHLORIDE

Videne

(DePuy) is a proprietary, non-prescription preparation of the ANTISEPTIC agent povidone-iodine. It can be used on the skin and is available as a dusting powder.
+▲ side-effects/warning: see
POVIDONE-IODINE

Videx

(Bristol-Myers) is a proprietary, prescription-only preparation of the ANTIVIRAL drug didanosine. It can be used in the treatment of AIDS and is available as tablets.
+▲ side-effects/warning: see DIDANOSINE

Vidopen

(Berk) is a proprietary, prescription-only preparation of the broad-spectrum ANTIBACTERIAL and (PENICILLIN) ANTIBIOTIC drug ampicillin. It can be used to treat systemic bacterial infections, infections of the upper respiratory tract, of the ear, nose and throat and the urinogenital tracts. It is available as capsules.
+▲ side-effects/warning: see
AMPICILLIN

vigabatrin

is an ANTI-EPILEPTIC drug, which is used to

V treat chronic epilepsy, especially in cases where other anti-epileptic drugs have not been effective. Administration is oral as tablets or a powder.

✚ side-effects: there may be fatigue, dizziness, drowsiness, depression, headache, nervousness and irritability, confusion, aggression, memory, visual and gastrointestinal disturbances; weight gain; psychotic episodes and excitation and agitation in children.

▲ warning: administer with caution to patients with kidney impairment, or where there is a history of psychosis or behavioural problems.

○ Related entry: Sabril

Villescon

(Boehringer Ingelheim) is a proprietary, prescription-only COMPOUND PREPARATION of the weak STIMULANT prolintane, VITAMIN B group and VITAMIN C. It can be used to treat debility or fatigue and is available as a liquid.

✚▲ side-effects/warning: see PROLINTANE

viloxazine hydrochloride

is a TRICYCLIC-related ANTIDEPRESSANT drug. It is less SEDATING than many other antidepressants and dosage must be carefully monitored to maintain the optimum effect for each patient. It is administered orally in the form of tablets.

✚▲ side-effects/warning: see under AMITRIPTYLINE HYDROCHLORIDE; but it has less sedative, anticholinergic and cardiovascular actions. Headache and nausea may occur.

○ Related entry: Vivalan

vinblastine sulphate

is a CYTOTOXIC DRUG and is one of the VINCA ALKALOIDS. It can be used as an ANTICANCER treatment of acute leukaemias, lymphomas and some solid tumours. Administration is by injection.

✚▲ side-effects/warning: see under CYTOTOXIC DRUGS; VINCA ALKALOIDS

○ Related entry: Velbe

Vinca alkaloids

are a type of CYTOTOXIC DRUG derived from the periwinkle *Vinca rosea*. They work by halting the process of cell replication and are thus used as ANTICANCER drugs, particularly for acute leukaemias, lymphomas and some solid tumours. Their toxicity inevitably causes some serious side-effects, in particular some loss of neural nerve function at the extremities, constipation and bloating, all of which may be severe.

See: VINBLASTINE SULPHATE;
VINCRISTINE SULPHATE;
VINDESINE SULPHATE

vincristine sulphate

is a CYTOTOXIC DRUG and one of the VINCA ALKALOIDS. It is used as an ANTICANCER drug, particularly in the treatment of acute leukaemias, lymphomas and some solid tumours. Administration is by injection.

✚▲ side-effects/warning: see under CYTOTOXIC DRUGS; VINCA ALKALOIDS. It causes little myelosuppression.

○ Related entry: Oncovin

vindesine sulphate

is a CYTOTOXIC DRUG and one of the VINCA ALKALOIDS. It is used as an ANTICANCER drug, particularly in the treatment of leukaemias, lymphomas and some solid tumours. Administration is by injection.

✚▲ side-effects/warning: see under CYTOTOXIC DRUGS; VINCA ALKALOIDS

○ Related entry: Eldisine

Vioform-Hydrocortisone

(Zyma Healthcare) is a proprietary, prescription-only COMPOUND PREPARATION of the CORTICOSTEROID drug hydrocortisone and the ANTIMICROBIAL drug clioquinol. It can be used to treat inflammatory skin disorders and is available as a water-based cream and an ointment.

✚▲ side-effects/warning: see CLIOQUINOL; HYDROCORTISONE

Viraferon

(Schering-Plough)is a proprietary, prescription-only preparation of the drug interferon (in the form alpha-2b, rbe). It can be used in the treatment of chronic active hepatitis B and chronic hepatitis. It is available in a form for injection.
+▲ side-effects/warning: see INTERFERON

Virazid

(Britannia) is a proprietary, prescription-only preparation of the ANTIVIRAL drug tribavirin. It can be used to treat severe bronchiolitis caused by the syncytial virus in infants and some other serious diseases (including lassa fever). It is available in a form for inhalation.
+▲ side-effects/warning: see TRIBAVIRIN

Virormone

(Paines & Byrne) is a proprietary, prescription-only preparation of the male SEX HORMONE testosterone (as testosterone propionate). In men, it can be used in hormone replacement therapy and for delayed puberty; in women, as an ANTICANCER drug for breast cancer. It is available in a form for injection.
+▲ side-effects/warning: see TESTOSTERONE

Virudox

(Bioglan) is a proprietary, prescription-only preparation of the ANTIVIRAL drug idoxuridine (in the organic solvent dimethyl sulphoxide; DMSO). It can be used to treat infections of the skin by herpes simplex or herpes zoster. It is available in a form for topical application.
+▲ side-effects/warning: see IDOXURIDINE

Visclair

(Sinclair) is a proprietary, non-prescription preparation of the MUCOLYTIC and EXPECTORANT drug methyl cysteine hydrochloride. It can be used to reduce the viscosity of sputum and thus facilitate expectoration in patients with chronic asthma or bronchitis. It is available as tablets.
+▲ side-effects/warning: see METHYL CYSTEINE HYDROCHLORIDE

Viscotears

(CIBA Vision) is a proprietary, non-prescription preparation of carbomer. It can be used as artificial tears where there is dryness of the eye due to disease (eg. ketanoconjunctivitis). It is available as a liquid gel for application to the eye.
+▲ side-effects/warning: see CARBOMER

Viskaldix

(Sandoz) is a proprietary, prescription-only COMPOUND PREPARATION of the BETA-BLOCKER drug pindolol and the DIURETIC drug clopamide. It can be used as an ANTIHYPERTENSIVE treatment for raised blood pressure and is available as tablets.
+▲ side-effects/warning: see CLOPAMIDE; PINDOLOL

Visken

(Sandoz) is a proprietary, prescription-only preparation of the BETA-BLOCKER drug pindolol. It can be used as an ANTIHYPERTENSIVE treatment for raised blood pressure and as an ANTI-ANGINA treatment to relieve symptoms and improve exercise tolerance. It can also be used as an ANTIMIGRAINE treatment to prevent attacks. It is available as modified-release tablets.
+▲ side-effects/warning: see PINDOLOL

Vista-Methasone

(Daniels) is a proprietary, prescription-only preparation of the CORTICOSTEROID and ANTI-INFLAMMATORY drug betamethasone (as sodium phosphate). It can be used to treat inflammation in the ear, eye, or nose and is available as drops.
+▲ side-effects/warning: see BETAMETHASONE

Vista-Methasone-N

(Daniel) is a proprietary, prescription-

V only COMPOUND PREPARATION of the ANTI-INFLAMMATORY and CORTICOSTEROID drug betamethasone (as sodium phosphate) and the ANTIBACTERIAL and (AMINOGLYCOSIDE) ANTIBIOTIC drug neomycin sulphate. It can be used to treat inflammation in the ear, eye, or nose and is available as drops.

✚▲ side-effects/warning: see BETAMETHASONE; NEOMYCIN SULPHATE

vitamin A

is another term for RETINOL.

vitamin B

is the collective term for a number of water-soluble vitamins, which are found particularly in dairy products, cereals and liver. See: CYANOCOBALAMIN; FOLIC ACID; NICOTINAMIDE; NICOTINIC ACID

vitamin C

See ASCORBIC ACID

vitamin D

occurs in four main forms, D_1, D_2, D_3 and D_4, which are produced in plants or in human skin by the action of sunlight. Vitamin D facilitates the absorption of calcium and, to a lesser extent, phosphorus from the intestine and therefore promotes good deposition into the bones. A deficiency of vitamin D therefore results in bone deficiency disorders, such as rickets in children. It is readily available in a normal, well-balanced diet and particularly good sources include eggs, milk, cheese and fish-liver oil, which can be used as a dietary supplement. Vitamin D deficiency is commonly found in communities eating unleavened bread, in the elderly and where certain diseases prevent proper absorption from food. The preferred therapeutic method (despite the cost) of replacing vitamin D in cases of severe deficiency is by using quantities of one of the synthetic vitamin D analogues, such as ALFACALCIDOL, CALCITRIOL,

DIHYDROTACHYSTEROL and ERGOCALCIFEROL. However, as with most vitamins, prolonged administration of large doses can produce adverse effects (hypervitaminosis).

✚ side-effects: there may be nausea, vomiting, anorexia, lassitude, diarrhoea, weight loss, sweating, headache, thirst, dizziness and vertigo.

▲ warning: an overdose may cause kidney damage. Calcium levels should be monitored and use with care in those who are breast-feeding (high levels of calcium may reach the baby).

vitamin E

See TOCOPHEROL

Vitamin E Suspension

(Cambridge) is a proprietary, prescription-only preparation of alpha tocopheryl acetate (a form of vitamin E). It can be used to treat vitamin E deficiency and is available in the form of an oral suspension.

✚▲ side-effects/warning: see ALPHA TOCOPHERYL ACETATE

vitamin K

is a fat-soluble vitamin that occurs naturally in two forms, vitamin K_1 (also called PHYTOMENADIONE) and vitamin K_2 and is an essential requirement for a healthy body. Vitamin K_1 is found in food and particularly good sources include fresh root vegetables, fruit, seeds, dairy products and meat. Vitamin K_2 is synthesized in the intestine by bacteria and this source supplements the dietary form. Vitamin K is necessary for blood-clotting factors and is also important for the proper calcification of bone.

Both forms of the vitamin require the secretion of bile salts by the liver and fat absorption from the intestine in order to be taken up into the body. For this reason, when treating vitamin K deficiency due to malabsorption disorders (eg. due to obstruction of the bile ducts or in liver disease) a synthetic form, vitamin K_3

(usually called MENADIOL SODIUM PHOSPHATE) is administered, because it is water-soluble and therefore effective when taken orally in such disease states. However, in adults, deficiency of vitamin K is rare because it is so readily available in a normal, balanced diet, but medical administration may be required in fat malabsorption states where the intestinal flora is disturbed by ANTIBIOTICS or certain ANTICOAGULANTS (eg. nicoumalone). Vitamin K is given routinely to newborn babies to prevent vitamin-K-deficiency bleeding. Chronic overdose due to vitamin supplements (hypervitaminosis) can be dangerous.

✚ side-effects: there may be liver damage if high doses are taken for a long period.

▲ warning: it should be administered with caution to patients who are pregnant, or susceptible to red-blood-cell haemolysis due to G6PD enzyme deficiency or vitamin E deficiency.

vitamins

are substances required in small quantities for growth, development and proper functioning of the metabolism. Because many of the vitamin cannot be synthesized by the body, they must be obtained from a normal, well-balanced diet. The lack of any one vitamin causes a specific deficiency disorder, which may be treated by the use of vitamin supplements.

Vivalan

(Zeneca) is a proprietary, prescription-only preparation of the TRICYCLIC-related ANTIDEPRESSANT drug viloxazine hydrochloride. It can be used to treat depressive illness, particularly where a less SEDATIVE effect is required. It is available as tablets.

✚▲ side-effects/warning: see VILOXAZINE HYDROCHLORIDE

Vividrin

(Novex) is a proprietary, prescription-only preparation of the ANTI-ALLERGIC drug

sodium cromoglycate. It can be used to treat allergic conjunctivitis and is available as eye-drops, an eye ointment and a nasal spray. (It is available without a prescription subject to certain conditions of quantity and use.)

✚▲ side-effects/warning: see SODIUM CROMOGLYCATE

Vivotif

(Evans) is a proprietary, prescription-only VACCINE preparation of typhoid vaccine as a *live* attenuated oral vaccine. It is available as capsules.

✚▲ side-effects/warning: see TYPHOID VACCINE

Volital

(LAB) is a proprietary, prescription-only preparation of the weak STIMULANT pemoline. It can be used to treat hyperkinesis (hyperactivity) in children and is available as tablets.

✚▲ side-effects/warning: see PEMOLINE

Volmax

(DF) is a proprietary, prescription-only preparation of the BETA-RECEPTOR STIMULANT drug salbutamol (as salbutamol sulphate). It can be used as a BRONCHODILATOR in reversible obstructive airways disease, as an ANTI-ASTHMATIC treatment in severe acute asthma and for the alleviation of symptoms of chronic bronchitis and emphysema. It is available as tablets.

✚▲ side-effects/warning: see SALBUTAMOL

Volraman

(Eastern) is a proprietary, prescription-only preparation of the (NSAID) NON-NARCOTIC ANALGESIC and ANTIRHEUMATIC drug diclofenac sodium. It can be used to treat arthritic and rheumatic pain, other musculoskeletal disorders and acute gout. It is available as tablets.

✚▲ side-effects/warning: see DICLOFENAC SODIUM

V Voltarol

(Geigy) is a proprietary, prescription-only preparation of the (NSAID) NON-NARCOTIC ANALGESIC and ANTIRHEUMATIC drug diclofenac sodium. It can be used to treat arthritic and rheumatic pain and other musculoskeletal disorders. It is available as tablets, modified-release tablets (*Voltarol 75 mg SR, Voltarol Retard*), suppositories, paediatric suppositories and in a form for injection.

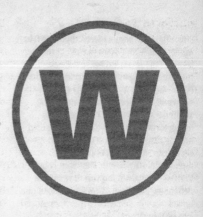

+▲ side-effects/warning: see DICLOFENAC SODIUM

Voltarol Emulgel

(Geigy) is a proprietary, prescription-only preparation of the (NSAID) NON-NARCOTIC ANALGESIC drug diclofenac sodium (as diethylammonium), which also has COUNTER-IRRITANT, or RUBEFACIENT, actions. It can be used for the symptomatic relief of underlying muscle or joint pain and is available as a gel for topical application to the skin. It is not normally used on children, except on medical advice.

+▲ side-effects/warning: see DICLOFENAC SODIUM; but adverse effects on topical application are limited.

Voltarol Optha

(CIBA Vision) is a proprietary, prescription-only preparation of the (NSAID) NON-NARCOTIC ANALGESIC drug diclofenac sodium. It can be used by topical application to inhibit contraction of the pupil of the eye and is available as eye-drops.

+▲ side-effects/warning: see DICLOFENAC SODIUM

VZIG

See VARICELLA-ZOSTER IMMUNOGLOBULIN (VZIG)

warfarin sodium

is an ANTICOAGULANT drug. It can be used
to prevent the formation of clots in heart
disease, after heart surgery (especially
following implantation of prosthetic heart
valves) and venous thrombosis and
pulmonary embolism. Administration is
oral in the form of tablets.
✚ side-effects: haemorrhaging.
▲ warning: it should be administered with
care to patients with certain kidney or liver
disorders and after recent operations. It
should not be used by patients with severe
hypertension, bacterial endocarditis, peptic
ulcer, or who are pregnant.
✿ Related entries: Marevan; Warfarin
WBP

Warfarin WBP

(Boehringer Ingelheim) is a proprietary,
prescription-only preparation of the
synthetic ANTICOAGULANT drug warfarin
sodium. It can be used to prevent the
formation of clots in heart disease, after
heart surgery (especially following
implantation of prosthetic heart valves)
and venous thrombosis and pulmonary
embolism. It is available as tablets.
✚▲ side-effects/warning: see WARFARIN
SODIUM

Warticon

(Perstorp) is a proprietary, prescription-
only preparation of the KERATOLYTIC agent
podophyllotoxin. It can be used by topical
application to treat and remove penile
warts and is available as a solution.
✚▲ side-effects/warning: see under
PODOPHYLLUM

Warticon Fem

(Perstorp) is a proprietary, prescription-
only preparation of the KERATOLYTIC agent
podophyllotoxin. It can be used to treat
and remove warts on the external genitalia
of women. It is available as a solution for
topical application.
✚▲ side-effects/warning: see under
PODOPHYLLUM

Waxsol

(Norgine) is a proprietary, non-
prescription preparation of docusate
sodium. It can be used for the dissolution
and removal of earwax and is available as
ear-drops.
✚▲ side-effects/warning: see DOCUSATE
SODIUM

Welldorm

(Smith & Nephew) is a proprietary,
prescription-only preparation of the
HYPNOTIC drug chloral hydrate (in the
form of chloral betaine). It can be used to
treat short-term insomnia in children and
the elderly and is available as tablets and
an elixir.
✚▲ side-effects/warning: see CHLORAL
HYDRATE

Wellferon

(Wellcome) is a proprietary, prescription-
only preparation of interferon (in the form
alpha-N1, 1ns). It can be used as
ANTICANCER drug in the treatment of hairy
cell leukaemia and chronic active hepatitis
B. It is available in a form for injection.
✚▲ side-effects/warning: see
INTERFERON

Wellvone

(Wellcome) is a proprietary, prescription-
only preparation of the ANTIPROTOZOAL
drug atovaquone. It can be used to treat
pneumonia caused by the protozoan
micro-organism *Pneumocystis carinii* in
patients whose immune system has been
suppressed. It is available as tablets.
✚▲ side-effects/warning: see
ATOVAQUONE

white soft paraffin

is used as a base for OINTMENTS and is
also incorporated into EMOLLIENT
preparations.
✿ Related entries: E45 Cream; Lacri-
Lube; Unguentum Merck; Vaseline
Dermacare; zinc and salicylic acid
paste, BP; zinc paste

W

W | **Whitfield's Ointment**
See BENZOIC ACID OINTMENT, COMPOUND, BP

wool alcohol
See WOOL FAT

wool fat
which contains lanolin, is a greasy preparation of hydrous wool fat in a yellow soft paraffin base. It is used as a protective BARRIER CREAM on cracked, dry or scaling skin and encourages hydration.
+▲ side-effects/warning: see under LANOLIN. Local reactions may occur in sensitive people.
✪ Related entries: E45 Cream; Hewletts Cream; Lubrifilm; Massé Breast Cream; Panda Baby Cream & Castor Oil Cream with Lanolin; simple eye ointment; Sprilon

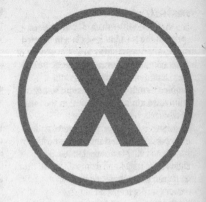

xamoterol

is a SYMPATHOMIMETIC and a weak BETA$_1$-RECEPTOR STIMULANT drug. It can be used as a CARDIAC STIMULANT in the treatment of heart conditions where moderate stimulation of the force of heartbeat is required, such as chronic moderate heart failure. Administration is oral in the form of tablets.

✚ side-effects: there may be headache, dizziness, hypotension and bronchospasm; there are some reports of palpitations and chest pains, rashes and cramps.

▲ warnings: it should not be given to patients with severe heart failure, when breast-feeding, or where certain other drugs are being used (especially cardiac glycosides and beta-receptor stimulant drugs for bronchoconstriction). Administer with caution in pregnancy, obstructive airways disease and certain heart and kidney disorders. Treatment will usually be initiated in hospital where full evaluation can be made.

❂ Related entry: Corwin

Xanax

(Upjohn) is a proprietary, prescription-only preparation of the BENZODIAZEPINE drug alprazolam. It can be used as an ANXIOLYTIC for the short-term treatment of anxiety and is available as tablets.

✚▲ side-effects/warning: see ALPRAZOLAM

xanthine-oxidase inhibitor

is an ENZYME INHIBITOR drug. It works by inhibiting the enzyme in the body that synthesizes uric acid and so can be used in the treatment of gout (because gout is caused by the deposition of uric acid crystal in the tissues). The most widely used xanthine-oxidase inhibitor is ALLOPURINOL, which is administered for the long-term treatment of gout.

Xanthomax

(Ashbourne) is a proprietary, prescription-only preparation of the ENZYME INHIBITOR allopurinol, which is a XANTHINE OXIDASE INHIBITOR. It can be used to treat excess uric acid in the blood and so prevent renal stones and attacks of gout. It is available as tablets.

✚▲ side-effects/warning: see ALLOPURINOL

Xatral

is a proprietary, prescription-only preparation of the ALPHA-ADRENOCEPTOR BLOCKER drug alfuosin. It can be used to treat urinary retention (eg. in benign prostatic hyperplasia) because of its SMOOTH MUSCLE RELAXANT properties. It is available as tablets.

✚▲ side-effects/warning: see ALFUOSIN

xipamide

is a DIURETIC drug of the THIAZIDE-related class. It can be used in ANTIHYPERTENSIVE treatment (either alone or in conjunction with other drugs) and also in congestive HEART FAILURE TREATMENT and associated oedema (accumulation of fluid in the tissues). Administration is oral in the form of tablets.

✚▲ side-effects/warning: see under BENDROFLUAZIDE. Also, there may be mild dizziness, gastrointestinal upsets and giddiness.

❂ Related entry: Diurexan

Xuret

(Galen) is a proprietary, prescription-only preparation of the THIAZIDE-like DIURETIC drug metolazone. It can be used, either alone or in conjunction with other drugs, as an ANTIHYPERTENSIVE. It is available as tablets.

✚▲ side-effects/warning: see METOLAZONE

Xylocaine

(Astra) is a series of proprietary, mainly prescription-only preparations of the LOCAL ANAESTHETIC drug lignocaine hydrochloride. They can be used for inducing anaesthesia or relieving pain by a variety of methods of application and at a number of sites. Some preparations include adrenaline as a SYMPATHOMIMETIC

X

and VASOCONSTRICTOR. Solutions and
forms for injection are available only on
prescription (including dental cartridges);
ointment, gel and spray preparations are
available without prescription.
+▲ side-effects/warning: see LIGNOCAINE
HYDROCHLORIDE

Xylocard

(Astra) is a proprietary, prescription-only
preparation of the LOCAL ANAESTHETIC drug
lignocaine hydrochloride. It can be used
as an ANTI-ARRHYTHMIC to treat
irregularities in the heartbeat, especially
after a heart attack and is available in a
form for injection.
+▲ side-effects/warning: see LIGNOCAINE
HYDROCHLORIDE

xylometazoline hydrochloride

is an alpha-adrenoceptor stimulant and
SYMPATHOMIMETIC drug with
VASOCONSTRICTOR properties, which is why
it is mainly used as a NASAL DECONGESTANT.
It is available as nose-drops and as a nasal
spray. It is also a constituent of some eye-
drop preparations that are used to treat
allergic conjunctivitis.
+▲ side-effects/warning: see under
EPHEDRINE HYDROCHLORIDE
**✪ Related entries: Otrivine Adult
Formula Drops; Otrivine Adult Formula
Spray; Otrivine Children's Formula
Drops; Otrivine-Antistin; Resiston One;
Rynacrom Compound**

Xyloproct

(Astra) is a proprietary, prescription-only
COMPOUND PREPARATION of the
CORTICOSTEROID drug hydrocortisone and
the LOCAL ANAESTHETIC drug lignocaine
hydrochloride (with aluminium acetate).
It can be used by topical application to
treat haemorrhoids and is available as an
ointment and as suppositories.
+▲ side-effects/warning: see
HYDROCORTISONE; LIGNOCAINE

HYDROCHLORIDE

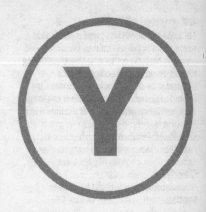

8Y

(BPL) is a proprietary, prescription-only preparation of dried human factor VIII fraction, which acts as a HAEMOSTATIC drug to reduce or stop bleeding in the treatment of disorders in which bleeding is prolonged and potentially dangerous (mainly haemophilia A). It is available in a form for intravenous infusion or injection

✚▲ side-effects/warning: see FACTOR VIII FRACTION, DRIED

Yel/Vac

is an abbreviation for YELLOW FEVER VACCINE

yellow fever vaccine

(Yel/Vac) is a VACCINE used for IMMUNIZATION consisting of a protein suspension containing *live*, but weakened (attenuated), yellow fever viruses that are cultured in chick embryos. Immunity lasts for at least ten years. The disease is still prevalent in parts of tropical Africa and northern South America. Administration is by subcutaneous injection.

✚▲ side-effects/warning: see under VACCINE. It should not be administered to those who are pregnant.

◯ Related entry: Arilvax

yellow soft paraffin

is used as a base for OINTMENTS and is also incorporated into EMOLLIENT preparations that are used for skin treatments.

◯ Related entries: LUBRIFILM; SIMPLE EYE OINTMENT

Yomesan

(Bayer) is a proprietary, non-prescription preparation of the ANTHELMINTIC drug niclosamide. It can be used to treat infestation by tapeworms and is available as chewable tablets.

✚▲ side-effects/warning: see NICLOSAMIDE

Yutopar

(Duphar) is a proprietary, prescription-only preparation of the BETA-ADRENOCEPTOR STIMULANT drug ritodrine hydrochloride. It can be used to prevent or delay premature labour and is available as tablets or in a form for intravenous infusion.

✚▲ side-effects/warning: see RITODRINE HYDROCHLORIDE

Z

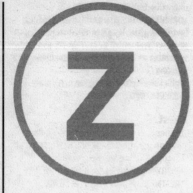

Zaditen

(Sandoz) is a proprietary, prescription-only preparation of the drug keftotifen (as hydrogen fumarate). It can be used as an ANTI-ASTHMATIC and is available as capsules, tablets and an elixir.

✚▲ side-effects/warning: see KEFTOTIFEN

Zadstat

(Lederle) is a proprietary, prescription-only preparation of the (AZOLE) ANTIMICROBIAL drug metronidazole, which has ANTIPROTOZOAL and ANTIBACTERIAL properties. It can be used to treat anaerobic infections, including those that may occur following surgery, vaginitis, dental infections and mouth ulcers. The antiprotozoal activity is effective against the organisms that cause amoebic dysentery, giardiasis and trichomoniasis. It is available as tablets and suppositories.

✚▲ side-effects/warning: see METRONIDAZOLE

Zagreb antivenom

(Regent) is a prescription-only, proprietary ANTIVENOM preparation. It can be used as an ANTIDOTE to the poison from an adder's bite. However, the systemic effects of the venom are rarely serious enough to warrant the use of the antivenom. It is available in a form for injection.

✚▲ side-effects/warning: see ANTIVENOM

zalcitabine

(DDC) is an ANTIVIRAL drug, which can be used in the treatment of AIDS patients who are intolerant to, or have not benefited from, the drug zidovudine. Administration is oral as tablets.

✚ side-effects: peripheral neuropathy, nausea, vomiting, mouth ulcers, anorexia, diarrhoea or constipation, abdominal pain, headache, dizziness, rash and other disorders.

▲ warning: it should not be used in patients with peripheral neuropathy, or who are breast-feeding. Administer with care where there is a history of pancreatitis or impaired

liver or kidney function.
○ Related entry: Hivid

Zantac

(Glaxo) is a proprietary, prescription-only preparation of the H₂-ANTAGONIST and ULCER-HEALING DRUG ranitidine hydrochloride. It can be used to treat benign peptic ulcers (in the stomach or duodenum), gastro-oesophageal reflux, dyspepsia and associated conditions. It is available as tablets, effervescent tablets, a syrup and in a form for infusion or injection.
✛▲ side-effects/warning: see RANITIDINE

Zantac 75

(Warner Wellcome) is a proprietary non-prescription preparation of the H₂-ANTAGONIST drug ranitidine (as hydrochloride). It can be used for the short-term relief of heartburn, dyspepsia and excess stomach acid. It is available as tablets.
✛▲ side-effects/warning: see RANITIDINE

Zarontin

(Parke-Davis) is a proprietary, prescription-only preparation of the ANTICONVULSANT and ANTI-EPILEPTIC drug ethosuximide. It can be used to treat absence (petit mal), myoclonic and some other types of seizure. It is available as capsules and a syrup.
✛▲ side-effects/warning: see ETHOSUXIMIDE

Zavedos

(Pharmacia) is a proprietary, prescription-only preparation of the (CYTOTOXIC) ANTICANCER drug idarubicin hydrochloride. It can be used to treat various cancers, particularly leukaemias and breast cancer. It is available as capsules and in a form for injection.
✛▲ side-effects/warning: see IDARUBICIN HYDROCHLORIDE

Zestoretic

(Zeneca) is a proprietary, prescription-only COMPOUND PREPARATION of the ACE INHIBITOR lisinopril and the (THIAZIDE) DIURETIC drug hydrochlorothiazide. It can be used as an ANTIHYPERTENSIVE and is available as tablets in two strengths, *Zestoretic 10* and *Zestoretic 20*.
✛▲ side-effects/warning: see HYDROCHLOROTHIAZIDE; LISINOPRIL

Zestril

(Zeneca) is a proprietary, prescription-only preparation of the ACE INHIBITOR lisinopril. It can be used as an ANTIHYPERTENSIVE and in HEART FAILURE TREATMENT. It is available as tablets.
✛▲ side-effects/warning: see LISINOPRIL

zidovudine

(azidothymidine; AZT) is an ANTIVIRAL drug that is used in the treatment of AIDS. Formerly, it was used for the treatment of advanced AIDS, but is now considered useful, by some, for the early forms of HIV virus infections before the full AIDS syndrome develops, including HIV-positive individuals who do not show symptoms of AIDS. It works by inhibiting the HIV virus and therefore delays progression of the disease, but does not cure it.
Administration is either oral as capsules or a syrup, or in a form for intravenous infusion.
✛ side-effects: there are many and may include disturbances in various blood cells, often to a degree requiring blood transfusions; nausea and vomiting, gastrointestinal disturbances, loss of appetite, headache, rashes, fever and sleep disturbances.
▲ warning: it should not be used where there is depression of neutrophils or haemoglobin, or when breast-feeding. Administer with care to those who are pregnant, have kidney or liver impairment, or are elderly. Avoid alcohol as its effects may be enhanced. Blood tests should be carried out.
○ Related entry: Retrovir

Zimovane

(Rhône-Poulenc Rorer is a proprietary,

S

Z non-prescription preparation of the
HYPNOTIC drug zopiclone. It can be used
for the short-term treatment of insomnia
and is available as tablets.
+▲ side-effects/warning: see ZOPICLONE

Zinacef

(Glaxo) is a proprietary, prescription-only
preparation of the ANTIBACTERIAL and
(CEPHALOSPORIN) ANTIBIOTIC drug
cefuroxime. It can be used to treat
bacterial infections and to prevent
infection during and following surgery. It
is available in a form for injection.
+▲ side-effects/warning: see CEFUROXIME

Zinamide

(Merck, Sharp & Dohme) is a proprietary,
prescription-only preparation of the
ANTIBACTERIAL drug pyrazinamide. It can
be used as an ANTITUBERCULAR drug,
usually in combination with other
antitubercular drugs and is available as
tablets.
+▲ side-effects/warning: see
PYRAZINAMIDE

zinc and salicylic acid paste, BP

(Lassar's paste) is a non-proprietary, non-
prescription preparation of the
ASTRINGENT agent zinc oxide and the
KERATOLYTIC agent salicylic acid, along
with starch in white soft paraffin. It can be
used in the treatment of psoriasis.
+▲ side-effects/warning: see
SALICYLIC ACID; WHITE SOFT PARAFFIN;
ZINC OXIDE

zinc oxide

is a mild ASTRINGENT agent, which is used
primarily to treat skin disorders such as
nappy rash, urinary rash and eczema. It is
available (without prescription) in any of
a number of compound forms: as a cream
with arachis oil, oleic acid and wool fat, or
with ichthammol and wool fat; as an
ointment and as an ointment with castor
oil; as a dusting powder with starch and

talc; as a paste with starch and white soft
paraffin, or with starch and zinc and
salicylic acid paste.
✪ Related entries: Anugesic-HC;
Anusol; Anusol-HC; Caladryl Cream;
Caladryl Lotion; calamine cream,
aqueous, BP; Germoline Ointment;
Germoloids; Hemocane; Hewletts
Cream; Morhulin Ointment;
Panda Baby Cream & Caster Oil Cream
with Lanolin; Sprilon; Ster-Zac Bath
Concentrates; Sudocrem Antiseptic
Cream; Vasogen Cream; zinc and
salicylic acid paste, BP; zinc paste

zinc paste

is a non-proprietary, ASTRINGENT
compound made up of zinc oxide and
white soft paraffin (and starch).
It is used as a base to which other
active constituents can be added,
especially within impregnated bandages.
Of all such pastes that are compounded to
treat and protect the lesions of skin
diseases such as eczema and psoriasis,
zinc paste is the standard type. There are
also pastes combining other active
substances, including *zinc and
ichthammol cream* and ZINC AND
SALICYLIC ACID PASTE, BP.
+▲ side-effects/warning: see under WHITE
SOFT PARAFFIN; ZINC OXIDE

zinc sulphate

is one form in which zinc supplements can
be administered in order to make up a
ZINC deficiency in the body. There are
several proprietary preparations that are
all different in form, though all are
adminsitered orally. In solution, zinc
sulphate is also used as an ASTRINGENT and
wound cleanser and also in eye-drops.
✚ side-effects: there may be abdominal pain
or mild gastrointestinal upsets.
✪ Related entries: Cicatrin; Efalith;
Polyfax; Tribiotic

zinc undecenoate

See UNDECENOIC ACID

Z

Zineryt

(Yamanouchi) is a proprietary, prescription-only preparation of the ANTIBACTERIAL and (MACROLIDE) ANTIBIOTIC drug erythromycin. It can be used to treat acne and is available as a solution for topical application.

+▲ side-effects/warning: see ERYTHROMYCIN

Zinnat

(Glaxo) is a proprietary, prescription-only preparation of the ANTIBACTERIAL and (CEPHALOSPORIN) ANTIBIOTIC drug cefuroxime. It can be used to treat bacterial infections and to prevent infection during and following surgery. It is available as tablets, sachets and an oral suspension.

+▲ side-effects/warning: see CEFUROXIME

Zirtek

(UCB Pharma) is a proprietary, prescription-only preparation of the ANTIHISTAMINE drug cetirizine. It can be used to treat the symptoms of allergic disorders such as hay fever and urticaria. It is available as tablets and an oral solution.

+▲ side-effects/warning: see CETIRIZINE

Zita

(Eastern) is a proprietary preparation of the H$_2$-ANTAGONIST and ULCER-HEALING DRUG cimetidine. It is available on prescription or without a prescription in a limited amount and for short-term uses only. It can be used to treat benign peptic ulcers (in the stomach or duodenum), gastro-oesophageal reflux, dyspepsia and associated conditions. It is available as tablets.

+▲ side-effects/warning: see CIMETIDINE

Zithromax

(Richborough) is a proprietary, prescription-only preparation of the ANTIBACTERIAL and (MACROLIDE) ANTIBIOTIC drug azithromycin. It can be used to treat and prevent many forms of infection and is usually used as an alternative to penicillin-type antibiotics in patients who are allergic to penicillin, or whose infections are resistant to penicillin. It is available as capsules and an oral suspension.

+▲ side-effects/warning: see AZITHROMYCIN

Zocor

(Merck, Sharp & Dohme) is a proprietary, prescription-only preparation of the the LIPID-LOWERING DRUG simvastatin. It can be used in hyperlipidaemia to reduce the levels, or change the proportions, of various lipids in the bloodstream. It is available as tablets.

+▲ side-effects/warning: see SIMVASTATIN

Zofran

(Glaxo) is a proprietary, prescription-only preparation of the ANTI-EMETIC and ANTINAUSEANT drug ondansetron. It can be used to give relief from nausea and vomiting, especially in patients receiving radiotherapy or chemotherapy and where other drugs are ineffective. It is available as tablets or in a form for intravenous injection or infusion.

+▲ side-effects/warning: see ONDANSETRON

Zoladex

(Zeneca) is a proprietary, prescription-only preparation of goserelin, which is an analogue of the pituitary HORMONE gonadorelin. It can be used as an ANTICANCER drug for cancer of the prostate gland, breast and for uterine endometriosis. It is available in a form for implantation into the abdominal wall (with a syringe supplied).

+▲ side-effects/warning: see GOSERELIN

zolpidem tartrate

is a newly introduced HYPNOTIC drug, which works in the same way as the BENZODIAZEPINE drugs. It can be used for the short-term treatment of insomnia. Administration is oral as tablets.

+ side-effects: diarrhoea, nausea, vomiting,

Z

dizziness, vertigo, headache, drowsiness during the day, memory disturbances, nocturnal restlessness, nightmares, confusion, depression, double vision and other visual disturbances, tremor, unsteady gait and falls.
▲ warning: it should not be administered to patients with pulmonary insufficiency, respiratory depression, severe liver impairment, myasthenia gravis, or who are pregnant or breast-feedings. Administer with care to those with depression, a history of alcohol or drug abuse, or liver or kidney disorders. Drowsiness may impair the performance of skilled tasks such as driving.
○ Related entry: Stilnoct

Zonulysin

(Henleys) is a proprietary, prescription-only preparation of the enzyme chymotrypsin. It can be used to dissolve a suspensory ligament of the lens of the eye to aid surgical remove of the lens because of a cataract. It is available in a form for injection.
✚▲ side-effects/warning: see CHYMOTRYPSIN

Zopiclone

(Lagap) is a proprietary, non-prescription preparation of the HYPNOTIC drug zopiclone. It can be used for the short-term treatment of insomnia and is available as tablets.
✚▲ side-effects/warning: see ZOPICLONE

zopiclone

is a newly introduced HYPNOTIC drug, which works in the same way as the BENZODIAZEPINE drugs. It can be used for the short-term treatment of insomnia. Administration is oral as tablets.
✚ side-effects: nausea, vomiting, gastrointestinal disturbances, a bitter or metallic taste in the mouth, drowsiness, light-headedness and affects co-ordination the next day, dizziness, depression, sensitivity reactions including rashes, amnesia, hallucinations, irritability and behavioural disturbances including aggression.
▲ warning: administer with care to patients

with liver impairment, psychiatric disorders, who have a history of drug abuse, or who are pregnant or breast-feeding. Avoid prolonged use. It may cause drowsiness and impair the performance of skilled tasks such as driving.
○ Related entries: Zimovane; Zopiclone

Zoton

(Lederle) is a proprietary, prescription-only preparation of the PROTON-PUMP INHIBITOR lansoprazole. It can be used as an ULCER-HEALING DRUG and for associated conditions and is available as capsules.
✚▲ side-effects/warning: see LANSOPRAZOLE

Zovirax

(Wellcome) is a proprietary, prescription-only preparation of the ANTIVIRAL drug acyclovir. It can be used to treat infection by herpes simplex and herpes zoster viruses. It is available as tablets, an oral suspension, an eye ointment, a cream and in a form for intravenous infusion. (A non-prescription ointment preparation for the treatment of cold sores is also available.)
✚▲ side-effects/warning: see ACYCLOVIR

Zovirax Cold Sore Cream

(Wellcome) is a proprietary, non-prescription preparation of the ANTIVIRAL drug acyclovir. It can be used to treat herpes simplex on the lip and face (cold sores) and is available as a cream.
✚▲ side-effects/warning: see ACYCLOVIR

zuclopenthixol acetate

is an ANTIPSYCHOTIC drug that is chemically one of the thioxanthenes, which have similar general actions to the PHENOTHIAZINE DERIVATIVES. It is used for the short-term management of acute psychotic and mania disorders or the exacerbation of chronic psychotic disorders. Administration is oral in the form of tablets. See also ZUCLOPENTHIXOL DECANOATE.
✚▲ side-effects/warning: see under

CHLORPROMAZINE HYDROCHLORIDE. Avoid its use in patients with porphyria.
○ Related entry: Clopixol Acuphase

zuclopenthixol decanoate

is an ANTIPSYCHOTIC drug that is chemically one of the thioxanthenes, which have similar general actions to the PHENOTHIAZINE DERIVATIVES. It is used for the long-term maintenance of schizophrenia and other psychotic disorders and is administered by depot deep intramuscular injection.
+▲ side-effects/warning: see under CHLORPROMAZINE HYDROCHLORIDE; but is less sedating. Avoid its use in patients with porphyria.
○ Related entries: Clopixol, Clopixol Conc.

zuclopenthixol dihydrochloride

is an ANTIPSYCHOTIC drug that is chemically one of the thioxanthenes, which have similar general actions to the PHENOTHIAZINE DERIVATIVES. It can be used to treat patients with psychotic disorders, such as schizophrenia and is particularly effective for agitated and aggressive behaviour. Administration is either oral as tablets or by depot deep intramuscular injection.
+▲ side effects/warning: see under CHLORPROMAZINE HYDROCHLORIDE. Avoid its use in patients with porphyria.
○ Related entry: Clopixol

Zumenon

(Duphar) is a proprietary, prescription-only preparation of the OESTROGEN of oestradiol. It can be used in HRT and is available as tablets in a calendar pack.
+▲ side-effects/warning: see OESTRADIOL

Zydol

(Searle) is a proprietary, prescription-only preparation of the (OPIOID) NARCOTIC ANALGESIC drug tramadol hydrochloride. It can be used to relieve pain, but seems to differ from typical opioids in its mode of action. It is available as capsules and in a form for injection.
+▲ side-effects/warning: see TRAMADOL HYDROCHLORIDE

Zyloric

(Wellcome) is a proprietary, prescription-only preparation of the ENZYME INHIBITOR allopurinol, which is a XANTHINE OXIDASE INHIBITOR. It can be used to treat excess uric acid in the blood and so prevent renal stones and attacks of gout. It is available as tablets.
+▲ side-effects/warning: see ALLOPURINOL

Z